Antibiotics, Chemotherapeutics, and Antibacterial Agents for Disease Control

Antibiotics, Chemotherapeutics, and Antibacterial Agents for Disease Control

ENCYCLOPEDIA REPRINT SERIES

Editor: Martin Grayson

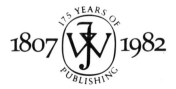

1807 1982

A WILEY-INTERSCIENCE PUBLICATION

JOHN WILEY & SONS

NEW YORK · CHICHESTER · BRISBANE · TORONTO · SINGAPORE

Printed in the United States of America

10 9 8 7 6 5 4 3 2 1

CONTENTS

EDITORIAL STAFF

Editorial Board: **Herman F. Mark,** Polytechnic Institute of New York
Donald F. Othmer, Polytechnic Institute of New York
Charles G. Overberger, University of Michigan
Glenn T. Seaborg, University of California, Berkeley

Executive Editor: **Martin Grayson**
Associate Editor: **David Eckroth**
Production Supervisor: **Michalina Bickford**
Editors: **Galen J. Bushey**   **Loretta Campbell**   **Caroline L. Eastman**
Anna Klingsberg   **Lorraine van Nes**

CONTRIBUTORS

Frederick J. Antosz, *The Upjohn Company, Kalamazoo, Michigan,* Antibiotics, ansama-crolides
Julius Berger, *Hoffmann-La Roche Inc., Nutley, New Jersey,* Antibiotics, phenazines
Alexander Bloch, *Roswell-Park Memorial Institute, Buffalo, New York,* Antibiotics, nucleosides
James H. Boothe, *Lederle Laboratories Division, American Cyanamid Company, Pearl River, New York,* Antibiotics, tetracyclines
Peter J. L. Daniels, *Schering-Plough Corporation, Bloomfield, New Jersey,* Antibiotics, aminoglycosides

Leonard Doub, *Warner Lambert-Parke Davis Research Laboratories, Detroit, Michigan,* Antibacterial agents, sulfonamides

Frank F. Ebetino, *Norwich Pharmacal Company, Division of Morton-Norwich Products, Inc., Norwich, New York,* Antibacterial agents, nitrofurans

Thomas E. Eble, *The Upjohn Company, Kalamazoo, Michigan,* Antibiotics, lincosaminides

John Ehrlich, *Detroit Institute of Technology, Grosse Pointe, Michigan,* Antibiotics, chloramphenicol and its analogues

Ashit K. Ganguly, *Schering Corp., Bloomfield, New Jersey,* Antibiotics, oligosaccharides

George E. Gifford, *University of Florida, Gainesville, Florida,* Chemotherapeutics, antiviral

William Gump, *Consultant, Upper Montclair, New Jersey,* Disinfectants and antiseptics

Joseph J. Hlavka, *Lederle Laboratories Division, American Cyanamid Company, Pearl River, New York,* Antibiotics, tetracyclines

John R. E. Hoover, *Smith Kline & French Laboratories, Philadelphia, Pennsylvania,* Antibiotics, β-lactams

James W. Ingalls, *Arnold & Marie Schwartz College of Pharmacy and Health Sciences, Brooklyn, New York,* Chemotherapeutics, anthelmintic

H. G. Klein, *Klein Medical International, New York, New York,* Antibiotics, survey

George Y. Lesher, *Sterling-Winthrop Research Institute, Rensselaer, New York,* Antibacterial agents, synthetic, nalidixic acid and other quinolone carboxylic acids

Alan K. Mallams, *Schering-Plough Corporation, Bloomfield, New Jersey,* Antibiotics, macrolides; Antibiotics, polyenes

Edgar J. Martin, *Food and Drug Administration, Rockville, Maryland,* Chemotherapeutics, antiprotozoal

Charles J. Masur, *Lederle Laboratories, American Cyanamid Company, Pearl River, New York,* Chemotherapeutics, antimitotic

C. Glen Mayhall, *Medical College of Virginia, Richmond, Virginia,* Chemotherapeutics, antimycotic and antirickettsial

Claude H. Nash, *Smith Kline & French Laboratories, Philadelphia, Pennsylvania,* Antibiotics, β-lactams

William Pearl, *Lederle Laboratories, American Cyanamid Company, Pearl River, New York,* Chemotherapeutics, antimitotic

D. Perlman[†], *University of Wisconsin, Madison, Wisconsin,* Antibiotics, peptides

Bing T. Poon, *Walter Reed Army Institute of Research, Washington, D.C.,* Chemotherapeutics, antiprotozoal

Smith Shadomy, *Medical College of Virginia, Richmond, Virginia,* Chemotherapeutics, antimycotic and antirickettsial

John W. Westley, *Hoffmann-La Roche Inc., Nutley, New Jersey,* Antibiotics, polyethers

Howard C. Zell, *Food and Drug Administration, Rockville, Maryland,* Chemotherapeutics, antiprotozoal

[†] Deceased.

PREFACE

This is the first of a new series of carefully selected reprints from the world-renowned Kirk-Othmer *Encyclopedia of Chemical Technology* designed to provide specific audiences with articles grouped by a central theme. The comprehensive, authoritative collection presented in this volume deals with chemical agents used in the control and treatment of the major disease classes: cancer, viral and bacterial diseases, fungal and rickettsial infections, parasitic diseases and substances used for disinfection and antisepsis. Health and medical professionals, pharmaceutical and medicinal chemists, biochemists and many others concerned with investigating, prescribing or administering antibiotic and chemotherapeutic agents will find this book to be an invaluable resource and reference tool. The authors are noted experts from the principal pharmaceutical companies and biomedical research institutes. The articles have been reviewed in every case by competent specialists in each field. The full text and extensive bibliographies, charts and figures of the original articles have been reproduced here unchanged. Cross references to other articles in the original Encyclopedia have been retained to facilitate peripheral searching where further details are required. All the useful features of the Encyclopedia have been retained, including: Chemical Abstracts Service Registry Numbers, simultaneous use of the international (SI) and English units, and thorough indexing of each article by automated retrieval and sorting from a machine-readable composition system. Coverage is complete and up to date. The articles have been edited carefully for clarity, readability, and technical accuracy with special regard to this area by the Associate Editor of the Encyclopedia, Dr. David Eckroth.

Later volumes in this series will range over the enormous variety of the Kirk-Othmer Encyclopedia to satisfy the particular information needs of professional and technical readers who do not have quick access to the 25-volume original work or who wish to maintain a desk-top collection for ready reference in their field. Many of these volumes are also expected to serve as supplementary course readings and research reference tools for teaching professionals and their students. The editor anticipates that many of the requests for these specialized collections received in the past will now be fulfilled and the books will serve a useful information function.

M. GRAYSON

NOTE ON CHEMICAL ABSTRACTS SERVICE REGISTRY NUMBERS AND NOMENCLATURE

Chemical Abstracts Service (CAS) Registry Numbers are unique numerical identifiers assigned to substances recorded in the CAS Registry System. They appear in brackets in the *Chemical Abstracts* (CA) substance and formula indexes following the names of compounds. A single compound may have many synonyms in the chemical literature. A simple compound like phenethylamine can be named β-phenylethylamine or, as in *Chemical Abstracts*, benzeneethanamine. The usefulness of the *Encyclopedia* depends on accessibility through the most common correct name of a substance. Because of this diversity in nomenclature careful attention has been given the problem in order to assist the reader as much as possible, especially in locating the systematic CA index name by means of the Registry Number. For this purpose, the reader may refer to the CAS Registry Handbook-Number Section which lists in numerical order the Registry Number with the *Chemical Abstracts* index name and the molecular formula; eg, **458-88-8,** Piperidine, 2-propyl-, (S)-, $C_8H_{17}N$; in the *Encyclopedia* this compound would be found under its common name, coniine [*458-88-8*]. The Registry Number is a valuable link for the reader in retrieving additional published information on substances and also as a point of access for such on-line data bases as Chemline, Medline, and Toxline.

In all cases, the CAS Registry Numbers have been given for title compounds in articles and for all compounds in the index. All specific substances indexed in *Chemical Abstracts* since 1965 are included in the CAS Registry System as are a large number of substances derived from a variety of reference works. The CAS Registry System identifies a substance on the basis of an unambiguous computer-language description of its molecular structure including stereochemical detail. The Registry Number is a machine-checkable number (like a Social Security number) assigned in sequential order to each substance as it enters the registry system. The value of the number lies in the fact that it is a concise and unique means of substance identification, which is independent of, and therefore bridges, many systems of chemical nomenclature. For polymers, one Registry Number is used for the entire family; eg, polyoxyethylene (20) sorbitan monolaurate has the same number as all of its polyoxyethylene homologues.

Registry numbers for each substance will be provided in the third edition cumulative index and appear as well in the annual indexes (eg, Alkaloids shows the Registry Number of all alkaloids (title compounds) in a table in the article as well, but the intermediates have their Registry Numbers shown only in the index). Articles such as Analytical methods, Batteries and electric cells, Chemurgy, Distillation, Economic evaluation, and Fluid mechanics have no Registry Numbers in the text.

Cross-references are inserted in the index for many common names and for some systematic names. Trademark names appear in the index. Names that are incorrect, misleading or ambiguous are avoided. Formulas are given very frequently in the text to help in identifying compounds. The spelling and form used, even for industrial names, follow American chemical usage, but not always the usage of *Chemical Abstracts* (eg, *coniine* is used instead of *(S)-2-propylpiperidine*, *aniline* instead of *benzenamine*, and *acrylic acid* instead of *2-propenoic acid*).

There are variations in representation of rings in different disciplines. The dye industry does not designate aromaticity or double bonds in rings. All double bonds and aromaticity are shown in the *Encyclopedia* as a matter of course. For example, tetralin has an aromatic ring and a saturated ring and its structure appears in the

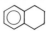

Encyclopedia with its common name, Registry Number enclosed in brackets, and parenthetical CA index name, ie, tetralin, [*119-64-2*] (1,2,3,4-tetrahydronaphthalene). With names and structural formulas, and especially with CAS Registry Numbers the aim is to help the reader have a concise means of substance identification.

CONVERSION FACTORS, ABBREVIATIONS, AND UNIT SYMBOLS

SI Units (Adopted 1960)

A new system of measurement, the International System of Units (abbreviated SI), is being implemented throughout the world. This system is a modernized version of the MKSA (meter, kilogram, second, ampere) system, and its details are published and controlled by an international treaty organization (The International Bureau of Weights and Measures) (1).

SI units are divided into three classes:

BASE UNITS

length	meter[†] (m)
mass[‡]	kilogram (kg)
time	second (s)
electric current	ampere (A)
thermodynamic temperature[§]	kelvin (K)
amount of substance	mole (mol)
luminous intensity	candela (cd)

[†] The spellings "metre" and "litre" are preferred by ASTM; however "-er" are used in the Encyclopedia.

[‡] "Weight" is the commonly used term for "mass."

[§] Wide use is made of "Celsius temperature" (t) defined by

$$t = T - T_0$$

where T is the thermodynamic temperature, expressed in kelvins, and $T_0 = 273.15$ K by definition. A temperature interval may be expressed in degrees Celsius as well as in kelvins.

xiii

SUPPLEMENTARY UNITS

plane angle	radian (rad)
solid angle	steradian (sr)

DERIVED UNITS AND OTHER ACCEPTABLE UNITS

These units are formed by combining base units, supplementary units, and other derived units (2–4). Those derived units having special names and symbols are marked with an asterisk in the list below:

Quantity	Unit	Symbol	Acceptable equivalent
*absorbed dose	gray	Gy	J/kg
acceleration	meter per second squared	m/s^2	
*activity (of ionizing radiation source)	becquerel	Bq	1/s
area	square kilometer	km^2	
	square hectometer	hm^2	ha (hectare)
	square meter	m^2	
*capacitance	farad	F	C/V
concentration (of amount of substance)	mole per cubic meter	mol/m^3	
*conductance	siemens	S	A/V
current density	ampere per square meter	A/m^2	
density, mass density	kilogram per cubic meter	kg/m^3	g/L; mg/cm^3
dipole moment (quantity)	coulomb meter	C·m	
*electric charge, quantity of electricity	coulomb	C	A·s
electric charge density	coulomb per cubic meter	C/m^3	
electric field strength	volt per meter	V/m	
electric flux density	coulomb per square meter	C/m^2	
*electric potential, potential difference, electromotive force	volt	V	W/A
*electric resistance	ohm	Ω	V/A
*energy, work, quantity of heat	megajoule	MJ	
	kilojoule	kJ	
	joule	J	N·m
	electron volt†	eV†	
	kilowatt-hour†	kW·h†	

† This non-SI unit is recognized by the CIPM as having to be retained because of practical importance or use in specialized fields (1).

Quantity	Unit	Symbol	Acceptable equivalent
energy density	joule per cubic meter	J/m^3	
*force	kilonewton	kN	
	newton	N	$kg \cdot m/s^2$
*frequency	megahertz	MHz	
	hertz	Hz	$1/s$
heat capacity, entropy	joule per kelvin	J/K	
heat capacity (specific), specific entropy	joule per kilogram kelvin	$J/(kg \cdot K)$	
heat transfer coefficient	watt per square meter kelvin	$W/(m^2 \cdot K)$	
*illuminance	lux	lx	lm/m^2
*inductance	henry	H	Wb/A
linear density	kilogram per meter	kg/m	
luminance	candela per square meter	cd/m^2	
*luminous flux	lumen	lm	$cd \cdot sr$
magnetic field strength	ampere per meter	A/m	
*magnetic flux	weber	Wb	$V \cdot s$
*magnetic flux density	tesla	T	Wb/m^2
molar energy	joule per mole	J/mol	
molar entropy, molar heat capacity	joule per mole kelvin	$J/(mol \cdot K)$	
moment of force, torque	newton meter	$N \cdot m$	
momentum	kilogram meter per second	$kg \cdot m/s$	
permeability	henry per meter	H/m	
permittivity	farad per meter	F/m	
*power, heat flow rate, radiant flux	kilowatt	kW	
	watt	W	J/s
power density, heat flux density, irradiance	watt per square meter	W/m^2	
*pressure, stress	megapascal	MPa	
	kilopascal	kPa	
	pascal	Pa	N/m^2
sound level	decibel	dB	
specific energy	joule per kilogram	J/kg	
specific volume	cubic meter per kilogram	m^3/kg	
surface tension	newton per meter	N/m	
thermal conductivity	watt per meter kelvin	$W/(m \cdot K)$	
velocity	meter per second	m/s	
	kilometer per hour	km/h	
viscosity, dynamic	pascal second	$Pa \cdot s$	
	millipascal second	$mPa \cdot s$	
viscosity, kinematic	square meter per second	m^2/s	

Quantity	Unit	Symbol	Acceptable equivalent
	square millimeter per second	mm^2/s	
volume	cubic meter	m^3	
	cubic decimeter	dm^3	L(liter) (5)
	cubic centimeter	cm^3	mL
wave number	1 per meter	m^{-1}	
	1 per centimeter	cm^{-1}	

In addition, there are 16 prefixes used to indicate order of magnitude, as follows:

Multiplication factor	Prefix	Symbol	Note
10^{18}	exa	E	
10^{15}	peta	P	
10^{12}	tera	T	
10^{9}	giga	G	
10^{6}	mega	M	
10^{3}	kilo	k	
10^{2}	hecto	h[a]	[a] Although hecto, deka, deci, and centi
10	deka	da[a]	are SI prefixes, their use should be
10^{-1}	deci	d[a]	avoided except for SI unit-mul-
10^{-2}	centi	c[a]	tiples for area and volume and
10^{-3}	milli	m	nontechnical use of centimeter,
10^{-6}	micro	μ	as for body and clothing
10^{-9}	nano	n	measurement.
10^{-12}	pico	p	
10^{-15}	femto	f	
10^{-18}	atto	a	

For a complete description of SI and its use the reader is referred to ASTM E 380 (4) and the article Units and Conversion Factors which will appear in a later volume of the *Encyclopedia*.

A representative list of conversion factors from non-SI to SI units is presented herewith. Factors are given to four significant figures. Exact relationships are followed by a dagger. A more complete list is given in ASTM E 380-79(4) and ANSI Z210.1-1976 (6).

Conversion Factors to SI Units

To convert from	To	Multiply by
acre	square meter (m^2)	4.047×10^3
angstrom	meter (m)	1.0×10^{-10}†
are	square meter (m^2)	1.0×10^{2}†
astronomical unit	meter (m)	1.496×10^{11}
atmosphere	pascal (Pa)	1.013×10^{5}
bar	pascal (Pa)	1.0×10^{5}†
barn	square meter (m^2)	1.0×10^{-28}†

† Exact.

To convert from	To	Multiply by
barrel (42 U.S. liquid gallons)	cubic meter (m^3)	0.1590
Bohr magneton (μ_β)	J/T	9.274×10^{-24}
Btu (International Table)	joule (J)	1.055×10^3
Btu (mean)	joule (J)	1.056×10^3
Btu (thermochemical)	joule (J)	1.054×10^3
bushel	cubic meter (m^3)	3.524×10^{-2}
calorie (International Table)	joule (J)	4.187
calorie (mean)	joule (J)	4.190
calorie (thermochemical)	joule (J)	4.184[†]
centipoise	pascal second (Pa·s)	1.0×10^{-3}[†]
centistoke	square millimeter per second (mm^2/s)	1.0[†]
cfm (cubic foot per minute)	cubic meter per second (m^3/s)	4.72×10^{-4}
cubic inch	cubic meter (m^3)	1.639×10^{-5}
cubic foot	cubic meter (m^3)	2.832×10^{-2}
cubic yard	cubic meter (m^3)	0.7646
curie	becquerel (Bq)	3.70×10^{10}[†]
debye	coulomb·meter (C·m)	3.336×10^{-30}
degree (angle)	radian (rad)	1.745×10^{-2}
denier (international)	kilogram per meter (kg/m)	1.111×10^{-7}
	tex[‡]	0.1111
dram (apothecaries')	kilogram (kg)	3.888×10^{-3}
dram (avoirdupois)	kilogram (kg)	1.772×10^{-3}
dram (U.S. fluid)	cubic meter (m^3)	3.697×10^{-6}
dyne	newton (N)	1.0×10^{-5}[†]
dyne/cm	newton per meter (N/m)	1.0×10^{-3}[†]
electron volt	joule (J)	1.602×10^{-19}
erg	joule (J)	1.0×10^{-7}[†]
fathom	meter (m)	1.829
fluid ounce (U.S.)	cubic meter (m^3)	2.957×10^{-5}
foot	meter (m)	0.3048[†]
footcandle	lux (lx)	10.76
furlong	meter (m)	2.012×10^{-2}
gal	meter per second squared (m/s^2)	1.0×10^{-2}[†]
gallon (U.S. dry)	cubic meter (m^3)	4.405×10^{-3}
gallon (U.S. liquid)	cubic meter (m^3)	3.785×10^{-3}
gallon per minute (gpm)	cubic meter per second (m^3/s)	6.308×10^{-5}
	cubic meter per hour (m^3/h)	0.2271
gauss	tesla (T)	1.0×10^{-4}
gilbert	ampere (A)	0.7958
gill (U.S.)	cubic meter (m^3)	1.183×10^{-4}
grad	radian	1.571×10^{-2}
grain	kilogram (kg)	6.480×10^{-5}
gram force per denier	newton per tex (N/tex)	8.826×10^{-2}

[†] Exact.
[‡] See footnote on p. xiv.

To convert from	To	Multiply by
hectare	square meter (m^2)	$1.0 \times 10^{4\dagger}$
horsepower (550 ft·lbf/s)	watt (W)	7.457×10^2
horsepower (boiler)	watt (W)	9.810×10^3
horsepower (electric)	watt (W)	$7.46 \times 10^{2\dagger}$
hundredweight (long)	kilogram (kg)	50.80
hundredweight (short)	kilogram (kg)	45.36
inch	meter (m)	$2.54 \times 10^{-2\dagger}$
inch of mercury (32°F)	pascal (Pa)	3.386×10^3
inch of water (39.2°F)	pascal (Pa)	2.491×10^2
kilogram force	newton (N)	9.807
kilowatt hour	megajoule (MJ)	$3.6^\dagger$
kip	newton (N)	4.48×10^3
knot (international)	meter per second (m/s)	0.5144
lambert	candela per square meter (cd/m^2)	3.183×10^3
league (British nautical)	meter (m)	5.559×10^3
league (statute)	meter (m)	4.828×10^3
light year	meter (m)	9.461×10^{15}
liter (for fluids only)	cubic meter (m^3)	$1.0 \times 10^{-3\dagger}$
maxwell	weber (Wb)	$1.0 \times 10^{-8\dagger}$
micron	meter (m)	$1.0 \times 10^{-6\dagger}$
mil	meter (m)	$2.54 \times 10^{-5\dagger}$
mile (statute)	meter (m)	1.609×10^3
mile (U.S. nautical)	meter (m)	$1.852 \times 10^{3\dagger}$
mile per hour	meter per second (m/s)	0.4470
millibar	pascal (Pa)	1.0×10^2
millimeter of mercury (0°C)	pascal (Pa)	$1.333 \times 10^{2\dagger}$
minute (angular)	radian	2.909×10^{-4}
myriagram	kilogram (kg)	10
myriameter	kilometer (km)	10
oersted	ampere per meter (A/m)	79.58
ounce (avoirdupois)	kilogram (kg)	2.835×10^{-2}
ounce (troy)	kilogram (kg)	3.110×10^{-2}
ounce (U.S. fluid)	cubic meter (m^3)	2.957×10^{-5}
ounce-force	newton (N)	0.2780
peck (U.S.)	cubic meter (m^3)	8.810×10^{-3}
pennyweight	kilogram (kg)	1.555×10^{-3}
pint (U.S. dry)	cubic meter (m^3)	5.506×10^{-4}
pint (U.S. liquid)	cubic meter (m^3)	4.732×10^{-4}
poise (absolute viscosity)	pascal second (Pa·s)	$0.10^\dagger$
pound (avoirdupois)	kilogram (kg)	0.4536
pound (troy)	kilogram (kg)	0.3732
poundal	newton (N)	0.1383
pound-force	newton (N)	4.448
pound per square inch (psi)	pascal (Pa)	6.895×10^3
quart (U.S. dry)	cubic meter (m^3)	1.101×10^{-3}

† Exact.

To convert from	To	Multiply by
quart (U.S. liquid)	cubic meter (m^3)	9.464×10^{-4}
quintal	kilogram (kg)	$1.0 \times 10^{2\dagger}$
rad	gray (Gy)	$1.0 \times 10^{-2\dagger}$
rod	meter (m)	5.029
roentgen	coulomb per kilogram (C/kg)	2.58×10^{-4}
second (angle)	radian (rad)	4.848×10^{-6}
section	square meter (m^2)	2.590×10^6
slug	kilogram (kg)	14.59
spherical candle power	lumen (lm)	12.57
square inch	square meter (m^2)	6.452×10^{-4}
square foot	square meter (m^2)	9.290×10^{-2}
square mile	square meter (m^2)	2.590×10^6
square yard	square meter (m^2)	0.8361
stere	cubic meter (m^3)	$1.0^\dagger$
stokes (kinematic viscosity)	square meter per second (m^2/s)	$1.0 \times 10^{-4\dagger}$
tex	kilogram per meter (kg/m)	$1.0 \times 10^{-6\dagger}$
ton (long, 2240 pounds)	kilogram (kg)	1.016×10^3
ton (metric)	kilogram (kg)	$1.0 \times 10^{3\dagger}$
ton (short, 2000 pounds)	kilogram (kg)	9.072×10^2
torr	pascal (Pa)	1.333×10^2
unit pole	weber (Wb)	1.257×10^{-7}
yard	meter (m)	$0.9144^\dagger$

Abbreviations and Unit Symbols

Following is a list of commonly used abbreviations and unit symbols appropriate for use in the *Encyclopedia*. In general they agree with those listed in *American National Standard Abbreviations for Use on Drawings and in Text (ANSI Y1.1)* (6) and *American National Standard Letter Symbols for Units in Science and Technology (ANSI Y10)* (6). Also included is a list of acronyms for a number of private and government organizations as well as common industrial solvents, polymers, and other chemicals.

Rules for Writing Unit Symbols (4):

1. Unit symbols should be printed in upright letters (roman) regardless of the type style used in the surrounding text.

2. Unit symbols are unaltered in the plural.

3. Unit symbols are not followed by a period except when used as the end of a sentence.

4. Letter unit symbols are generally written in lower-case (eg, cd for candela) unless the unit name has been derived from a proper name, in which case the first letter of the symbol is capitalized (W,Pa). Prefix and unit symbols retain their prescribed form regardless of the surrounding typography.

5. In the complete expression for a quantity, a space should be left between the numerical value and the unit symbol. For example, write 2.37 lm, *not* 2.37lm, and 35 mm, *not* 35mm. When the quantity is used in an adjectival sense, a hyphen is often used, for example, 35-mm film. *Exception:* No space is left between the numerical value and the symbols for degree, minute, and second of plane angle, and degree Celsius.

6. No space is used between the prefix and unit symbols (eg, kg).

7. Symbols, not abbreviations, should be used for units. For example, use "A," not "amp," for ampere.

8. When multiplying unit symbols, use a raised dot:

$$N \cdot m \text{ for newton meter}$$

In the case of W·h, the dot may be omitted, thus:

$$Wh$$

An exception to this practice is made for computer printouts, automatic typewriter work, etc, where the raised dot is not possible, and a dot on the line may be used.

9. When dividing unit symbols use one of the following forms:

$$m/s \; or \; m \cdot s^{-1} \; or \; \frac{m}{s}$$

In no case should more than one slash be used in the same expression unless parentheses are inserted to avoid ambiguity. For example, write:

$$J/(mol \cdot K) \; or \; J \cdot mol^{-1} \cdot K^{-1} \; or \; (J/mol)/K$$

but *not*

$$J/mol/K$$

10. Do not mix symbols and unit names in the same expression. Write:

$$joules \; per \; kilogram \; or \; J/kg \; or \; J \cdot kg^{-1}$$

but *not*

$$joules/kilogram \; nor \; joules/kg \; nor \; joules \cdot kg^{-1}$$

ABBREVIATIONS AND UNITS

A	ampere
A	anion (eg, H*A*); mass number
a	atto (prefix for 10^{-18})
AATCC	American Association of Textile Chemists and Colorists
ABS	acrylonitrile–butadiene–styrene
abs	absolute
ac	alternating current, *n*.
a-c	alternating current, *adj*.
ac-	alicyclic
acac	acetylacetonate
ACGIH	American Conference of Governmental Industrial Hygienists
ACS	American Chemical Society
AGA	American Gas Association
Ah	ampere hour
AIChE	American Institute of Chemical Engineers
AIME	American Institute of Mining, Metallurgical, and Petroleum Engineers
AIP	American Institute of Physics
alc	alcohol(ic)
Alk	alkyl
alk	alkaline (not alkali)
amt	amount
amu	atomic mass unit
ANSI	American National Standards Institute
AO	atomic orbital
AOAC	Association of Official Analytical Chemists
AOCS	American Oil Chemist's Society

APHA	American Public Health Association
API	American Petroleum Institute
aq	aqueous
Ar	aryl
ar-	aromatic
as-	asymmetric(al)
ASH-RAE	American Society of Heating, Refrigerating, and Air Conditioning Engineers
ASM	American Society for Metals
ASME	American Society of Mechanical Engineers
ASTM	American Society for Testing and Materials
at no.	atomic number
at wt	atomic weight
av(g)	average
AWS	American Welding Society
b	bonding orbital
bbl	barrel
bcc	body-centered cubic
Bé	Baumé
BET	Brunauer-Emmett-Teller (adsorption equation)
bid	twice daily
Boc	t-butyloxycarbonyl
BOD	biochemical (biological) oxygen demand
bp	boiling point
Bq	becquerel
C	coulomb
°C	degree Celsius
C-	denoting attachment to carbon
c	centi (prefix for 10^{-2})
c	critical
ca	circa (approximately)
cd	candela; current density; circular dichroism
CFR	Code of Federal Regulations
cgs	centimeter–gram–second
CI	Color Index
cis-	isomer in which substituted groups are on same side of double bond between C atoms

cl	carload
cm	centimeter
cmil	circular mil
cmpd	compound
CNS	central nervous system
CoA	coenzyme A
COD	chemical oxygen demand
coml	commercial(ly)
cp	chemically pure
cph	close-packed hexagonal
CPSC	Consumer Product Safety Commission
cryst	crystalline
cub	cubic
D-	denoting configurational relationship
d	differential operator
d-	dextro-, dextrorotatory
da	deka (prefix for 10^1)
dB	decibel
dc	direct current, $n.$
d-c	direct current, $adj.$
dec	decompose
detd	determined
detn	determination
Di	didymium, a mixture of all lanthanons
dia	diameter
dil	dilute
DIN	Deutsche Industrie Normen
dl-; DL-	racemic
DMA	dimethylacetamide
DMF	dimethylformamide
DMG	dimethyl glyoxime
DMSO	dimethyl sulfoxide
DOD	Department of Defense
DOE	Department of Energy
DOT	Department of Transportation
dp	dew point
DP	degree of polymerization
DPH	diamond pyramid hardness
dstl(d)	distill(ed)
dta	differential thermal analysis
(E)-	entgegen; opposed
e	dielectric constant (unitless number)
e	electron

ECU	electrochemical unit		grd	ground
ed.	edited, edition, editor		Gy	gray
ED	effective dose		H	henry
EDTA	ethylenediaminetetraacetic acid		h	hour; hecto (prefix for 10^2)
emf	electromotive force		ha	hectare
emu	electromagnetic unit		HB	Brinell hardness number
en	ethylene diamine		Hb	hemoglobin
eng	engineering		hcp	hexagonal close-packed
EPA	Environmental Protection Agency		hex	hexagonal
epr	electron paramagnetic resonance		HK	Knoop hardness number
			HRC	Rockwell hardness (C scale)
			HV	Vickers hardness number
eq.	equation		hyd	hydrated, hydrous
esp	especially		hyg	hygroscopic
esr	electron-spin resonance		Hz	hertz
est(d)	estimate(d)		^{i}(eg, Pr^i)	iso (eg, isopropyl)
estn	estimation		i-	inactive (eg, i-methionine)
esu	electrostatic unit		IACS	International Annealed Copper Standard
exp	experiment, experimental		ibp	initial boiling point
ext(d)	extract(ed)		IC	inhibitory concentration
F	farad (capacitance)		ICC	Interstate Commerce Commission
F	faraday (96,487 C)			
f	femto (prefix for 10^{-15})		ICT	International Critical Table
FAO	Food and Agriculture Organization (United Nations)		ID	inside diameter; infective dose
			ip	intraperitoneal
			IPS	iron pipe size
fcc	face-centered cubic		IPT	Institute of Petroleum Technologists
FDA	Food and Drug Administration			
FEA	Federal Energy Administration		IPTS	International Practical Temperature Scale (NBS)
fob	free on board		ir	infrared
fp	freezing point		IRLG	Interagency Regulatory Liaison Group
FPC	Federal Power Commission			
FRB	Federal Reserve Board		ISO	International Organization for Standardization
frz	freezing			
G	giga (prefix for 10^9)		IU	International Unit
G	gravitational constant = 6.67×10^{11} N·m^2/kg^2		IUPAC	International Union of Pure and Applied Chemistry
g	gram		IV	iodine value
(g)	gas, only as in H_2O(g)		iv	intravenous
g	gravitational acceleration		J	joule
gem-	geminal		K	kelvin
glc	gas-liquid chromatography		k	kilo (prefix for 10^3)
g-mol wt; gmw	gram-molecular weight		kg	kilogram
			L	denoting configurational relationship
GNP	gross national product			
gpc	gel-permeation chromatography		L	liter (for fluids only)(5)
			l-	$levo$-, levorotatory
GRAS	Generally Recognized as Safe		(l)	liquid, only as in NH_3(l)

LC_{50}	conc lethal to 50% of the animals tested	μ	micro (prefix for 10^{-6})
LCAO	linear combination of atomic orbitals	N	newton (force)
		N	normal (concentration); neutron number
LCD	liquid crystal display	N-	denoting attachment to nitrogen
lcl	less than carload lots		
LD_{50}	dose lethal to 50% of the animals tested	n (as n_D^{20})	index of refraction (for 20°C and sodium light)
LED	light-emitting diode	^{n} (as Bu^n),	normal (straight-chain structure)
liq	liquid		
lm	lumen	n-	
ln	logarithm (natural)	n	neutron
LNG	liquefied natural gas	n	nano (prefix for 10^9)
log	logarithm (common)	na	not available
LPG	liquefied petroleum gas	NAS	National Academy of Sciences
ltl	less than truckload lots		
lx	lux	NASA	National Aeronautics and Space Administration
M	mega (prefix for 10^6); metal (as in MA)		
		nat	natural
M	molar; actual mass	NBS	National Bureau of Standards
$\overline{M}_w$	weight-average mol wt		
$\overline{M}_n$	number-average mol wt	NF	*National Formulary*
m	meter; milli (prefix for 10^{-3})	NIH	National Institutes of Health
m	molal		
m-	meta	NIOSH	National Institute of Occupational Safety and Health
max	maximum		
MCA	Chemical Manufacturers' Association (was Manufacturing Chemists Association)		
		nmr	nuclear magnetic resonance
		NND	New and Nonofficial Drugs (AMA)
MEK	methyl ethyl ketone		
meq	milliequivalent	no.	number
mfd	manufactured	NOI- (BN)	not otherwise indexed (by name)
mfg	manufacturing		
mfr	manufacturer	NOS	not otherwise specified
MIBC	methyl isobutyl carbinol	nqr	nuclear quadruple resonance
MIBK	methyl isobutyl ketone	NRC	Nuclear Regulatory Commission; National Research Council
MIC	minimum inhibiting concentration		
		NRI	New Ring Index
min	minute; minimum	NSF	National Science Foundation
mL	milliliter	NTA	nitrilotriacetic acid
MLD	minimum lethal dose	NTP	normal temperature and pressure (25°C and 101.3 kPa or 1 atm)
MO	molecular orbital		
mo	month		
mol	mole	NTSB	National Transportation Safety Board
mol wt	molecular weight		
mp	melting point	O-	denoting attachment to oxygen
MR	molar refraction		
ms	mass spectrum	o-	ortho
mxt	mixture	OD	outside diameter

OPEC	Organization of Petroleum Exporting Countries	r-f	radio frequency, *adj.*
		rh	relative humidity
		RI	Ring Index
o-phen	*o*-phenanthridine	rms	root-mean square
OSHA	Occupational Safety and Health Administration	rpm	rotations per minute
		rps	revolutions per second
owf	on weight of fiber	RT	room temperature
Ω	ohm	^{s} (eg, Bu^s); *sec-*	secondary (eg, secondary butyl)
P	peta (prefix for 10^{15})		
p	pico (prefix for 10^{-12})		
p-	para	S	siemens
p	proton	(*S*)-	sinister (counterclockwise configuration)
p.	page		
Pa	pascal (pressure)	*S*-	denoting attachment to sulfur
pd	potential difference		
pH	negative logarithm of the effective hydrogen ion concentration	*s-*	symmetric(al)
		s	second
		(s)	solid, only as in $H_2O(s)$
phr	parts per hundred of resin (rubber)	SAE	Society of Automotive Engineers
p-i-n	positive-intrinsic-negative	SAN	styrene–acrylonitrile
pmr	proton magnetic resonance	sat(d)	saturate(d)
p-n	positive-negative	satn	saturation
po	per os (oral)	SBS	styrene–butadiene–styrene
POP	polyoxypropylene	sc	subcutaneous
pos	positive	SCF	self-consistent field; standard cubic feet
pp.	pages		
ppb	parts per billion (10^9)	Sch	Schultz number
ppm	parts per million (10^6)	SFs	Saybolt Furol seconds
ppmv	parts per million by volume	SI	Le Système International d'Unités (International System of Units)
ppmwt	parts per million by weight		
PPO	poly(phenyl oxide)		
ppt(d)	precipitate(d)	sl sol	slightly soluble
pptn	precipitation	sol	soluble
Pr (no.)	foreign prototype (number)	soln	solution
pt	point; part	soly	solubility
PVC	poly(vinyl chloride)	sp	specific; species
pwd	powder	sp gr	specific gravity
py	pyridine	sr	steradian
qv	quod vide (which see)	std	standard
R	univalent hydrocarbon radical	STP	standard temperature and pressure (0°C and 101.3 kPa)
(*R*)-	rectus (clockwise configuration)	sub	sublime(s)
r	precision of data	SUs	Saybolt Universal seconds
rad	radian; radius	syn	synthetic
rds	rate determining step	^{t} (eg, Bu^t), *t-*, *tert-*	tertiary (eg, tertiary butyl)
ref.	reference		
rf	radio frequency, *n.*		

T	tera (prefix for 10^{12}); tesla (magnetic flux density)	USDA	United States Department of Agriculture
t	metric ton (tonne); temperature	USP	*United States Pharmacopeia*
		uv	ultraviolet
TAPPI	Technical Association of the Pulp and Paper Industry	V	volt (emf)
		var	variable
tex	tex (linear density)	*vic-*	vicinal
T_g	glass-transition temperature	vol	volume (not volatile)
tga	thermogravimetric analysis	vs	versus
THF	tetrahydrofuran	v sol	very soluble
tlc	thin layer chromatography	W	watt
TLV	threshold limit value	Wb	Weber
trans-	isomer in which substituted groups are on opposite sides of double bond between C atoms	Wh	watt hour
		WHO	World Health Organization (United Nations)
TSCA	Toxic Substance Control Act	wk	week
TWA	time-weighted average	yr	year
Twad	Twaddell	(Z)-	zusammen; together; atomic number
UL	Underwriters' Laboratory		

Non-SI (Unacceptable and Obsolete) Units		*Use*
Å	angstrom	nm
at	atmosphere, technical	Pa
atm	atmosphere, standard	Pa
b	barn	cm^2
bar[†]	bar	Pa
bbl	barrel	m^3
bhp	brake horsepower	W
Btu	British thermal unit	J
bu	bushel	m^3; L
cal	calorie	J
cfm	cubic foot per minute	m^3/s
Ci	curie.	Bq
cSt	centistokes	mm^2/s
c/s	cycle per second	Hz
cu	cubic	exponential form
D	debye	C·m
den	denier	tex
dr	dram	kg
dyn	dyne	N
dyn/cm	dyne per centimeter	mN/m
erg	erg	J
eu	entropy unit	J/K
°F	degree Fahrenheit	°C; K
fc	footcandle	lx
fl	footlambert	lx
fl oz	fluid ounce	m^3; L
ft	foot	m
ft·lbf	foot pound-force	J
gf den	gram-force per denier	N/tex

[†] Do not use bar (10^5Pa) or millibar (10^2Pa) because they are not SI units, and are accepted internationally only for a limited time in special fields because of existing usage.

Non-SI (Unacceptable and Obsolete) Units		*Use*
G	gauss	T
Gal	gal	m/s^2
gal	gallon	m^3; L
Gb	gilbert	A
gpm	gallon per minute	(m^3/s); (m^3/h)
gr	grain	kg
hp	horsepower	W
ihp	indicated horsepower	W
in.	inch	m
in. Hg	inch of mercury	Pa
in. H_2O	inch of water	Pa
in.-lbf	inch pound-force	J
kcal	kilogram-calorie	J
kgf	kilogram-force	N
kilo	for kilogram	kg
L	lambert	lx
lb	pound	kg
lbf	pound-force	N
mho	mho	S
mi	mile	m
MM	million	M
mm Hg	millimeter of mercury	Pa
mμ	millimicron	nm
mph	miles per hour	km/h
μ	micron	μm
Oe	oersted	A/m
oz	ounce	kg
ozf	ounce-force	N
η	poise	Pa·s
P	poise	Pa·s
ph	phot	lx
psi	pounds-force per square inch	Pa
psia	pounds-force per square inch absolute	Pa
psig	pounds-force per square inch gauge	Pa
qt	quart	m^3; L
°R	degree Rankine	K
rd	rad	Gy
sb	stilb	lx
SCF	standard cubic foot	m^3
sq	square	exponential form
thm	therm	J
yd	yard	m

BIBLIOGRAPHY

1. The International Bureau of Weights and Measures, BIPM (Parc de Saint-Cloud, France) is described on page 22 of Ref. 4. This bureau operates under the exclusive supervision of the International Committee of Weights and Measures (CIPM).
2. *Metric Editorial Guide (ANMC-78-1)* 3rd ed., American National Metric Council, 1625 Massachusetts Ave. N.W., Washington, D.C. 20036, 1978.
3. *SI Units and Recommendations for the Use of Their Multiples and of Certain Other Units (ISO 1000-1981)*, American National Standards Institute, 1430 Broadway, New York, N. Y. 10018, 1981.
4. Based on *ASTM E 380-79 (Standard for Metric Practice)*, American Society for Testing and Materials, 1916 Race Street, Philadelphia, Pa. 19103, 1979.
5. *Fed. Regist.*, Dec. 10, 1976 (41 FR 36414).
6. For ANSI address, see Ref. 3.

R. P. LUKENS
American Society for Testing and Materials

ANTIBACTERIAL AGENTS, SYNTHETIC

NALIDIXIC ACID AND OTHER QUINOLONE CARBOXYLIC ACIDS

Quinolone carboxylic acids are an emerging group of compounds with useful antibacterial activity. The title *quinolone* is used for simplicity although several of the compounds in the group are *aza* derivatives of quinolones.

Totally synthetic antibacterial agents that have proven clinically useful are rare. The sulfonamides (qv), the nitrofurans (qv), and the newer group of compounds covered in this section, other than an assorted group of antitubercular agents (see Chemotherapeutics, antibacterial), are the only examples. Work with the sulfonamides and nitrofurans appears to have matured. The introduction of new sulfonamides for human clinical use in the United States has dropped noticeably in the last decade (Fig. 1). Only four nitrofuran derivatives have been introduced in the United States (between 1954 and 1961). Nothing new has appeared in this area despite a strong continuing synthetic effort.

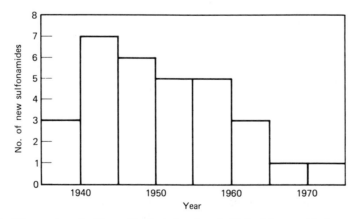

Figure 1. The number of sulfonamides introduced to the United States each five years.

1

The first compound of the quinolone type, introduced to the United States in 1964, is nalidixic acid (**1**) (1–6). Three others have been introduced more recently, piromidic acid (**2**) (7–9) (1972, Japan), pipemidic acid (**3**) (10–18) (1975, France), and oxolinic acid (**4**) (19–23) (1975, United States) (Table 1).

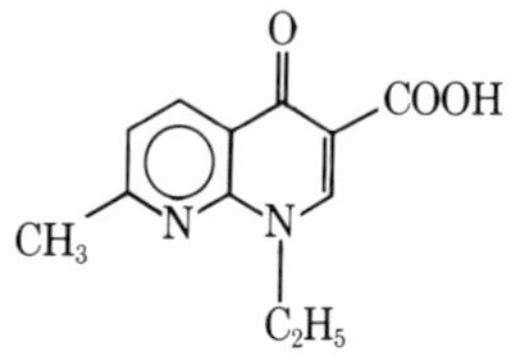

(**1**) 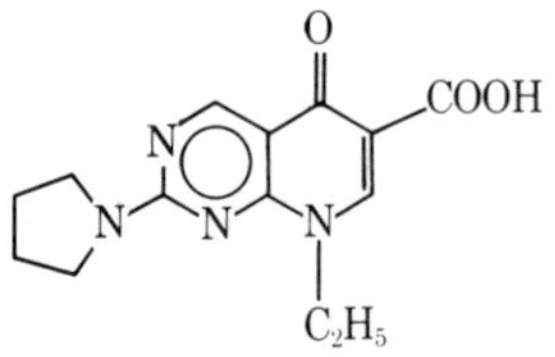   (**2**)

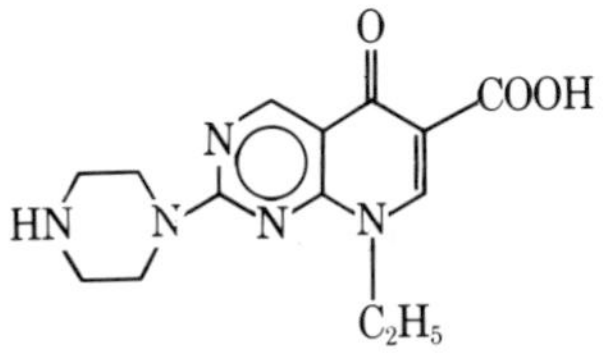

(**3**) 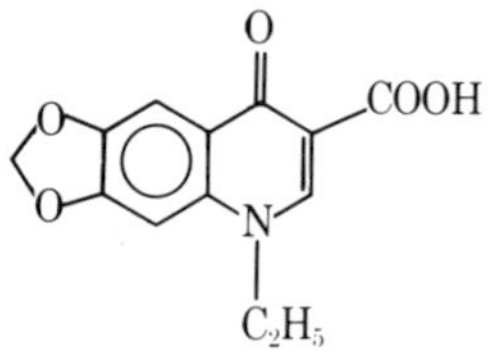   (**4**)

They all have a range of gram-negative antibacterial activity and the ability to concentrate in the urine after oral administration; they have thus proven useful as agents against urinary tract infections [(**1**) (1,5–6), (**2**) (7–9), (**3**) (10,12–17), and (**4**) (19,21–23)]. Comparison of the clinical utility of these four agents cannot be made because data are not yet available for the latter three.

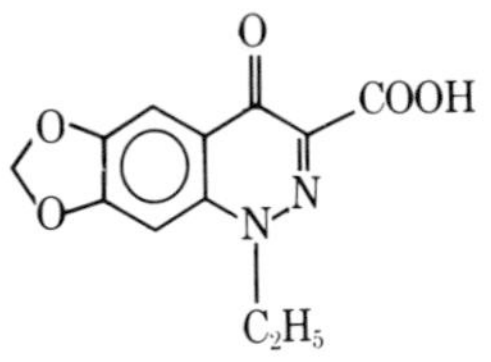

(**5**) 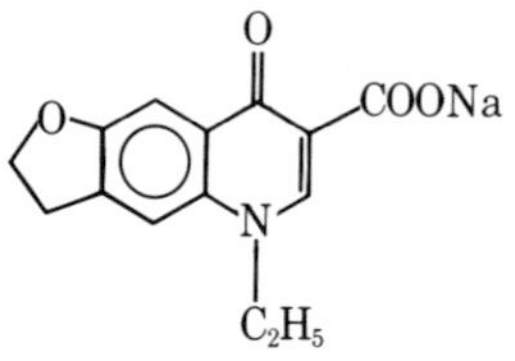   (**6**)

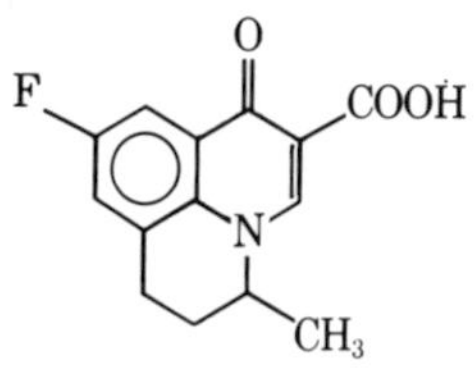

(**7**) 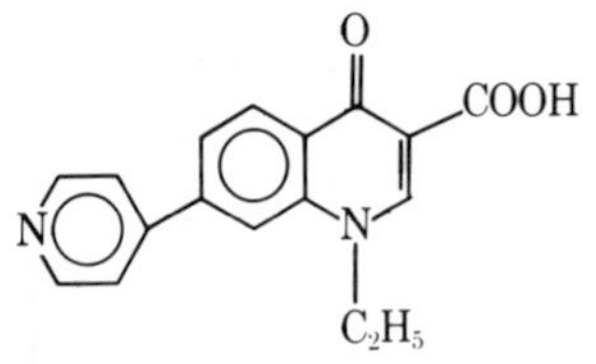   (**8**)

Structure and Activity

The obvious common structural feature of these compounds is a fused 1-alkyl-1,4-dihydro-4-oxo-3-pyridinecarboxylic acid (**9**), except for cinoxacin (**5**).

Table 1.   Manufacturer and Trade Names of Quinolone Carboxylic Acids

Quinolone carboxylic acid	CAS Registry Number	Trade names[a]	Manufacturer
Commercial products			
nalidixic acid (1)	[389-08-2]	Betaxina, Dixiben, Kusnarin, Nalidixin, Nalix, Negabatt, *NegGram,* Negram, Nevigramon, Nicelate, Nogram, Specifin, Uralgin, Uriclar, Urodixin, Urogram, Uroneg, Valuren, Wintomylon	Winthrop Laboratories (Division of Sterling Drug, Inc.)
piromidic acid (2)	[19562-30-2]	Panacid	Dainippon Pharmaceutical Co., Ltd. (Japan)
pipemidic acid (3)	[51940-44-4]	Pipram	Laboratoire Roger Bellon (France)
oxolinic acid (4)	[14698-29-4]	Ossian, Pietil, Prodoxal, Vritrate, Urotrate, *Utibid*	Warner-Lambert Co.
Under development			
cinoxacin (5)	[28657-80-9]		Eli Lilly and Co.
droxacin sodium (6)	[57363-13-0]		Schering A.G. (Germany)
flumequine (7)	[42835-25-6]		Riker Laboratories, Inc. (Subsidiary of Minnesota Mining and Manufacturing Co.)
rosoxacin (8)	[40034-42-2]		Sterling Drug, Inc.

[a] The italicized trade name is the one used in the USA by the manufacturer.

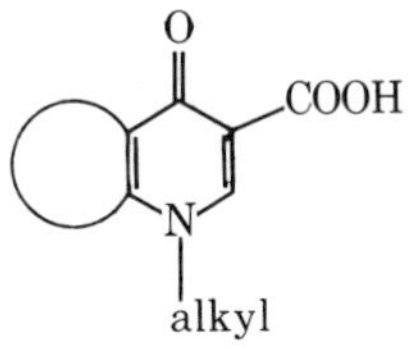

(9)

Some generalizations about the effect of structural changes and the resulting antibacterial activity of these molecules have been collected in Table 2.

As can be seen in this table, hydrogen at the 1-position results in inactive compounds, but certain of these 1-unsubstituted quinolones have useful anticoccidial activity (25). The portion fused to the pyridone ring apparently offers more room for variation and would seem to be where future modifications will be made that will result in useful additions to this group of antibacterial agents. These antibacterial agents are chemically quite stable and are readily soluble in aqueous base.

The United States Adopted Name Council (USAN) has recently assigned the suffix oxacin for nonproprietary names of drugs belonging to this class of antibacterial agents.

Table 2.   Effect on Antibacterial Activity of Structural Changes of 1-Alkyl-1,4-Dihydro-4-Oxo-3-Pyridinecarboxylic Acid

Function	Replaced with	In vitro activity[a]
4-oxo	=S[b], =NR[c], or transfer 4-oxo to the 2-position[d]	−
3-carboxylic acid	H[e], CH$_3$, NR$_2$, COOR[f], CONR$_2$[f], CN, CONHOH, (CH$_2$)$_n$COOH (n = 1 or 2), CH=CHCOOH, CHO, COCH$_3$, CH$_2$OH, SO$_3$H, SO$_2$NR$_2$, or 5-tetrazolyl	−
2-H	CH$_3$, COOH, or COOC$_2$H$_5$	−
1-alkyl	CH$_3$, C$_2$H$_5$, CH=CH$_2$, C$_3$H$_7$, CH(CH$_3$)$_2$, CH$_2$CH=CH$_2$, or CH$_2$C≡CH[g]	+
	CH$_2$CF$_3$[h], CH$_2$CN, OCH$_3$[i], CH$_2$OCH$_3$[h], CH$_2$SCH$_3$[j], CH$_2$CH$_2$OH[j], CH$_2$CH$_2$Cl, or CH$_2$CH$_2$CN	+
	H, C$_5$H$_{11}$, and higher alkyls, CH$_2$C$_6$H$_5$, CH$_2$COOH, or CH$_2$CH$_2$NR$_2$[g]	−

[a] −, little or no activity; +, activity.
[b] This and all unreferenced material is from unpublished work of the author and co-authors.
[c] R = H or lower alkyl.
[d] From Ref. 19.
[e] From Ref 7.
[f] From Refs. 7 and 19.
[g] All from Refs. 10, 19, and 24.
[h] From Ref. 24.
[i] From Ref. 26.
[j] From Refs. 10, 19, and 24.

Preparation

The preparation of these antibacterial agents involves a portion of the Gould-Jacobs synthetic sequence (27). The initial step in the preparation of nalidixic acid (**1**) is the reaction of 2-amino-6-methylpyridine (**10**) with diethyl ethoxymethylene-malonate (**11**) under mild conditions to give diethyl [[(6-methyl-2-pyridinyl)amino]methylene] propanedioic acid (**12**) which is thermally cyclized to ethyl 4-hydroxy-7-methyl-1,8-naphthyridine-3-carboxylate (**13**) in a method described by Lappin (28). Subsequent alkylation to ethyl 1-ethyl-1,4-dihydro-7-methyl-4-oxo-1-naphthyridine-3-carboxylate (**14**) and hydrolysis to nalidixic acid (**1**) are straightforward high-yield reactions (1–4).

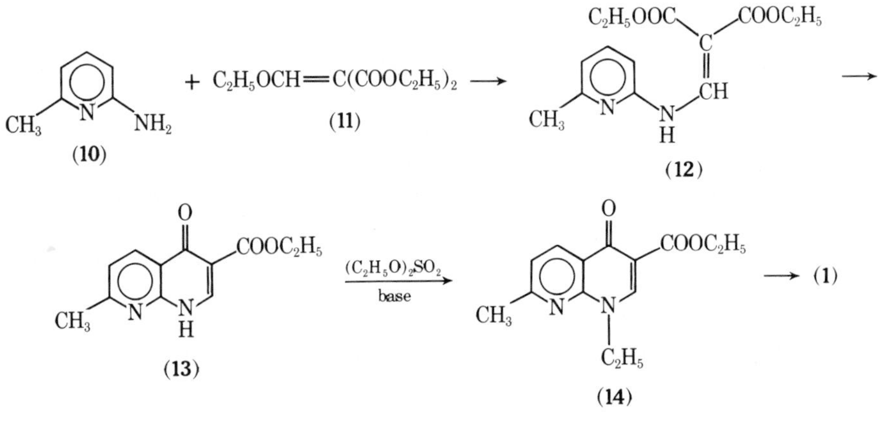

Oxolinic acid (4) is prepared in a similar manner from 1,3-benzodioxol-5-amine (15) (19–20).

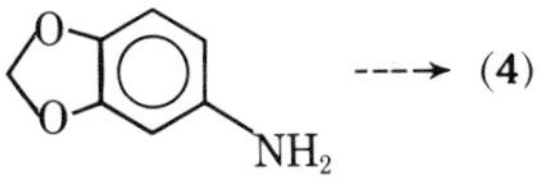

(15)

Piromidic acid (2) requires the preparation of a commercially unavailable pyrimidine intermediate (16). This is obtained by a recognized procedure (7–8).

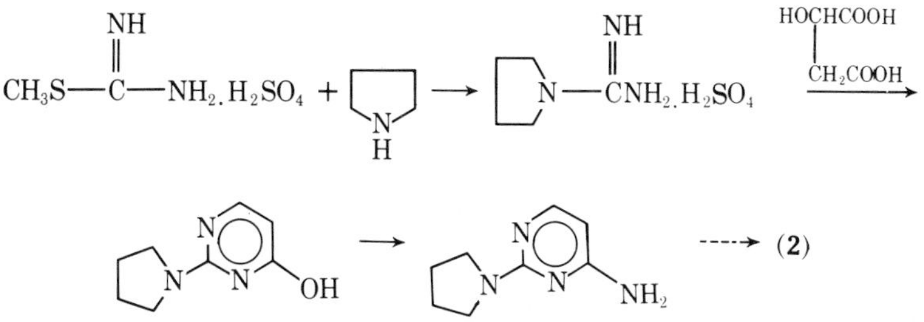

(16)

2-(1-pyrrolidinyl)-4-pyrimidinol   4-amino-2-(1-pyrrolidinyl)-pyrimidine

Pipemidic acid (3) requires the preparation of a pyrimidine intermediate (17) (10–11,13,15).

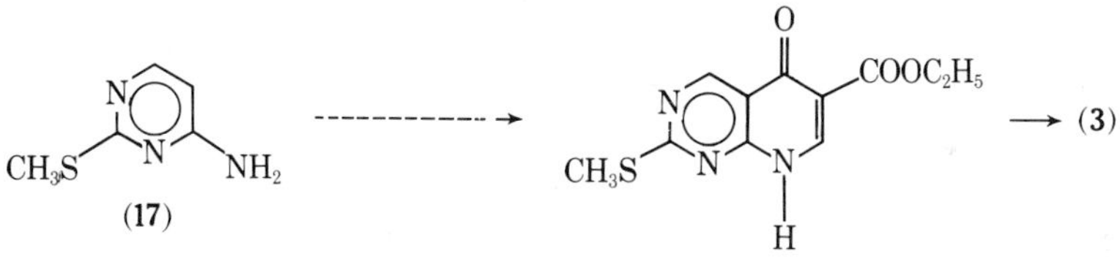

(17)

2-(methylthio)-4-pyrimidinamine   ethyl 5,8-dihydro-2-(methylthio)-5-oxo-pyrido[2,3-d]pyrimidine-6-carboxylate

Metabolism and Toxicity

The metabolism of these drugs has been reviewed (29).

The reported toxicity of quinolone carboxylic acids in mice is given in Table 3.

Resistance

A continuing problem in the field of chemotherapy is the development of resistance. There are, in a broad sense, two types of resistance. One is chromosomal, where one or more individuals in a large population of an organism may have the genetic (DNA) ability to circumvent the lethal effects of a drug; when exposed to this drug, these resistant organisms will survive and may multiply, generating a new resistant population. The other type of resistance is due to a resistance factor (R factor) (30); certain organisms have been found to contain a plasmid, a genetic (DNA) element essentially independent of the chromosome, that carries the codes for resistance to one or more antibacterial agents. The ominous aspect of these R factor plasmids is

Table 3.   Toxicity of Quinolone Carboxylic Acids in Mice

Compound	LD$_{50}$, g/kg				
	Per os oral	Intravenous	Subcutaneous	Intraperitoneal	Ref.
nalidixic acid (1)	3.3	0.18	0.5		1
	1.5–2.1	0.1–0.2	2.0	0.9–1.1	9
piromidic acid (2)	>4	0.3	>4	>4	9
pipemidic acid (3)	>16	0.7	2.2		12
oxolinic acid (4)	>6				21

that they can be transferred with the resistance characteristics to non R factor bacteria of like or of different species. The new R factor-containing organism can then lead to a new resistant population.

Nalidixic acid (1) is susceptible to chromosomal resistance as demonstrated in clinical studies but not to R factor resistance (31–32) (a relatively rare effect that appears to be true for the nitrofuran agents as well). It is a reasonable assumption that all the quinolone carboxylic acids are susceptible only to chromosomal resistance. These compounds have been shown to be cross resistant with each other, a common phenomenon among related agents, especially with chromosomal resistance.

There has been some concern expressed in the medical literature that nalidixic acid and, by association, the related agents develop resistance so rapidly that they may not be too useful (33). The rebuttal to this has been that these studies were not well controlled, that less than the recommended dosage of the drug was used (34) and that overall resistance to nalidixic acid has not shown a noticeable increase over the years it has been in use, as have agents that are susceptible to R factor resistance, ie, sulfonamides, penicillins, and other antibiotics (32,35).

Mode of Action

The mode of antibacterial action of these agents is of considerable theoretical interest as well as practical importance. Studies that are far from complete, indicate that nalidixic acid (and almost certainly the other drugs of this type) selectively inhibit the synthesis of bacterial DNA (24,36).

New Agents

Quinolone carboxylic acids represent a developing class of antibacterial agents. This can best be illustrated by the fact that besides the four compounds being marketed, there are at least four more under advanced study, cinoxacin (5) (37), droxacin sodium (6) (38), flumequine (7) (39), and rosoxacin (8) (40). These newer compounds are also intended as agents against urinary tract infections; however, the last compound, rosoxacin (8), in early work, shows promise of having broader utility, ie, systemic antibacterial activity.

BIBLIOGRAPHY

1. G. Y. Lesher, E. J. Froelich, M. D. Gruett, J. H. Bailey, and R. P. Brundage, *J. Med. Pharm. Chem.* **5,** 1063 (1962).

2. G. Y. Lesher, *Proc. 3rd Int. Congr. Chemother., Stuttgart*, **2**, 1367 (1963).
3. U.S. Pat. 3,149,104 (Sept. 16, 1964), G. Y. Lesher and M. D. Gruett (to Sterling Drug, Inc.).
4. U.S. Pat. 3,590,036 (June 29, 1971), G. Y. Lesher and M. D. Gruett (to Sterling Drug, Inc.).
5. W. H. Deitz, J. H. Bailey, and E. J. Froelich, *Antimicrob. Agents Annu.* 583 (1963).
6. E. J. Froelich and W. H. Deitz in Ref. 2, p. 1370.
7. S. Minami, T. Shono, and J. Matsumoto, *Chem. Pharm. Bull.* **19**, 1426, 1482 (1971).
8. U.S. Pat. 3,673,184 (June 27, 1972), S. Minami, T. Shono, M. Shimizu, and Y. Takase (to Dainippon Pharmaceutical Co., Ltd.).
9. M. Shimizu, S. Nakamura, and Y. Takase, *Antimicrob. Agents Annu.* 117 (1970).
10. J. Matsumoto and S. Minami, *J. Med. Chem.* **18**, 74 (1975).
11. U.S. Pat. 3,887,557 (June 3, 1975), S. Minami, J. Matsumoto, K. Kawaguchi, S. Michio, M. Shimizu, Y. Takase, and S. Nakamura (to Dainippon Pharmaceutical Co., Ltd.).
12. M. Shimizu, S. Nakamura, Y. Takase, and N. Kurobe, *Antimicrob. Agents Chemoth.* **7**, 441 (1975).
13. Ger. Pat. 2,338,325 (Feb. 7, 1974), M. Pesson (to Laboratoire Roger Bellon).
14. M. Pesson, P. De Lajudie, M. Antoine, S. Chabassier, D. Richer, and P. Girard, *C. R. Acad. Sci. Ser. C.* **278**, 1169 (1974).
15. M. Pesson, M. Antoine, S. Chabassier, S. Geiger, P. Girard, D. Richer, P. De Lajudie, E. Horvath, B. Leriche, and S. Patte, *Eur. J. Med. Chem. Chim. Ther.* **9**, 585, 591 (1974).
16. M. Shimizu, Y. Takase, S. Nakamura, H. Katae, A. Minami, K. Nakata, S. Inoue, M. Ishiyama, and Y. Kubo, *Antimicrob. Agents Chemother.* **8**, 132 (1975).
17. M. Shimizu, Y. Takase, S. Nakamura, H. Katae, A. Minami, K. Nakata, and N. Kurobe, *Antimicrob. Agents Chemother.* **9**, 569 (1976).
18. C. Orpianesi, C. Vitali, and C. Nuara, *Farmaco Ed. Prat.* **31**, 35 (1976).
19. D. Kaminsky and R. I. Meltzer, *J. Med. Chem.,* **11**, 160 (1968).
20. U.S. Pat. 3,287,458 (Nov. 22, 1966), D. Kaminsky and R. I. Meltzer (to Warner-Lambert Co.).
21. F. J. Turner, S. M. Ringel, J. F. Martin, P. J. Storino, J. M. Daly, and B. S. Schwartz, *Antimicrob. Agents Annu.* **1967**, 475.
22. D. Klein and J. M. Matsen, *Antimicrob. Agents Chemother.* **9**, 649 (1976).
23. H. Neussel and G. Linzenmeier, *Chemotherapy (Basel)* **18**, 253 (1973).
24. W. A. Goss and T. M. Cook in J. W. Corcoran and F. E. Hahn, eds., *Mechanism of Action of Antimicrobial and Antitumor Agents, Antibiotics*, Vol. III, Springer-Verlag New York, Inc., New York, 1975, pp. 174–196.
25. J. F. Ryley and M. S. Betts in S. Garattini, A. Goldin, F. Hawking, and I. J. Kopin, eds., *Adv. Pharmacol. Chemother.* **11**, 256 (1973).
26. T. Komatsu, A. Izawa, and Y. Eda, *Chemotherapy (Tokyo)* **21**, 1881 (1973); Jpn. Kokai 75,117,909 (Sept. 16, 1975), T. Komatsu, A. Izawa, Y. Eda, Y. Taira, T. Nabagome, and H. Agui; Jpn. Kokai 75,117,908 (Sept. 16, 1975), T. Komatsu, A. Izawa, Y. Eda, Y, Taira, and T. Nabagome.
27. R. G. Gould and W. A. Jacobs, *J. Am. Chem. Soc.* **61**, 2890 (1939); C. C. Price and R. M. Roberts, *J. Am. Chem. Soc.* **68**, 1204, 1255 (1946); R. C. Elderfield, *Heterocyclic Compounds*, Vol. IV, John Wiley & Sons, Inc., New York, 1952, p. 38.
28. G. R. Lappin, *J. Am. Chem. Soc.* **70**, 3348 (1948).
29. J. Edelson, C. Davison, and D. P. Benziger, *Drug Metab. Rev.* **6**, 105 (1977).
30. T. Watanabe, *N. Engl. J. Med.* **275**, 888 (1966); J. E. Davies and R. Rownd, *Science* **176**, 758 (1972).
31. H. S. Carr and H. S. Rosenkranz, *Chemotherapy (Basel)* **21**, 41 (1975); T. W. Maier, L. Zubrzycki, M. B. Coyle, M. Chila, and P. Warner, *J. Bacteriol.* **124**, 834 (1975); J. K. Moller, A. L. Bak, P. Bulow, C. Christiansen, G. Christiansen, and A. Stenderup, *Scand. J. Infect. Dis.* **8**, 112 (1976)); H. C. Neu, C. E. Cherubin, and E. D. Longo, *2nd International Symposium on Drug-Inactivation and Enzyme Antibiotic Resistance* 473, 1975.
32. R. C. Cooksey, E. R. Bannister, and W. E. Farrar, Jr., *Antimicrob. Agents Chemoth.* **7**, 396 (1975).
33. M. Buchbinder, J. C. Webb, L. V. Anderson, and W. R. McCabe, *Antimicrob. Agents Annu.* 308 (1963); A. R. Ronald, M. Turck, and R. G. Petersdord, *N. Engl. J. Med.* **275**, 1081 (1966); H. Clark, N. K. Brown, J. F. Wallace, and M. Turck, *Am. J. Med. Sci.* **261**, 145 (1971).
34. T. A. McAllister, J. G. Alexander, C. Dulake, A. Percival, J. M. H. Boyce, and P. J. Wormald, *Postgrad. Med. J. Suppl.* **47**, 7 (1971); T. A. Stamey and J. Bragonge, *J. Am. Med. Assoc.* **236**, 1857 (1976).
35. M. Nadaud, C. Suc, and L. Lapchine, *Rev. Med. Toulouse* **11**, 537 (1975); H. C. Neu, C. E. Cherubin, E. D. Longo, B. Flouton, and J. Winter, *J. Infect. Dis.* **132**, 617 (1975); F. Legler, *Arztl. Praxis* **58**, 2425 (1975).

36. R. Okazaki, T. Okazaki, K. Sakabe, K. Sugimoto, and A. Sugino, *Proc. Nat. Acad. Sci. U.S.A.,* **59,** 598 (1968); R. E. Moses and C. C. Richardson, *Proc. Nat. Acad. Sci. U.S.A.* **67,** 674 (1970); J. A. Wechsler and J. D. Gross, *Mol. Gen. Genet.* **113,** 273 (1971); J. Neuhard and E. Thomassen, *Eur. J. Biochem.* **20,** 36 (1971); A. Puga and I. Tessman, *J. Mol. Biol.* **75,** 99 (1973); G. J. Bourguignon, M. Levitt, and R. Sternglanz, *Antimicrob. Agents Chemother.* **4,** 479 (1973); S. Hayes and W. Szybalski, *Fed. Proc. Fed. Amer. Soc. Exp. Biol.* **32,** 529 (1973); P. K. Schneck, W. L. Staredenbauer, and P. H. Hofschneider, *Eur. J. Biochem.* **38,** 130 (1973); C. A. Michels, J. Blamire, B. Goldfinger, and S. Marmur, *Antimicrob. Agents Chemother.* **3,** 562 (1973); W. E. Hill and W. L. Fangman, *J. Bacteriol.* **116,** 1329 (1973); G. T. Javor, *J. Bacteriol.* **120,** 282 (1974); Y. Sakakibara and J. Tomizawa, *Proc. Nat. Acad. Sci. U.S.A.* **71,** 802 (1974); T. J. Simon, W. E. Masker, and P. C. Hanawalt, *Biochem. Biophys. Acta,* **349,** 271 (1974); J. J. Dermody, G. J. Bourguignon, P. D. Foglesong, and R. Sternglanz, *Biochem. Biophys. Res. Commun.* **61,** 1340 (1974); J. F. de Castro, J. F. O. Carvalho, N. Moussatché, and F. T. de Castro, *Antimicrob. Agents Chemother.* **7,** 487 (1975); G. C. Crumplin and J. T. Smith, *Antimicrob. Agents Chemother.* **8,** 251 (1975); M. Nishida, Y. Mishima, J. Kawada, and K. L. Yielding, *Antimicrob. Agents Chemother.* **8,** 384 (1975); G. C. Crumplin and J. T. Smith, *Nature (London)* **260,** 643 (1976).

37. U.S. Pat. 3,669,965 (June 13, 1972), W. W. White (to Eli Lilly and Co.); W. E. Wick, D. A. Preston, W. A. White, and R. S. Gordee, *Antimicrob. Agents Chemother.* **4,** 415 (1973); S. Kurtz and M. Turck, *Antimicrob. Agents Chemother.* **7,** 370 (1975); R. N. Jones and P. C. Fuchs, *Antimicrob. Agents Chemother.* **10,** 146 (1976).

38. R. Albrecht, *Justus Liebigs Ann. Chem.* **762,** 55 (1972); U.S. Pat. 3,773,769 (Nov. 20, 1973), R. Albrecht, J. J. Kessler, and E. Schroeder (to Schering A.G.).

39. U.S. Pat. 3,883,522 (May 13, 1975), J. F. Ferster (to Riker Laboratories, Inc.); U.S. Pat. 3,969,463 (July 13, 1976), J. F. Ferster (to Riker Laboratories, Inc.); G. Stilwell, K. Holmes, and M. Turck, *Antimicrob. Agents Chemother.* **7,** 483 (1975); S. R. Rohlfing, J. F. Gerster, and D. C. Kvam, *Antimicrob. Agents Chemother.* **10,** 20 (1976).

40. U.S. Pat. 3,753,993 (Aug. 13, 1973), G. Y. Lesher and P. M. Carabateas (to Sterling Drug, Inc.).

GEORGE Y. LESHER
Sterling-Winthrop Research Institute

NITROFURANS

Antibacterial nitrofurans are a class of synthetic compounds characterized by the presence of the 5-nitro-2-furanyl group:

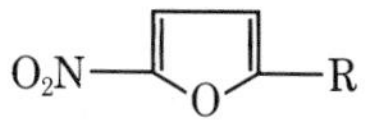

In the most prominent members each R substituent includes an azomethine (—CH=N—) linkage attached to the furan ring.

The antimicrobial activity of nitrofurans was first reported by Stillman, Scott, and Clampit in 1943 (1), and independently by Dann and Möller (2). Dodd and Stillman (3) investigated a number of derivatives and concluded that the presence of a nitro group in the 5-position of the molecule conferred antibacterial activity on such derivatives. These initial reports stimulated the synthesis of approximately 4000 members of this class and the publication of more than 10,000 articles on nitrofurans. A number of nitrofurans have attained commercial utility as antibacterial agents in human and veterinary medicine because of their broad spectrum activity, relatively mild toxicity, and low tendency to develop resistant bacterial strains.

Chemical Properties

Most nitrofurans are relatively stable crystalline solids; however, they will darken on prolonged exposure to strong alkali and light. They are relatively insoluble in water and have characteristic ultraviolet absorption, a useful property in many sensitive analytical procedures. Nitrofuran derivatives undergo chemical reactions typical of the side chain. Chemical reduction leads to aminofurans (4) and furan ring-opened products (5–6). The nitro group can be displaced by methoxy (7–8), halogen (9), azido, alkylmercapto, and phenylsulfonyl groups (10). Photochemical hydroxylation of 5-nitro-2-furancarboxaldehyde leads to 4-hydroxy derivatives (11).

The General References include extensive reviews of the physical, chemical, biological, and chemotherapeutic properties of the nitrofurans.

Preparation

Most of the commercialized nitrofurans are derivatives of 5-nitro-2-furancarboxaldehyde or its diacetate. These compounds were first prepared by Gilman and Wright (12) by the action of fuming nitric acid in excess acetic anhydride (acetyl nitrate) at low temperatures on 2-furancarboxaldehyde [98-01-1] (furfural) or its diacetate, followed by conversion of an intermediate 2-acetoxy-2,5-dihydrofuran (13) with pyridine. This process was later improved by the use of concentrated nitric acid (14–15) and acidic catalysts such as phosphorous pentoxide, -trichloride and -oxychloride (16), and sulfuric acid (17). Orthophosphoric acid, p-toluenesulfonic acid, arsenic acid, boric acid, stibonic acid, and others have also been shown to be beneficial additives for the nitration of furfural with acetyl nitrate. Hydrolysis of 5-nitro-2-furancarboxaldehyde diacetate with aqueous acids generates the aldehyde which is commonly used without isolation.

The use of 5-nitro-2-furancarboxaldehyde oxime, which was prepared by low temperature, mixed-acid nitration of 2-furancarboxaldehyde oxime, as a source of the free aldehyde has been reported (18).

Alternatively, the 2-furancarboxaldehyde derivatives with the R substituent in place have been nitrated to give the desired antibacterial agents (19).

Nitrofurazone. Condensation of 5-nitro-2-furancarboxaldehyde with semicarbazide produces nitrofurazone, 2-[(5-nitro-2-furanyl)methylene]hydrazinecarboxamide (15) (Table 1), the first nitrofuran to be used clinically. Nitrofurazone is a topical antibacterial agent and a systemic agent for bacterial diseases in poultry and swine. Condensation of the aldehyde with semioxamazide affords nifuraldezone [3270-71-1], aminooxoacetic acid [(5-nitro-2-furanyl)methylene]hydrazide (20), useful in the treatment of calf scours (dysentery).

Furazolidone. Furazolidone, 3-[[(5-nitro-2-furanyl)methylene]amino]-2-oxazolidinone, is manufactured (15,21) by the condensation of 3-amino-2-oxazolidinone, prepared from 2-hydrazinoethanol (22) and diethyl carbonate, with 5-nitro-2-furancarboxaldehyde. By similar processes furaltadone [139-91-3], 5-(4-morpholinyl-

Table 1.   Structures of Representative Antibacterial Nitrofurans

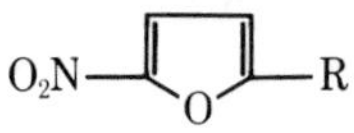

$$O_2N \underset{O}{\overline{}} R$$

Name	CAS Registry No.	R
nitrofurazone	[59-87-0]	—CH=NNHCONH₂
furazolidone	[67-45-8]	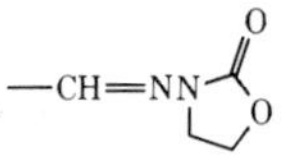 —CH=NN (oxazolidinone)
nitrofurantoin	[67-20-9]	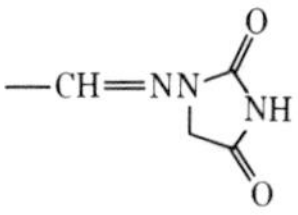 —CH=NN (imidazolidinedione)
nifuroxime	[6236-05-1]	—CH=N\OH (anti)
Z-furan	[710-25-8]	—CH=CH—C(=O)—NH₂
nitrofurfuryl methyl ether	[586-84-5]	—CH₂—O—CH₃
nitrovin	[2315-20-0]	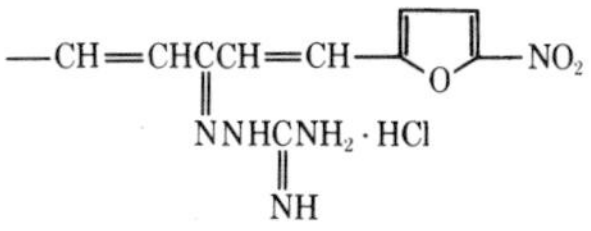 —CH=CHCCH=CH—(furan)—NO₂, NNHCNH₂·HCl, NH
furalazine, R′ = H	[556-12-7]	—CH=CH—(triazine)—NHR′
acetylfuratrizine, R′ = CH₃CO—	[1789-26-0]	
Furium	[531-82-8]	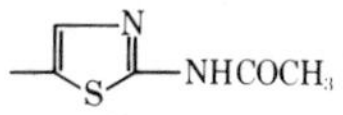 (thiazole)—NHCOCH₃
nitrofurathiazide	[61143-06-4]	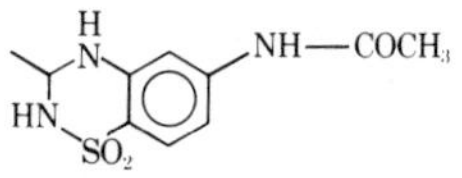 (structure with NH—COCH₃, HN, SO₂)

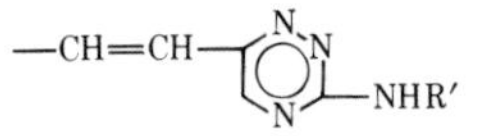

methyl)-3-[[(5-nitro-2-furanyl)methylene]amino]-2-oxazolidinone (23), and nifuratel [4936-47-4], 5-[(methylthio)methyl]-3-[[(5-nitro-2-furanyl)methylene]amino]-2-oxazolidinone (24) are prepared starting with substituted hydrazinopropanols. Furazolidone is used for gastrointestinal and vaginal infections in humans and for a wide variety of bacterial and protozoal infections in poultry and swine. Furaltadone is utilized in veterinary medicine for the treatment of bovine mastitis and for *E. coli* and control of *Salmonella* in chickens. Nifuratel is effective against bacterial and trichomonal infections.

Nitrofurantoin. Nitrofurantoin, 1-[[(5-nitro-2-furanyl)methylene]amino]-2,4-imidazolidinedione, is obtained from the reaction of 1-amino-2,4-imidazolidinedione and 5-nitro-2-furancarboxaldehyde diacetate in aqueous acid (15,25). The aminoimidazolidinedione is obtained by treating an excess of hydrazine hydrate with sodium hydroxide and chloroacetic acid, followed by reaction with an alkali cyanate and then cyclization in mineral acid. Condensation of ethyl chloroacetate with acetone semicarbazone in the presence of alcoholic sodium alkoxide, followed by cyclization in acid also yields the aminoimidazolidinedione (26).

Crystallization of nitrofurantoin from a suitable solvent, such as nitromethane, produces a macrocrystalline form (27); treatment of nitrofurantoin with sodium hydroxide or sodium alkoxides produces the soluble sodium salt [54-87-5] (28). Hydroxymethylation with formaldehyde yields urfadyn [1088-92-2], 3-(hydroxymethyl)-1-[[(5-nitro-2-furanyl)methylene]amino]-2,4-imidazolidinedione (29). Nitrofurantoin is useful in the treatment of bacterial urinary tract infections. Urfadyn, which reverts to nitrofurantoin, has similar utility.

Nifuroxime. The antioxime, nifuroxime (1,13), of 5-nitro-2-furancarboxaldehyde is active against many bacteria and fungi, particularly against *Candida albicans*. The acethydrazone, nihydrazone [67-28-7], acetic acid [(5-nitro-2-furanyl)methylene]-hydrazide (20), is effective against poultry coccidiosis and it has antibacterial properties.

Z-Furan. Z-Furan, 3-(5-nitro-2-furanyl)-2-propenamide (30), a Japanese food preservative, is readily prepared by Perkin reaction of 5-nitro-2-furancarboxaldehyde diacetate, followed by PCl$_5$ chlorination and amination with ammonia. A second nitrofuran, also used as a food preservative in Japan until it was withdrawn in 1974 because of mutagenic activity, is furylfuramide [3688-53-7], α-[(5-nitro-2-furanyl)-methylene]-2-furanacetamide. Furylfuramide was prepared by a similar reaction sequence involving 5-nitro-2-furancarboxaldehyde and 2-furanacetic acid (31).

Nitrofurfuryl Methyl Ether. Nitrofurfuryl methyl ether, 2-(methoxymethyl)-5-nitrofuran, synthesis starts with the methyl iodide alkylation of 2-furanmethanol, followed by nitration (15). This topical drug is especially effective against dermatomycoses.

Nitrovin. 2-[3-(5-Nitro-2-furanyl)-1-[2-(5-nitro-2-furanyl)ethenyl]-2-propenylidene]hydrazinecarboximidamide hydrochloride, nitrovin, has bacteriostatic and bactericidal action and is employed in many countries as a growth promotant in chickens (32). Acetone is combined with two equivalents of 5-nitro-2-furancarboxaldehyde to produce a pentadienone that is condensed with aminoguanidine to give nitrovin (33).

Furalazine. On heating nitrovin in butanol or dimethylformamide at 100–130°C a cyclic triazine is formed: 6-[2-(5-nitro-2-furanyl)ethenyl]-1,2,4-triazine-3-amine, furalazine, (34). An improved synthesis of furalazine starting with the condensation product of 5-nitro-2-furancarboxaldehyde and acetone, 4-(5-nitro-2-furanyl)-3-buten-2-one, has been reported (35). Oxidation of the butenone with selenium dioxide and condensation of the resulting pyruvaldehyde hydrate with aminoguanidine bicarbonate gives furalazine. Furalazine hydrochloride [3012-10-0], its N-acetyl derivative, acetylfuratrizine (36), and the N,N-bis(hydroxymethyl) derivative [794-93-4], Panfuran S, formed by addition of formaldehyde (37), are systemic antibacterial agents.

Furium. Among the large number of nitrofurans synthesized, several compounds containing the R substituent as part of a heterocyclic ring have emerged with clinical utility. Furium, N-[4-(5-nitro-2-furanyl)-2-thiazolyl]acetamide, commercialized in Italy, exhibits activity against bacilli and pathogenic enterobacteria (38). It is prepared by condensation of thiourea and 2-bromo-1-(5-nitro-2-furanyl)ethanone [15057-21-3], followed by acetylation of the resulting aminothiazole with acetic anhydride in pyridine (39). A similar condensation with ethylenethiourea leads to furazolium chloride [5118-17-2], 6,7-dihydro-3-(5-nitro-2-furanyl)-5H-imidazo[2,1-b]thiazol-4-ium chloride (40). Furazolium chloride is an effective broad spectrum antibacterial agent for the prevention or treatment of topical infections in horses and dogs.

Nitrofurathiazide. Nitrofurathiazide, 6-acetylamino-3,4-dihydro-3-(5-nitro-2-furanyl)-2H-1,2,4-benzothiadiazine 1,1-dioxide, is prepared by condensation of 5-nitro-2-furancarboxaldehyde with 4-acetylamino-2-aminobenzenesulfonamide (41). Nitrofurathiazide exhibits antibacterial activity and is used in combination with other drugs in treating acute or chronic otitis externa of dogs and cats.

A review (42) of the chemotherapeutic properties of nitrofurazone, furazolidone, and nitrofurantoin includes physical properties; antimicrobial activity; mode of action; bacterial resistance; absorption, distribution, and excretion; clinical use; and adverse reactions. For other reviews covering the side effects and toxicity of nitrofurans see the General References.

BIBLIOGRAPHY

"Nitrofurans" in ECT 2nd ed., Vol. 13, pp. 853–857, K. J. Hayes, Norwich Pharmacal Co.

1. U.S. Pat. 2,319,481 (May 18, 1943), W. B. Stillman, A. B. Scott, and J. M. Clampit (to Norwich Pharmacal Co.).
2. O. Dann and E. F. Möller, Ber. **80,** 23 (1947).
3. M. C. Dodd and W. B. Stillman, J. Pharmacol. Exp. Ther. **82,** 11 (1944).
4. F. F. Ebetino, J. J. Carroll, and G. Gever, J..Med. Pharm. Chem. **5,** 513 (1962).
5. F. L. Austin, Chem. Ind., 523 (1957).
6. J. J. Gavin, F. F. Ebetino, R. Freedman, and W. E. Waterbury, Arch. Biochem. Biophys. **113,** 399 (1966).
7. J. Olivard and J. P. Heotis, J. Org. Chem. **33,** 2552 (1968).
8. L. J. Powers, J. Pharm. Sci. **60,** 1425 (1971).
9. H. R. Snyder, Jr., and P. H. Seehausen, J. Heterocycl. Chem. **10,** 385 (1973).
10. F. Lieb and K. Eiter, Justus Liebigs Ann. Chem. **761,** 130 (1972).
11. J. Olivard, G. M. Rose, G. M. Klein, and J. P. Heotis, J. Med. Chem. **19,** 729 (1976).
12. H. Gilman and G. F. Wright, J. Am. Chem. Soc. **52,** 2550, 4165 (1930).
13. A. P. Dunlop and F. N. Peters, "The Furans," ACS Monograph Series No. 119, Reinhold Publishing Corp., New York, 1953, pp. 141–169, 725, 727.
14. U.S. Pat. 2,490,006 (Nov. 29, 1949), W. Kimel, J. H. Coleman, and W. B. Stillman (to Eaton Laboratories, Inc.).
15. H. J. Sanders, R. T. Edmunds, and W. B. Stillman, Ind. Eng. Chem. **47,** 358 (1955).
16. U.S. Pat. 2,502,114 (Mar. 28, 1950), M. Witte and C. J. Lind (to Allied Chemical & Dye Corp.).
17. Jpn. Kokai 4377 (Dec. 16, 1950), J. Yoshida and co-workers.

18. U.S. Pat. 2,927,110 (Mar. 1, 1960), G. Gever and C. J. O'Keefe (to Norwich Pharmacal Co.).
19. U.S. Pat. 2,898,335 (Aug. 4, 1959), J. G. Michels (to Norwich Pharmacal Co.).
20. U.S. Pat. 2,416,234 (Feb. 18, 1947), W. B. Stillman and A. B. Scott (to Eaton Laboratories, Inc.).
21. U.S. Pat. 2,742,462 (Apr. 17, 1956), G. Gever (to Norwich Pharmacal Co.).
22. U.S. Pat. 2,660,607 (Nov. 24, 1953), G. Gever (to Eaton Laboratories, Inc.).
23. U.S. Pat. 2,802,002 (Aug. 6, 1957), G. Gever (to Norwich Pharmacal Co.).
24. U.S. Pat. 3,288,787 (Nov. 29, 1966), G. Massarolli (to Inphar S.A.).
25. U.S. Pat. 2,610,181 (Sept. 9, 1952), K. J. Hayes (to Eaton Laboratories, Inc.); U.S. Pat. 2,779,786 (Jan. 29, 1957), J. H. Coleman, W. Hayden, Jr., and C. J. O'Keefe (to Norwich Pharmacal Co.).
26. U.S. Pat. 2,990,402 (June 27, 1961), D. Jack and G. Sutno (to Smith, Kline & French Laboratories, Ltd.).
27. U.S. Pat. 3,401,221 (Sept. 10, 1968), A. R. Borgmann, K. J. Hayes, H. E. Paul, and M. F. Paul (to Norwich Pharmacal Co.).
28. U.S. Pat. 3,007,846 (Nov. 7, 1961), G. Gever and J. G. Vincent, Jr. (to Norwich Pharmacal Co.).
29. U.S. Pat. 3,446,802 (May 27, 1969), J. G. Michels (to Norwich Pharmacal Co.).
30. T. Takahashi, H. Saikachi, T. Sasaki, K. Suzuki, and E. Moritani, *J. Pharm. Soc. Jpn.* **69,** 286 (1949).
31. H. Saikachi and A. Tanaka, *J. Pharm. Soc. Jpn.* **83,** 147 (1963).
32. U.S. Pat. 3,264,112 (Aug. 2, 1966), Y. Kodama, T. Fujiwara, and T. Inagaki (to Toyama Chemical Industries Co., Ltd.).
33. Jpn. Kokai 2673 (July 18, 1952), H. Uota and co-workers (to Toyama Chemical Industries Co., Ltd.); Jpn. Kokai 2974 (Aug. 7, 1952), H. Uota and A. Kuriyama (to Toyama Chemical Industries Co., Ltd.).
34. U.S. Pat. 3,159,625 (Dec. 1, 1964), Y. Kodama, I. Saikawa, T. Maeda, A. Takai, and I. Takamichi (to Toyama Chemical Industries Co., Ltd.).
35. U.S. Pat. 3,349,086 (Oct. 24, 1967), Fr. Pat. 1,377,650 (Nov. 6, 1964), R. R. G. Haber (to ABIC Chemical Laboratories, Ltd.).
36. A. Takai and I. Saikawa, *J. Pharm. Soc. Jpn.* **84,** 9 (1964).
37. Ref. 36, p. 16.
38. K. Miura and H. K. Reckendorf, *Progress in Medicinal Chemistry,* Vol. 5, Plenum Press, New York, 1967, p. 320.
39. U.S. Pat. 2,992,225 (July 11, 1961), D. E. Dickson (to Abbott Laboratories).
40. U.S. Pat. 3,169,970 (Feb. 16, 1965), H. R. Snyder, Jr. (to Norwich Pharmacal Co.).
41. U.S. Pat. 3,155,654 (Nov. 3, 1964), Fr. Pat. M1831 (June 24, 1963), M. H. Sherlock (to Schering Corp.).
42. R. E. Chamberlain, *J. Antimicrob. Chemother.* **2,** 325 (1976).

General References

A. P. Dunlop and F. N. Peters, "The Furans," *ACS Monograph Series No. 119,* Reinhold Publishing Corp., New York, 1953, pp. 141–169, 725, 727.
H. E. Paul and M. F. Paul in R. J. Schnitzer and F. Hawking, eds., *Experimental Chemotherapy,* Vol. 2, Academic Press, Inc., New York, 1964, pp. 207–370; Vol. 4, 1966, pp. 521–536.
K. Miura and H. K. Reckendorf in G. P. Ellis and G. B. West, eds., *Progress in Medicinal Chemistry,* Vol. 5, Plenum Press, New York, 1967, pp. 320–381.
H. Kala and D. Ausborn, *Pharmazie* **26,** 121–135, 193–207 (1971).
E. Grunberg and E. H. Titsworth, *Annu. Rev. Microbiol.* **27,** 317–346 (1973).

FRANK F. EBETINO
Norwich Pharmacal Company
Division of Morton-Norwich Products, Inc.

SULFONAMIDES

Sulfa drugs are sulfonamides derived from sulfanilamide (p-aminobenzenesulfonamide). Substitution on the sulfonamide nitrogen is referred to as N^1-substitution, and substitution on the p-amino group as N^4-substitution. The therapeutically active derivatives usually are N^1-substituted (Table 1). The structures of sulfanilamide (1) and sulfadiazine (4) illustrate these relations.

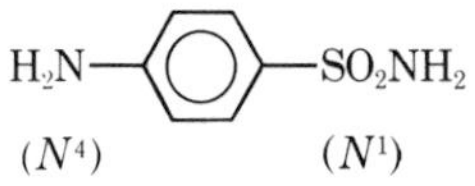

The fact that sulfa drugs are antibacterial agents separates them sharply from the diuretic, hypoglycemic, and uricosuric sulfonamide drugs. It has become customary to include with the sulfa drugs certain related antibacterials in which the formal structural divergence from sulfanilamide is considerable, such as Prontosil (29), which is converted *in vivo* to sulfanilamide and mafenide (26). One important class of sulfanilamide analogues are not sulfonamides; they are the antibacterial sulfones (eg, dapsone (27)).

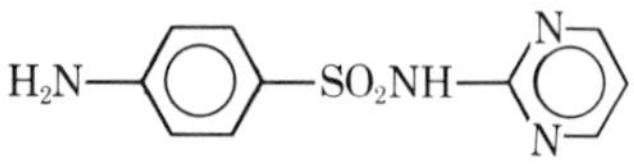

The action of the sulfa and sulfone drugs is bacteriostatic rather than bactericidal and, with some exceptions, is thought to arise from a derangement of the metabolic conversion of p-aminobenzoic acid (PABA) to the folic acid-related vitamins (5a,6) (see Vitamins). The sulfa drugs are still immensely important although they have been largely displaced by antibiotics (qv) from their original application in systemic disease treatment. They provide a principal treatment of urinary-tract disease for which they are not only cheaper than the antibiotics, but may actually be considered superior by some physicians. The sulfa drugs have some application in the treatment of the fungus-related nocardiosis and in the prophylaxis of rheumatic fever under certain circumstances (7a). Certain sulfa drug relatives are used empirically to treat ulcerative colitis although the basis of their action is not understood (7a). The related sulfones have become an accepted treatment for leprosy and have extensive worldwide use for this purpose (see Chemotherapeutics, antibacterial and antimycotic).

A list of sulfa drugs with their structural formulas and some physical properties is given in Table 1. These compounds include all currently important drugs, a few experimental drugs not yet marketed in the United States, and a few drugs no longer used but historically important. A complete list of all sulfa drugs would be much longer. Following sulfanilamide (1), Table 1 lists the principal classes of derivatives, the N^1-heterocyclic derivatives, (2) through (19); the N^1-acyl derivatives, (20) and (21); the N^1-acyl-N^1-heterocyclic derivative, (22); and the N^4-acyl derivatives, (23) and (24). The remaining compounds, (25) through (29), are not sulfa drugs in the strictest sense but are closely related.

Northey describes over 5000 sulfanilamide derivatives, their preparation, properties, trade names, and biologic applications up through 1944 in his review (5). Several thousand additional derivatives have been made since 1944 but no comparable review is available. For mode of action see Seydel (6), for a definitive medical overview to 1960 see Weinstein, Madoff and Samet (7), for a review of the experimental antibacterial aspects with some historical background see Neipp (8), Zbinden (9), and Anand (10), and for pharmacology and toxicology see Bagdon (11) and Rieder (2).

The discovery and development of the sulfa drugs is a landmark in modern medicine. They were the first drugs to control systemic bacterial disease and they still find important application for this purpose. The success of the sulfa drugs in the previously unrewarding treatment of bacterial disease made the immensely expensive effort reasonable that led to penicillin and later the broad-spectrum antibiotics (12). During clinical use it was noted that certain sulfa drugs had unexpected pharmacological effects. These effects, perfected in various derivatives, became the main properties of important new classes of diuretics, hypoglycemics, and uricosurics (drugs for treating gout) (13).

In a sense the sulfa drugs were an outgrowth of Paul Ehrlich's ideas of the mechanism of action of chemotherapeutic agents and can be traced to him through the unsuccessful early efforts of Julius Morgenroth, R. Levey, Michael Heidelberger and of Walter A. Jacobs. The studies that mark the actual beginning of the sulfa drugs were those of the team Fritz Mietzsch and Joseph Klarer, chemists, and Gerhard Domagk, pharmacologist, at I. G. Farbenindustrie in Germany from 1930 to 1935. These studies culminated in Prontosil (29) (sulfamidochrysoidine; p-[(2,4-diaminophenyl)azo]benzenesulfonamide), the first drug to cure bacterial septicemias. A very important factor in this discovery was the use of an animal infection to test for activity; Prontosil (H. Bayer, Leverkusen) is inactive in the test tube. It was established (14) that sufanilamide, which could be formed from Prontosil in the body, was responsible for the activity of that drug. This discovery marked the beginning of a worldwide research effort in the synthesis and testing of sulfanilamide derivatives (5b). This vast effort, in less than 10 yr, produced over 5000 derivatives listed in Northey's review (5). The primary aim of this early work was to find more active compounds with a broader spectrum. This objective was reached in the N^1-heterocyclic-substituted sulfanilamides exemplified by (2), (3), and (4). Maximum activity was reached in these compounds which was not surpassed substantially by later derivatives.

Nevertheless, most of the early N^1-heterocyclic substituted sulfanilamides are now obsolete (9); only the sulfapyrimidines (4) and (8) remain, and these are diminishing in use. The second-generation sulfa drugs that now dominate the market are also N^1-heterocyclic-substituted sulfanilamides. Although usually not more active, these are less toxic or have pharmacologic advantages (9).

During that time the N^1-substituted sulfanilamides were becoming widely accepted for the treatment of systemic disease caused by common bacteria, another class of derivatives showed promise in mycobacterial infections. These were congeners of bis-(p-aminophenyl)sulfone, often referred to as 4,4'-diaminodiphenylsulfone, or DDS (27). In contrast to the direction of progress in the sulfonamides, sulfone derivatives did not find wide use but today the parent sulfone, dapsone (27), is the treatment of choice for the ancient scourge, leprosy (15–17).

Table 1. Selected Major Sulfa Drugs and Related Compounds

No.	Generic or common name	Structure	CAS Registry Number	mp, °C[a]	Approximate solubility in water at 25°C, mg/100 mL[a]	Approximate half-life, h[b]	pK_a[b]
(1)	sulfanilamide	$H_2NC_6H_4SO_2NH_2$	[16-74 1]	164.5–166.5	750	6.8	10.08.
(2)	sulfapyridine	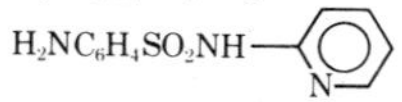 $H_2NC_6H_4SO_2NH$—	[144-83-2]	191–193	30		8.43[c]
(3)	sulfathiazole	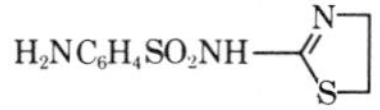 $H_2NC_6H_4SO_2NH$—	[72-14-0]	200–204	60	3.8	7.25
(4)	sulfadiazine	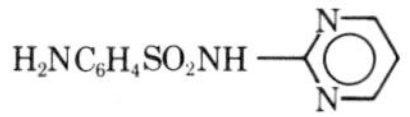 $H_2NC_6H_4SO_2NH$—	[68-35-9]	252–256	8	16.7	6.52
(5)	sulfachloropyridazine	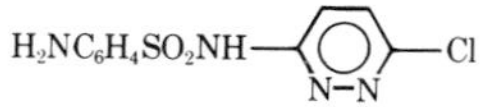 $H_2NC_6H_4SO_2NH$—	[80-32-0]		ca 90[d] at pH 5.5	8.0	6.10
(6)	sulfadimethoxine	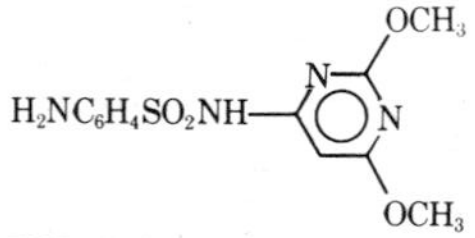 $H_2NC_6H_4SO_2NH$—	[122-11-2]	201–203	<4.6	ca 33	6.32
(7)	sulfaethidole	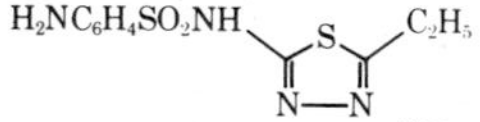 $H_2NC_6H_4SO_2NH$—	[94-19-9]	185–186	25	4.8	5.65
(8)	sulfamethazine	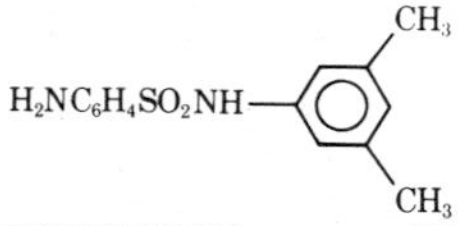 $H_2NC_6H_4SO_2NH$—	[57-68-1]	176	ca 100	7.0	7.37[c]
(9)	sulfamethizole	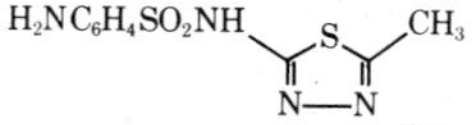 $H_2NC_6H_4SO_2NH$—	[144-82-1]	208	25	short	5.45
(10)	sulfamethoxazole	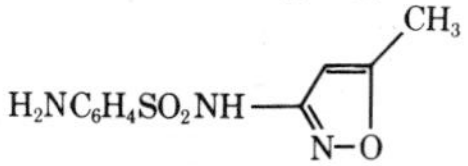 $H_2NC_6H_4SO_2NH$—	[723-46-6]	167		11.0	6.03
(11)	sulfamethoxypyridazine	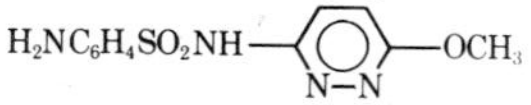 $H_2NC_6H_4SO_2NH$—	[80-35-3]	182–183	110 at pH 5	40.0	7.20
(12)	sulfameter	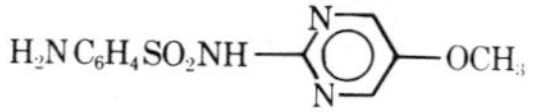 $H_2NC_6H_4SO_2NH$—	[651-06-9]	214–216		36.6	7.02

16

No.	Name	Structure	CAS Registry No.	mp, °C	Solubility	pKa	pKa
(13)	sulfamoxole	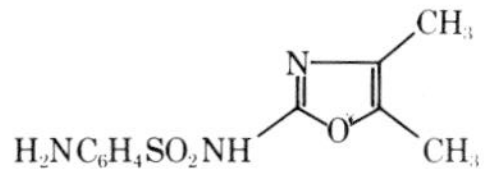 $H_2NC_6H_4SO_2NH$ (isoxazole, CH_3, CH_3)	[729-99-7]	193–194		10.6	7.40
(14)	sulfaphenazole	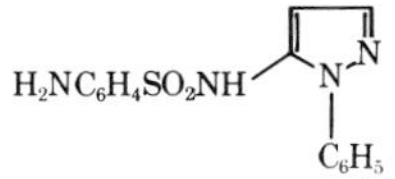 $H_2NC_6H_4SO_2NH$ (C_6H_5)	[526-08-9]	179–183		10.0	6.09
(15)	sulfapyrazine	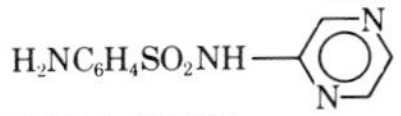 $H_2NC_6H_4SO_2NH$ (pyrazine)	[116-44-9]	250–254	5		6.04^c
(16)	sulfaquinoxaline	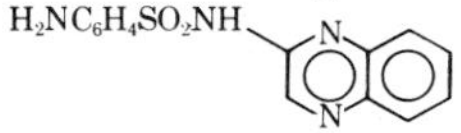 $H_2NC_6H_4SO_2NH$ (quinoxaline)	[59-40-5]	247–248	<0.75		
(17)	sulfisomidine	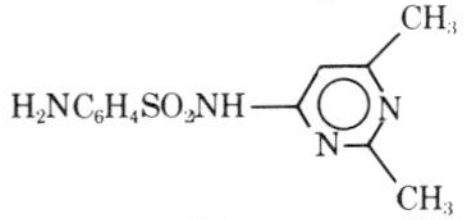 $H_2NC_6H_4SO_2NH$ (CH_3, CH_3)	[515-64-0]	243	ca 200	7.4	7.57
(18)	sulfisoxazole	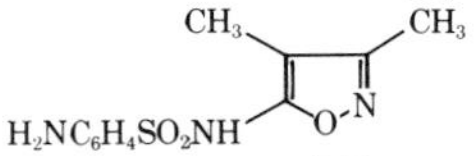 CH_3, CH_3, $H_2NC_6H_4SO_2NH$ (isoxazole)	[127-69-5]	194	350 at pH 6	6.0	5.0
(19)	sulfacytine	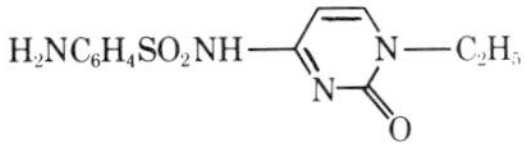 $H_2NC_6H_4SO_2NH$ (N–C_2H_5)	[17784-12-2]	167–168	109 at pH 5	4	6.9
(20)	sulfacetamide	$H_2NC_6H_4SO_2NHCOCH_3$	[144-80-9]	182–184	>670	7.0	5.78 (base)
(21)	sulfaguanidine	$H_2NC_6H_4SO_2NHC(:NH)NH_2$	[57-67-0]	190–193	100		
(22)	N^1-acetylsulfisoxazole	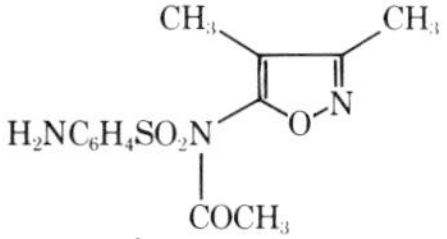 $H_2NC_6H_4SO_2N$ (COCH$_3$)	[80-74-0]	192–195	7		
(23)	succinylsulfathiazole	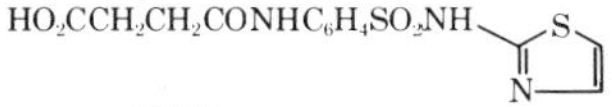 $HO_2CCH_2CH_2CONHC_6H_4SO_2NH$ (thiazole)	[116-43-8]	184–186	(soluble pH 7)		(acid)
(24)	phthalylsulfathiazole	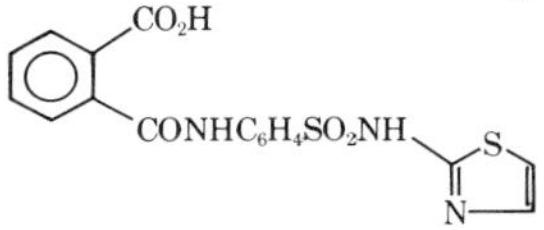 CO_2H, $CONHC_6H_4SO_2NH$ (thiazole)	[85-73-4]	240–250 effervesces 272–277 dec	(soluble pH 7		(acid)

Table 1 *(continued)*

No.	Generic or common name	Structure	CAS Registry Number	mp, °C[a]	Approximate solubility in water at 25°C mg/100 mL[a]	Approximate half-life, hr[b]	pK_a[b]
(25)	salicylazosulfapyridine	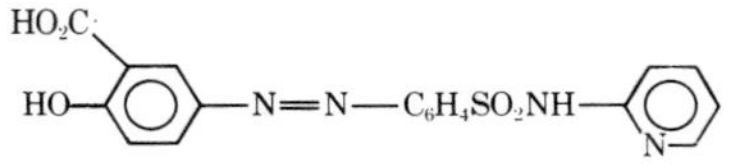	[*599-79-1*]	240–245	(soluble pH 7)		(acid)
(26)	mafenide (homosulfanilamide)	$H_2NCH_2C_6H_4SO_2NH_2$	[*138-39-6*]	153 (HCl salt 256)	(salt soluble)		(acid)
(27)	dapsone (4,4′-diaminodiphenyl sulfone, DDS)	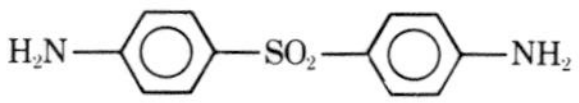	[*80-08-0*]	175–176	(soluble)		(base)
(28)	acedapsone (4,4′-diacetamino-diphenyl sulfone, DADDS)	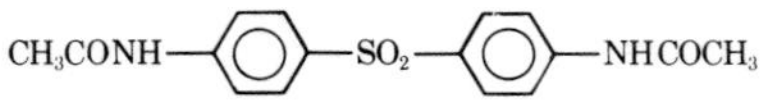	[*77-46-3*]	282–285	(nearly insoluble)		neutral
(29)	Prontosil (sulfamidochrysoidine)	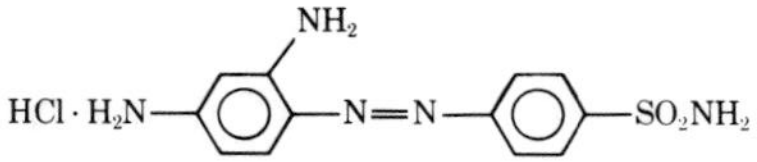	[*103-12-8*]		(soluble)		

[a] Unless otherwise noted, source of data ref. 1.
[b] Unless otherwise noted, source of data ref. 2.
[c] From ref 3.
[d] From ref. 4.

Therapeutic Aspects

Systemic Infections. It was in the treatment of bacterial septicemias (blood stream infections) that the sulfa drugs had their spectacular beginning; they have been effective in internal infections, both septicemias and other tissue infections, that are due to *Streptococci,* pneumococci, *Staphylococci,* meningococci gonococci, *Hemophilis influenza*, and the fungus-related *Nocardia* (5e,7). From the time penicillin was introduced, ca 1944, the sulfa drugs have been increasingly displaced from this important field by the antibiotics (7b,8b). Now they are rarely the treatment of choice, and it is controversial whether they should be supplanted altogether by antibiotics except perhaps in rheumatic fever prophylaxis and in nocardiosis (15–17). Nevertheless their low cost, convenience (by oral dosing), and traditional acceptance keep them significant drugs for the treatment of systemic disease, particularly in Europe.

Outside the United States, sulfas are used especially in combination with the antifolic drug trimethoprim. This is a synergistic combination of sulfamethoxazole (**10**) and trimethoprim. Both drugs have a half-life of approximately 11 h, thus when dosed in a fixed mixture give a constant proportion of one drug to the other in the blood stream. This proportion is adjusted in the dose to give maximum synergistic effects (**18**).

Urinary Tract Infections. Despite the rise of the antibiotics, the sulfa drugs have kept an important place in this field. Indeed, the view of many investigators is that the sulfa drugs are the treatment of choice, especially in acute infections of the urinary tract (7c,8c). There is near consensus that short-acting soluble drugs are best in urinary tract disease. Advocates of short-acting drugs point to the high levels in the urine assured by the quick throughput of these drugs (8c). This is probably the prevailing view among practitioners, as the short-acting drugs sulfisoxazole (**18**), sulfamethizole (**9**), and sulfisoimidine (**17**) dominate the entire United States sulfa drug market (9). Recently, sulfacytine (**19**), another short-acting sulfa drug, was introduced (19).

For chronic urinary tract infection the combination sulfamethoxazole–trimethoprim has been introduced to the United States market. No other usage has yet been allowed in its United States application, ie, it is not recommended for systemic bacterial disease or acute urinary tract disease (20).

Physical and Chemical Properties

The sulfa drugs are white or nearly-white powders melting above 150°C. The azo and nitro derivatives may be yellow. These compounds are not very soluble in cold water but are somewhat soluble in alcohol or acetone. Sulfanilamide (**1**), sulfaguanidine (**21**), sulfacetamide (**20**), and mafenide (**26**) are fairly soluble in hot water (Table 1). N^4-Acetylation generally lowers solubility, but there are exceptions (Table 2).

These drugs are weak acids, the more important ones generally have a pK_a in the range 5–8. With this acidity the sulfa drugs are generally soluble in basic aqueous solutions. The N^1-acyl substituted and some N^1-heterocyclic substituted sulfas, are highly soluble as salts at body pH, eg, sulfactamide (**20**) ($pK_a = 5.38$) and sulfisoxazole (**18**) ($pK_a = 5.0$). The N^4-acyl derivatives succinylsulfathiazole (**23**), phthalylsulfathiazole (**24**) and salicylazosulfapyridine (**25**) contain a free carboxyl and are entirely soluble at pH 7. As the pH is lowered, the solubility of the N^1-substituted sulfanilamides reaches a minimum, usually in the pH range 3–5. This minimum corresponds

Table 2. Renal Safety and Solubility (21)

| Drug | Solubility at 37°C at pH 5.5, mg/100 mL | | Safety |
	Free drug[a]	N^4-Acetyl drug	
sulfanilamide (1)	1500	530	very good
sulfathiazole (3)	98	7	very poor
sulfadiazine (4)	13	20	poor
sulfamethazine (9)	75	115	good
sulfapyrazine (15)	5	5	very poor
sulfisoxazole (18)	100 est[b]	50 est[b]	good
sulfacetamide (20)	1100	215	very good

[a] In general these values are higher than the solubilities given in Table 1 because of the higher temperature. However, some inconsistencies are apparent and are typical of the poor reproducibility of this determination.

[b] From ref. 21b.

to the solubility of the molecular species and approximates the intrinsic solubility in water as given in Table 1. The sulfa drugs, with a free amino group are weak bases, all of about the same strength (approx $pK_a = 2$). Consequently, with a further decrease of pH to that of a moderately strong acid, the sulfa drugs dissolve as the cations. They are usually freely soluble in aqueous strong mineral acids such as hydrochloric or sulfuric acid. The sulfa drugs generally are stable in strong alkali and strong acid but there are exceptions. Their solubilities have been studied widely, particularly in body fluids or in buffered solutions, in order to understand their behavior in the body (5d,2,21). The binding of sulfa drugs to blood proteins is important in theoretical interpretations of their systemic activity (11a).

The amino group is readily diazotized with nitrous acid and this is a basis for its assay. Aldehydes react with the amino group to form anils and other condensation products. The yellow product formed with 4-(dimethylamino)benzaldehyde is useful for the visualization of sulfa drugs with free amino groups in thin-layer and paper chromatography. Acylation of the amino group occurs readily with agents such as acetic or phthalic anhydride.

Theoretical Aspects

Biological Mechanism of Action. It is generally agreed that the sulfa drugs act primarily by holding back growth (bacteriostatic) rather than by destroying the pathogen (bactericidal). The sulfa drugs inhibit bacteria *in vitro* only if the growth medium is free of inactivating materials, notably peptones and *p*-aminobenzoic acid (PABA) derivatives. Had *in vitro* activity been a prerequisite, neither Prontosil (inactive even in the absence of antagonists) nor its degradation product sulfanilamide would have been tried as a drug, and the rise of bacterial chemotherapy would have been delayed. Prontosil itself, and the many sulfanilamide derivatives have been compared in experimental animal infections to determine the superior variants (5).

With the successful entry of the antibiotics into clinical medicine, a curious contrast developed. The applicability of an antibiotic in a given clinical case could be checked quickly and accurately by *in vitro* tests on the particular infecting organism. However, because of the requirement for stringently simplified media to test sulfonamides, no comparable *in vitro* testing was done. Besides, there was disagreement as to the significance of therapy in the results of such *in vitro* tests that had been done (8e). This situation may be changing; there is now evidence that there may be a correlation between the clinical effectiveness of sulfa drugs and their bacteriostatic effect against the isolated bacteria in simplified media (10).

The Woods-Fildes theory postulates that PABA is an essential metabolite for the bacteria that are affected (22). The primary action of the sulfa drugs is assumed to be a competitive inhibition of one or more enzyme reactions involving PABA. Subsequent work has shown the principal role of PABA to be that of a building block for folic acid and related vitamins (primarily folinic acid). The sulfa drugs prevent this synthesis and are, therefore, toxic to those bacteria that must synthesize their own folic acid vitamins. Mammals cannot synthesize these vitamins and thus depend on food sources; consequently, sulfa drugs are not toxic to them in this sense.

The mechanism of action of sulfa drugs has been the subject of intensive studies since their development. Four good reviews are those of Seydel (6), Anand (10), Rogers (23) and Hitchings (18). The only rule that holds with certainty is that ultimately the primary amino group is necessary for biological action (N^4-derivatives must be hydrolyzed to be active). This amino group appears to react with a pterin compound (or precursor) involved in the formation of the essential metabolite folinic acid from PABA. This competing reaction may be nonenzymatic, and involve the accompanying Schiff base with pterinaldehyde, or the reaction may be with a simpler aldehyde fragment. The competing reaction (aldehyde or not) may, as originally suggested by Woods, be at an enzyme receptor site that normally handles PABA. However, impressive evidence favors nonenzymatic action as being more important (6).

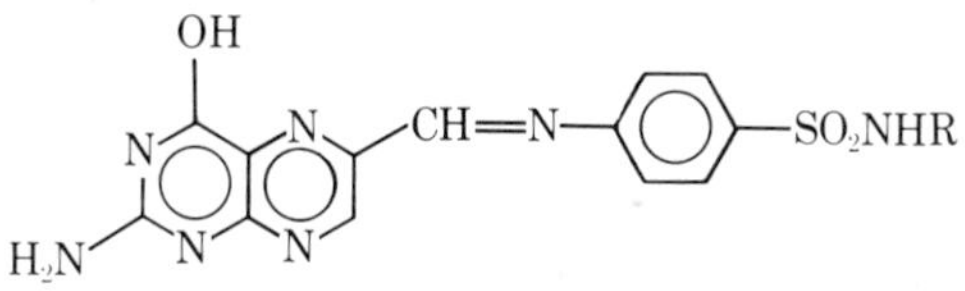

a pterinaldehyde—sulfa drug condensation product

The sulfa drugs inhibit an early step or steps in the biosynthetic chain to folic acid derivatives; there exist other drugs, so-called antifolics, which inhibit other closely sequential steps in this same biosynthesis. Pyrimethamine (**30**) and trimethoprim (**31**) are prominent examples of such drugs.

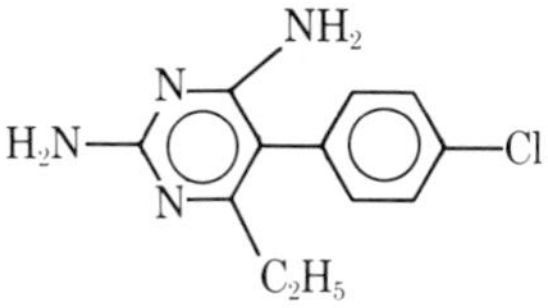

(**30**)

pyrimethamine

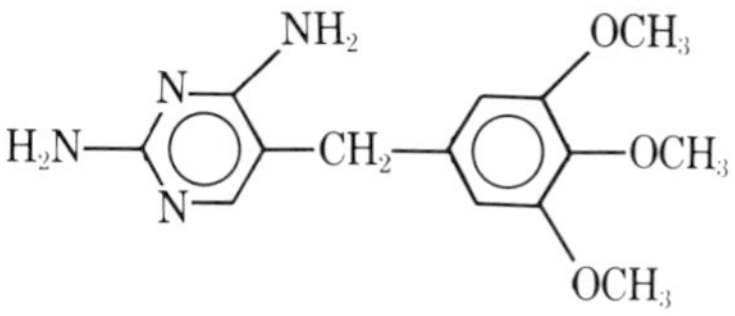

(**31**)

trimethoprim

Combinations of sulfas with (**30**) and (**31**) give effects greater than either drug alone; ie, they are synergistic. This is characteristic of two drugs acting in the same metabolic pathway (18).

There have been numerous attempts to organize into one theory the great array of facts that have come from the synthesis and testing of thousands of analogues (5a,6,10). The earliest was the theory of Bell and Roblin which posited a direct relationship between activity and the electronegativity of the sulfone portion of the sulfonamide group as deduced from the pK_a. Activity has been correlated with basicity of the amino group, with dipole moment, with spectral data, and has been calculated quantum mechanically (6).

Structure-Activity Relationship. The vast field of sulfanilamide-related compounds has been reviewed in depth (5,6,10). If attention is limited to those compounds whose bacteriostatic activity is reversed by PABA, the following formulas summarize the features essential to highest activity:

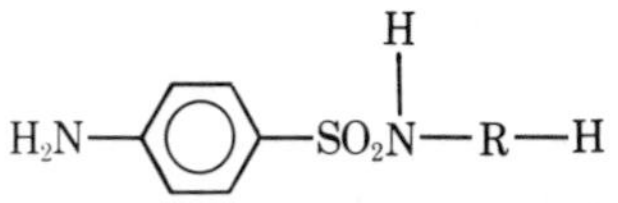

a sulfonamide 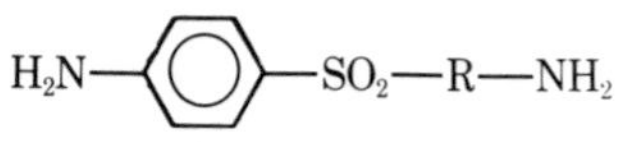   a sulfone

Each structure has a p-aminobenzenesulfonyl group unsubstituted either in the ring or on the amino group. In the best sulfonamides, R is heterocyclic but can be isocyclic or acyl. In the sulfones, R can be phenylene or a heterocycle; the parent dapsone (R = C_6H_4) is the most highly active.

One compound defies the above rules. It is the important tuberculostatic compound PAS (p-aminosalicylic acid). Although it is not a sulfa drug at all, it shares the same mechanism of action since it is reversed by PABA (24). The narrow structural limits above, are thus, not inviolable since PAS has neither a sulfonyl group nor an unsubstituted benzene ring. However, PAS may be exceptional in all ways. It is highly bacteriostatic but most specific in its action to *Mycobacteria* and often only to virulent ones at that (24).

Violation of the above structure–activity rules does occasionally give active compounds by a different mechanism. Separation of the amino group from the ring by a methyl group in mafenide (**26**), or its replacement by an amidine group (in methyl p-amidinophenyl sulfone), gives active compounds whose action has no known metabolite antagonist (5h).

Preparation and Manufacture

By far the most usual method of preparing sulfa drugs is by the reaction of N-acetylsulfanilyl chloride (ASC) with the appropriate amine (5c). Extra amine or a suitable base is used to neutralize the hydrochloric acid freed in the reaction.

$$CH_3CONHC_6H_4SO_2Cl + RNH_2 \xrightarrow{base} CH_3CONHC_6H_4SO_2NHR$$

The resulting acetyl product is usually hydrolyzed with aqueous alkali to the free amino compound. On occasion certain other N-acylsulfanilyl chlorides may be used. p-Nitrobenzenesulfonyl chloride can be used instead of ASC; the intermediate nitro sulfa drug can then be converted to the free amino compound by reduction instead of hydrolysis. The nitro intermediate is much more expensive than ASC, thus, this route is rarely used. ASC is very cheaply obtained by the chlorosulfonation of acetanilide and is a basic raw material for most sulfa drugs.

N^1-Heterocyclic Sulfanilamides. Sulfanilamide itself is manufactured as above by the reaction of ASC with excess concentrated aqueous ammonia and hydrolysis of the product. Most heterocyclic amines are less reactive and the condensation with ASC is usually done in anhydrous media in the presence of an acid-binding agent. The anhydrous conditions avoid a hydrolytic destruction of ASC. Commonly the solvent and acid-binding roles are filled by pyridine alone or by mixtures of acetone and pyridine. Tertiary amines (eg, triethylamine) can be substituted for pyridine. Excess of reactant amine can also be used as the acid-binding agent but since these amines are usually expensive, efficient recovery procedures must be available. The majority of N^1-heterocyclic substituted sulfanilamides are made by the above simple condensation with ASC and hydrolysis.

Sulfisómidine (**17**) is prepared by a variation of this route because of the different character of the amino group in the 4-position in pyrimidines. Two mol of ASC are condensed with one mol of 4-amino-2,6-dimethylpyrimidine in the presence of triethylamine as hydrogen chloride acceptor. The resulting bis(acetylsulfanilyl) derivative is readily hydrolyzed to (**17**). A similar bis(acetylsulfanilyl) derivative has been employed in the synthesis of sulfathiazole (**3**) (5a) and sulfamoxole (**13**) (25) but the direct 1:1 reaction is probably preferable in these latter cases.

Occasionally N^1-heterocyclic sulfanilamides are prepared by an alternative condensation. The sulfonamide nitrogen of sulfanilamide or N^4-acetylsulfanilamide condenses with an active heterocyclic halide in the presence of an acid-binding agent to form the sulfa drug. Sulfapyridine (**2**) (from 2-chloropyrazine) , sulfadiazine (**4**) (from 2-halopyrimidine), and sulfapyrazine (**15**) (from 2-halopyrazine) have been prepared by this method (5c). The most important application, however, is probably in the synthesis of sulfachloropyridazine (**5**) and sulfamethoxypyridazine (**11**) (26).

Cl—⟨N—N⟩—Cl + H₂NC₆H₄SO₂NH₂ $\xrightarrow{\text{K}_2\text{CO}_3}$ H₂NC₆H₄SO₂NH—⟨N—N⟩—Cl $\xrightarrow{\text{NaOCH}_3}$

(1)   (5)

H₂NC₆H₄SO₂NH—⟨N—N⟩—OCH₃ ⸜

(11)

Finally, N^1-heterocyclic derivatives in some cases can be formed by a ring closure of a simpler sulfanilamide derivative. Sulfadiazine, sulfamethazine, sulfamerazine, and sulfathiazole have been prepared by this method, in addition to their having been synthesized from aminoheterocycle and ASC. The synthesis of sulfamethazine (**8**) from sulfaguanidine (**21**) and acetylacetone is an example.

H₂NC₆H₄SO₂NHC(:NH)NH₂ + CH₃COCH₂COCH₃ ⟶ H₂NC₆H₄SO₂NH—⟨N=, N=, CH₃, CH₃⟩

(21)

(8)

N^1-Acylsulfanilamides. Of this once numerous class of sulfa drugs, only two examples have remained important in the United States. Sulfacetamide (**20**) is prepared by acetylating N^4-acetylsulfanilamide with acetic anhydride or with acetyl chloride in pyridine. The resulting N^1,N^4-diacetylsulfanilamide can be hydrolyzed selectively with mild alkali to the desired product (20). Its isolation and purification from regenerated sulfanilamide is easy because of the greater acidity of sulfacetamide. Sulfaguanidine (21) is prepared by condensing ASC with guanidine in the presence of sodium hydroxide. The N^4-acetyl group may be removed by acid or alkaline hydrolysis.

N^1-Heterocyclic-N^4-Acylsulfanilamides. The two important examples in this class are succinylsulfathiazole (23) and phthalylsulfathiazole (24). They are best prepared by fusing sulfathiazole with either succinic anhydride or phthalic anhydride as required.

N^1-Heterocyclic-N^1-Acetylsulfanilamides. A straightforward but expensive preparation of these compounds starts with the heterocyclic amine (RNH$_2$) and p-nitrobenzenesulfonyl chloride and involves acetylating the nitro sulfa drug (27).

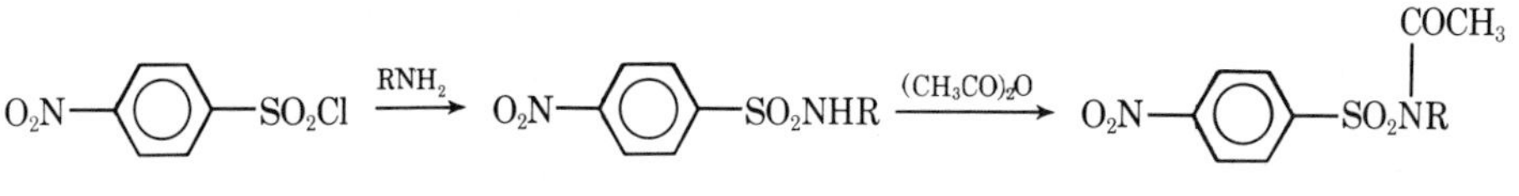

The resulting compound is reduced under very mild conditions to give the required product.

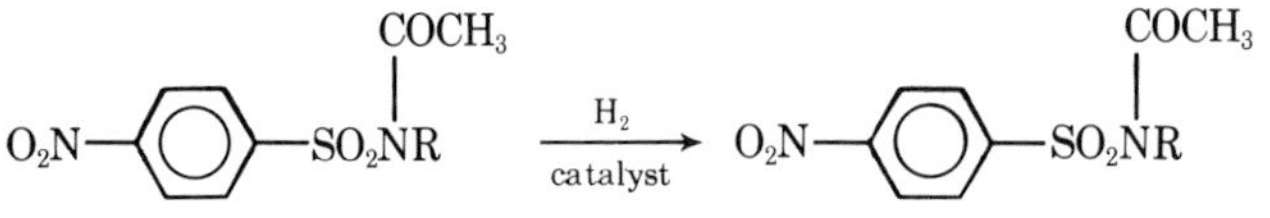

To avoid use of the expensive p-nitrobenzenesulfonyl chloride, other approaches have been developed (28,29). N^1-Acetyl sulfisoxazole can be prepared by these methods.

Miscellaneous Compounds. Salicylazosulfapyridine (25) can be prepared by diazotizing sulfapyridine (2) and coupling it to salicyclic acid (30). Mafenide (26) has been synthesized by chlorosulfonating N-benzylacetamide, reaction of the resultant α-acetamido-p-toluenesulfonyl chloride with ammonia, and finally, hydrolyzing to remove the acetyl group. Dapsone (27) has been prepared by numerous methods (5c,15). Excess sodium sulfide with 1-chloro-4-nitrobenzene gives high yields of 4-amino-4′-nitrodiphenyl sulfide:

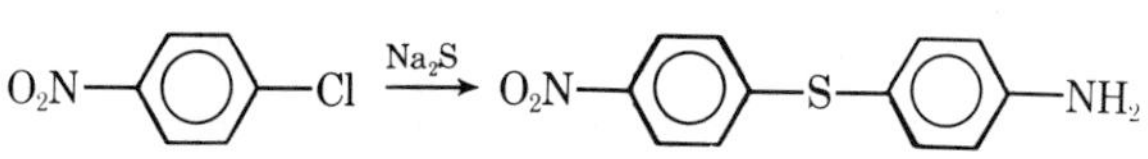

This sulfide, after acetylation to protect the amino group, can be oxidized with hydrogen peroxide to the sulfone, then the nitro group is reduced to amino and, finally, acidic or basic hydrolysis yields the product bis(p-aminophenyl) sulfone (27).

$$O_2NC_6H_4SC_6H_4NHCOCH_3 \xrightarrow{H_2O_2} O_2NC_6H_4SO_2C_6H_4NHCOCH_3 \xrightarrow[H^+ \text{ or } OH^-]{H_2} H_2NC_6H_4SO_2C_6H_4NH_2 \quad (27)$$

Amination of bis(4-chlorophenyl sulfone at a high temperature and under pressure is claimed to be a good method.

$$ClC_6H_4SO_2C_6H_4Cl \xrightarrow[\text{ca } 200°C]{\text{NH}_3} H_2NC_6H_4SO_2C_6H_4NH_2$$

$$(27)$$

Economic Aspects

The production of sulfa drugs increased rapidly after their introduction; spurred on by the military needs of World War II, it reached a maximum of 9000 metric tons in 1943. An abrupt drop to less than half this amount occurred in 1944, concomitant with the commercial development of antibiotics. This led to the belief that the sulfa drugs would be quickly replaced, or at least reduced to a very low level of consumption. Their output has, however, been maintained close to the 1944 level, in spite of a very rapid increase in the production of antibiotics. An increased veterinary use, as well as their low cost and general effectiveness, has helped to hold a market for the sulfa drugs. Selected United States production figures of sulfa drugs and antibiotics are shown in Table 3.

Since the total production of sulfa drugs has stabilized since 1944, it might appear that the field had become static. This is far from being the case. Sulfathiazole (3), at 1800 metric tons in 1946, was 40% of the entire sulfa drug production. By 1953 this drug had dropped to about 15% and at present is practically obsolete. A similar drop has occurred with most of the main drugs of 1946. In contrast, sulfisoxazole (18), a safer soluble derivative, not available in 1946, is currently the major sulfa drug in the United States (9a). To some extent the stabilization and even resurgence of the sulfa drugs in recent years come from a recognition that they are not only cheap but, for uncomplicated urinary tract disease, may be superior to antibiotics (7a).

Analysis

For most sulfa drugs having a free p-amino group, assay is readily carried out by titration with nitrous acid (31a). For assaying sulfa drugs in body fluids the Bratton-Marshall method is used (32). The basis for this method is the diazotization of the aromatic amino group, followed by coupling with N-naphthylethylenediamine and estimation of the color. After hydrolysis in acid, such fluids give an added color response for N^4-acetyl derivatives which may have been formed *in vivo*. The difference between color readings before and after hydrolysis measures the extent of N^4-acetylation. A variety of simple chemical and physical tests have been used to identify individual sulfa drugs (32b). The multiplicity of metabolic conjugates of sulfa drugs, as well as the deliberate use of mixtures of sulfa drugs in therapy, have given rise to great difficulties in identification and assay. Chromatographic separation is invaluable

Table 3.   **United States Production of Sulfa Drugs and Antibiotics, Metric Tons** [a]

Drug	1943	1946	1952	1956	1966	1975
total sulfa drugs	9077	4630	5249	3462	4944	2122
sulfathiazole	not given	1828	657	[b]	[b]	[b]
total antibiotics	0	34.5	1349	1784	8756	8312
penicillins	0	32	608	572	1897	3129

[a] From ref. 31.

[b] Probably negligible.

in such complex cases. Separations have been made on paper, and by the use of thin-layer chromatography (33).

Toxicity. A small percentage of patients treated with sulfa drugs have developed symptoms of toxicity such as drug fever, rashes, mild peripheral neuritis, and mental disturbances. The incidence of these reactions may vary considerably from drug to drug. In general, toxicity is higher with higher blood levels and thus often accompanies poor excretion or overdosing (21). In 1966 the FDA required that the two long-acting sulfa drugs sulfamethoxypyridazine (11) and sulfadimethoxine (6) carry a label warning that the drugs had been implicated in deaths due to Stevens-Johnson syndrome (an extremely severe dermatologic reaction) (34).

A more common and generally recognized toxic effect of sulfa drugs is their potential to damage the kidney. The metabolic acetylation of sulfa drugs adds a degree of complexity to the control and prevention of this toxicity. Usually, but not always, the N^4-acetylated drug is less soluble than the parent. Some soluble sulfa drugs, unlikely themselves to precipitate, are converted extensively to the N^4-acetyl derivatives whose solubility lies in a range thought to be dangerous. Lehr arbitrarily selects a solubility of ca 70 mg/100 mL at pH 5.5 and 37°C as the lower limit of safety (21). Sulfathiazole (3) is a drug that illustrates this situation. Judged retrospectively from its solubility of 98 mg/100 mL, sulfathiazole should be safe. But because of the lower solubility of its acetyl derivative, only 7 mg/100 mL, it was found to cause blockage of the kidneys by crystalline deposits (21a). Kidney toxicity is an important factor in the obsolescence of this effective drug. Table 2 summarizes the solubility and presumed safety data of some sulfa drugs and acetylated derivatives. The solubility safety limit of ca 70 mg/100 mL would have uncertain application to long-acting drugs. Their slow excretion guarantees that high concentrations will not be reached in the urine from ordinary doses of these drugs.

The danger of kidney blockage is reduced by increasing the fluid intake and by administering sodium bicarbonate. These two measures simultaneously dilute the excreted drug and increase its solubility by alkalinizing the urine. The threat of this toxicity is also reduced by administering mixtures of drugs (21). The therapeutic efficacy of a mixture is presumably equal to the sum of its components but the solubilities of the components are independent so that effective levels can be maintained with less likelihood of precipitation. One example, sold as a triple sulfonamide mixture, contained the three sulfa drugs sulfadiazine, sulfamerazine, and sulfamethazine. Numerous other mixtures were sold at one time. Some disadvantages of sulfa mixtures have also been pointed out (8d).

BIBLIOGRAPHY

"Sulfonamides" in *ECT* 1st ed., Vol. 13, pp. 312–316; and "Sulfa Drugs" in *ECT* 1st ed., Vol. 13, pp. 271–285, by M. E. Hultquist, Research Division, American Cyanamid Company; "Sulfonamides" in *ECT* 2nd ed., Vol. 19, pp. 255–261; and "Sulfonamides (Sulfa Drugs)" in *ECT* 2nd ed., Vol. 19, pp. 261–279, by Leonard Doub, Parke, Davis & Company.

1. M. Windholz, ed., *The Merck Index*, 9th ed., Merck & Co. Inc., Rahway, N. J., 1976.
2. J. Rieder, *Arzneim.-Forsch.* **13,** 81, Pts. I–III (1936).
3. P. H. Bell and R. O. Roblin, *J. Am. Chem. Soc.* **64,** 2905 (1942).
4. U.S. Pat. 2,833,761 (1958), D. M. Murphy and R. G. Shepherd.
5. E. H. Northey, *The Sulfonamides and Allied Compounds*, Reinhold Publishing Corp., New York, 1948; (a) Chap. XI, pp. 466–516; (b) pp. 1–6; (c) except where noted, from pp. 11–20; (d) pp. 458–459; (e) pp. 517–577; (f) p. 340; (g) pp. 252–253; (h) pp. 510–511.

6. J. K. Seydel, *J. Pharm. Sci.* **57,** 1455 (1968).
7. L. Weinstein, M. A. Madoff, and C. M. Samet, *N. Engl. J. Med.* **263,** 793, 842, 900, 952 (1960); (a) pp. 900–905; (b) p. 793; (c) pp. 952–957.
8. L. Neipp in R. J. Schnitzer and F. Hawking, eds., *Experimental Chemotherapy,* Vol. II, Academic Press, Inc., New York, 1964, pp. 169–249; (a) pp. 178–179; (b) p. 170; (c) pp. 175–176; (d) pp. 176–177; (e) pp. 231–235.
9. G. Zbinden in R. F. Gould, ed., *Molecular Modification in Drug Design, Adv. Chem. Ser.* **45,** 25 (1964).
10. N. Anand in J. W. Corcoran and F. E. Hahn, eds., *Antibiotics,* Vol. III, Springer-Verlag, New York, 1975, pp. 668–698; (a) p. 673.
11. R. E. Bagdon in R. J. Schnitzer and F. Hawking, eds., *Exp. Chemother.* Vol. II, Academic Press, Inc., New York, 1964, pp. 249–306; (a) pp. 290–292; (b) p. 301; (c) p. 282.
12. The sulfa drugs rarely get this credit. It is in part acknowledged by G. T. Stewart, *The Penicillin Group of Drugs,* Elsevier Publishing Co., New York, 1965, pp. 8–9.
13. M. Tishler in R. F. Gould, ed., *Molecular Modification in Drug Design, Advan. Chem. Ser.* **45,** 5 (1964).
14. J. Tréfouël, J. Tréfouël, F. Nitti, and D. Bovet, *Compt. Rend. Soc. Biol.* **121,** 756 (1935).
15. L. Doub in W. H. Hartung, ed., *Med. Chem.,* Vol. V, John Wiley & Sons, Inc., New York, 1961, pp. 352–354.
16. S. G. Browne, *Brit. Med. J.* III, 725 (**1968**).
17. G. Middlebrook and R. J. Dubos in R. J. Dubos, ed., *Bacterial and Mycotic Infections of Man,* 3rd ed., J. B. Lippincott Co., Philadelphia, Pa., 1958, pp. 305–306.
18. G. H. Hitchings and J. J. Burchall in F. F. Nord, ed., *Adv. in Enzymol.* Vol. 27, Interscience, New York, 1975, pp. 417–468.
19. L. Doub, U. Krolls, J. M. Vandenbelt, and M. Fisher, *J. Med. Chem.* **13,** 242 (1970).
20. B. B. Huff, ed., *Physicians Desk Reference* 30th ed., The Medical Economics Co., Rahway, N. J., 1976, p. 683.
21. D. Lehr, *Ann. N. Y. Acad. Sci.* **69,** 417 (1958); (a) p. 418; (b) 430.
22. D. D. Woods and P. Fildes, *J. Soc. Chem. Ind. (London)* **59,** 133 (1940).
23. H. J. Rogers in R. J. Schnitzer and F. Hawking, eds., *Experimental Chemotherapy,* Vol. II, Academic Press, Inc., New York, 1964, pp. 45–56.
24. G. P. Youmans and A. S. Youmans in R. J. Schnitzer and F. Hawking, eds., *Experimental Chemotherapy,* Vol. II, Academic Press, Inc., New York, 1964, pp. 445–447.
25. Brit. Pat. 819,019 (August 26, 1959), (to Nordmark-Werke Gesellschaft, Hamburg).
26. J. H. Clark, J. P. English, C. R. Jansen, H. W. Marson, M. M. Rogers, and W. E. Taft, *J. Am. Chem. Soc.* **80,** 890 (1958).
27. Northey (5c) does not discuss this class of derivatives. The information given in this section is from general background of the author and partially extrapolated from cited sources.
28. U.S. Pat. 2,974,137 (March 7, 1961), G. T. Fitchett, J. E. Gordon, and R. G. Shepherd, (to American Cyanamid Co., New York).
29. U.S. Pat. 2,721,200 (April 18, 1955), M. Hoffer, (to Hoffmann-LaRoche, Nutley, N. J.).
30. U.S. Pat. 2,396,145 (March 5, 1946), A. Askelof, N. Svartz, and H. C. Willstaedt, (to Aktiebolaget Pharmacia).
31. United States Tariff Commission, *Synthetic Organic Chemicals, United States Production and Sales,* U.S. Government Printing Office, Washington, D.C.; used in Table 3, *1941–1943,* TC Publication 153, 1946; *Preliminary for 1946,* 1947; *1956,* TC Publication 200, 1957; *Preliminary for 1966,* 1967; *Preliminary for 1975,* 1976.
32. *The U.S. Pharmacopeia,* 19th Revision, 1975, (a) p. 626; (b) pp. 475–481.
33. T. Bićan-Fišter and V. Kajganović, *J. Chromatography* **16,** 503 (1964). (These authors cite earlier literature on paper-chromatographic separations.)
34. Washington News Section, *J. Am. Med. Assoc.* **195,** 27 (1966).

LEONARD DOUB
Warner Lambert-Parke Davis Research Laboratories

ANTIBIOTICS

SURVEY

"Out of the earth shall come thy salvation."—Selman A. Waksman

Antibiotics are chemical substances produced by various species of microorganisms and other living systems· that are capable in small concentrations of inhibiting the growth of or killing bacteria and other microorganisms.

Antibiotics are intermediates or end products of microbial metabolism. In the soil, where many microorganisms live, the waste products of one species may be quite toxic to another, or in other cases, they may be supportive to the growth of neighboring organisms. The term antibiosis (against life) applies to the antagonistic effect.

A substance can be classified as an antibiotic agent although it is without effect *in vivo* (within the body) or too toxic to permit its use in the body. *In vitro* (outside the body) activity alone is sufficient to indicate antibiotic activity. However, only if the substance is effective in the presence of body fluids and is sufficiently nontoxic to tissue cells to permit safe administration, can it possibly be a therapeutic agent. Owing to their property of destroying microorganisms *in vivo,* many antibiotics have rapidly found practical applications in combating infectious diseases. Important antibiotics produced in the United States are listed in Table 1.

The study of antibiotics is based mainly on microbiological and biochemical methods, which distinguish them from similar compounds obtained by chemical synthesis. Today, out of the several thousand antibiotics produced biosynthetically, chemical synthesis has succeeded in only a few instances and only a few of these antibiotics have therapeutic value (see Antibacterial agents; Chemotherapeutics).

History

Few developments in the history of medicine have had such a profound effect upon human life and society as the development of the power to control infections due to microorganisms.

Although true antibiotics were recognized in folk medicine as long as 2500 years

Table 1.   Important Antibiotics Produced in the United States (1976)

amikacin [39831-55-5]
bacitracin [1405-87-4]
candicidin [1403-17-4]
capreomycin [11003-38-6]
cephalosporins
   cefazolin [25953-19-9]
   cephaloglycine [3577-01-3]
   cephaloridine [50-59-9]
   cephalothin [153-61-7]
   cephapirin sodium [24356-60-3]
   cephradine [3882-53-3]
chloramphenicol [56-75-7]
colistin (polymyxin) [1066-17-7]
cycloserine [68-41-7]
dactinomycin [50-76-0]
erythromycin [114-07-8]
fusidic acid [6990-06-3]
gentamicin [1403-66-3]
gramicidin [113-73-5]
kanamycin [59-01-8]
lincomycins
   clindamycin [18323-44-9]
   lincomycin [154-21-2]
neomycin [1404-04-2]
oleandomycins
   oleandomycin [3922-90-5]
   troleandomycin [2751-09-9]
paromomycin [7542-37-2]

penicillins
   amoxicillin [26787-78-0]
   ampicillin [69-53-4]
   carbenicillin [4697-36-3]
   carbenicillin, indanyl ester [26605-69-6]
   cloxacillin [61-72-3]
   dicloxacillin [3116-76-5]
   hetacillin [3511-16-8]
   methacillin [132-92-3]
   nafcillin [985-16-0]
   oxacillin [66-79-5]
   penicillin G (benzylpenicillin) [61-33-6]
   penicillin V (phenoxymethylpenicillin) [87-08-1]
   phenethicillin [132-93-4]
rifampin [13292-46-1]
spectinomycin [1695-77-8]
staphylomycin [11006-76-1]
streptomycins
   dihydrostreptomycin [128-46-1]
   streptomycin [57-92-1]
tetracyclines
   chlortetracycline [57-62-5]
   demeclocycline [127-33-3]
   deoxycycline [564-25-0]
   methacycline [914-00-1]
   minocycline [10118-90-8]
   oxytetracycline [79-57-2]
   tetracycline [60-54-8]
tyrothricin [1404-88-2]
vancomycin [1404-90-6]
viomycin [32988-50-4]

ago when the Chinese reported the medicinally beneficial effects of moldy bean curd, it was not until the nineteenth century when Pasteur founded the science of bacteriology that it became possible to study these substances systematically. Pasteur noted the antagonism of some growing organisms for other groups, when he studied the rate of growth of different species of bacteria in 1877. A few years later in 1889, Vuillemin coined the term antibiosis to denote antagonism between living creatures. The first extensive therapeutic application of the principle took place in Germany in 1898 by Emmerich, professor of bacteriology and hygiene at the University of Munich. He extracted a substance from cultures of *B. pyocyaneus* (pyocyanase), which destroyed the bacilli of anthrax, diptheria, typhoid fever, and bubonic plague. Unknown at the time, the product actually contained two substances now recognized as antibiotics. Unfortunately, this crude mixture was not satisfactory for the intended chemotherapeutic uses, and after nearly fifteen years of clinical experience, it was abandoned. Pyocyanase must be recognized, nevertheless, for the fact that it was the first antibiotic preparation to be extensively tested in the clinic.

Thirty years later, in 1928, Alexander Fleming, working in England, noted that a mold with which a plate culture of staphylococci had been contaminated destroyed the bacteria. He isolated the mold, grew it in pure culture, and showed that a filtrate from the culture medium in which it grew killed a great variety of microorganisms and was not toxic to small animals. Since the mold was a strain of *Penicillium* (*P. notatum*), he named the antibacterial substance penicillin. For lack of time and money, Fleming did not pursue the investigation further, but simply placed his discovery on the shelf in the hope that someday it would be carried on. A decade later his hope was realized when two other Englishmen, Chain and Florey, expanded Fleming's investigations and developed an antibiotic preparation for human use (1). In the summer of 1941, Chain and Florey came to the United States with a request for assistance to the US Government for the manufacture of penicillin. After a tremendous cooperative effort, which included the United States pharmaceutical industry, penicillin became commercially available. This event marked the beginning of the antibiotic era.

At about the same time, Dubos, working at the Rockefeller Institute, described a series of microbial products to which he gave the name tyrothricin (2). Further investigation showed that his preparation contained two major materials, gramicidin and tyrocidine [8011-61-8]; both were found useful in treating infections in humans. Similar investigations were underway at Rutgers University, where Waksman made a systematic search for antimicrobial substances in a group of soil-inhabiting *Streptomyces*. Waksman and his associates reported the isolation of actinomycin [1402-38-6] in 1940, streptothricin [5822-34-4] in 1942, streptomycin in 1943, and neomycin in 1949. The discovery of streptomycin, which was found to be particularly useful in treating bacterial infections, especially tuberculosis, greatly stimulated the search for useful antibiotics among *Streptomyces*. This group of microorganisms is the source of many of the currently used antibiotics.

The word antibiotic was first introduced in 1942 by Waksman. Prior to that time, however, antimicrobial substances produced by microorganisms were called toxins, lysins, or bacteriostatic or bacteriolytic agents.

Chloromycetin (chloramphenicol), the first of the so-called broad spectrum antibiotics of commercial importance, was first isolated by Ehrlich in 1947. The following year, Duggar described aureomycin [57-62-5], an antibiotic obtained from cultures of *Streptomyces aureofaciens*. This event opened up the search and the discovery of the important class of antibiotics called the tetracyclines. Following these discoveries, the pace of new discoveries accelerated. Table 2 lists the year of discovery of the most important antibiotics.

Nomenclature

Antibiotics, and in general all drug products that are marketed are identified by three names. Two of these names are based on the structure of the antibiotic, and the third, or trade name, is given to the drug by the manufacturer. The three names are: (*1*) the conventional chemical name or a name descriptive of the chemical structure of the compound based on rules of standard nomenclature; (*2*) the generic name, a shorter, established name, which is the name most commonly used in the scientific literature and which may or may not be an abbreviated form of the chemical name; and (*3*) the trade name or brand name, which is the name given to the antibiotic by the manufacturer to distinguish it from competitive products. In cases in which the complete structure of the antibiotic has not been elucidated only the generic name, not the chemical name, is used.

In general, the generic name is preferred to identify an antibiotic, and this name is used here. An example of this system of nomenclature is shown below.

Table 2.   Years Of Discovery Of Important Antibiotics

Antibiotic	Year of discovery
penicillin	1929
tyrothricin {gramicidin / tyrocidine	1939
griseofulvin	1939
streptomycin	1943
bacitracin	1945
chloramphenicol	1947
polymyxin	1947
chlortetracycline	1948
cephalosporin C, N, P	1948
neomycin	1949
oxytetracycline	1950
nystatin	1950
erythromycin	1952
novobiocin	1955
kanamycin	1957
fusidic acid	1960
ampicillin	1961
cephalothin	1962
lincomycin	1962
gentamicin	1963
carbenicillin	1964
cephalexin	1967
clindamycin	1968

chemical name	4-dimethylamino-1,4,4a,5,5a,6,11,12a-octahydro-3,6,10,12,12a-pentahydroxy-6-methyl-1,11-dioxo-2-naphthacenecarboxamide
generic name	tetracycline [60-54-8]
trade names	Achromycin (Lederle), Panmycin (Upjohn), Sumycin (Squibb), Tetracyn (Pfizer), Tetrex (Bristol), etc

Classification Of Antibiotics

Chemically, the antibiotics belong to various groups of compounds. In general, they are low molecular weight compounds, exhibiting a variety of chemical structures, elemental composition, and physical–chemical properties. Although the chemical characterization of antibiotics has been extensive, a good chemical classification is not yet possible.

In addition to chemical structure, antibiotics have been classified according to microbial source and mechanism of action. The first classification, based on microbial source, suffers from the drawback that it is much too broad. More than one-half of the antibiotics discovered to date are produced by *Actinomyces*. This group includes, among others, streptomycin, the tetracyclines, chloramphenicol, the macrolide family (erythromycin), and the antifungal polyene antibiotics such as nystatin (3), see below. Chemotherapeutic drugs are known to interfere with a number of vulnerable sites in the cell wall, according to Joklik and Smith (4). They are known to interfere with cell wall synthesis, membrane function, protein synthesis, nucleic acid metabolism, and intermediary metabolism. A classification based on mechanism of action suffers from the fact that some agents may have more than one primary site of attack or mechanism of action.

Garrod, Lambert, and O'Grady (5) have classified antibiotics on the basis of general similarity of chemical structure, although a large number of antibiotics were left unclassified. Following their classification, the antibiotics that are manufactured and distributed today can be divided into the following groups.

Penicillin and Related Antibiotics. All members of this group have a β-lactam ring in their structure. This group includes the natural penicillins, the semisynthetic penicillins, and the cephalosporins.

Aminoglycoside Antibiotics. All members of this group have amino sugars in glycosidic linkage. This group comprises the streptomycins, neomycin, kanamycin, paromomycin, gentamicin, tobramycin [32986-56-4], and amikacin.

Macrolide Antibiotics. They all consist of a macrocyclic lactone ring to which sugars are attached. This group comprises erythromycin, oleandomycin, and spiromycin [8025-81-8].

Tetracycline Antibiotics. The tetracyclines are derivatives of the polycyclic naphthacenecarboxamide. This group consists of tetracycline, chlortetracycline, demeclocycline, oxytetracycline, and minocycline.

Chloramphenicol. This antibiotic is in a class of itself. It is a nitrobenzene derivative of dichloroacetic acid.

Peptide Antibiotics. These antibiotics form a large group, but very few have found therapeutic application. These antibiotics are composed of peptide-linked amino acids which commonly include both D- and L-forms. Antibiotics in this category include bacitracin, gramicidin, and the polymyxins.

Antifungal Antibiotics. This group has two main subgroups: (1) polyenes which contain a large ring with a conjugated double-bond system. Over fifty polyene antibiotics have been discovered, the most important of which are nystatin [1400-61-9] and amphotericin B [1397-89-3]; and (2) other antifungal antibiotics including 5-fluorocytosine [2022-85-7], clotrimazole [23953-75-1], and griseofulvin [126-07-8] (see Fungicides; Industrial antimicrobial agents).

Unclassified. These antibiotics have varied structures and are not classified among the main groups described above. Antibiotics in this group include cycloserine, fusidic acid, novobiocin [303-81-1], prasinomycin [12687-95-5], spectinomycin, and vancomycin.

Additional antibiotic categories from Garrod's unclassified category are possible. For example, the antibiotics lincomycin and clindamycin could be placed in a separate class called the lincosaminides and the antibiotic rifampin in the ansamacrolides. Those categories of antibiotics that will be discussed in detail in later sections are the aminoglycosides, ansamacrolides, β-lactams, chloramphenicols, lincosaminides, macrolides, nucleosides, oligosaccharides, phenazines, polyenes, polyethers, peptides, and the tetracyclines. Foye (6) discusses the chemistry of the individual antibiotics.

Production

Several thousand antibiotics are known, but only a relative handful have reached production and commercial importance. According to Foye (6), only a few, perhaps

0.3%, of the many antibiotics mentioned in the scientific literature are now used in medicine and agriculture. Although no definitive international list of all the antibiotics that are produced commercially is available, see Table 1 for a list of most of the important antibiotics produced in the United States in 1976.

A number of antibiotics are produced abroad, but not yet in the United States. Examples of these antibiotics are epicillin [26774-90-3], flucloxacillin [5250-39-5], and cyclacillin [3485-14-1]. Griseofulvin, produced overseas, is available in the United States.

Methods of Production. All but a few antibiotics are the complete products of microbial synthesis. The exceptions are the semisynthetic penicillins, the cephalosporins, and the tetracyclines, in addition to clindamycin [18323-44-9], and dihydrostreptomycin [128-46-1], which are made by chemical manipulation of microbially produced antibiotics. Chloramphenicol and cycloserine are antibiotics of chemotherapeutic interest manufactured entirely by chemical synthesis. Virtually all other antibiotics are produced on a large scale by microbial processes or by procedures involving these processes in the intermediate steps.

Since almost all antibiotics are made by aerobic fermentation processes, a number of similarities in the processes used in their production exist. The general outline of these methods is fairly well known although the industrial concerns producing antibiotics have been reluctant to publish details of their processes.

The technique involves growing the microorganism in totally enclosed stainless steel or nickel–chrome alloy tanks having a capacity as high as 113.6 m^3 (30,000 gal). The vessels are fitted with aerating and agitating devices and cooling coils or jackets, or both, for accurate temperature control. The medium may be sterilized in a separate cooker and then pumped into the sterile culture vessels, or may be sterilized *in situ*. Large inoculum levels, sometimes as much as 10% of the volume of the fermentation have been reported. Careful choice and control of incubation temperatures, pH control, and continuous addition of energy sources are usually helpful in keeping the fermentation process operating efficiently.

The fermentation medium is devised to stimulate maximum antibiotic production. In general, the medium contains: a carbohydrate such as glucose, sucrose, lactose, or starch; a simple nitrogen source such as urea or ammonium sulfate; or a more complex nitrogen source such as soybean meal, cornsteep liquor, or whey. In addition, various salts may be added to the fermentation medium. Product formation is stimulated by the addition of a compound that the microorganism can incorporate into the final product. For example, the addition of phenylacetic acid to the fermentation medium in the production of penicillin results in the production of benzylpenicillin, in which a benzyl side chain is incorporated in the final product.

When the microorganisms have made all the product they can, as shown by assay of the samples removed from the fermentor at periodic intervals, the contents of the fermentation are drawn off and harvested. The first step in the recovery of the product is the removal of the microorganisms from the fermented broth, either by filtration or centrifugation. The cells, if they do not contain appreciable quantities of the products, are generally discarded. Usually, the antibiotic is recovered from the fermentation broth by solvent extraction, ion-exchange chromatography, or by precipitation, or a combination of these recovery techniques.

Some antibiotics, such as the semisynthetic penicillins and cephalosporins, are produced from intermediates. For example, the key intermediate for the production of most of the cephalosporins is 7-aminocephalosporanic acid [957-68-6], which is formed by hydrolysis of cephalosporin C [61-24-5] produced by fermentation.

Economic Aspects

Antibiotics are produced in plants located in most of the developed countries of the world, with the greatest concentration in the more heavily industrialized nations, such as the United States, Japan, the Federal Republic of Germany, Italy, and the United Kingdom. Production figures for most countries are not readily available. The United States Government publishes detailed yearly statistics on the production and sale of antibiotics. In the United States, antibiotics as a group are the single most important bulk medicinal chemical produced according to data published by the US Tariff Commission and the US International Trade Commission (7). A comparison of the production and sales of antibiotics compared with all medicinal chemicals is shown in Table 3 for the years 1973 through 1975. The sales value of bulk antibiotics as a percentage of sales of all bulk medicinal chemicals rose from 28% in 1973 to 37% in 1975.

Note the discrepancy between the production and sales figures for antibiotics in each year. The reason for this difference is that sales include only those bulk antibiotics sold to other companies by the manufacturer. The sales figures do not include bulk antibiotics used captively by the manufacturer to produce antibiotics in finished dosage forms. Thus the difference between production and sales of antibiotics of 5.1 kt in 1975 represents the quantity of bulk antibiotics used captively by the manufacturer.

The production and sale of bulk antibiotics for medicinal use (both human and veterinary) and for animal feeds and other nonmedical use for the years 1971 through 1975 are shown in Table 4. Production and sales in 1975 of bulk antibiotics in metric tons for nonmedicinal use almost equaled production for medicinal use. However, dollar sales of antibiotics for medicinal use was six times greater because of the significantly higher unit value.

United States manufacturer's shipments of antibiotic preparations in dosage form in 1974 was 736 million dollars in human-use drugs and 92 million dollars in veterinary antibiotic preparations, according to data from the Bureau of Census (8). Data for the year 1974 for human-use antibiotic preparations are shown in Table 5. This table also provides a breakdown of this category into systemic antibiotics (administered orally or parenterally) and topical antibiotics (applied on the skin surface). Broad- and medium-spectrum antibiotics accounted for about two-thirds of total

Table 3. Production and Sales of Medicinal Chemicals and Antibiotics

Category	1973 Medicinal chemicals, total	1973 Antibiotics[a]	1974 Medicinal chemicals, total	1974 Antibiotics[a]	1975 Medicinal chemicals, total	1975 Antibiotics[a]
production, kilotons	106.0	9.4	111.8	9.3	94.5	8.3
sales, kilotons	81.3	3.6	80.5	3.8	67.3	3.2
millions of dollars	582.4	164.0	814.8	254.5	772.0	287.9

[a] Total antibiotics for human and veterinary use.

Table 4.   Production and Sales of Bulk Antibiotics for Medicinal and Nonmedicinal Use [a]

	Production, kilotons			Sales, kilotons			Sales, millions of dollars		
	Medicinal	Nonme-dicinal	Total	Medicinal	Nonme-dicinal	Total	Medicinal	Nonme-dicinal	Total
1971	4.9	3.2	8.1	1.9	1.2	3.1	104.7	32.1	136.8
1972	4.4	3.1	7.5	1.6	0.9	2.5	115.9	23.4	139.3
1973 [b]	5.7	3.7	9.4	n.a.	n.a.	3.6	n.a.	n.a.	164.0
1974	6.0	3.4	9.4	2.4	1.3	3.7	211.8	42.6	254.4
1975	4.3	4.0	8.3	1.7	1.6	3.3	240.4	47.4	287.8

[a] Includes animal-feed supplements.
[b] n.a. means not available.

manufacturer's shipments of systemic-use antibiotics. In 1974, antibiotic preparations accounted for 15% of the 5 billion dollar pharmaceutical market in the United States.

The market in the non-Communist nations for all ethical pharmaceuticals reached an estimated $30 billion in 1975. About 15% (4.5 billion dollars) were shipments of antibiotics. The two largest markets for antibiotics were Japan (950 million dollars) and the United States (750 million dollars), accounting for 38% of the non-Communist world's consumption of antibiotics. Argentina, Brazil, France, Italy, Mexico, Spain, the United Kingdom, and the Federal Republic of Germany were other major consuming nations.

American drug companies dominate the world market for antibiotics. Leading United States producers include Pfizer, Eli Lilly, Bristol-Myers, Upjohn, Schering-Plough, American Cyanamid, American Home Products, Abbott, Squibb, Warner-Lambert and Smith Kline. Worldwide shipments of antibiotics of each of these eleven producers during 1975 are shown in Table 6. Combined shipments of these producers totaled about 2.0 billion dollars or 44% of the world's antibiotic market. Several foreign companies, such as Glaxo, Beecham, Lepetit, Fujisawa, Bayer, and Hoechst, are major producers.

The three leading classes of antibiotics sold in the world market are the semisynthetic penicillins, the cephalosporins, and the penicillins. Although the cephalosporins were the newest class of antibiotics to be introduced, they have become

Table 5.   Manufacturer's Shipments in 1974 of Human-Use Antibiotic Preparations

Antibiotics	Millions of dollars
Systemic	
broad and medium spectrum [a]	502.2
penicillin (single)	
injectible	50.4
other forms	154.4
all others	14.3
Total	*721.3*
Topical	15.1
Total	*736.4*

[a] Single or in combination with other antibiotics, except penicillins.

Table 6.   Sales of Antibiotics of Leading United States Pharmaceutical Manufacturers in 1975

Company	Worldwide antibiotic sales, millions of dollars
Pfizer	415
Eli Lilly	401
Bristol-Myers	290
Schering-Plough	195
Upjohn	168
American Cyanamid (Lederle)	130
American Home Products (Wyeth)	125
Abbott	100
Squibb	90
Warner-Lambert	45
Smith Kline	40
Total	*1999*

in about ten years the second leading class of antibiotics. In 1975, sales of the leading classes of antibiotics were as follows: semisynthetic penicillins (950 million dollars), cephalosporins (825 million dollars), penicillins (700 million dollars), tetracyclines (550 million dollars), aminoglycosides (250 million dollars), erythromycins (200 million dollars), chloramphenicols (200 million dollars), and the lincomycins (120 million dollars). The cephalosporins, the aminoglycosides, and the semisynthetic penicillins are showing the fastest growth in use.

The market for antibiotics for human use in the United States can be divided into out-patient use and hospital use. The out-patient or pharmacy market accounted for an estimated 430 million dollars in 1975, whereas the hospital market probably reached 270 million dollars. Important antibiotics used in the out-patient market were the penicillins and ampicillins, and the tetracyclines. The hospital market for antibiotics is divided into two segments; oral and injectables. In the larger segment, the injectables, the leading classes of antibiotics were the cephalosporins, the aminoglycosides, the penicillins and ampicillins. In the oral segment of the hospital market, the cephalosporins predominate, followed by the penicillins, and ampicillins.

Government Control

In the United States, the Food and Drug Administration (FDA), by virtue of the 1962 Amendment of the Federal Food, Drug, and Cosmetic Act of 1938, requires all drug manufacturers to show, before any new drug product is approved for marketing, that the drug is both safe and effective. In order to meet these requirements, drug companies are required to undertake extensive and lengthy tests of the drug before applying for approval to the FDA to market a new drug (see Regulatory agencies).

The FDA also has the authority and responsibility to certify each batch of all antibiotic products before the manufacturer releases their product for distribution. Batch certification involves testing for potency and purity.

Uses

The primary uses of antibiotics are in the prevention and treatment of diseases in humans and animals. The application of antibiotics to animals was an outgrowth of the work in the human disease field. Certain antibiotics have found widespread use as animal-feed supplements to promote growth in livestock (see Pet and livestock feeds). Additionally, antibiotics had some use in food preservation and the spraying of crops to control specific crop diseases, but these applications have been abandoned.

Human use antibiotics are characterized by a selective spectrum of activity. Some affect primarily gram-positive bacteria, others inhibit gram-negative bacteria, and still others inhibit only certain fungi, yeasts, or protozoa. A few antibiotics inhibit both gram-positive and gram-negative bacteria and are called broad spectrum. Desired characteristics for antibacterial antibiotics include: selective and effective antibacterial activity; broad activity; function as a bactericide (kill bacteria) rather than bacteriostat (arrest bacterial growth without killing); does not easily produce resistance; absence of toxicity to kidney, liver, and central nervous system; ease of administration; and availability in oral and parenteral forms.

Physicians choose antibiotics to administer to patients by isolating the microorganism and determining its sensitivity to a variety of antimicrobial agents (drug susceptibility tests). The choice also depends on the patient's allergies and general physical condition, as well as the site of infection. For a review of the medical therapeutic applications of antibiotics see Goodman and Gilman (9).

BIBLIOGRAPHY

"Antibiotics" in *ECT* 2nd ed., Vol. 2, pp. 533–540, by W. E. Brown, The Squibb Institute for Medical Research.

1. E. Chain, H. W. Florey, and co-workers, *Lancet* **2,** 226 (1940); *Lancet* **2,** 177 (1941).
2. R. Dubos, *J. Exp. Med.* **70,** 1 (1939).
3. G. A. Wistreich and M. D. Lechtman, *Microbiology and Human Disease,* Glencoe Press, Beverly Hills, Calif., 1973, p. 338.
4. W. K. Joklik and D. T. Smith, *Zinnser Microbiology,* Appleton-Century-Crofts, New York, 1972, Chapt. 10.
5. L. P. Garrod, H. P. Lambert, and F. O'Grady, *Antibiotic and Chemotherapy,* 4th ed, Churchill Livingstone, London, Eng., 1973.
6. W. O. Foye, *Principles of Medicinal Chemistry,* Lea & Febiger, Philadelphia, Pa., 1974, Chapt. 31.
7. *Synthetic Organic Chemicals, United States Production and Sales of Medicinal Chemicals, U.S. Tariff Commission (1972–73), United States International Trade Commission (1974–1975),* U.S. Government Printing Office, Washington, D.C.
8. *Pharmaceutical Preparations, Except Biologicals, 1974, Current Industrial Reports, Series MA-28G(74)-1,* U.S. Department of Commerce, Bureau of the Census, Washington, D.C.
9. L. S. Goodman and A. Gilman, *The Pharmacological Basis of Therapeutics,* 5th ed., Macmillan Publishing Co., New York, 1975, Chapt. 55–61.

General References

Annual Report to Shareholders, Bristol-Myers Company, 1975, pp. 20–32.
H. M. Boettcher, *Wonder Drugs, A History of Antibiotics,* J. B. Lippincott Co., Philadelphia, Pa., 1964.
Economic Report on Antibiotics Manufacture, Federal Trade Commission, Washington, D.C., June 1958.
A. L. Elder, "The History of Penicillin Production," *Chem. Eng. Prog. Symp. Ser.* **66**(100), (1970).

H. G. Klein, *Rash of Discoveries, Competition in Antibiotics Is Spreading Fast,* Barron's, Dow Jones & Co., Princeton, N. J., Jan. 5, 1976, p. 11.

T. Korzybski and co-workers, *Antibiotics Origin, Nature and Properties,* Vols. I and II, Pergamon Press Ltd., London, Eng., 1967.

H. J. Peppler, *Microbial Technology,* Rheinhold Publishing Co., New York, 1967, Chapt. 11.

Annual Report to Shareholders, Squibb Corporation, 1974.

L. A. Underkofler and R. J. Hickey, *Industrial Fermentations,* Vol. II, Chemical Publishing Co., New York, 1954.

H. T. Clarke, J. R. Johnson, and R. Robinson, eds., *The Chemistry of Penicillins,* Princeton University Press, Princeton, N. J., 1949.

H. G. KLEIN
Klein Medical International

AMINOGLYCOSIDES

This clinically important group of antibiotics comprises the compounds commonly referred to as aminoglycoside antibiotics. The term aminoglycoside is too broad to apply to this group of compounds, since glycosides of aminosugars are component parts of a very large number of antibiotics belonging to several different classes. The best known members of the aminoglycoside family of antibiotics are streptomycin, neomycin, kanamycin, and gentamicin. All of these compounds contain an aminocyclitol unit as well as being aminoglycosides, and for this reason the term aminocyclitol antibiotic has been used more definitively for these substances (1). Nevertheless, the keyword aminoglycoside is so firmly entrenched that the term *aminoglycoside–aminocyclitol antibiotic* seems a reasonable compromise between accuracy and ease of recognition. Among related antibiotics considered in this section are a group of glycoside–aminocyclitol and aminoglycoside–cyclitol compounds, several of which also have commercial value.

Aminoglycoside–aminocyclitol antibiotics are valuable therapeutic agents and are among the oldest known antibiotics. The first member of the series, streptomycin, was isolated from a species of *Streptomyces* by Waksman in 1944 (2). Since that time many other aminoglycoside–aminocyclitols have been isolated as fermentation products of soil microorganisms, and more recently medicinally important semisynthetic derivatives have also been prepared. Currently, thirteen aminoglycoside–aminocyclitol antibiotics are available for therapeutic use in various parts of the world (see Table 1) with an estimated total sales of approximately a half-billion dollars. Gentamicin sales comprise about one half of this total. The majority of these substances are products of the fermentation of actinomycetes of the *Streptomyces* genus, although an important group, including the gentamicins, is derived from the *Micromonospora* species. Additionally, a few antibiotics of this class have now been isolated from other bacterial genera. In the case of *Micromonospora*-derived compounds, the terminal portion of their generic names are spelled micin to distinguish them from the mycins which are derived from *Streptomyces* species.

Table 1. Aminoglycoside–Aminocyclitol Antibiotics Used in Therapy

Antibiotic	Trade names[a]	Manufacturers[a]
streptomycin	Streptsulfat, Ampistrep	Antibioticos (Madrid, Spain)
		Dumex A/S (Copenhagen, Denmark)
		Fervet, S.p.A. (Milan, Italy)
		Gist-Brocades (Delft, Neth.)
		Glaxo Laboratories (Ulverston, UK)
		Hindustan Antibiotics Ltd. (Pimpri, India)
		Kaken Chemical Company (Tokyo, Japan)
		Kyowa Hakko Kogyo Company (Tokyo, Japan)
		Leo Pharmaceutical Products (Ballerup, Denmark)
		Meiji Seika Kaisha Ltd. (Tokyo, Japan)
		Merck and Company, Inc. (Rahway, N. J.)
		Novo Industri A/S (Bagsvaerd, Norway)
		Pfizer, Inc. (Groton, Conn.)
		Rhone Poulenc (Paris, France)
		E. R. Squibb and Sons (New Brunswick, N.J.)
neomycin (framycetin) (neomycin B)	Neocin, Neobiotic, Myciguent, Soframycin, Framygen	Biogal (Debrecen, Hungary)
		Nihon Kayaku Company (Tokyo, Japan)
		Novo Industri A/S (Bagsvaerd, Norway)
		S. B. Penick and Company (Orange, N.J.)
		Pierrel S.p.A. (Milan, Italy)
		Rhone Poulenc (Paris, France)
		Roussel-UCLAF (Romainville, France)
		E. R. Squibb and Sons (New Brunswick, N.J.)
		Takeda Chemical Industries (Osaka, Japan)
		The Upjohn Company (Kalamazoo, Mich.)
		Pfizer, Inc. (Groton, Conn.)
		American Cyanamid (Wayne, N. J.)
paromomycin (aminosidin)	Pargonyl, Humatin, Gabbromycin	Farmitalia (Milan, Italy)
		Parke-Davis (Detroit, Mich.)
kanamycin (kanamycin A)	Kantrex, Kanacyn	Banyu Pharmaceutical Company (Tokyo, Japan)
		Bristol Laboratories (Syracuse, N. Y.)
		Farmitalia, S.p.A. (Milan, Italy)
		Meiji Seika Kaisha (Tokyo, Japan)
		Nikken Chemicals Company (Tokyo, Japan)
		Pierrel, S.p.A. (Milan, Italy)
		Rhone Poulenc (Paris, France)

Table 1 (*continued*)

Antibiotic	Trade names[a]	Manufacturers[a]
aminodeoxykanamycin (kanamycin B)	Kanendomycin, Nekacyn, Bekanacyn	Meiji Seika Kaisha (Tokyo, Japan)
gentamicin (gentamicins C_1, C_2, and C_{1a})	Garamycin, Gentacin, Cidomycin, Refobacin	Schering Corp. (Bloomfield, N. J.)
		Chinoin (Budapest, Hungary)
sisomicin	Extramycin, Pathomycin	Schering Corp. (Bloomfield, N. J.)
		Bayer A.G. (Darmstadt, Ger.)
dihydrostreptomycin	Vibriomycin, Didromycin	
ribostamycin	Vistamycin	Meiji Seika Kaisha (Tokyo, Japan)
lividomycin (lividomycin A)	Livalline	Kowa Co. (Nagoya, Japan)
tobramycin	Nebcin, Obracin, Tobrasix	Eli Lilly and Co. (Indianapolis, Ind.)
dibekacin (DKB)	Panimycin, Dibekacin	Meiji Seika Kaisha (Tokyo, Japan)
amikacin (BB-K8)	Biklin, Briclin, Novamin	Banyu Pharmaceuticals (Tokyo, Japan)
		Bristol Laboratories (Syracuse, N. Y.)

[a] A number of the older antibiotics have many trade names and manufacturers, consequently, this list is not comprehensive.

All aminoglycoside–aminocyclitol antibiotics are relatively small, basic, water-soluble molecules which form stable acid addition salts; they are biosynthesized from carbohydrate components of their fermentation media. They are broad-spectrum antibiotics, active against both gram-positive and gram-negative bacteria as well as mycobacteria, none of them are absorbed well from the alimentary tract or when applied topically and hence must be administered parenterally for systemic use. Moreover, all have some potential for toxicity to the kidney (nephrotoxicity) and the inner ear (eighth nerve or ototoxicity) (3).

None of the aminoglycoside–aminocyclitol antibiotics are effective against anaerobic bacteria, or even against aerobic organisms growing under anaerobic conditions. They are primarily effective against aerobic gram negative bacilli such as *E. coli*, *Klebsiella*, *Proteus*, and *Enterobacter*. Some, but not all, are capable of inhibiting *Pseudomonas aeruginosa*. Although many of the agents are very active against *Staphylococcus aureus in vitro*, there is a dearth of information regarding their clinical effectiveness against serious infections caused by these organisms. None of the antibiotics are effective when used alone against streptococci. They have varying activities against *Mycobacterium tuberculosis*, with streptomycin being the most widely used of the drugs against this organism.

The aminoglycoside–aminocyclitol antibiotics are bactericidal, rather than bacteriostatic. The mechanism of killing involves uptake of the antibiotic followed by binding to bacterial ribosomes and inhibition of protein synthesis. Because of the complexity of events surrounding these processes, however, the exact mode of bacterial killing is still unsettled.

All aminoglycoside–aminocyclitol antibiotics encounter some problems of bacterial resistance, usually following several years of extensive use. A substantial amount is known about the biochemical mechanisms involved in resistance which are frequently associated with the presence in the bacterium of antibiotic-inactivating enzymes. An understanding of these resistance mechanisms at a molecular level has provided the chemist with a rationale for the preparation of semisynthetic variants having predictably broader spectra of activity than their naturally occurring precursors. With the exception of dihydrostreptomycin, which is made by chemical reduction of streptomycin, all clinically useful antibiotics of this class up to 1973 were naturally occurring. The most important recent entries in the field, however, have been semi-synthetic compounds (dibekacin, amikacin), and this trend is expected to continue in the future.

Chemical Aspects

The aminoglycoside–aminocyclitol antibiotics are a structurally diverse group of colorless, water-soluble, polyhydroxy-polyamino compounds with 300–800 molecular weights. Although some compounds in the series have been obtained crystalline, and the x-ray crystal structures of a few of these have been determined, the antibiotics in general are obtained as hydrated, amorphous solids without characteristic melting points, uv or ir absorption. In addition, the free bases are often obtained with varying degrees of carbonation. Optical rotation is of limited value for identification purposes since related compounds show very similar optical rotations. This combination of ill-defined physical properties has, in the past, made identification of these compounds troublesome and a number of these antibiotics have been rediscovered under new names before their identities with existing compounds were demonstrated. Recently, this problem has diminished with the availability of more modern physical techniques.

The most useful method of identifying aminoglycoside–aminocyclitol antibiotics has been traditionally by paper and thin layer chromatography and this remains an important technique (4). The newer methods of mass spectrometry (5–7), proton (8) and carbon-13 nmr spectroscopy (9–12), however, have made identification much simpler. This latter in particular is the method of choice for identification of compounds of this class. Gas–liquid chromatography of derivatized antibiotics has been reported (13–14); however, recent studies with high pressure liquid chromatography (15–16) suggest that this technique is likely to become a preferred method for the identification of aminoglycoside–aminocyclitols and for the analysis of their mixtures.

The chemistry of the aminoglycoside–aminocyclitol antibiotics has been the subject of comprehensive reviews (17–20) and a system of classification based on the type and substitution pattern of the aminocyclitol present has been proposed (1). The first antibiotic of this class to be discovered was streptomycin which contains the aminocyclitol streptidine [85-17-6] (1); the largest group of antibiotics however is that containing 2-deoxystreptamine [2037-48-1] (2). This group can be further subdivided into those antibiotics in which the deoxystreptamine is substituted on two adjacent hydroxyl groups (4,5-disubstituted 2-deoxystreptamine group), those antibiotics in which the deoxystreptamine is substituted on two nonadjacent hydroxyl groups (4,6-disubstituted 2-deoxystreptamine group), and those compounds having a mononosubstituted deoxystreptamine unit.

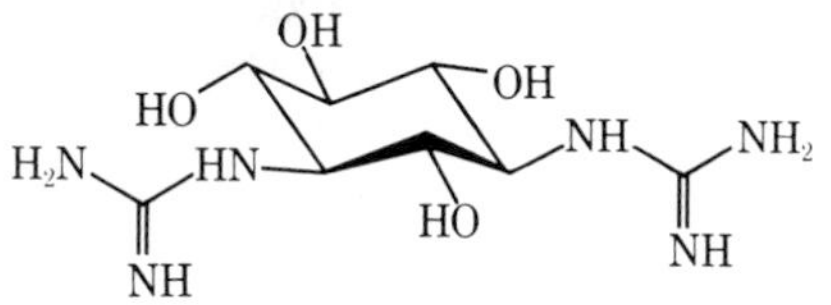

(1) streptidine 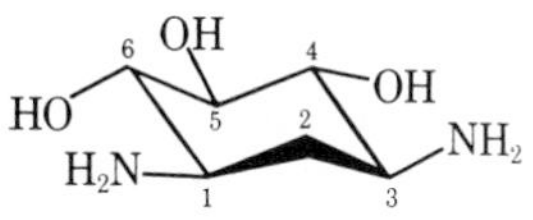   (2) 2-deoxystreptamine

Microbiologically produced compounds of these classes, their producing organisms and leading references are listed in Tables 2–5.

Structural Elucidation.   In most cases structural elucidation of aminoglycoside–aminocyclitol antibiotics has been accomplished via sequential acid hydrolysis to the component sugars and aminocyclitols. In earlier work, identification of the degradation fragments and the ways in which they were connected to form the antibiotic were determined by further painstaking oxidative degradation. This difficult phase of aminoglycoside structure determination is described in excellent reviews of the early streptomycin work by Lemieux and Wolfrom (78) and for the neomycins by Rinehart (17).

Structural studies on compounds discovered more recently, such as the gentamicins (**55–57**) (53), were carried out by similar degradative sequences except that in these cases the identities of the acid hydrolysis fragments could be obtained largely by modern spectroscopic techniques. Recently, in a favorable case, the structures of several novel gentamicins (**72–75**) were demonstrated entirely by spectroscopic means (63–64).

Biosynthesis

The biosynthesis of aminocyclitol antibiotics has recently been comprehensively reviewed (79). Glucose has been shown to provide the carbon skeletons of all subunits of the antibiotics so far studied; however, details of the steps involved are still unknown in almost all cases. A notable exception is the biosynthesis of the streptidine unit (**1**) of streptomycin (**3**), which has been shown to proceed from glucose-6-phosphate by cyclization and loss of inorganic phosphate to give *myo*-inositol (80).

One might expect that 2-deoxystreptamine (**2**) would be biosynthesized from glucose along similar lines to streptidine. This however does not appear to be the case since, eg, *myo*-inositol, an intermediate in streptidine biosynthesis, is not incorporated into the deoxystreptamine-containing antibiotic neomycin (79). Labeling experiments have shown that the positioning of the nitrogen functions with respect to the glucose precursor is different for streptidine and deoxystreptamine (81–82).

The biosynthesis of the sugar components of streptomycin has been investigated by a number of groups. The N-methyl-L-glucosamine moiety has been shown to arise from D-glucose. A number of the possible ways in which this transformation could take place have been ruled out by labeling experiments (83–84), leaving as the most likely route a remarkable series of epimerizations of the D-glucose precursor. Using a cell free extract of *S griseus*, the streptomycin producer, it has been shown that the thymidine diphosphate (dTDP) derivative of glucose is converted via the 4-oxo-4,6-dideoxyglucose derivative to dTDP-dihydrostreptose. This compound could then serve as a streptomycin precursor either via oxidation to a streptose derivative or via dihydrostreptomicin (85).

Other biosynthetic work has shown that, whereas the isolated, underivatized sugar components of antibiotics usually cannot serve directly as precursors for their antibiotics, the isolated aminocyclitol units can. This latter finding allowed workers at the University of Illinois to devise an important method of biosynthetically creating new antibiotics containing novel aminocyclitol units (32).

By appropriate screening of mutants of *S. fradiae,* the neomycin producer, strains were found which had lost the ability to biosynthesize 2-deoxystreptamine (D-mu-

Table 2. Aminocyclitol-Aminoglycosides Derived from Streptidine and Bluensidine

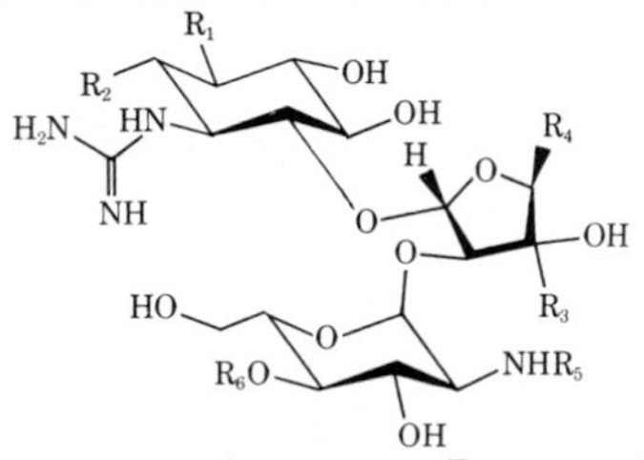

Structure	Name	CAS Registry No.	Producing organism	R_1	R_2	R_3	R_4	R_5	R_6	References
(3)	streptomycin	[57-92-1]	Streptomyces griseus	NHC(=NH)NH$_2$	OH	CHO	CH$_3$	CH$_3$	H	2,20–21
(4)	dihydrostreptomycin	[128-46-1]	S. humidus	NHC(=NH)NH$_2$	OH	CH$_2$OH	CH$_3$	CH$_3$	H	22
(5)	mannosidostreptomycin (streptomycin B)	[128-45-0]	S. griseus	NHC(=NH)NH$_2$	OH	CHO	CH$_3$	CH$_3$	α-D-mannopyranosyl	23
(6)	hydroxystreptomycin (reticulin)	[6835-00-3]	S. griseocarneus	NHC(=NH)NH$_2$	OH	CHO	CH$_2$OH	CH$_3$	H	24
(7)	N-demethylstreptomycin	[19022-67-4]		NHC(=NH)NH$_2$	OH	CHO	CH$_3$	H	H	25
(8)	mannisidohydroxystreptomycin	[28979-71-7]	Streptomyces 86	NHC(=NH)NH$_2$	OH	CHO	CH$_2$OH	CH$_3$	α-D-mannopyranosyl	26
(9)	bluensomycin (glebomycin)	[11011-72-6]	S. bluensis var. bluensis	OCONH$_2$	OH	CH$_2$OH	CH$_3$	CH$_3$	H	27–28
(10)	streptomutin A (2-deoxystreptomycin A)[a]	[58194-40-4]	S. griseus M1T-A5	NHC(=NH)NH$_2$	H	CHO	CH$_3$	CH$_3$	H	29–30

[a] Unnatural aminocyclitol prepared by mutational biosynthesis.

43

Table 3. Aminoglycoside–Aminocyclitol Antibiotics Containing a 4,5-Disubstituted 2-Deoxystreptamine Group

Structure	Name	CAS Registry No.	Producing organisms	R_1	R_2
(11)	neomycin B	[119-04-0]	S. fradiae	NH_2	OH
(12)	neomycin C	[66-86-4]	S. fradiae	NH_2	OH
(13)	neomycin LP-B	[54631-94-6]	S. fradiae	NH_2	OH
(14)	neomycin LP-C	[54617-40-2]	S. fradiae	NH_2	OH
(15)	hybrimycin A_1[a]	[22332-07-6]	S. fradiae	NH_2	OH
(16)	hybrimycin A_2[a]	[22400-60-8]	S. fradiae	NH_2	OH
(17)	hybrimycin B_1[a]	[22332-08-7]	S. fradiae	NH_2	OH
(18)	hybrimycin B_2[a]	[27425-78-1]	S. fradiae	NH_2	OH
(19)	paromomycin I (aminosidine, hydroxymycin, catenulin, zygomycin A_1)	[7542-37-2]	S. rimosus forma paromomycinus, S. pulveraceus	OH	OH
(20)	paromomycin II (zygomycin A_2)	[51795-47-2]	S. rimosus forma paromomycinus, S. pulveraceus	OH	OH
(21)	lividomycin A	[36441-41-5]	S. lividus	OH	H
(22)	lividomycin B	[37636-51-4]	S. lividus	OH	H
(23)	2230-C	[36019-37-1]	S. lividus	OH	OH
(24)	hybrimycin C_1[a]	[38965-79-6]	S. rimosus forma paromomycinus	OH	OH
(25)	hybrimycin C_2[a]	[39004-63-2]	S. rimosus forma paromomycinus	OH	OH
(26)	6-deoxyneomycin B[a]	[61430-98-6]	S. fradiae	NH_2	OH
(27)	6-deoxyneomycin C[a]	[61476-27-5]	S. fradiae	NH_2	OH
(28)	6-deoxyparomomycin I[a]	[61430-99-7]	S. rimosus forma paromomycinus	OH	OH
(29)	6-deoxyparomomycin II[a]	[61476-28-6]	S. rimosus forma paromomycinus	OH	OH
(30)	ribostamycin (SF-733)	[25546-65-0]	S. ribosidificus	NH_2	OH
(31)	2-hydroxyribostamycin[a]	[52198-59-1]	S. ribosidificus AF-1	NH_2	OH
(32)	2-epihydroxyribostamycin[a]	[52248-05-2]	S. ribosidificus AF-1	NH_2	OH
(33)	1 N-methylribostamycin[a]	[52275-05-5]	S. ribosidificus AF-1	NH_2	OH
(34)	3′,4′-dideoxyribostamycin[a]	[39535-80-3]	S. ribosidificus AF-1	NH_2	H
(35)	xylostacin (xylostamycin)	[50474-67-4]	Bacillus sp. Y-399	NH_2	OH
(36)	butirosin A	[34291-02-6]	Bacillus circulans	NH_2	OH
(37)	butirosin B	[34291-03-7]	B. circulans	NH_2	OH
(38)	2-hydroxybutirosin A[a]	[59867-75-3]	B. circulans	NH_2	OH
(39)	2-hydroxybutirosin B[a]	[59905-78-1]	B. circulans	NH_2	OH
(40)	4′-deoxybutirosin A (BU-1975 C_1)	[52760-38-0]	B. circulans	NH_2	H
(41)	4′-deoxybutirosin B (BU-1975 C_2)	[53185-10-7]	B. circulans	NH_2	H
(42)	BU-1709 E_1	[39471-56-2]	B. circulans	OH	OH
(43)	BU-1709 E_2	[39471-57-3]	B. circulans	OH	OH
(44)	LL-BM-408 α	[55781-25-4]	S. canus	OH	OH

Table 3 (continued)

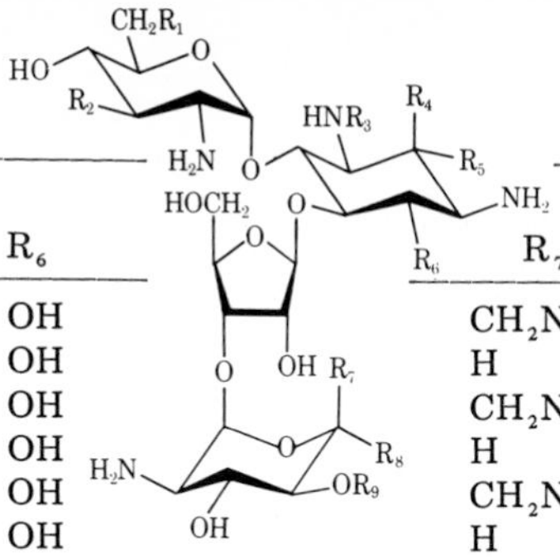

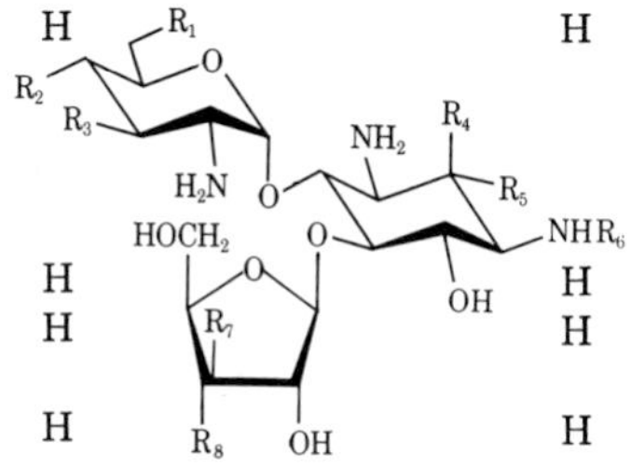

R_3	R_4	R_5	R_6	R_7	R_8	R_9	References
H	H	H	OH	CH_2NH_2	H	H	17
H	H	H	OH	H	CH_2NH_2	H	17
CH_3CO	H	H	OH	CH_2NH_2	H	H	31
CH_3CO	H	H	OH	H	CH_2NH_2	H	31
H	H	OH	OH	CH_2NH_2	H	H	32
H	H	OH	OH	H	CH_2NH_2	H	32
H	OH	H	OH	CH_2NH_2	H	H	32
H	OH	H	OH	H	CH_2NH_2	H	32
H	H	H	OH	CH_2NH_2	H	H	33
H	H	H	OH	H	CH_2NH_2	H	17,34
H	H	H	OH	CH_2NH_2	H	α-D-manno-pyranosyl	35
H	H	H	OH	CH_2NH_2	H	H	36
H	H	H	OH	CH_2NH_2	H	α-D-manno-pyranosyl	37
H	H	OH	OH	CH_2NH_2	H	H	38
H	H	OH	OH	H	CH_2NH_2	H	38
H	H	H	H	CH_2NH_2	H	H	39
H	H	H	H	H	CH_2NH_2	H	39
H	H	H	H	CH_2NH_2	H	H	39
H	H	H	H	H	CH_2NH_2	H	39

R_3	R_4	R_5	R_6	R_7	R_8	References
OH	H	H	H	H	OH	40
OH	H	OH	H	H	OH	41
OH	OH	H	H	H	OH	41
OH	H	H	CH_3	H	OH	41
H	H	H	H	H	OH	41
OH	H	H	H	OH	H	42
OH	H	H	$COCH(OH)CH_2CH_2NH_2$	OH	H	43
OH	H	H	$COCH(OH)CH_2CH_2NH_2$	H	OH	43
OH	H	OH	$COCH(OH)CH_2CH_2NH_2$	OH	H	44
OH	H	OH	$COCH(OH)CH_2CH_2NH_2$	H	OH	44
OH	H	H	$COCH(OH)CH_2CH_2NH_2$	OH	H	45–46
OH	H	H	$COCH(OH)CH_2CH_2NH_2$	H	OH	45–46
OH	H	H	$COCH(OH)CH_2CH_2NH_2$	OH	H	47
OH	H	H	$COCH(OH)CH_2CH_2NH_2$	H	OH	47
OH	H	H	H	H	OH	48–49

[a] Unnatural aminocyclitol prepared by mutational biosynthesis.

45

Table 4. Aminoglycoside-Aminocyclitol Antibiotics Containing a 4,6-Disubstituted 2-Deoxystreptamine Group

Structure	Name	CAS Registry No.	Producing organisms	R_1	R_2
(45)	kanamycin A	[59-01-8]	S. kanamyceticus	H	NH_2
(46)	kanamycin B	[4696-76-8]	S. kanamyceticus	H	NH_2
(47)	kanamycin C	[2280-32-2]	S. kanamyceticus	H	NH_2
(48)	NK-1001	[31077-69-7]	S. kanamyceticus	H	OH
(49)	NK-1012-1	[31077-70-0]	S. kanamyceticus	H	OH
(50)	NK-1013-1	[31156-79-3]	S. kanamyceticus	H	$NHCOCH_3$
(51)	NK-1013-2	[31156-80-6]	S. kanamyceticus	H	NH_2
(52)	nebramycin factor 4	[37321-10-1]	S. tenebrarius	$CONH_2$	NH_2
(53)	nebramycin factor 5'	[37321-12-3]	S. tenebrarius	$CONH_2$	NH_2
(54)	tobramycin (nebramycin factor 6)	[32986-56-4]	S. tenebrarius	OH	NH_2
(55)	gentamicin C_1	[25876-10-2]	Micromonospora purpurea	NH_2	H
(56)	gentamicin C_2	[25876-11-3]	M. purpurea	NH_2	H
(57)	gentamicin C_{1a}	[26098-04-4]	M. purpurea	NH_2	H
(58)	2-hydroxy-gentamicin $C_1{}^a$	[60802-56-4]	M. purpurea 6B-3P	NH_2	H
(59)	2-hydroxy-gentamicin $C_2{}^a$	[60768-15-2]	M. purpurea 6B-3P	NH_2	H
(60)	5-deoxy-gentamicin $C_1{}^a$	[60768-21-0]	M. purpurea 6B-3P	NH_2	H
(61)	5-deoxy-gentamicin $C_2{}^a$	[60768-22-1]	M. purpurea 6B-3P	NH_2	H
(62)	5-deoxy-gentamicin $C_{1a}{}^a$	[60768-20-9]	M. Purpurea 6B-3P	NH_2	H
(63)	gentamicin C_{2a}	[59751-72-3]	M. purpurea	NH_2	H
(64)	gentamicin C_{2b} (sagamicin, XK-62-2)	[52093-21-7]	M. purpurea, Micromonospora MK62 and MK65	NH_2	H
(65)	gentamicin X_2	[36889-17-5]	M. purpurea	NH_2	OH
(66)	gentamicin B	[36889-15-3]	M. purpurea	OH	OH
(67)	gentamicin B_1	[36889-16-4]	M. purpurea	OH	OH
(68)	G-148	[49863-47-0]	M. rhodorangea	NH_2	OH
(69)	JI-20A	[51846-97-0]	M. purpurea JI-20	NH_2	OH
(70)	JI-20B	[51846-98-1]	M. purpurea JI-20	NH_2	OH

Table 4 (*continued*)

R_3	R_4	R_5	R_6	R_7	R_8	Stereochemistry at C-6'	References
OH	OH	NH_2	H	H			18,20
NH_2	OH	NH_2	H	H			18,20
NH_2	OH	OH	H	H			18,20
OH	OH	NH_2	H	H			50
NH_2	OH	NH_2	H	H			50
NH_2	OH	NH_2	H, $COCH_3$	$COCH_3$			50
NH_2	OH	NH_2	H, $COCH_3$	$COCH_3$			50
NH_2	OH	NH_2	H	H			51
NH_2	H	NH_2	H	H			51
NH_2	H	NH_2	H	H			52

R_1	R_2	R_3	R_4	R_5	R_6	R_7	Stereochemistry at C-6'	References
H		CH_3		$NHCH_3$	OH	H	R	53
H		CH_3		NH_2	OH	H	R	53
H		H		NH_2	OH	H		53
H		CH_3		$NHCH_3$	OH	OH	unknown	54−55
H		CH_3		NH_2	OH	OH	unknown	54−55
H		CH_3		$NHCH_3$	H	H	unknown	54−55
H		CH_3		NH_2	H	H	unknown	54−55
H		H		NH_2	H	H		54−55
H		CH_3		NH_2	OH	H	S	56
H		H		$NHCH_3$	OH	H		57−58
OH		H		OH	OH	H		53
OH		H		NH_2	OH	H		53,59
OH		CH_3		NH_2	OH	H	R	53
OH		CH_3		OH	OH	H	R	60
OH		H		NH_2	OH	H		61
OH		CH_3		NH_2	OH	H	S	61

Table 4 (*continued*)

Struct-ture	Name	CAS Registry No.	Producing organisms	R$_1$	R$_2$
(71)	gentamicin A	[13291-74-2]	M. purpurea	H	HO
(72)	gentamicin A$_1$	[55925-13-8]	M. purpurea	OH	H
(73)	gentamicin A$_2$	[55715-66-7]	M. purpurea	H	OH
(74)	gentamicin A$_3$	[55715-67-8]	M. purpurea	OH	H
(75)	gentamicin A$_4$	[55904-33-1]	M. purpurea	H	OH
(76)	seldomycin factor 1 (XK-88-1)	[56276-04-1]	S. hofunensis	H	OH
(77)	seldomycin factor 3 (XK-88-3)	[56276-05-2]	S. hofunensis	H	OH
(78)	seldomycin factor 5 (XK-88-5)	[56276-26-7]	S. hofunensis	H	OCH$_3$
(79)	Mu-2a[a,b]	[54797-14-7]	M. purpurea	H	OH
(80)	sisomicin (66-40)	[32385-11-8]	M. inyoensis	OH	CH$_3$
(81)	verdamicin	[49863-48-1]	M. grisea	OH	CH$_3$
(82)	G-52	[51909-61-6]	M. zionensis	OH	CH$_3$
(83)	66-40 B	[53797-16-3]	M. inyoensis	H	OH
(84)	66-40 D	[53759-50-5]	M. inyoensis	OH	H
(85)	Mu-1[a,b]	[54830-49-8]	M. inyoensis 1550F	OH	CH$_3$
(86)	Mu-1a[a,b]	[54830-50-1]	M. inyoensis 1550F	OH	CH$_3$
(87)	Mu-1b[a,b]	[54830-51-2]	M. inyoensis 1550F	OH	CH$_3$
(88)	Mu-2[a,b]	[54830-48-7]	M. inyoensis 1550F	OH	CH$_3$

Table 4 (*continued*)

R_3	R_4	R_5	R_6	R_7	R_8	References
$NHCH_3$	OH	OH	NH_2	OH	OH	62
$NHCH_3$	OH	OH	NH_2	OH	OH	63
OH	OH	OH	NH_2	OH	OH	64
$NHCH_3$	OH	OH	OH	OH	NH_2	63
$N(CHO)CH_3$	OH	OH	NH_2	OH	OH	63
OH	NH_2	OH	NH_2	OH	OH	65–66
OH	NH_2	OH	NH_2	OH	NH_2	65–66
NH_2	NH_2	OH	NH_2	H	NH_2	65,67
$NHCH_3$	OH	H	NH_2	OH	OH	68

R_3	R_4	R_5	R_6	R_7		References
CH_3	H	OH	H	H		69
CH_3	H	OH	H	CH_3		70–71
CH_3	H	OH	CH_3	H		72–73
CH_3	H	OH	H	H		74
CH_3	H	OH	H	H		74
CH_3	OH	OH	H	H		68
$COCH_3$	OH	OH	H	H		68
H	OH	OH	H	H		68
CH_3	H	H	H	H		68

[a] Unnatural aminocyclitols were prepared by mutational biosynthesis.

[b] The antibiotics Mu-1, 1b, 2, and 2a were originally referred to as mutamicins 1, 1a, etc. The names have been changed because mutamycin is the name of an antibiotic of another type.

Table 5. Aminoglycoside–Aminocyclitol Antibiotics Containing a Mono-Substituted 2-Deoxystreptamine Group

Structure	Name	CAS Registry No.	Producing organisms
(89)	apramycin (nebramycin factor 2)	[37321-09-8]	S. tenebrarius
(90)	oxyapramycin (nebramycin factor 7)	[56283-52-4]	S. tenebrarius
(91)	neamine (neomycin A)	[3947-65-7]	S. fradiae, S. tenebrarius, S. kanamyceticus
(92)	paromamine	[534-47-4]	S. kanamyceticus, S. tenebrarius, M. purpurea
(93)	NK-1003	[31077-71-1]	S. kanamyceticus
(94)	seldomycin factor 2 (4'-deoxyneamine)	[54333-78-7]	S. hofunensis
(95)	nebramine (3'-deoxyneamine)	[34051-04-2]	S. hofunensis
(96)	lividamine (3'-deoxy-paromamine)	[36019-33-7]	S. tenebarius
(97)	5-deoxybuti-rosamine[a]	[59867-74-2]	B. circulans
(98)	NK-1012-2 (3-amino-3-deoxyglucosyl-2-deoxy-streptamine)	[20744-51-8]	S. kanamyceticus
(99)	garamine	[49751-51-1]	M. purpurea, M. inyoensis

Table 5 (*continued*)

R_1		R_2	R_3	R_4	R_5	R_6	References

R_1	R_2	R_3	R_4	R_5	R_6	References
H						75
OH						76·

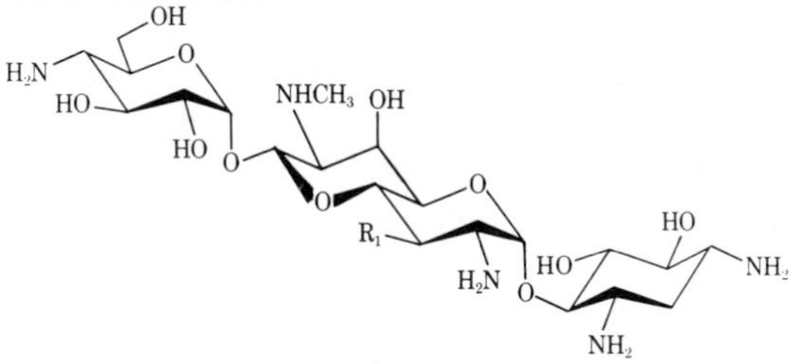

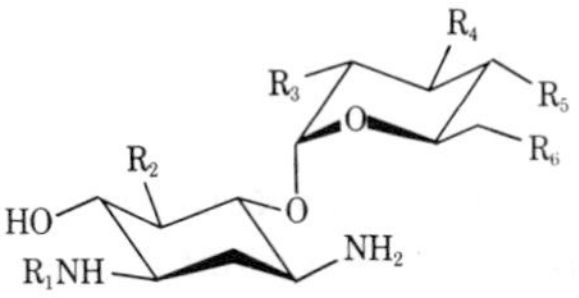 R_1	R_2	R_3	R_4	R_5	R_6	References
H	OH	NH_2	OH	OH	NH_2	17
H	OH	NH_2	OH	OH	OH	17,33
H	OH	OH	OH	OH	NH_2	50
H	OH	NH_2	OH	H	NH_2	66
H	OH	NH_2	H	OH	NH_2	52
H	OH	NH_2	H	OH	OH	76–77
$COCH(OH)CH_2CH_2NH_2$	H	NH_2	OH	OH	NH_2	44

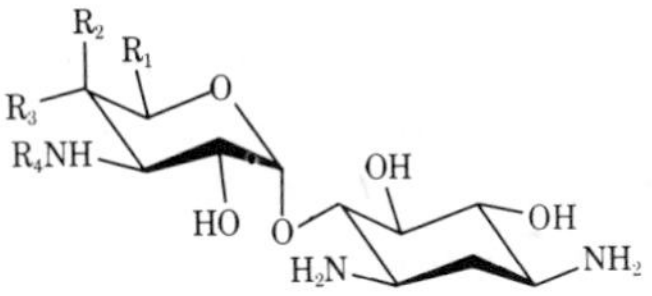 R_1	R_2	R_3	R_4			References
CH_2OH	H	OH	H			50
H	OH	CH_3	CH_3			69

[a] Unnatural aminocyclitol prepared by mutational biosynthesis.

51

tants). These mutants were able to produce neomycin only when deoxystreptamine was added exogenously (32). By adding aminocyclitols other than the natural one, the mutant organisms could be induced to elaborate novel antibiotics. In the case of the *S. fradiae* mutant these compounds were named hybrimycins (see Table 3). This process for preparing new antibiotics has been called mutasynthesis, the antibiotics so produced have been called mutasynthetics, and the aminocyclitols introduced mutasynthons (79). The alternative term, mutational biosynthesis, has also been applied to the process and the producing organisms have been called idiotrophs (29). Mutasynthesis has now been used to produce novel antibiotics related to streptomycin, neomycin, ribostamycin, butirosin, kanamycin, paromomycin, spectinomycin, gentamicin, and sisomicin. The mutasynthetics listed in Tables 2–5 are indicated by an appropriate footnote. The range of aminocyclitols bioconverted to new antibiotics by idiotrophs is often quite small (86), and the method has thus far suffered from the disadvantage that yields of new antibiotics have been too low for commercial exploitation.

Manufacture

Aminoglycoside–aminocyclitol antibiotics are produced by submerged aerobic fermentation of the appropriate producing organism (see Tables 2–5) in an aqueous nutrient medium containing assimilable carbon and nitrogen sources, inorganic ions, and occasionally some form of pH control (see Fermentation). The fermentations are usually carried out in very large vessels, often in excess of 40 m³ (10,000 gal), and utilize media composed principally of some combination of soybean meal, dextrin, starch, and glucose. A spore or mycelial preparation of the producing organism is grown through germination stages of increasing size until a 5–10% inoculum is obtained for the manufacturing step. The precise conditions of fermentation differ in detail for different antibiotics and manufacturers and specialized ingredients, such as yeast and meat extracts, cornsteep liquor, certain amino acids, trace elements, acids, bases, or calcium carbonate, are often advantageously added to germination or fermentation stages. Vigorous aeration and agitation are generally necessary, as well as temperature control, usually in the range of 25–38°C. After the fermentation cycle of 3–6 d, antibiotic activity is found partly in the broth and partly associated with the mycelium, from which it can be released by acidification. Isolation of the antibiotic is usually accomplished by filtration of the acidified broth, followed by extraction with an acidic ion-exchange resin. Elution with acid or base then gives the crude antibiotic, which is almost always obtained as a complex of closely related compounds. Purification may be by any of the well known techniques of chromatography, crystallization, or precipitation of insoluble salts. The yields obtained in commercial antibiotic fermentations are usually trade secrets but are probably as high as 15 g/L in favorable cases.

Antibacterial Activity and Uses

The microbiological properties and clinical uses of aminoglycosides have been extensively reviewed (3,87). The antibiotics of this class in clinical use are listed in Table 1.

Aminoglycoside–aminocyclitols are among the most potent antibiotics known. Their spectrum of activity covers most of the common gram-negative bacteria as well as *Staphylococcus*. Against *Streptococcus* they are relatively weak. They have no useful activity against anaerobic bacteria or fungi. The *in vitro* antibacterial activities of a number of important aminocyclitols are compared in Table 6. The results are expressed as the minimum inhibitory concentrations (MIC) required to prevent growth of the test organism. In Table 7 the comparative MIC values for a number of newer agents against sensitive gram-negative bacteria are given.

Antibiotics of the aminoglycoside class are an important clinical resource despite a liability to produce serious side effects. The justification for their use lies in the very wide range of pathogens which they inhibit, including many organisms which cannot be effectively treated by other agents. Their potential toxicity limits their systemic application in the United States and certain other countries to the treatment of serious infections in hospitalized patients who can be carefully monitored for side effects. In

Table 6. Mean[a] Minimum Inhibitory Concentrations (MIC) (µg/mL) of Aminoglycoside Antibiotics

Organism	No. of strains	Strepto-mycin	Neomycin	Kanamycin	Paromo-mycin	Gentamicin
Staphylococcus aureus	29	2	0.5	1	1	0.125
Streptococcus faecali	32	64	64	32	64	8
Escherichia coli	22	8	8	4	8	1
Klebsiella sp	20	4	2	2	2	1
Aerobacter sp	10	4	2	2	2	0.5
Proteus mirabilis	6	8	8	4	8	2
Proteus vulgaris	6	4	4	4	4	1
Proteus morganii	10	8	8	4	4	1
Proteus rettgeri	7	4	8	2	4	1
Pseudomonas aeruginosa	31	32	32	128	512	4
Salmonella sp	14	16	2	2	2	1
Shigella sp	17	8	8	4	8	2

[a] Tests mainly of recent isolates at Hammersmith Hospital by plate dilution method with 2-fold differences. Means are of $\log_2$ of MIC to the nearest $\log_2$. In the series, tested strains showing a clearly abnormal degree of resistance (sometimes following treatment with the antibiotic) were omitted from these calculations.

[b] Courtesy of Churchill Livingstone (88).

Table 7. Median Minimal Inhibitory Concentrations (µg/mL) of Aminoglycoside Antibiotics[a]

Organism	No. of strains	Gentamicin	Tobramycin	Amikacin	Netilmicin
Escherichia coli	9	0.25	0.5	1.0	0.25
Enterobacter sp	7	0.25	0.5	1.0	0.25
Klebsiella pneumoniae	8	0.25	0.25	1.0	0.25
Providencia sp	9	4.0	4.0	1.0	8.0
Pseudomonas aeruginosa	21	2.0	0.5	4.0	4.0
Serratia marcescens	9	0.5	2.0	2.0	1.0
Proteus, indole pos	9	1.0	1.0	2.0	1.0
Proteus, indole neg	3	1.0	2.0	1.0	2.0

[a] Aminoglycoside-sensitive strains only were used. Values were determined in Mueller-Hinton agar by standard dilution methods (89).

other parts of the world, however, systemic aminoglycoside therapy is used on an out-patient basis.

Aminoglycosides are usually given by intramuscular injection for systemic infections; they are rapidly absorbed and peak serum levels are attained in 30–90 min. The serum half-lives for most aminoglycosides are similar, averaging 2–3 h. In life-threatening situations, careful intravenous administration may be desirable. None of the aminoglycosides have any appreciable absorption following oral administration. Aminoglycosides are also used topically for wounds and to prevent infection in burn patients.

Excretion of the drug occurs almost exclusively through the kidney and high concentrations are found in urine. No significant metabolism of aminoglycosides occurs, the drugs being excreted unchanged.

The acute toxicity of aminoglycosides, usually cited as the intravenous 50% lethal dose (LD_{50}) in mice, is caused by neuromuscular blockade. This is an uncommon side effect during human therapy and is observed almost exclusively in patients receiving other neuromuscular blocking drugs. the most important toxicity involves the kidney (nephrotoxicity) and both the balance (vestibular) and hearing (cochlear) functions of the inner ear. Nephrotoxicity can be produced to some extent by all aminoglycoside–aminocyclitols and therapy must be undertaken cautiously. This is especially true in patients with existing renal insufficiency and when other potentially nephrotoxic drugs are being administered simultaneously. Careful monitoring of a patient's renal function provides early signs of incipient nephrotoxicity which is usually reversible when the drug is withdrawn. Very rarely a severe nephrotoxic reaction, resulting in loss of kidney function occurs. This rare reaction is sometimes reversible if, in the interim, the patient is supported by dialysis. Aminoglycosides vary in the incidence and type of ototoxicity they produce. Gentamicin is reported to cause more vestibular than cochlear toxicity, whereas the reverse has been reported for kanamycin (3). The incidence of cochlear toxicity and nephrotoxicity for neomycin is such that this drug is no longer recommended for systemic use in the United States. Severe damage to the inner ear is usually irreversible, although vestibular damage can be partially compensated for by other mechanisms.

Among the aminoglycosides, gentamicin (a mixture of gentamicins C_1 (55), C_2 (56), and C_{1a} (57)) presently occupies a position of preeminence due to its particularly broad spectrum, which includes the troublesome pathogen *Pseudomonas aeruginosa*, as well as many gram-negative organisms which have acquired resistance to kanamycin (45).

Gentamicin is a drug of choice for septicemia and serious infections of the central nervous system, urinary tract, respiratory tract, gastrointestinal tract, and skin, bone, and soft tissue (including burns) caused by sensitive gram-negative organisms. When *Pseudomonas aeruginosa* is the infectious organism involved, carbenicillin is often administered concomitantly, since synergism of these two antibiotics has been widely reported.

Despite the well-known hazards associated with aminoglycoside therapy, gentamicin has experienced dramatically increased usage during the last ten years (90). Aminoglycosides are not indicated in uncomplicated infections where potentially less toxic antibiotics can be used. Thus despite high *in vitro* activity, they are not normally used against staphylococcal infections, except in those rare cases when the strains are resistant to other antibiotics. Despite generally poor activity when used alone against streptococcal species, aminoglycosides show a useful synergy with penicillins against these organisms and penicillin-aminoglycoside combinations are the therapy of choice for serious enterococcal infections, especially endocarditis. Aminoglycosides have also been used in gonorrhea, although for sensitive gonococci, penicillin G is the drug of choice.

Streptomycin, kanamycin, and gentamicin all show good *in vitro* activity against *Mycobacterium tuberculosis*. Only streptomycin, however, is widely used for the treatment of tuberculosis; although kanamycin is used in Japan.

Kanamycin is used for many of the same indications as gentamicin, provided kanamycin-sensitive organisms are involved. The incidence of resistance to kanamycin is higher than for gentamicin and the drug is ineffective against *Pseudomonas aeruginosa*. The use of paromomycin (19) is restricted in the United States to oral treatment of intestinal amebiasis. Several of the clinically useful aminoglycosides are also used in veterinary medicine.

Among agents introduced into the clinic more recently, tobramycin (54) has greater potency against *Pseudomonas aeruginosa* than gentamicin but is otherwise similar. Sisomicin (80) and dibekacin [34493-98-6] (100) are generally similar to gentamicin, although the former compound is somewhat more potent. Amikacin [39831-55-5] (101), on the other hand, shows activity against many gentamicin-resistant organisms (19) and seems destined for an important place in therapy. Amikacin is less toxic than gentamicin but also less potent, requiring higher dose levels. A recent study (91) suggests that amikacin has no advantage in safety over gentamicin. A recently developed semisynthetic aminocyclitol netilmicin [56391-56-1] (102), now undergoing clinical trials, retains most of the potency of gentamicin and has a much broader spectrum of activity. Its most interesting property, however, is a substantially

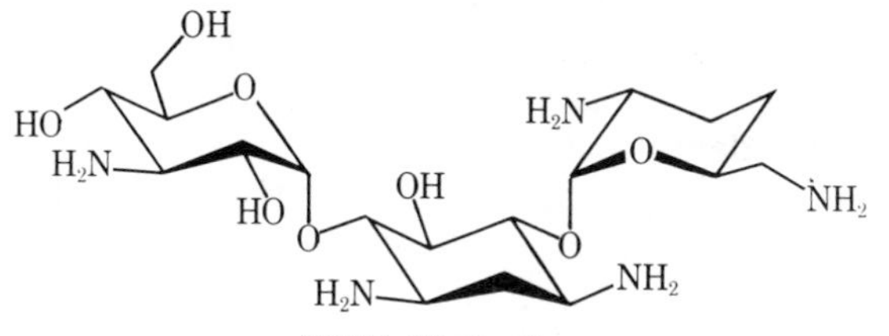

(100) dibekacin

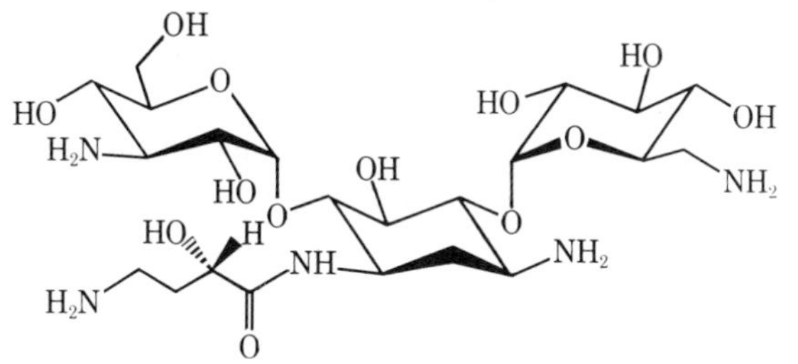

(101) amikacin

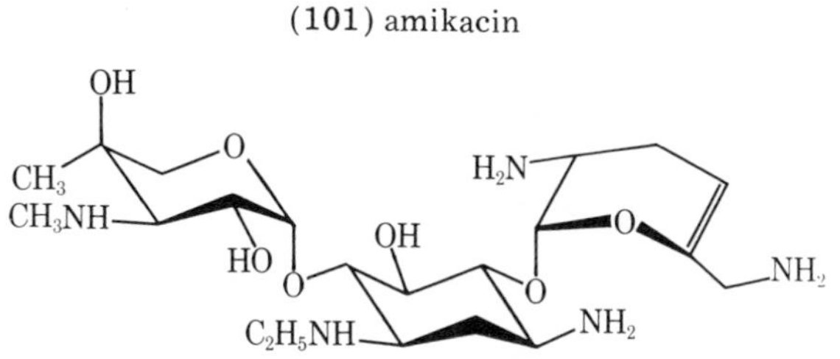

(102) netilmicin

improved chronic toxicity profile compared to gentamicin in laboratory animals (92).

Bacterial Resistance. All antibiotics, to variable extents, experience bacterial resistance to their inhibitory action. Aminoglycosides are no exception to this clinically important phenomenon and the biochemical basis for their resistance has been extensively examined. A number of structural features of the antibiotic molecules have been identified as being associated with resistance. This has led to the rational synthesis of aminoglycosides active against resistant bacteria. Several comprehensive reviews of the subject have appeared (19,93–94).

Three general mechanisms are known by which bacteria acquire resistance to aminoglycosides. One of these involves mutation of the organism leading to altered ribosomes which no longer bind the drug. A second mechanism results from reduced permeability of the bacterium to the drug, and the third, and most important mechanism, is mediated by bacterial enzymes, which inactivate the drug. Resistance due to ribosomal mutation is restricted to aminoglycoside–aminocyclitols of the streptomycin type. Claims of ribosomal resistance to gentamicin and kanamycin have not been confirmed and are probably erroneous. Ribosomal resistance to streptomycin has been shown to occur via spontaneous mutation, resulting in a single amino acid change in one of the 21 proteins of the small ribosomal subunit. Such altered ribosomes are incapable of binding streptomycin (94). Bacterial resistance due to mutation affecting ribosomes is relatively rare and such strains are usually sensitive to other aminoglycoside antibiotics.

Bacterial resistance due to reduced permeability to aminoglycosides probably accounts for less than 20% of the total incidence of clinical resistance. There has, however, been one report of an institution experiencing an exceeding high percentage of resistant *P. aeruginosa* strains operating by this mechanism (95). Evidence has been presented that streptomycin and gentamicin are taken up into *E. coli* and *P. aeruginosa* by an energy-dependent process of active accumulation (95–96). Permeability-resistant strains apparently lack this facility for active accumulation. Permeability-resistant organisms are usually resistant to all aminoglycosides and must be treated with antibiotics of a different class.

The most common and, therefore, the most important mode of resistance to aminoglycosides, involves modification of the antibiotic by bacterial enzymes to give an inactive product. The enzymes responsible for aminoglycoside inactivation are coded for by small, self-replicating, extra-chromosomal loops of DNA (plasmids) known as R-factors. R-factors are often able to transfer their genetic information to other bacteria by a process known as conjugation; they are infectious and can be re-

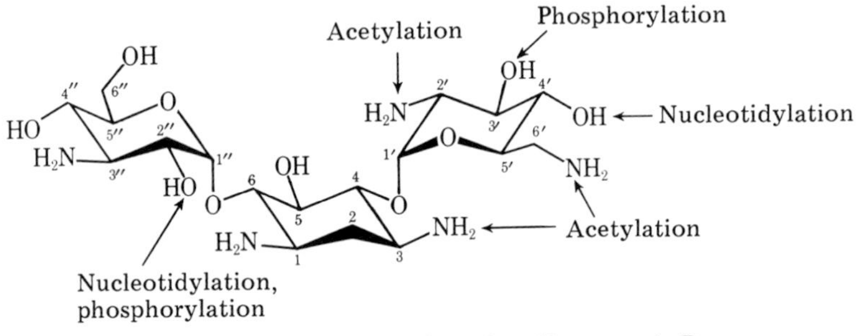

Figure 1. Enzymatic modification of kanoamycin B.

sponsible for the spread of antibiotic resistance. The first case of inactivation of an aminoglycoside to be studied involved a kanamycin-resistant strain of *E. coli*. H. Umezawa and co-workers (97) showed that resistance was associated with enzymic transfer of an acetyl group from acetyl CoA to give the inactive product 6'-*N*-acetyl-kanamycin A. Since this initial finding, other types of bacterial enzymatic inactivation of aminoglycosides have been discovered. These involve, besides *N*-acetylation, *O*-phosphorylation, and *O*-nucleotidylation. As an example, the presently known modes of inactivation of kanamycin B, a representative of the 4,6-disubstituted 2-deoxy-streptamine class of compounds, are shown in Figure 1. Although kanamycin B can be inactivated in an impressive number of ways, it should be pointed out that this compound is still a useful antibiotic. The principal reason for this is that inactivating enzymes are far from ubiquitous; some in fact being quite rare. Thus 6'-*N*-acetyl-transferase enzymes are uncommon in clinical isolates and in some cases, where present, they specify a level of resistance too low to be clinically significant. 2'-*N*-Acetylation is also an uncommon mode of resistance found only in *Providencia* and *Proteus* species to date. 4'-*O*-Nucleotidylation and 2''-*O*-phosphorylation have so far occurred only in strains of *Staphylococcus aureus*, for which aminoglycoside therapy is not usually indicated. On the other hand, 3'-*O*-phosphorylation is a common mode of resistance which presents clinical problems not only for the kanamycins, but also for neomycin and ribostamycin. Very many strains of *P. aeruginosa* appear to possess this enzyme (93). Clearly, antibiotics like the gentamicins (55–57), which lack 3'- and 4'-hydroxyl groups, are not affected by resistance mechanisms operating at these centers. Acetylation of the 3-nitrogen of the deoxystreptamine ring is also a resistance mechanism of some clinical importance. Although specifying resistance to a number of aminoglycosides, it is most troublesome in strains of *Pseudomonas aeruginosa* resistant to gentamicin. 2''-*O*-Nucleotidylation is a resistance mechanism of clinical concern for the kanamycins, tobramycin, and gentamicin; it occurs most commonly in the *Enterobacteriacea*.

Recent studies with newly isolated, resistant bacterial strains make it clear that, for each position of modification of an aminoglycoside molecule, there may exist one

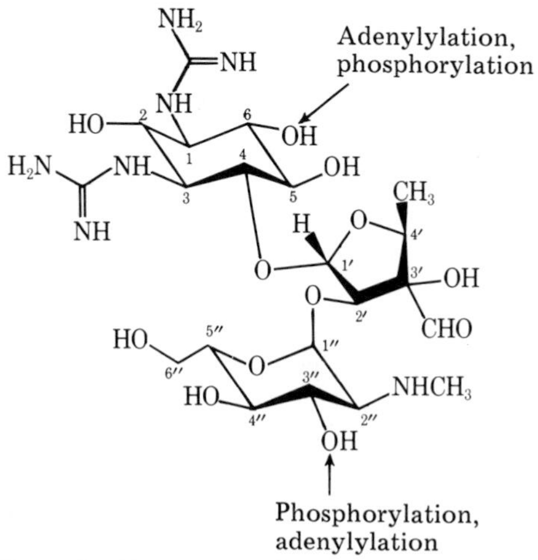

Figure 2.   Enzymatic modification of streptomycin.

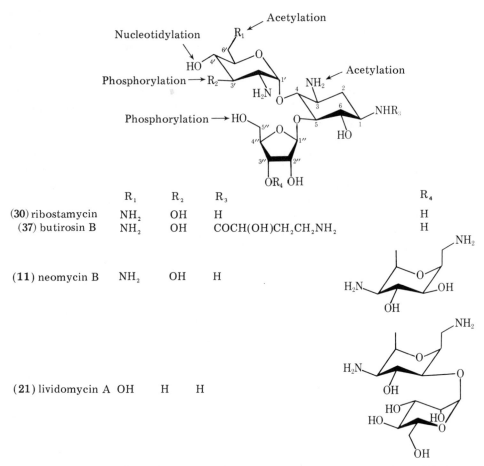

	R_1	R_2	R_3		R_4
(30) ribostamycin	NH_2	OH	H		H
(37) butirosin B	NH_2	OH	$COCH(OH)CH_2CH_2NH_2$		H
(11) neomycin B	NH_2	OH	H		
(21) lividomycin A	OH	H	H		

Figure 3. Enzymatic modification of some 4,5-disubstituted 2-deoxystreptamine antibiotics.

or more enzymes which differ in their substrate ranges. For example, 3-N-acetyl-transferases have been isolated for which gentamicin but not tobramycin are efficient substrates; other enzymes can use both antibiotics as substrates. A whole range of 6'-N-acetyltransferases have been described (98–99).

In Figure 2, the presently known modes of bacterial enzymatic inactivation of streptomycin are shown. Of these the 3″-O-phosphotransferase enzyme is commonly found in clinically resistant strains. The 6-O-nucleotidyltransferase has been found only in $S.$ $aureus$ and the 6-O-phosphotransferase, found in a resistant strain of $P.$ $aeruginosa$, was shown to phosphorylate dihydrostreptomicin (4) rather inefficiently.

As in the case of the kanamycins, phosphorylation of the 4,5-disubstituted deoxystreptamine class (Figure 3) is the most clinically important of the inactivation mechanisms. Three types of enzymes are known which can phosphorylate the 3'-hydroxyl group of aminoglycosides. The first of these is able to phosphorylate the kanamycins, neomycins, ribostamycin, etc, at the 3'-position and compounds such as lividomycin, which lacks a 3'-hydroxyl group, can be phosphorylated at the 5″-position. This enzyme, however, is unable to phosphorylate compounds having an α-hydroxy-γ-aminobutyric acid (HABA) substituent at 1-N, such as butirosin or the semisynthetic aminoglycoside amikacin. The second phosphotransferase enzyme is able to phosphorylate only at the 3'-position (ie, kanamycins, neomycins, but not lividomycin), but is able to phosphorylate butirosin (93–94). A third type of enzyme reported recently (100) has the combined substrate ranges of both the other enzymes.

The nomenclature of the aminoglycoside modifying enzymes is somewhat confused in the literature. Enzymes were initially named for the first antibiotic found to be a substrate, eg, kanamycin acetyltransferase (KAT). As other substrates for the same enzymes were discovered these names became redundant. They are, nevertheless, still widely used in the literature. A proposal for a more rational nomenclature of these enzymes has been put forward (101) and is gaining acceptance. Table 8 lists the enzymes by their names, abbreviations, and most important substrates. The enzyme systematic names are similar to the trivial ones given in Table 8 but incorporate the name of the donor molecules, usually ATP or acetyl CoA.

It is clear that in bacteria possessing R-factors specifying aminoglycoside modifying enzymes, these enzymes are required for resistance, since the same strains cured of their R-factors are drug-sensitive. It has been shown, however, that in whole bacteria the amount of drug inactivation which takes place is almost immeasurably small, unlike, eg, certain β-lactamase enzymes which are capable of inactivating large amounts of penicillins. It has been suggested that a very small amount of enzyme-modified aminoglycoside present in the bacterial inner membrane, somehow effectively prevents accumulation of lethal amounts of antibiotic; the basic mechanism of resistance specified by modifying enzymes is inhibition of transport of aminoglycoside antibiotic into the cell (109).

Semisynthetic Aminoglycoside–Aminocyclitols. With the recognition that bacterial resistance could be linked to specific structural features of aminoglycoside molecules came a tremendous impetus to prepare semisynthetic derivatives incapable of enzymatic inactivation. This approach has yielded two semisynthetic aminoglycosides, amikacin and dibekacin, already in clinical use and at least one other, netilmicin, in clinical trials. Reviews covering this aspect of aminoglycoside work have appeared (18–20).

The most straightforward approach to improving the spectrum of activity of natural aminoglycoside–aminocyclitols has been to remove or sterically hinder sites of enzymatic modification. Gentamicin C_1 (**55**), as shown in Figure 4, provides an example from nature of such desirable structural modification. Lacking the hydroxyl groups at the 3'- and 4'-positions, gentamicin C_1 cannot be modified by APH(3') and ANT(4') enzymes (see Table 8) and is active against bacteria harboring these enzymes. The presence of C- and N-methyl groups around the 6'-position also prevents inactivation by AAC(6') enzymes (see Table 8), presumably due to steric hindrance. Chemical modification at the 3'-, 4'-, and 6'-positions of a number of aminoglycosides have been carried out, principally by H. Umezawa, S. Umezawa, and their co-workers. 3'-Deoxykanamycin A [*35906-65-1*] (**103**), prepared by total synthesis by S. Umezawa, possesses excellent activity against kanamycin-resistant bacteria containing APH(3') enzymes, as does the naturally occurring 3'-deoxykanamycin B (**54**, tobramycin). 3'-O-Methyl-kanamycin A [*35906-62-8*] (**104**), however, has little activity. 3',4'-Dideoxykanamycin B (**100,** dibekacin) has predictable activity against APH(3')- and ANT(4')-containing bacteria and is now used clinically. 6'-N-Methylkanamycin A

Table 8.   Proposed Rational Nomenclature of Aminoglycoside–Aminocyclitol Modifying Enzymes[a]

Enzyme activity	Enzyme trivial name	Abbreviation	Reference
Phosphorylation			
phosphorylation of 3″-hydroxyl of streptomycin and dihydrostreptamicin	aminoglycoside 3″-phosphotransferase	APH(3″)	93
phosphorylation of 6-hydroxyl of dihydrostreptomycin	aminoglycoside 6-phosphotransferase	APH(6)	102
phosphorylation of the 3′-hydroxyl of kanamycins, neomycins ribostamycin (not butirosins), and the 5″-hydroxyl of lividomycins	aminoglycoside 3′-phosphotransferase I	APH(3′)-I	93
phosphorylation of the 3′-hydroxyl of kanamycins, neomycins, ribostamycin, and butirosins	aminoglycoside 3′-phosphotransferase II	APH(3′)-II	93
phosphorylation of the 3′-hydroxyl of kanamycins, neomycins, ribostamycin, butirosins, and the 5″-hydroxyl of lividomycins	aminoglycoside 3′-phosphotransferase-III	APH(3′)-III	100
phosphorylation of the 5″-hydroxyl of ribostamycin	aminoglycoside 5″-phosphotransferase	APH(5″)	103
phosphorylation of the 2″-hydroxyl of gentamicins and kanamycins	aminoglycoside 2″-phosphotransferase	APH(2″)	104
Nucleotidylation			
adenylylation of 3″-hydroxyl of streptomycin and dihydrostreptomycin	aminoglycoside 3″-adenylyltransferase	AAD(3″)	93
adenylylation of 6-hydroxyl of streptomycin	aminoglycoside 6-adenylyltransferase	AAD(6)	105
nucleotidylation of 2″-hydroxyl of gentamicins, kanamycins, tobramycin, dibekacin, and sisomicin (not amikacin, netilmicin)	aminoglycoside 2″-nucleotidyltransferase	ANT(2″)	93
nucleotidylation of 4′-hydroxyl of kanamycins, tobramycin, lividomycin, neomycins, butirosins, ribostamycin, and amikacin	aminoglycoside 4′-nucleotidyltransferase	ANT(4′)	106
Acetylation			
acetylation of 6′-amino of neomycins, kanamycins, gentamicin C_{1a}, sisomicin, amikacin, dibekacin, and ribostamycin	aminoglycoside 6′-acetyltranferase[b]	AAC(6′)	93
acetylation of 3-amino of gentamicins, sisomicin (not tobramycin, dibekacin, amikacin, or netilmicin)	aminoglycoside 3-acetyltransferase I	AAC(3)-I	93
acetylation of 3-amino of gentamicins, sisomicin tobramycin, dibekacin, neomycin, and netilmicin (not amikacin)	aminoglycoside 3-acetyl transferase II	AAC(3)-II	107
acetylation of 2′-amino of gentamicins, sisomicin, tobramycin, butirosin, and dibekacin	aminoglycoside 2′-acetyltransferase	AAC(2′)	108

[a] Ref. 101.

[b] There is more than one type of aminoglycoside 6′-acetyltransferase (98–99). The uniqueness of some of the enzymes described in the published literature, however, is not clear.

[40371-46-8] (105) has been synthesized and is active against AAC(6′)-containing bacteria, and 6′-*N*-methyl-3″,-dideoxykanomycin B [40371-47-9] (106) has a very similar spectrum of activity to gentamicin C_1 (18,93). A novel and efficient method

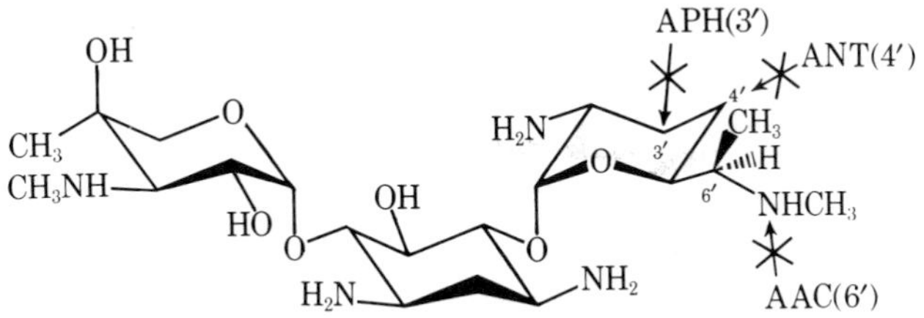

Figure 4.   Gentamicin C_1 (**55**).

for preparing 3'-deoxyaminoglycosides, via their enzymatically modified 3'-O-phosphates, has been described recently (110).

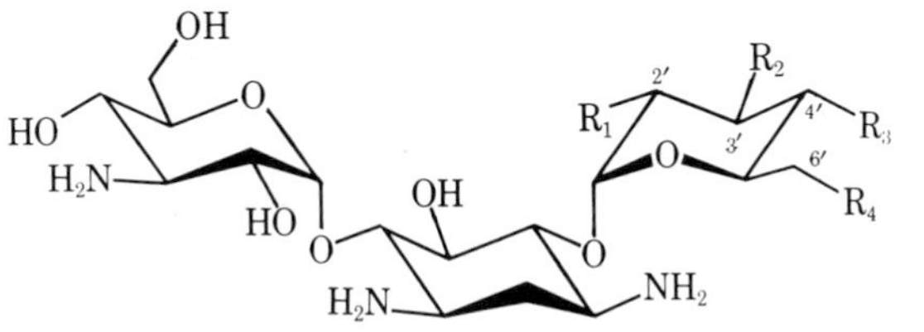

		R_1	R_2	R_3	R_4
(100)	3',4'-dideoxykanamycin B	NH_2	H	H	NH_2
(103)	3'-deoxykanamycin A	OH	H	OH	NH_2
(104)	3'-O-methylkanamycin A	OH	OCH_3	OH	NH_2
(105)	6'-N-methylkanamycin A	OH	OH	OH	$NHCH_3$
(106)	6'-N-methyl-3',4'-dideoxykanamycin B	NH_2	H	H	$NHCH_3$

Similar semisynthetic deoxy derivatives have been made from compounds of the 4,5-disubstituted deoxystreptamine class. In the case of ribostamycin (**30**), removal of the 3'- and 4'-hydroxyl groups gave a derivative (**107**) resistant to the action of APH(3')-II enzymes but not APH(3')-I enzymes which are able to phosphorylate the 5''-hydroxyl group of this compound. Taking this logic one step further, 3',4',5''-trideoxyribostamicin [*39535-84-7*] (**108**) was prepared but turned out to be a very weak antibiotic, as were 5''-deoxylividomycin A [*39039-99-1*] and 5''-amino-5''-deoxylividomycin A [*38907-28-7*]. 3'-Deoxyneomycin B [*51587-90-7*] has been prepared from lividomycin B (**22**) and, although exhibiting substantial potency against sensitive bacteria, the compound was predictably weak against bacteria possessing APH(3')-I enzymes (18,93).

2''-Deoxygentamicin C_2 [*51785-93-4*] (**109**) has been prepared and found, as expected, to show activity against bacteria producing the ANT(2'') enzyme. The compound however was otherwise less potent than its precursor antibiotic (111). 4''-Deoxygentamicin C_1 [*51587-74-7*] (**110**) was almost inactive (112). A relatively large number of gentamicin-like aminoglycosides have been prepared from garamine (**99**) by glycoside synthesis (113–117). The biology of these compounds however has not yet been published.

The most potentially useful semisynthetic aminoglycosides have resulted from work with 1-N-substituted derivatives. Butirosins A (**36**) and B (**37**) are naturally occurring compounds of this type. Butirosin B differs from ribostamicin (**30**) only in

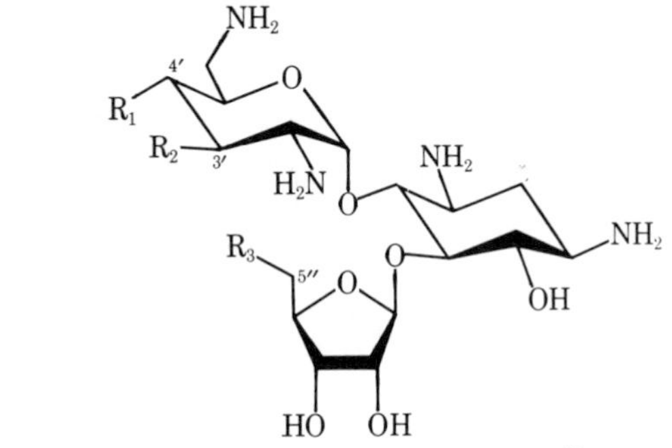

		R_1	R_2	R_3
(30)	ribostamycin	OH	OH	OH
(107)	3′,4′-dideoxyribostamycin	H	H	OH
(108)	3′,4′,5″-trideoxyribostamycin	H	H	H

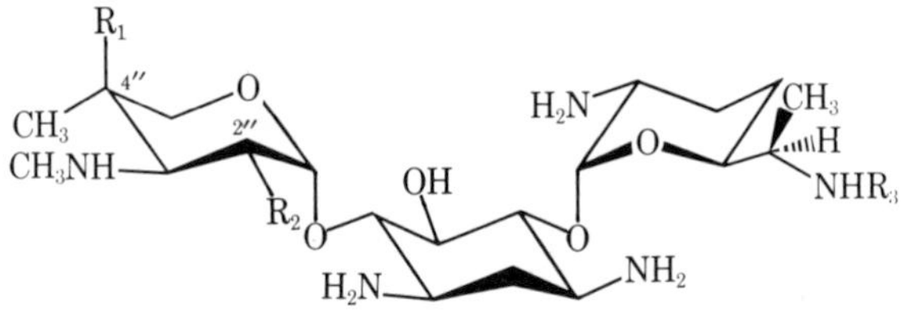

		R_1	R_2	R_3
(109)	2″-deoxygentamicin C$_2$	OH	H	H
(110)	4″-deoxygentamicin C$_1$	H	OH	CH$_3$

the presence of an (S)-α-hydroxy-γ-aminobutyric acid (HABA) substituent at 1-nitrogen. The presence of this HABA substituent confers activity on butirosin B against *P. aeruginosa*, as well as organisms containing enzymes of the APH(3′)-I type. This activity is not shown by ribostamicin. A large number of derivatives of the butirosins have been reported. 5″-Amino-5″-deoxybutirosin A [*49863-03-8*] (111) showed greater potency than the parent compound (118); however, in a fairly extensive study in which many different 1-*N*-substituents were exchanged for the HABA group of butirosin A, only the lower homologue, the (S)-α-hydroxy-β-aminopropionyl derivative, showed activity similar to the parent compound (119). The 3′,4′-dideoxy derivatives of butirosins A [*53318-76-6*] (112) and B [*42242-66-0*] (113) have been prepared and showed predictably improved activity against bacteria containing 3′-*O*-phosphorylating enzymes (18,120). The best compound of this type, however, appears to be 5″-amino-3′,4′,5″-trideoxybutirosin A [*56182-07-1*] (114), prepared independently by two groups, which has outstanding potency and spectrum of activity (121–122).

Kawaguchi and co-workers (123) made a substantial breakthrough when they prepared the 1*N*-HABA derivative of kanamycin A. This antibiotic, now named amikacin (101), not only showed predictably good activity against *Pseudomonas aeruginosa*, but also inhibited bacteria containing all 3′-*O*-phosphorylating, 3-*N*-acetylating and 2″-*O*-nucleotidylating enzymes. Amikacin is a substrate for only the relatively rare 6′-*N*-acetylating and 4′-*O*-nucleotidylating enzymes, and is consequently the broadest-spectrum aminoglycoside in use today (124). Since the synthesis of amikacin, 1*N*-hydroxyaminoacyl derivatives of many aminoglycosides have been made, including kanamycin B, 3′,4′-dideoxykanamycin B [*34493-98-6*], tobramycin, paromomycin I,

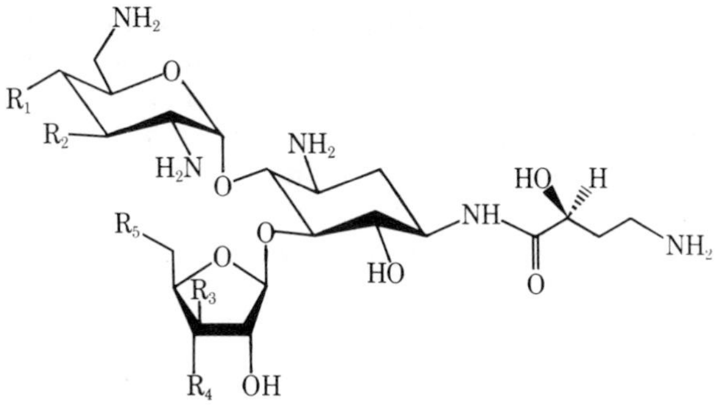

		R_1	R_2	R_3	R_4	R_5
(36)	butirosin A	OH	OH	OH	H	OH
(37)	butirosin B	OH	OH	H	OH	OH
(111)	5''-amino-5''-deoxybutirosin A	OH	OH	OH	H	NH$_2$
(112)	3',4'-dideoxybutirosin A	H	H	OH	H	OH
(113)	3',4'-dideoxybutirosin B	H	H	H	OH	OH
(114)	5''-amino-3',4',5'-trideoxybutirosin A	H	H	OH	H	NH$_2$

neamine, lividomycin A (18), gentamicin C_1 (125), gentamicin C_{1a}, sisomicin (126), 6'-N-alkylkanamycins (127) and 6'-N-methyl-3',4'-dideoxykanamycin B [40371-47-9] (128). All of these compounds show advantages over their 1-N-unsubstituted analogues in terms of the breadth of organisms they inhibit. In an investigation of alternative 1-N-substituents of kanamycin A, no derivative was found with better activity than amikacin; simple 1-N-acyl derivatives of kanamycin had relatively weak activity (129). In contrast, the 1-N-acetyl derivative of sisomicin [59712-05-9] (80) showed quite good activity (126).

A series of 1-N-alkyl and substituted alkyl derivatives of gentamicins (55–57) and sisomicin (80) have been reported by Wright and co-workers (130). These compounds exhibited activity against many organisms resistant to the parent antibiotics. One of these compounds, netilmicin (102), was selected for further study (131) and shown to possess a remarkably low toxic potential in laboratory animals, as well as good potency and spectrum of activity (132). The compound is undergoing clinical trials.

The total synthesis of a number of natural aminoglycosides has been achieved. Much of this work has been reviewed (18). More recently S. Umezawa reported the total synthesis of dihydrostreptomicin (133) and its 3''-deoxy derivative [26086-49-7]. The latter compound showed expectedly improved activity over the parent antibiotic (134).

Related Compounds

A number of antibiotics which are not strictly aminoglycoside–aminocyclitols are conveniently considered here because of some commonality in structure or biological properties with the latter compounds.

Spectinomycin [1695-77-8] (115), formerly called actinospectacin, is produced by *Streptomyces spectabilis*. Its unique fused ring structure was reported by its discoverers (135); details of the stereochemistry, however, were ascertained by x-ray crystallography (136). Dihydrospectinomycin [28048-39-7] (116) has also been isolated from the same microorganism (137). Unlike other aminocyclitol antibiotics, spectinomycin is bacteriostatic rather than bactericidal. It was recently released for clinical use for the treatment of gonorrhea. Bacterial resistance to spectinomycin has been shown in *E. coli* to be due to ribosomal mutation. Spectinomycin is also a substrate for streptomycin 3″-adenylyltransferase [AAD(3″)] and resistance may also be found due to this mechanism. The site of adenylylation is thought to be the 6-hydroxyl group of spectinomycin (94). A few chemically modified spectinomycins have been prepared but these lacked advantage over spectinomycin itself (138–139). Spectinomycin is manufactured by the Upjohn Company and marketed under the name Trobicin.

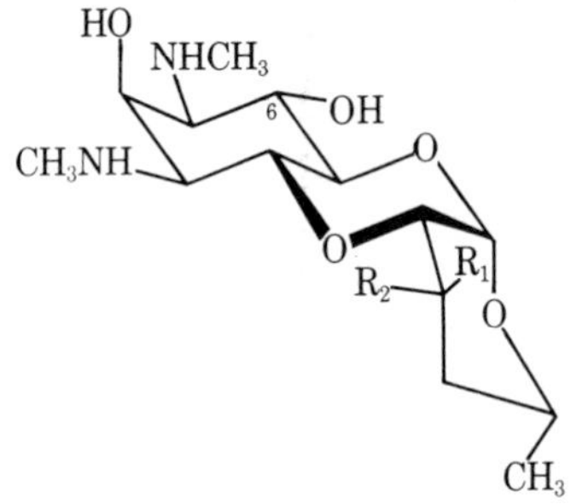

(115) spectinomycin hydrate R$_1$ = R$_2$ = OH
(116) dihydrospectinomycin R$_1$ = OH, R$_2$ = H

Kasugamycin [*6980-18-3*] (117), produced by *S. kasugaensis,* is bactericidal and includes *Pseudomonas* in its spectrum of organisms inhibited (140). Its importance, however, lies in its powerful action against *Pericularia oryzae*, the causative organism of rice blast disease. It is manufactured for this purpose by several Japanese companies. A number of semisynthetic kasugamycins have been prepared. One of these, BL-A2 [*26289-10-1*] (118), was found to be more active than its parent, especially against *Pseudomonas* (141–142). A related compound, minosaminomycin [*51746-09-9*] (119), has been isolated from *Streptomyces* No. MA514-A1 (143). Its structure was

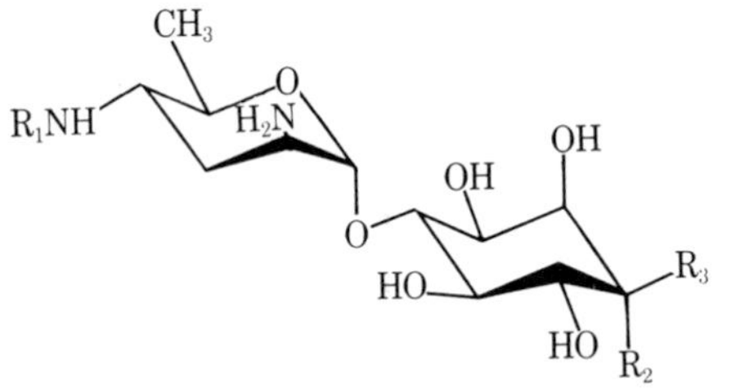

	R$_1$	R$_2$	R$_3$
(117) kasugamycin	—C—COOH, ‖ NH	OH	H
(118) BL-A2	—C—CH$_3$, ‖ NH	OH	H
(119) minosaminomycin	H	H	

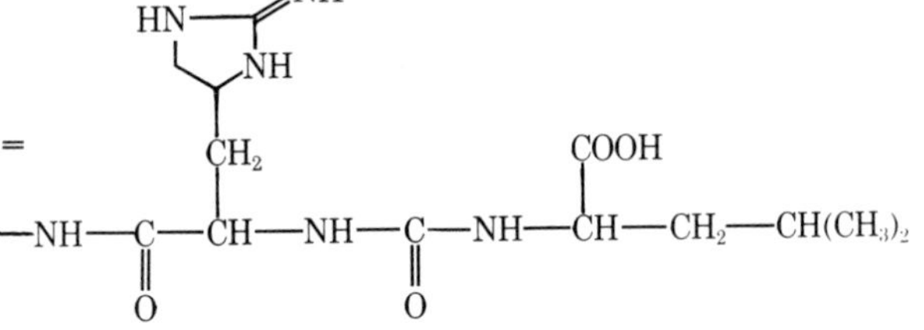

determined by Iinuma and co-workers (144). Minosaminomycin inhibits *Mycobacteria;* its mechanism of action has been discussed (145).

Investigation of the products of fermentation of *Streptomyces hygroscopicus* resulted in the isolation of a monoaminocyclitol antibiotic, hygromycin A [6379-56-2] (120). The structure of this compound was proposed in 1957 (146), although some points of stereochemistry have only recently been resolved (147). A more important antibiotic isolated from the same source was hygromycin B (121) which was shown to have excellent anthelmintic activity. This compound, manufactured by Eli Lilly & Co., is a veterinary product used principally against *Ascaris* in swine. Destomycin, manufactured by Meiji Seika Kaisha, Ltd., in Japan, is a related compound used for similar indications (see Chemotherapeutics, anthelmintic). The presently known members of the hygromycin–destomycin group of aminocyclitol antibiotics are listed in Table 9.

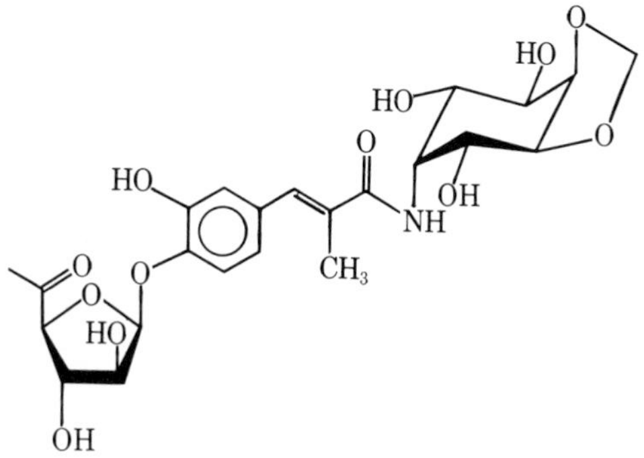

(120) hygromycin A

Validamycin A [37248-47-8] (129) and validamycin E [12650-71-4] (130) contain a novel unsaturated monoaminocyclitol called valienamine. They are produced by *Streptomyces hygroscopicus* var *limoneus* (153) and have been found effective against certain fungi pathogenic to plants. Validamycin is manufactured by Takeda Chemical Industries, Osaka, Japan. The structure of validamycin A was elucidated by Horii and Kameda (154).

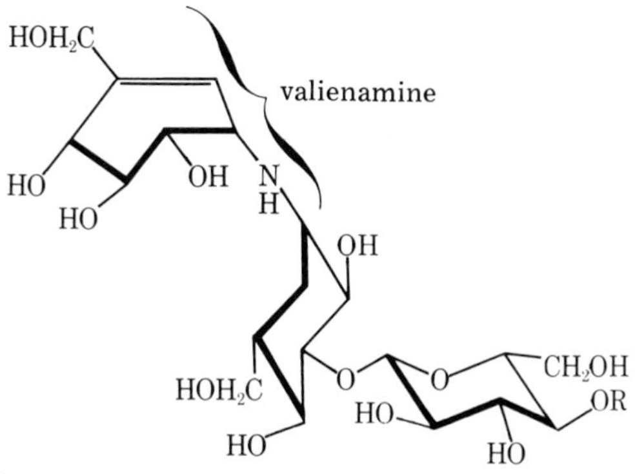

(129) validamycin A   R = H
(130) validamycin B   R = α-D-glucopyranosyl

Table 9. Compounds Related to Hygromicin B

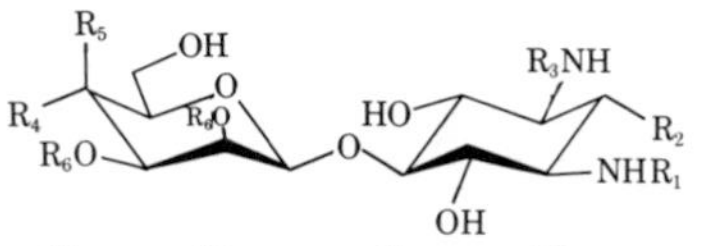

Structure	Name	CAS Registry Number	Producing organism	R_1	R_2	R_3	R_4	R_5	R_6	Reference
(121)	hygromycin B	[31282-04-9]	S. hygroscopicus	H	H	CH₃	H	OH	DAOE[a]	148
(122)	destomycin A	[14918-35-5]	S. rimofaciens	CH₃	H	H	H	OH	DAOE[a]	149
(123)	destomycin B	[11005-98-4]	S. rimofaciens	CH₃	H	CH₃	OH	H	EDOE[b]	149
(124)	destomycin C	[55651-94-0]	S. rimofaciens	CH₃	H	CH₃	H	OH	DAOE[a]	150
(125)	A-396-I (SS-56D)	[31357-30-9]	Streptoverticillium eurocidicus	H	H	H	H	OH	DAOE[a]	151
(126)	SS-56A	[39471-53-9]	S. eurocidicus	H	H	H	OH	H	H	152
(127)	SS-56B	[39471-54-0]	S. eurocidicus	H	H	H	H	OH	H	152
(128)	SS-56C	[39471-55-1]	S. eurocidicus	H	OH	H	H	OH	DAOE[a]	152

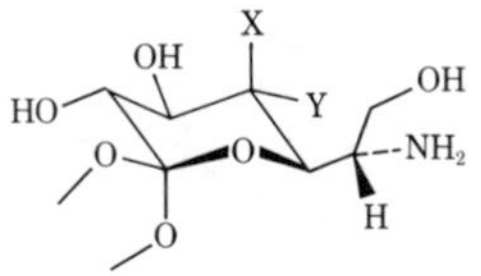

[a] DAOE = destomic acid ortho ester, X = OH; Y = H.
[b] EDOE = 4-epidestomic acid ortho ester, X = H; Y = OH.

Two novel aminoglycoside–aminocyclitols, fortimicin A [55779-06-1] (131) and fortimicin B [54783-95-8] (132) produced by *Micromonospora olivoasterospora,* were announced by Nara and co-workers (155). Their structures were demonstrated by Egan and co-workers (156) who showed that the compounds contained a unique 1,4-diaminocyclitol unit. Fortimicin A is an *N*-glycyl derivative of fortimycin B. The presence of the acyl substituent causes the conformational inversion shown in the formulas.

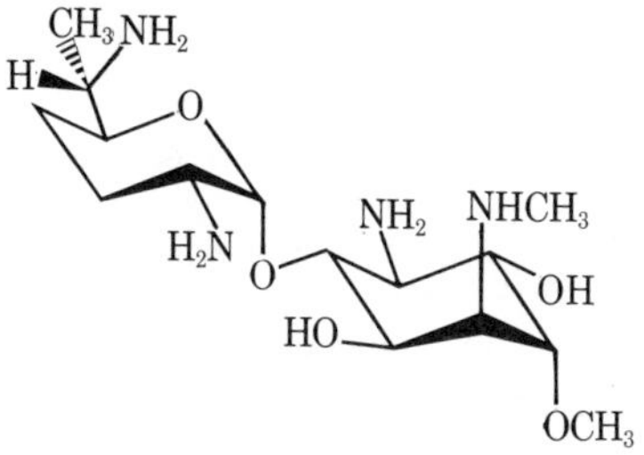

(131) fortimicin A 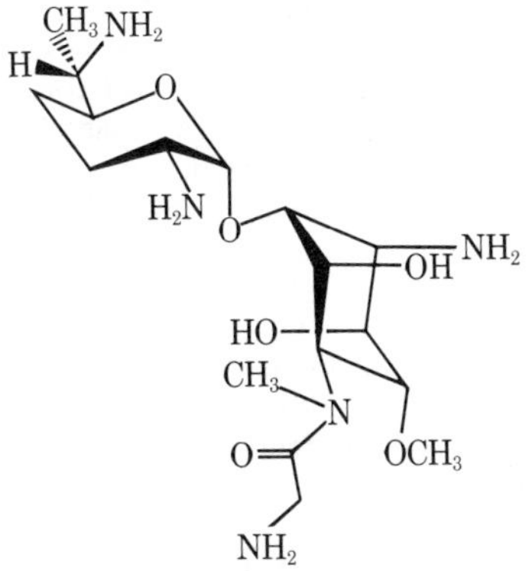   (132) fortimicin B

BIBLIOGRAPHY

"Streptomycin Antibiotics (Survey; Streptomycin; Neomycin)" in *ECT* 1st ed., Vol. 13, pp. 57–81 and 90–94, by S. A. Waksman and H. A. Lechevalier, Institute for Microbiology, Rutgers University; "Streptomycin and Related Antibiotics" in ECT 2nd ed., Vol. 19, pp. 33–48, by D. Perlman, University of Wisconsin.

1. K. L. Rinehart, Jr., *J. Infect. Dis.* 119, 345 (1969).
2. S. A. Waksman, *Science* 118, 259 (1953).
3. S. L. Rosenthal, *N. Y. State J. Med.* 75, 535 (1975).
4. G. H. Wagman and M. J. Weinstein, *Chromatography of Antibiotics,* American Elsevier Publishing Co., Inc., New York, 1973.
5. D. C. DeJongh, E. B. Hills, J. D. Hribar, S. Hanessian, and T. Chang, *Tetrahedron* 29, 2707 (1973).
6. S. Inouye, *Chem. Pharm. Bull.* 20, 2331 (1972).
7. P. J. L. Daniels, A. K. Mallams, J. Weinstein, and J. J. Wright, *J. Chem. Soc. Perkin Trans. 1* 1078 (1976).
8. H. Naganawa, S. Kondo, K. Maeda, and H. Umezawa, *J. Antibiot.* 24, 823 (1971).
9. J. B. Morton, R. C. Long, P. J. L. Daniels, R. W. Tkach, and J. H. Goldstein, *J. Am. Chem. Soc.* 95, 7464 (1973).
10. S. Omoto, S. Inouye, M. Kojima, and T. Niida, *J. Antibiot.* 26, 717 (1973).
11. P. K. Woo and R. D. Westland, *Carbohydr. Res.* 31, 27 (1973).
12. K. F. Koch, J. A. Rhoades, E. W. Hagaman, and E. Wenkert, *J. Am. Chem. Soc.* 96, 3300 (1974).
13. K. Tsuji and J. H. Robertson, *Anal. Chem.* 42, 1661 (1970).
14. S. Omoto, S. Inouye, and T. Niida, *J. Antibiot.* 24, 430 (1971).
15. D. L. Mays, R. J. Van Apeldoorn, and R. G. Lauback, *J. Chromatogr.* 120, 93 (1976).
16. J. Anhalt, *Antimicrob. Agents Chemother.* 11, 651 (1977).
17. K. L. Rinehart, Jr., *The Neomycins and Related Antibiotics,* John Wiley & Sons, Inc., New York, 1961.
18. S. Umezawa in R. S. Tipson and D. Horton, eds., *Advances in Carbohydrate Chemistry and Biochemistry,* Vol. 30, Academic Press, Inc., New York, 1974, p. 111.

19. K. E. Price, J. C. Godfrey, and H. Kawaguchi in D. Perlman, ed., *Advances in Applied Microbiology,* Vol. 18, Academic Press, Inc., New York, 1974, p. 191.
20. S. Umezawa in S. Mitsuhashi, ed., *Drug Action and Drug Resistance in Bacteria,* Vol. 2, University Park Press, Baltimore, Md., 1975, p. 3.
21. S. Neidle, D. Rogers, and M. B. Hursthouse, *Tetrahedron Lett.* 4725 (1968).
22. F. Kavanaugh, E. Grinnan, E. Allanson, and D. Tunin, *Appl. Microbiol.* **8,** 160 (1960).
23. J. Fried and H. E. Stavely, *J. Am. Chem. Soc.* **74,** 5461 (1952).
24. F. H. Stodola, O. L. Shotwell, A. M. Borud, R. G. Benedict, and A. C. Riley, Jr., *J. Am. Chem. Soc.* **73,** 2290 (1951).
25. H. Heding, *Acta Chem. Scand.* **23,** 1275 (1969).
26. F. Arcamone, G. Cassinelli, G. d'Amico, and P. Orezzi, *Experientia* **24,** 441 (1968).
27. B. Bannister and A. D. Argoudelis, *J. Am. Chem. Soc.* **85,** 234 (1963).
28. T. Miyaki, H. Tsukiura, M. Wakae, and H. Kawaguchi, *J. Antibiot. Ser. A.* **15,** 15 (1962).
29. K. Nagaoka and A. L. Demain, *J. Antibiot.* **28,** 627 (1975).
30. U.S. Pat. 3,956,275 (May 11, 1976), A. L. Demain and K. Nagaoka (to Massachusetts Institute of Technology).
31. W. S. Chilton, *Diss. Abstr.* **24,** 4990 (1964).
32. W. T. Shier, K. L. Rinehart, Jr., and D. Gottlieb, *Proc. Nat. Acad. Sci. U.S.A.* **63,** 198 (1969).
33. T. H. Haskell, J. C. French, and Q. R. Bartz, *J. Am. Chem. Soc.* **81,** 3481 (1959).
34. K. L. Rinehart, Jr., M. Hichens, A. D. Argoudelis, W. S. Chilton, H. E. Carter, M. Georgiadis, C. P. Schaffner, and R. T. Schillings, *J. Am. Chem. Soc.* **84,** 3218 (1962).
35. T. Mori, T. Ichiyanagi, H. Kondo, K. Takunaga, T. Oda, and K. Munakata, *J. Antibiot. Ser. A* **24,** 339 (1971).
36. T. Mori, Y. Kyotani, I. Watanabe, and T. Oda, *J. Antibiot.* **25,** 149 (1972).
37. Ref. 36, p. 317.
38. W. T. Shier, P. C. Schaefer, D. Gottlieb, and K. L. Rinehart, Jr., *Biochemistry* **13,** 5073 (1974).
39. J. Cleophax, S. D. Gero, J. Leboul, M. Akhtar, J. E. G. Barnett, and C. J. Pearce, *J. Am. Chem. Soc.* **98,** 7110 (1976).
40. E. Akita, T. Tsuruoka, N. Ezaki, and T. Niida, *J. Antibiot.* **23,** 173 (1970).
41. M. Kojima and A. Satoh, *J. Antibiot.* **26,** 784 (1973).
42. S. Horii, I. Nogami, N. Mizokami, Y. Arai, and M. Yoneda, *Antimicrob. Agents Chemother.* **5,** 578 (1974); T. H. Haskell, R. Rodebaugh, N. Plessas, D. Watson, and R. D. Westland, *Carbohydr. Res.* **28,** 263 (1973); H. Tsukiura, K. Fujisawa, M. Konishi, K. Saito, K. Numata, H. Ishikawa, T. Miyaki, K. Tomita, and H. Kawaguchi, *J. Antibiot.* **26,** 351 (1973).
43. P. W. K. Woo, H. W. Dion, and Q. R. Bartz, *Tetrahedron Lett.* **1971,** 2625.
44. H. D. Taylor and H. Schmitz, *J. Antibiot.* **29,** 532 (1976).
45. H. Kawaguchi, K. Tomita, T. Hoshiya, T. Miyaki, K. Fujisawa, M. Kimeada, K. Numata, M. Konishi, H. Tsukiura, M. Hatori, and H. Koshiyama, *J. Antibiot.* **27,** 460 (1974).
46. M. Konishi, K. Numata, S. Shimoda, H. Tsukiura, and H. Kawaguchi, *J. Antibiot.* **27,** 471 (1974).
47. H. Tsukiura, K. Saito, S. Kobaru, M. Konishi, and H. Kawaguchi, *J. Antibiot.* **26,** 386 (1973).
48. J. P. Kirby, D. B. Borders, and G. E. Van Lear, Abstracts, *168th National Meeting of the American Chemical Society, Atlantic City, N.J., Sept. 1974, MICR 23.*
49. U.S. Pat. 3,928, 317 (Dec. 23, 1975), J. P. Kirby, D. B. Borders, and J. H. Korshalla (to American Cyanamid Company).
50. M. Murase, T. Ito, S. Fukatsu, and H. Umezawa, "Progress in Antimicrobial and Cancer Chemotherapy," *Proceedings of the 6th International Congress on Chemotherapy,* Vol. II, University Park Press, Baltimore, Md., 1970, p. 1098.
51. K. F. Koch, F. A. Davis, and J. A. Rhoades, *J. Antibiot.* **26,** 745 (1973).
52. K. F. Koch and J. A. Rhoades, *Antimicrob. Agents Chemother.* **1970,** 309 (1971).
53. P. J. L. Daniels in Ref. 20, p. 77.
54. D. Rosi, W. A. Goss, and S. J. Daum, *J. Antibiot.* **30,** 88 (1977).
55. S. J. Daum, D. Rosi, and W. A. Goss, *J. Antibiot.* **30,** 98 (1977).
56. U.S. Pat. 3,984,395 (Oct. 5, 1976), P. J. L. Daniels and J. A. Marquez (to Schering Corporation).
57. R. S. Egan, R. L. De Vault, S. L. Mueller, M. I. Levenberg, A. C. Sinclair, and R. S. Stanaszek, *J. Antibiot.* **28,** 29 (1975).
58. P. J. L. Daniels, C. Luce, T. L. Nagabhushan, R. S. Jaret, D. Schumacher, H. Reimann, and J. Ilavsky, *J. Antibiot.* **28,** 35 (1975).
59. J. Weinstein, D. J. Cooper, and P. J. L. Daniels, Abstract 9 *12th Interscience Conference on Antimicrobial Agents and Chemotherapy, Atlantic City, N. J., Oct. 1972.*

60. P. J. L. Daniels, A. S. Yehaskel, and J. B. Morton, Abstract 137 *13th Interscience Conference on Antimicrobial Agents and Chemotherapy, Washington, D.C., Sept. 1973.*
61. U.S. Pat. 3,903,072 (Sept. 2, 1975), J. Ilavsky, A. P. Bayan, W. Charney, and H. Reimann (to Schering Corporation).
62. H. Maehr and C. P. Schaffner, *J. Am. Chem. Soc.* **92**, 1697 (1970).
63. T. L. Nagabhushan, W. N. Turner, P. J. L. Daniels, and J. B. Morton, *J. Org. Chem.* **40**, 2830 (1975).
64. T. L. Nagabhushan, P. J. L. Daniels, R. S. Jaret, and J. B. Morton, *J. Org. Chem.,* **40**, 2835 (1975).
65. S. Sato, S. Takasawa, M. Yamamoto, R. Okachi, I. Kawamoto, T. Iida, A. Morikawa, and T. Nara, *J. Antibiot.* **30**, 25 (1977).
66. R. S. Egan, A. C. Sinclair, R. L. DeVault, J. B. McAlpine, S. L. Mueller, P. C. Goodley, R. S. Stanaszek, M. Cirovic, and R. J. Mauritz, *J. Antibiot.* **30**, 31 (1977).
67. J. B. McAlpine, A. C. Sinclair, R. S. Egan, R. L. DeVault, R. S. Stanaszek, M. Cirovic, S. L. Mueller, P. C. Goodley, R. J. Mauritz, and N. E. Wideburg *J. Antibiot.* **30**, 39 (1977).
68. R. T. Testa, G. H. Wagman, P. J. L. Daniels, and M. J. Weinstein, *J. Antibiot.* **27**, 917 (1974).
69. H. Reimann, D. J. Cooper, A. K. Mallams, R. S. Jaret, A. Yehaskel, M. Kugelman, H. F. Vernay, and D. Schumacher, *J. Org. Chem.* **39**, 1451 (1974).
70. M. J. Weinstein, G. H. Wagman, J. A. Marquez, R. T. Testa, and J. A. Waitz, *Antimicrob. Agents Chemother.* **7**, 246 (1975).
71. P. J. L. Daniels and A. S. Yehaskel in Ref. 60, Paper 135.
72. J. A. Marquez, G. H. Wagman, R. T. Testa, J. A. Waitz, and M. J. Weinstein, *J. Antibiot.* **29**, 483 (1976).
73. P. J. L. Daniels, R. S. Jaret, T. L. Nagabhushan, and W. N. Turner, *J. Antibiot.* **29**, 488 (1976).
74. D. H. Davies, D. Greeves, A. K. Mallams, J. B. Morton, and R. T. Tkach, *J. Chem. Soc. Perkin Trans. 1* 814 (1975).
75. S. O'Connor, L. K. T. Lam, N. D. Jones, and M. O. Chaney, *J. Org. Chem.* **41**, 2087 (1976).
76. D. E. Dorman, J. W. Paschal, and K. E. Merkel, *J. Am. Chem. Soc.* **98**, 6885 (1976).
77. T. Oda, T. Mori, and Y. Kyotani, *J. Antibiot.* **24**, 503 (1971).
78. R. U. Lemieux and M. L. Wolfrom, *Advances in Carbohydrate·Chemistry,* Vol. 3, Academic Press, Inc., New York, 1948, p. 337.
79. K. L. Rinehart, Jr., and R. M. Strochane, *J. Antibiot.* **29**, 319 (1976).
80. J. B. Walker, *Lloydia* **34**, 363 (1971).
81. K. L. Rinehart, Jr., J. M. Malik, R. S. Nystrom, R. M. Strochane, S. T. Truit, M. Taniguchi, J. P. Rolls, W. J. Haak, and B. A. Ruff, *J. Am. Chem. Soc.* **96**, 2263 (1974).
82. M. H. G. Munro, M. Taniguchi, K. L. Rinehart, Jr., D. Gottieb, T. H. Stoudt, and T. O. Rogers, *J. Am. Chem. Soc.* **97**, 4782 (1975).
83. M. Silverman and S. V. Rieder *J. Biol. Chem.* **235**, 1251 (1960).
84. J. Bruton, W. H. Horner, and G. A. Russ, *J. Biol. Chem.* **242**, 813 (1967).
85. R. Ortmann, U. Matern, H. Grisebach, P. Stadler, V. Sinnwell, and H. Paulsen, *Eur. J. Biochem.* **43**, 265 (1974); B. Kniep and H. Grisebach, *FEBS Lett.* **65**, 44 (1976).
86. W. T. Shier, S. Ogawa, M. Hichens, and K. L. Rinehart, Jr., *J. Antibiot.* **26**, 551 (1973).
87. A. Kucers and N. Mck. Bennett, *The Use of Antibiotics,* J. B. Lippincott Company, Philadelphia, Pa., 1975.
88. L. P. Garrod, H. P. Lambert, and F. O'Grady, *Antibiotic and Chemotherapy,* 4th ed., Churchill Livingstone, Edinburgh, Eng., 1973.
89. G. Miller, private communication, Schering Laboratories.
90. W. L. Hewitt, *Postgrad. Med. J. Suppl.* **50** (7), 55 (1974).
91. C. R. Smith, K. L. Baughman, C. Q. Edwards, J. F. Rogers, and P. S. Lietman, *N. Eng. J. Med.* **296**, 349 (1977).
92. G. H. Miller, G. Arcieri, M. J. Weinstein, and J. A. Waitz, *Antimicrob. Agents Chemother.* **10**, 827 (1976).
93. H. Umezawa in R. S. Tipson and D. Horton, eds., *Advances in Carbohydrate Chemistry and Biochemistry,* Vol. 30, Academic Press, Inc., New York, 1974, p. 183.
94. R. Benveniste and J. Davies, *Ann. Rev. Biochem.* **42**, 471 (1973).
95. L. E. Bryan, H. M. Van Den Elzen, and M. S. Shahrabadi in S. Mitsuhashi and H. Hashimoto, eds., *Microbial Drug Resistance,* University Park Press, Baltimore, Md., 1975, p. 475.
96. L. E. Bryan and H. M. Van Den Elzen, *Antimicrob. Agents Chemother.* **9**, 928 (1976).
97. H. Umezawa, M. Okanishi, R. Utahara, K. Maeda, and S. Kondo, *J. Antibiot.* **20**, 136 (1976).

98. H. Kawabe, S. Kondo, H. Umezawa, and S. Mitsuhashi, *Antimicrob. Agents Chemother.* **7,** 494 (1975).
99. M. Haas, S. Biddlecome, J. Davies, C. E. Luce, and P. J. L. Daniels, *Antimicrob. Agents Chemother.* **9,** 945 (1976).
100. Y. Umezawa, M. Yagisawa, T. Sawa, T. Takeuchi, H. Umezawa, H. Matsumoto, and T. Tazaki, *J. Antibiot.* **28,** 845 (1975).
101. S. Mitsuhashi in S. Mitsuhashi, L. Rosival and V. Krčméry, eds., *Drug-Inactivating Enzymes and Antibiotic Resistance,* Springer-Verlag, Berlin, 1975, p. 115.
102. M. Kida, T. Asako, M. Yoneda, and S. Mitsuhashi in Ref. 95, p. 441.
103. M. Kida, S. Igarasi, T. Okutani, T. Asako, K. Hiraga and S. Mitsuhashi, *Antimicrob. Agents Chemother.* **5,** 92 (1974).
104. T. L. Nagabhushan, A. B. Cooper, P. J. L. Daniels, J. Davies, and B. Hoffman, Abstr. 21, *17th Interscience Conference on Antimicrobial Agents and Chemotherapy, New York, Oct. 1977.*
105. I. Suzuki, N. Takahashi, S. Shirato, H. Kawabe, and S. Mitsuhashi in Ref. 95, p. 463.
106. F. LeGoffic, A. Martel, M. L. Capmau, B. Baca, P. Goebel, H. Chardon, C. J. Soussy, J. Duval, and D. H. Bouanchaud, *Antimicrob. Agents Chemother.* **10,** 258 (1976).
107. S. Biddlecome, M. Haas, J. Davies, G. H. Miller, D. F. Rane, and P. J. L. Daniels, *Antimicrob. Agents Chemother.* **9,** 951 (1976).
108. M. Chevereau, P. J. L. Daniels, J. Davies, and F. LeGoffic, *Biochemistry* **13,** 598 (1974).
109. J. E. Davies and R. E. Benveniste, *Ann. N.Y. Acad. Sci.* **235,** 130 (1974).
110. T. Okutani, T. Asako, K. Yoshioka, K. Hiraga, and M. Kida, *J. Am. Chem. Soc.* **99,** 1278 (1977).
111. P. J. L. Daniels, J. Weinstein, R. W. Tkach, and J. Morton, *J. Antibiot.* **27,** 150 (1974).
112. A. K. Mallams, H. F. Vernay, D. F. Crowe, G. Detre, M. Tanabe, and D. M. Yasuda, *J. Antibiot.* **26,** 782 (1973).
113. M. Kugelman, A. K. Mallams, H. F. Vernay, D. F. Crowe, and M. Tanabe, *J. Chem. Soc. Perkin Trans. 1* 1088 (1976).
114. M. Kugelman, A. K. Mallams, H. F. Vernay, D. F. Crowe, G. Detre, M. Tanabe, and D. M. Yasuda, *J. Chem. Soc. Perkin Trans. 1* 1097 (1976).
115. M. Kugelman, A. K. Mallams, and H. F. Vernay *J. Chem. Soc. Perkin Trans. 1* 1113 (1976).
116. M. Kugelman, A. K. Mallams, and N. F. Vernay, *J. Chem. Soc. Perkin Trans. 1* 1126 (1976).
117. A. K. Mallams, S. Saluja, D. F. Crowe, G. Detre, M. Tanabe, and D. M. Yasuda, *J. Chem. Soc. Perkin Trans. 1* 1135 (1976).
118. T. P. Culbertson, D. R. Watson, and T. H. Haskell, *J. Antibiot.* **26,** 790 (1973).
119. T. H. Haskell, R. Rodebaugh, N. Plessas, D. Watson, and R. D. Westland, *Carbohydr. Res.* **28,** 263 (1973).
120. H. Saeki, Y. Shimada, Y. Ohashi, M. Tajima, S. Sugawara, and E. Ohki, *Chem. Pharm. Bull.* **22,** 1145 (1974).
121. P. W. K. Woo, *J. Antibiot.* **28,** 522 (1975).
122. H. Saeki, Y. Shimada, E. Ohki, and S. Sugawara, *J. Antibiot.* **28,** 530 (1975).
123. H. Kawaguchi, T. Naito, S. Nakagawa, and K. Fujisawa, *J. Antibiot.* **25,** 695 (1972).
124. *J. Infect. Dis.* **134**(S), 242 (1976).
125. P. J. L. Daniels, J. Weinstein, and T. L. Nagabhushan, *J. Antibiot.* **27,** 889 (1974).
126. J. J. Wright, A. Cooper, P. J. L. Daniels, T. L. Nagabhushan, D. Rane, W. N. Turner, and J. Weinstein, *J. Antibiot.* **29,** 714 (1976).
127. H. Umezawa, K. Iinuma, S. Kondo, and K. Maeda, *J. Antibiot.* **28,** 483 (1975).
128. H. Umezawa, K. Iinuma, S. Kondo, M. Hamada, and K. Maeda, *J. Antibiot.* **28,** 340 (1975).
129. T. Naito, S. Nakagawa, Y. Narita, S. Toda, Y. Abe, M. Oka, H. Yamashita, T. Yamasaki, K. Fujisawa, and H. Kawaguchi, *J. Antibiot.* **27,** 815 (1974).
130. J. J. Wright, Abstract 91, *15th Interscience Conference on Antimicrobial Agents and Chemotherapy, Washington, D.C., Sept. 1975.*
131. J. J. Wright, *J. Chem. Soc. Chem. Commun.* 206 (1976).
132. G. H. Miller, G. Arcieri, M. J. Weinstein, and J. A. Waitz, *Antimicrob. Agents Chemother.* **10,** 827 (1976).
133. S. Umezawa, T. Yamasaki, Y. Kubota, and T. Tsuchiya, *Bull. Chem. Soc. Jpn.* **48,** 563 (1975).
134. H. Sano, T. Tsuchiya, S. Kobayashi, M. Hamada, S. Umezawa, and H. Umezawa, *J. Antibiot.* **29,** 978 (1976).
135. P. F. Wiley, A. D. Argoudelis, and H. Hoeksema, *J. Am. Chem. Soc.* **85,** 2652 (1963).
136. T. G. Cochran, D. J. Abraham, and L. L. Martin, *J. Chem. Soc. Chem. Commun.* 494 (1972).
137. H. Hoeksema and J. C. Knight, *J. Antibiot.* **28,** 240 (1975).

138. W. Rosenbrook, Jr., and R. E. Carney, *J. Antibiot.* **28,** 953 (1975).
139. W. Rosenbrook, Jr., R. E. Carney, R. S. Egan, R. S. Stanaszek, M. Cirovic, T. Nishinaga, K. Mochida, and Y. Mori, *J. Antibiot.* **28,** 960 (1975).
140. Y. Suhara, K. Maeda, H. Umezawa, and M. Ohno, *Tetrahedron Letts.* 1239 (1966).
141. M. J. Cron, R. E. Smith, I. R. Hooper, J. G. Keil, E. A. Ragan, R. H. Schreiber, G. Schwab, and J. C. Godfrey, *Antimicrob. Agents Chemother.* **1969,** 219 (1970).
142. M. Misiek, D. R. Chisholm, F. Leitner and K. E. Price in Ref. 141, p. 225.
143. M. Hamada, S. Kondo, T. Yokoyama, K. Miura, K. Iinuma, H. Yamamoto, K. Maeda, T. Takeuchi, and H. Umezawa, *J. Antibiot.* **27,** 81 (1974).
144. K. Iinuma, S. Kondo, K. Maeda, and H. Umezawa, *J. Antibiot.* **28,** 613 (1975).
145. K. Suzukake, M. Hori, Y. Uehara, K. Inuma, M. Hamada, and H. Umezawa, *J. Antibiot.* **30,** 132 (1977).
146. R. L. Mann and D. O. Woolf, *J. Am. Chem. Soc.* **79,** 120 (1957).
147. K. Kakinuma, S. Kitahara, K. Watanabe, Y. Sakagami, T. Fukuyasu, M. Shimura, M. Ueda, and Y. Sekizawa, *J. Antibiot.* **29,** 771 (1975).
148. R. L. Mann and W. W. Bromer, *J. Am. Chem. Soc.* **80,** 2714 (1958).
149. ·S. Kondo, K. Iinuma, H. Naganawa, M. Shimura, and Y. Sekizawa, *J. Antibiot.* **28,** 79 (1975).
150. M. Shimura, Y. Sekizawa, K. Iinuma, H. Naganawa, and S. Kondo, *J. Antibiot.* **28,** 83 (1975).
151. J. Shoji and Y. Nakagawa, *J. Antibiot.* **23,** 569 (1970).
152. S. Inouye, T. Shomura, H. Watanabe, K. Totsugawa, and T. Niida, *J. Antibiot.* **26,** 374 (1973).
153. T. Iwasa, H. Yamamoto, and M. Shibata, *J. Antibiot.* **23,** 595 (1970).
154. S. Horii and Y. Kameda, *J. Chem. Soc. Chem. Commun.* 747 (1972).
155. T. Nara, R. Okachi, M. Yamamoto, I. Kawamoto, K. Takayama, S. Takasawa, T. Sato, and S. Sato, Abstract 56, *16th Interscience Conference on Antimicrobial Agents and Chemotherapy, Chicago, Ill., Oct. 1976.*
156. R. S. Egan, J. R. Martin, J. Tadanier, R. S. Stanaszek, S. L. Mueller, P. Collum, A. W. Goldstein, R. L. Devault, A. C. Sinclair, E. E. Fager, and L. A. Mitshcer in Ref. 155, Abstract 58.

PETER J. L. DANIELS
Schering-Plough Corporation

ANSAMACROLIDES

The ansamycins are a family of antibiotics characterized by an aliphatic *ansa*-bridge which connects two nonadjacent positions of an aromatic nucleus. The name was originally suggested by Prelog (1) and is based on the term ansa compounds coined by Lüttringhaus (2). The ansamacrolides can be divided into two groups based on the aromatic nucleus present. One group contains a naphthoquinone and the other a benzoquinone nucleus. The naphthoquinoid ansamycins comprise the majority of the known ansamacrolides and include the streptovaricins, rifamycins, tolypomycins, halomicins, and naphthomycin. The benzoquinoid ansamacrolides include geldanamycin and the maytansinoids. Table 1 lists the naturally occurring ansamycins along with some of their physical properties and Table 2 lists the biological activities of the ansamacrolides.

Table 1. Properties of the Ansamacrolides

Ansamacrolide	CAS Registry No.	Producing organism	Molecular formula	Melting point, °C	$[\alpha]_D$[a]	uv max, nm (log ε)[b]	Refs.
Naphthoquinoid							
streptovaricin A	[23344-16-3]	*Streptomyces spectabilis*	$C_{42}H_{53}NO_{16}$	233–243	+610	245 (4.58), 262 (sh, 4.47), 320 (4.08), 430 (4.06)	3
streptovaricin B	[11031-82-6]	*Streptomyces spectabilis*	$C_{42}H_{53}NO_{15}$	187–189	+576	245 (4.54), 262 (sh, 4.46), 320 (4.05), 430 (4.03)	3
streptovaricin C	[23344-17-4]	*Streptomyces spectabilis*	$C_{40}H_{51}NO_{14}$	189–191	+602	245 (4.57), 262 (sh, 4.49), 320 (4.11), 430 (4.05)	3
streptovaricin D	[32164-26-4]	*Streptomyces spectabilis*	$C_{40}H_{51}NO_{13}$	172–175	+590.3	246 (4.43), 265 (sh, 4.39), 320 (3.99), 430 (3.73)	3
streptovaricin E	[35413-63-9]	*Streptomyces spectabilis*	$C_{40}H_{49}NO_{14}$	198–202	+412.3	246 (4.44), 272 (4.39), 320 (4.10), 430 (3.83)	3
streptovaricin F	[35512-37-9]	*Streptomyces spectabilis*	$C_{39}H_{47}NO_{14}$	222–224	+488[c]		3
streptovaricin G	[11031-85-9]	*Streptomyces spectabilis*	$C_{40}H_{51}NO_{15}$	190–192	+473	245 (4.55), 267 (4.43), 320 (4.08), 430 (3.96)	3
streptovaricin J	[52275-61-3]	*Streptomyces spectabilis*	$C_{42}H_{53}NO_{15}$	177–180	+436	245 (4.49), 260 (sh, 4.42), 310 (sh, 4.05), 428 (3.99)	3
streptovaricin K	[23344-16-3]	*Streptomyces spectabilis*	$C_{42}H_{53}NO_{16}$	162–165	−11[d]	223 (555)[e], 304 (275)[e], 425 (220)[e,f]	4
rifamycin B	[13929-35-6]	*Nocardia mediterranei* n. sp.	$C_{39}H_{49}NO_{14}$	160–164 dec	+71.5[g]	226 (365)[e], 273 (440)[e], 370 (60)[e,h]	5–6
rifamycin O	[14487-05-9]	*Streptomyces tolypophorus* No. 4107 A₂	$C_{39}H_{47}NO_{14}$	160 dec	+462	277 (4.46), 330 (3.97), 390 (3.74)	5–7
rifamycin S	[13553-79-2]	*Nocardia mediterranei* n. sp.	$C_{37}H_{45}NO_{12}$	146–147	−4[d]	223 (586)[e], 314 (322)[e], 445 (204)[e,f]	5–8
rifamycin SV	[6998-60-3]	*Nocardia mediterranei* mutant ATCC 21271	$C_{37}H_{47}NO_{12}$	140 dec	+325[d]		5–9
rifamycin Y	[15271-73-5]	*Nocardia mediterranei*	$C_{39}H_{47}NO_{15}$			298 (4.30), 412 (4.24)[i]	10
rifamycin L	[26117-02-2]	*Nocardia mediterranei*	$C_{39}H_{49}NO_{14}$				11
rifamycin W	[53904-81-7]	*Nocardia mediterranei* mutant 126	$C_{35}H_{45}NO_{11}$	152–153 dec		239 (4.56), 255 (sh), 285 (sh), 350 (4.09), 540 (3.73)[j]	12–13
tolypomycin Y	[23412-26-2]	*Streptomyces tolypophorus*	$C_{43}H_{54}N_2O_{14}$	120	+326[c]	232 (4.46), 290 (4.38), 337 (4.10), 370–430 (sh)	6
halomicin B	[54356-09-1]	*Micromonospora halophytica*	$C_{43}H_{58}N_2O_{12}$	178–182	+73.1[d]	238 (4.62), 298 (4.15), 415 (4.31)[d]	14–15
naphthomycin	[55557-40-9]	*Streptomyces collinus* Lindenbein (Tü 105)	$C_{40}H_{46}ClNO_9$	ca 200	+432	235, 281, 360 (sh)	16
Benzoquinoid							
geldanamycin	[30562-34-6]	*Streptomyces hygroscopicus* var. *geldanus* var. *nova* (UC-5208)	$C_{29}H_{40}N_2O_9$	252–255	+55	255 (4.21), 304 (4.29), 400 (2.99)[d]	17

Name	CAS No.	Formula	mp (°C)	[α]	UV absorption	Ref.
maytansine	[35486-53-8]	$C_{34}H_{46}ClN_3O_{10}$	171–172	−145	233 (4.47), 243 (sh, 4.43), 254 (4.43), 282 (3.76), 290 (3.74)	18
maytanprine	[38997-09-0]	$C_{35}H_{48}ClN_3O_{10}$	169–170	−125		19
maytanbutine	[38997-10-3]	$C_{36}H_{50}ClN_3O_{10}$	170–171	−122		19
maytanvaline	[52978-27-5]	$C_{37}H_{52}ClN_3O_{10}$	175–176.5	−135	233 (4.46), 243 (sh, 4.42), 254 (4.43), 281 (3.72), 288 (3.73)	20
maysine	[52978-28-6]	$C_{28}H_{35}ClN_2O_7$	137–141	−173[c]	226 (4.46), 241 (sh, 4.37), 252 (sh, 4.24), 280 (3.63), 289 (sh, 3.59)	20
normaysine	[52978-29-7]	$C_{27}H_{33}ClN_2O_7$	187–188	−217[c]	229 (4.65), 242 (sh, 4.56), 252 (sh, 4.44), 280 (sh, 3.77), 290 (sh, 3.72)	20
maysenine	[52978-30-0]	$C_{27}H_{33}ClN_2O_6$	184–185	−57[c]	234 (4.64), 243 (4.73), 252 (sh, 4.62), 271 (4.37), 300 (sh, 3.98)	20
colubrinol	[50657-35-5]	$C_{36}H_{50}ClN_2O_{11}$	194–196	−94		21
colubrinol acetate	[50499-79-1]	$C_{38}H_{52}ClN_2O_{12}$	179–182	−127		21
maytanacine	[57103-69-2]	$C_{30}H_{39}ClN_2O_9$	234–237	−119	233 (4.48), 242 (sh, 4.43), 252 (4.45), 281 (3.74), 289 (3.74)	22
maytansinol	[57103-68-1]	$C_{28}H_{37}ClN_2O_9$	173–174.5	−309	232 (4.51), 244 (sh, 4.49), 252 (4.50), 281 (3.76), 288 (3.75)	22

Species:
- maytansine — *Maytenus ovatus* Loes.
- maytanprine — *Maytenus buchananii* (Loes.) R. Wilczek
- maytanbutine — *Maytenus buchananii* (Loes.) R. Wilczek
- maytanvaline — *Maytenus buchananii* (Loes.) R. Wilczek
- maysine — *Maytenus buchananii* (Loes.) R. Wilczek
- normaysine — *Maytenus buchananii* (Loes.) R. Wilczek
- maysenine — *Maytenus buchananii* (Loes.) R. Wilczek
- colubrinol — *Colubrina texensis* Gray (Rhamnaceae)
- colubrinol acetate — *Colubrina texensis* Gray (Rhamnaceae)
- maytanacine — *Putterlickia verrucosa* Szysyl. (Celastraceae)
- maytansinol — *Putterlickia verrucosa* Szysyl. (Celastraceae)

[a] Determined in $CHCl_3$ unless noted otherwise.
[b] Determined in ethanol unless noted otherwise.
[c] Determined in ethanol.
[d] Determined in methanol.
[e] Reported as $E^{1\%}_{1cm}$.
[f] Determined in phosphate buffer, pH 7.3.
[g] Determined in dioxane.
[h] Determined in acetate buffer, pH 4.62.
[i] Determined at pH 7.38.
[j] Determined in 0.1 M NaOH.

Table 2. Biological Activities of Ansamacrolides

Name	Biological activity
streptovaricins	antibacterial (gram-positive and mycobacterial)
	antiviral
	inhibitors of reverse transcriptase
rifamycins	antibacterial (gram-positive, gram-negative, and
	mycobacteria)
	antiviral
	inhibitors of reverse transcriptase
tolypomycins	antibacterial (gram-positive)
halomicins	antibacterial (gram-positive)
naphthomycin	antibacterial (gram-positive)
	vitamin K antagonist
geldanamycins	antiprotozoal
	inhibitors of reverse transcriptase
maytansinoids	antileukaemic, antitumor

NAPHTHOQUINOIDS

Streptovaricins

Isolation and Structure Proof. The streptovaricins are produced by *Streptomyces spectabilis* n. sp., an actinomycete isolated from a soil sample collected in Dallas, Texas (23–24). The streptovaricin complex is isolated from the fermentation broth by extraction with ethyl acetate followed by precipitation with hexane (25). The partially crystalline precipitate is a bright yellow–orange material composed of nine major components and a variety of minor components. Separation and purification of the streptovaricins can be achieved by countercurrent distribution or column chromatography on silica gel. Substance B 44 P, isolated from *Streptomyces* No. B 44-P1, was shown to be identical with the streptovaricins (26).

Chemical degradation studies were carried out on streptovaricins A and C, which are the major components of the crude complex. Streptovaricin A consumes two moles of sodium periodate to yield varicinal A [*21913-68-8*] (1), which accounts for the aliphatic portion of the molecule and prestreptovarone [*58074-37-6*] (2), which accounts for the aromatic chromophore of the streptovaricins. Streptovaricin G is the only other streptovaricin that yields prestreptovarone upon treatment with sodium periodate. Treatment of streptovaricins A, B, C, E, and G with sodium periodate and osmium tetroxide yields streptovarone [*36108-44-8*] (3), which is also produced by the reaction of prestreptovarone with sodium periodate and osmium tetroxide (4,27). A number of aliphatic products were isolated from the oxidation of streptovaricin C and its derivatives (28). The relationship between these oxidation products and varicinal A was established by nmr spectroscopy. The structures of the individual streptovaricins were established on the basis of the isolated oxidation products and a thorough nmr study including decoupling experiments (Figure 1).

The relationships among the various streptovaricins were shown by the following reactions: streptovaricin E is converted to streptovaricin C upon treatment with sodium

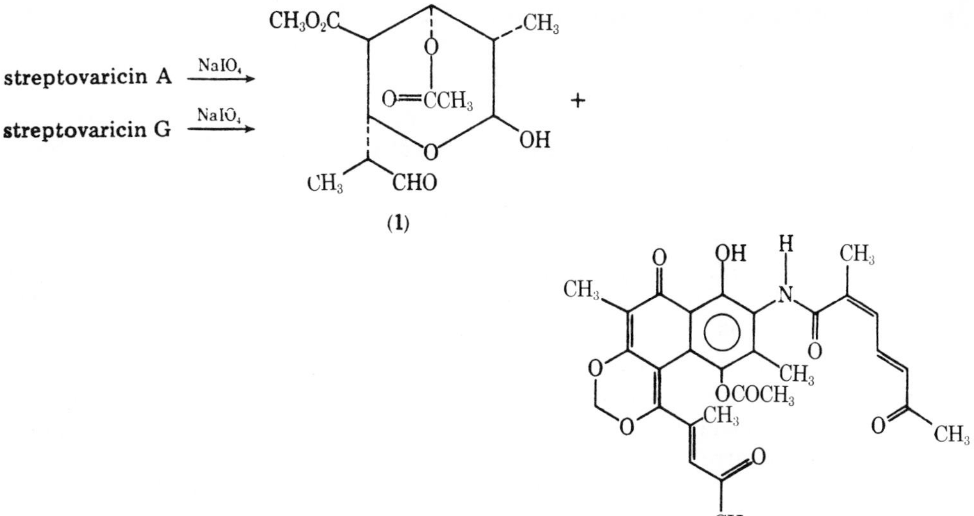

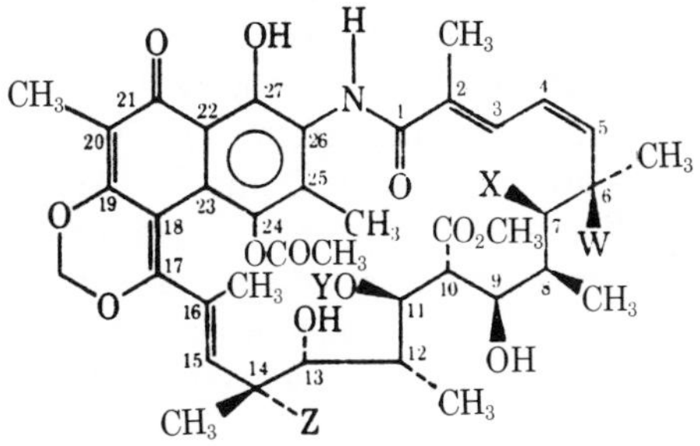

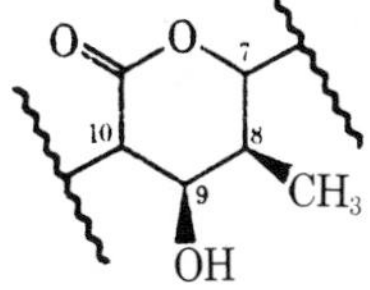

streptovaricin	W	X	Y	Z
A	OH	OH	COCH₃	OH
B	H	OH	COCH₃	OH
C	H	OH	H	OH
D	H	OH	H	H
E	H	O=	H	OH
G	OH	OH	H	OH
J	H	OCOCH₃	H	OH
K	OH	OCOCH₃	H	OH

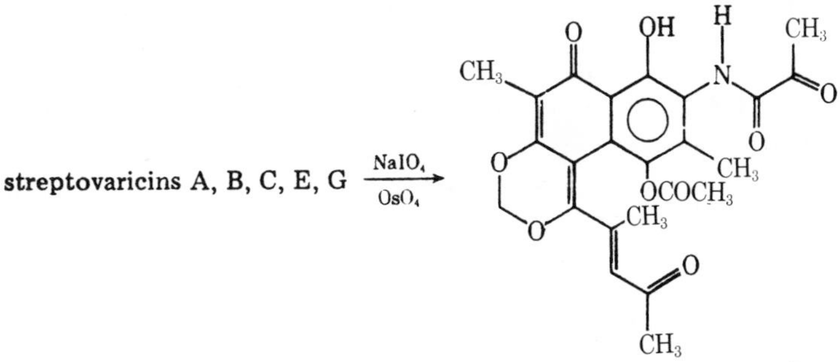

streptovaricin F_G

W = OH
Y = H
Z = OH

Figure 1. Structures of the streptovaricins.

75

borohydride; streptovaricins A, G, and K yield the same triacetate derivative upon acetylation; streptovaricins B, C, and J yield the same tri- and tetraacetate derivatives upon acetylation; streptovaricin G is converted to streptovaricin F_G by treatment with base (4).

The structures of the streptovaricins were confirmed by x-ray crystallographic studies (29–30). The absolute configuration of the *ansa*-bridge is 6R, 7R, 8R, 9R, 10S, 11S, 12R, 13S, and 14R with a helicity of P (31). Complete mass spectral (4,32) and ^{13}C nmr studies have been reported (33).

Chemical Properties. All of the streptovaricins except streptovaricin D react with one mole of sodium periodate to yield the corresponding streptovals (4) (4). The streptovaricins undergo thermal isomerization to the corresponding atropisostreptovaricin (34). In the natural streptovaricins the *ansa*-bridge lies above the aromatic nucleus but in the atropisostreptovaricins the *ansa*-bridge lies below the aromatic nucleus. Most spectral properties of the isomers are nearly identical, but the optical rotations, though of approximately equal magnitude, are of opposite sign. The circular dichroism curves of the isomers are nearly mirror images of each other. If pyridine is used as the solvent, lactonized streptovaricins are obtained similar to streptovaricin F_G as well as the atropisostreptovaricins. Treatment of streptovaricin C or D with oxygenated concentrated ammonia–methanol solution yields damavaricin C [58849-86-8] or D [59556-95-5] (5) through loss of the enol acetate and methylenedioxy groups (35). The damavaricins are related to the naturally occurring rifamycin W, and damavaricin D has recently been isolated from the streptovaricin complex. Besides damavaricins C and D, the basic methanolysis yields the corresponding atropisodamavaricins and lactonized damavaricins. The streptovaricins form acetonides and are hydrogenated to mixtures of dihydro and tetrahydro derivatives (4).

Biological Activity. The streptovaricins are active mainly against gram-positive organisms, with very good activity against *Mycobacterium tuberculosis, M. leprae* and *Staphylococcus aureus* infections in animals (23,36). The streptovaricins are labile in alkaline solutions, losing practically all activity in three days at pH 7.8. This loss in activity is associated with a decrease in the absorbance at 435 nm which can be used to measure the stability of the streptovaricins. Biological activity is also lost in acidic media but at a much slower rate. The order of antibacterial activity is streptovaricins A and G > streptovaricins B and C > streptovaricins D and J > streptovaricin E ≫ streptovaricin F_G [35512-45-9] (3). The totally acetylated streptovaricins lose their antibacterial activity. Lactonization greatly reduces any biological activity a streptovaricin possesses. The antibacterial activities of the atropisostreptovaricins are about the same as the natural isomers. Although the damavaricins retain biological activity, they are not as active as the corresponding streptovaricins. The streptovals are also inactive as antibacterial agents (4).

The streptovaricins also inhibit the reverse transcriptase of some RNA oncogenic viruses that may be involved in the process of viral transformation. The order of activity against the reverse transcriptase of Rauscher leukemia virus is streptovaricin G triacetate and streptovaricin C tri- and tetraacetates ≃ streptovaricin D > streptovaricins J, C, B, and G > streptovaricins E, A, and, F_G (3). The atropisostreptovaricins again have similar activities to the corresponding natural isomers. The streptovals exhibit greatly improved activity against reverse transcriptase relative to the corresponding streptovaricin. The damavaricins also inhibit reverse transcriptase (4).

The streptovaricins have also been shown to inhibit cowpox virus plaque formation (36).

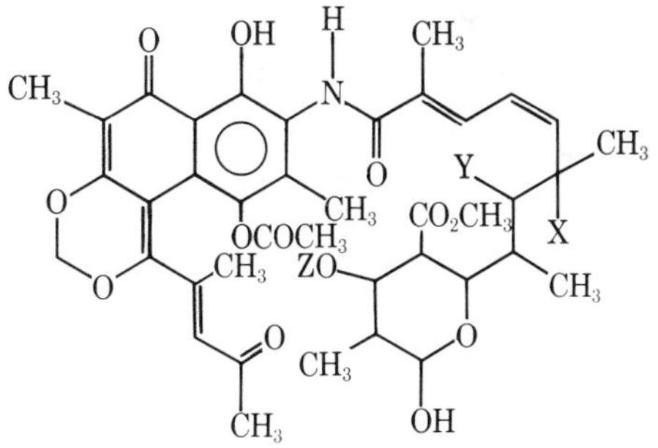

(4)

streptoval A	[60760-75-0]	X = Y = OH; Z = COCH₃
streptoval B	[60735-99-1]	X = H; Y = OH; Z = COCH₃
streptoval C	[54955-14-5]	X = Z = H; Y = OH
streptoval E	[60736-00-7]	X = Z = H; Y = O=
streptoval G	[60736-02-9]	X = Y = OH; Z = H
streptoval J	[60736-03-0]	X = Z = H; Y = COCH₃

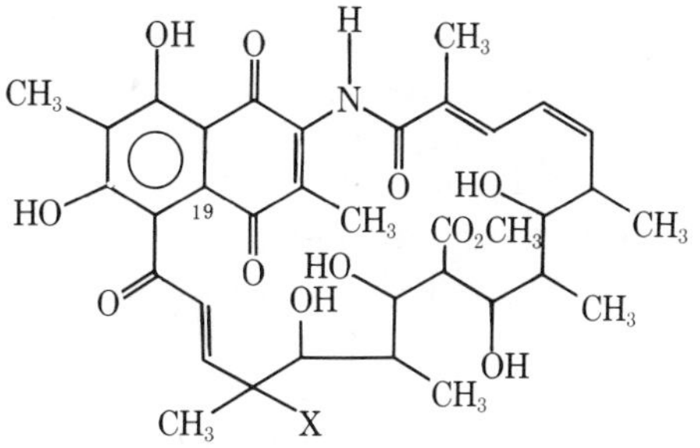

(5)

damavaricin C	X = OH
damavaricin D	X = H

Clinical studies with streptovaricins have been very limited. The major toxicity reported in the clinical studies has been gastrointestinal disturbances. However, indications are that the toxicity is not due to the individual streptovaricins but to some impurity in some fermentation lots (36).

Assay Methods. The primary assay for the streptovaricins is the microbiological assay using the agar diffusion method or a turbidimetric procedure; both methods employ *Mycobacterium ranae* as the test organism (23). The streptovaricins can also be identified by paper chromatography (23,39) or thin-layer chromatography (3).

Derivatives. Very few derivatives of the streptovaricins have been prepared. One group of derivatives are the 19-O-substituted damavaricins many of which exhibit greater antibacterial activity than the parent streptovaricin (37). Many of these derivatives also inhibited tumor cell growth (38).

Rifamycins

Isolation and Structure Proof. The rifamycins were first isolated from a fermentation broth of *Nocardia mediterranei* (the producing organism was originally identified as *Streptomyces mediterranei*) an actinomycete isolated from a soil sample collected in France. The microorganism produces at least five substances having biological activity and designated rifamycins A through E. The rifamycins were originally designated as rifomycins but the name was changed to avoid confusion with the commercial name of other antibiotic drugs. The complex can be isolated by extracting the filtrate broth with ethyl acetate followed by precipitation with petroleum ether. Only rifamycin B, which accounts for 10–15% of the crude complex, can be isolated easily as a stable, crystalline compound. Because of its acidic nature, rifamycin B can be separated from the other rifamycins by extracting the ethyl acetate solution with a pH 6.5–7.5 buffer, acidifying the aqueous solution and extracting with ethyl acetate. Concentrating the ethyl acetate extract yields rifamycin B as a yellow crystalline substance (5,40–41).

Because of difficulties encountered in the separation and the stability of the individual rifamycins, studies were started to find ways to increase the yield of individual components of the complex. A mutant of *N. mediterranei* was isolated which produced mainly a mixture of rifamycins C and D (42). However, it was found that by adding sodium diethylbarbiturate to the fermentation medium of *N. mediterranei,* rifamycin B was practically the only substance formed. It was shown that 5,5-diethylbarbituric acid was not a precursor of the rifamycins and that it probably inhibited the normal metabolic pathway of *N. mediterranei.* A study of other barbituric acid derivatives indicated that lipophilic groups and disubstitution in the 5-position were required for the inhibitory effect (43–44). Work on the other rifamycins was abandoned in favor of the easily isolable and stable rifamycin B.

Rifamycin B is oxidized to the more active rifamycin O upon standing in solution. This reaction also occurs when rifamycin B is treated with a variety of oxidizing agents such as hydrogen peroxide. Rifamycin O can be reconverted to rifamycin B by treatment with ascorbic acid. Rifamycin O in turn can be hydrolyzed to the even more active rifamycin S with the expulsion of glycolic acid. Rifamycin S can be reduced with ascorbic acid to rifamycin SV. Rifamycin SV can be oxidized to rifamycin S (5,45–46). Although rifamycins O and S were originally chemical derivatives of rifamycin B, microorganisms have been found that produce these rifamycins naturally.

The structures of the rifamycins were arrived at by chemical degradation studies (1,4,47–48) and confirmed by x-ray crystallographic studies (49–51) (Figure 2).

The absolute configuration of the *ansa*-bridge is 6S, 7S, 8R, 9R, 10R, 11S, 12R, and 13S (52). Studies of ^{13}C nmr (4,12–13,53–55) and ir (55) have been reported for several rifamycins.

Biological Activity.   The rifamycins are biologically active against gram-positive microorganisms and mycobacteria, particularly *M. tuberculosis* (5,57–60). At higher concentrations the rifamycins are also active against gram-negative bacteria. The rifamycins also show antiviral activity (61–62) and inhibit reverse transcriptase (63–65).

Although rifamycin B has undergone clinical trials showing good therapeutic activity in biliary tract infections, the trials were abandoned when it was found that Rifamycin B could be transformed into the more active rifamycin SV (5). Rifamycin SV is effective against a variety of infections including those of the skin, ear, nose, throat, liver, biliary tract, as well as being active against tuberculosis and leprosy (58). Rifamycin SV, as its sodium salt, is commercially available as a solution (Rifacin, Lepetit) containing sodium ascorbate, polyvinylpyrrolidone, lidocaine hydrochloride,

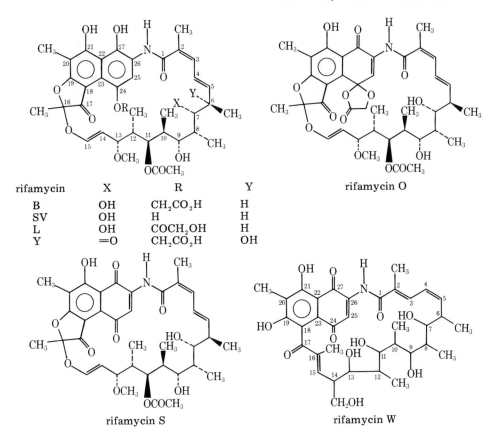

Figure 2. Structures of the rifamycins.

preservative, and stabilizers. Sodium rifamycin SV is poorly absorbed when given orally which is probably due to its conversion in the stomach to the free acid which is not very soluble in aqueous solutions.

Chemical Properties and Derivatives. There have been thousands of derivatives of the rifamycins prepared in the attempt to obtain a broader-spectrum antibiotic as well as one with good oral absorption. Rifamycins B, O, and S have served as starting materials for large groups of derivatives.

Treatment of rifamycin B with amines, hydrazines, and alcohols yield (6) the corresponding amides, hydrazides, and esters, respectively (4,5,66).

$$X = NR_2, \ NHNR_2, \ OR$$
$$X = N(CH_2CH_3)_2 = \text{rifamide}$$

The tertiary amides are more active than the esters or the primary and secondary amides (5,67). The most active of the group is the N,N-diethyl derivative known as rifamide [2750-76-7] (68). The antibiotic is active against gram-positive bacteria, especially *Staphylococcus, Streptococcus*, and *Pneumococcus* strains, with very low toxicity (69–71). Very good activity was exhibited against *M. tuberculosis*. No cross-resistance with other antibiotics was observed. Variable blood levels are obtained when rifamide is administered orally but high levels are obtained at all dosages for 6–8 h when administered intramuscularly.

Rifamycin O reacts with a variety of aromatic amines, hydrazides, amidrazones, and aminoguanidines to give quinonimine derivatives (7). All of the derivatives show good activity against gram-positive bacteria. The condensation product with amino-guanidine (rifamycin AG) is a broad-spectrum antibiotic possessing good activity against gram-positive, gram-negative bacteria, and *M. tuberculosis*. However, rifamycin AG is poorly absorbed due to its low solubility in aqueous solutions (5,72).

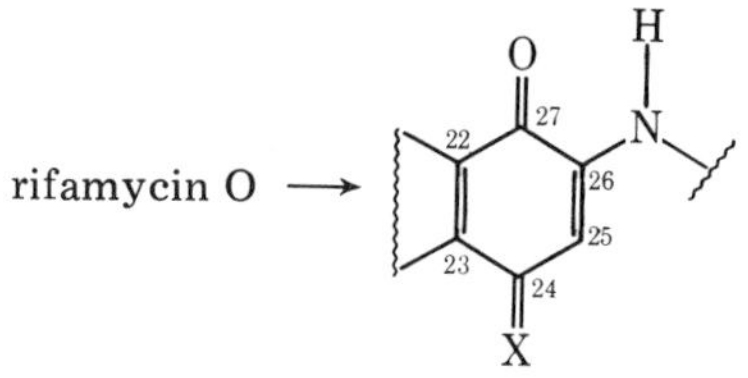

rifamycin O $\longrightarrow$

(7)

X = N-aryl
X = N-NHCO-aryl
X = NNHC-aryl
        ‖
        NH
X = NNHC-NHR
        ‖
        NH

Reaction of rifamycin S with a variety of *o*-phenylenediamines and *o*-amino-phenols produces a series of phenazines (8) and phenoxazines (9), respectively, which proved to be very active biologically but disrupted liver function. Rifazine [10238-70-7] ((8) R = H) is the simplest of the phenazines (73–76).

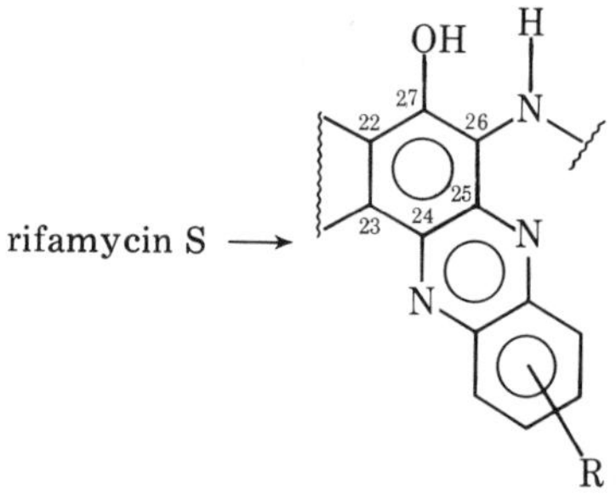

rifamycin S $\longrightarrow$

(8) 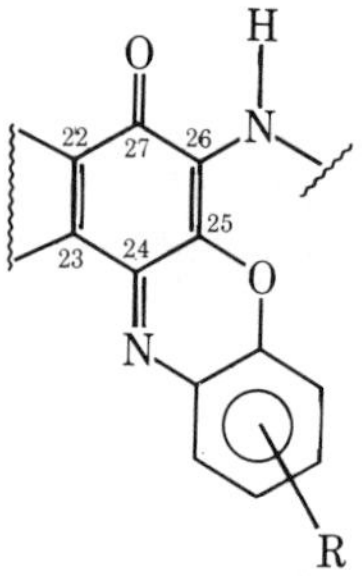   (9)

Rifamycin S also undergoes conjugate addition reactions to the quinone ring by a variety of nucleophiles including ammonia, primary and secondary amines, mercaptans, carbanions, and enamines giving the C-25 substituted derivatives of rifamycin

SV (10) (74,77–78). Many of the derivatives show excellent antibacterial properties (75,79,80). The 25-cyclic amino derivatives of rifamycin SV also inhibit the polymerases of RNA tumor viruses (80–81).

rifamycin SV →

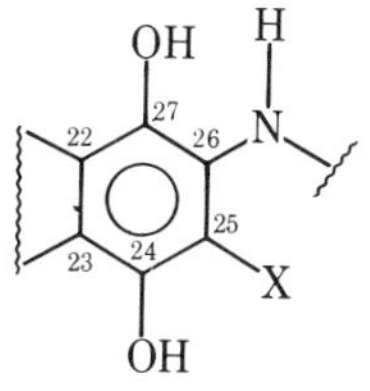

(10)

X = NRR'
X = SR
X = CHRR'
X = Cl, Br, CN

Treatment of rifamycin S with formaldehyde and secondary amines yields via a Mannich reaction the 25-aminomethyl derivatives (11), which are not of therapeutic interest (82). However, upon oxidation in acidic medium, the aminomethyl derivatives yield 25-formylrifamycin SV (rifaldehyde) (12). Treatment of rifaldehyde with amines, hydrazines, hydroxylamines, and hydrazides yields a number of derivatives of the 25-formyl group having excellent biological activity (83–85). The most therapeutically useful derivative is the N-amino-N'-methylpiperazine hydrazone of rifaldehyde [13292-22-3] (12) known as rifampin in the United States and rifampicin elsewhere. Rifampicin [13292-46-1] (13) ($C_{43}H_{58}N_4O_{12}$) is an orange–yellow crystalline solid mp 183–188°C (dec), $\lambda_{max}^{ethanol}$ 237 (ϵ 33,200), 255 (ϵ 32,100), 334 (ϵ 27,000), 475 nm (ϵ 15,400) (85).

Rifampicin is active against a variety of gram-positive and gram-negative bacteria; however resistance develops rapidly if it is used alone (87–88). Rifampicin finds its greatest use in the treatment of tuberculosis (88–91). Because resistance develops rapidly, rifampicin is normally given in combination with other antituberculosis drugs,

rifamycin S →

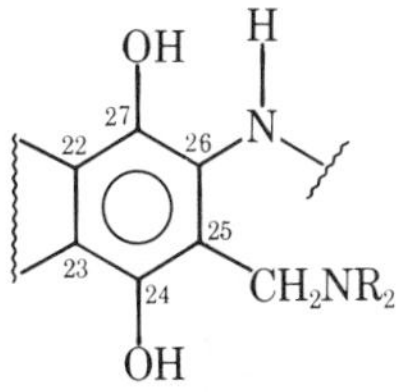

(11)

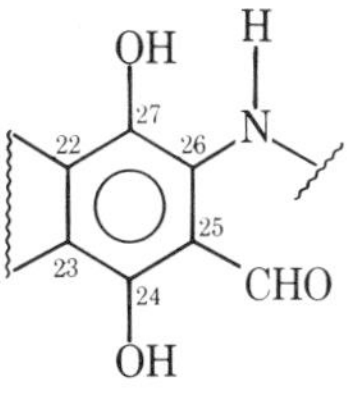

rifaldehyde
(12)

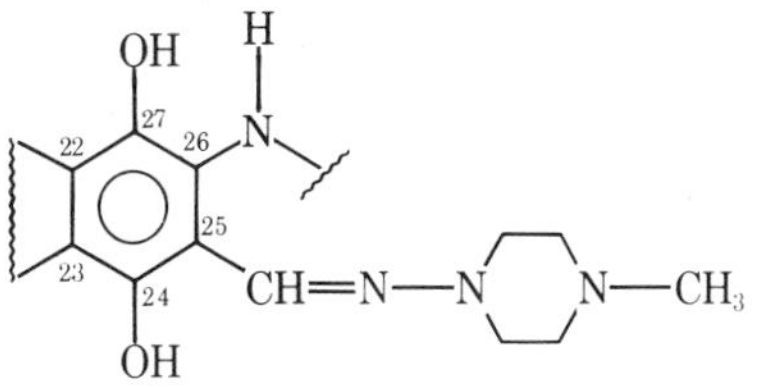

rifampicin
(13)

eg, isoniazid. Good serum levels are attained when rifampicin is administered orally, with very few side effects. No cross-resistance was observed with other antibiotics (88,90,92).

Rifampicin also has shown antiviral activity but at levels five hundred to one thousand times greater than required for antibacterial activity (61–62,88,93). Rifampicin also shows promise in the treatment of leprosy (88). A large number of rifampicin-like derivatives are potent inhibitors of reverse transcriptase (80,94–98).

A number of oxime derivatives of rifaldehyde have been prepared. Many of these derivatives exhibit good activity against rifampicin-resistant organisms (99). Structure–activity relationships for the oximes have been studied (100).

Assay Methods.   A large number of assays exist for the determination of the various rifamycins. Rifamycin SV and rifampicin can be determined by a microbiological assay using *Sarcina lutea* ATCC 9341 as the test organism (58,88), and rifampicin can be determined using *S. aureus* 560 (101). Rifamycins B, S, and SV can be separated by electrophoresis on agar gel and determined microbiologically using *B. subtilis* or *S. lutea* (102). Spectrophotometric assays exist for the rifamycins (58,88,103–104). Rifamycins B, O, S, and SV can be determined via polarography (105) or by amperometric titration (106). Rifamycins B, O, S, and SV can be separated by thin-layer chromatography on silica gel or by paper chromatography (107). Fluorimetric assays exist for rifamycin B (108) and rifampicin (101).

Tolypomycins

Tolypomycin Y was isolated from a fermentation broth of *Streptomyces tolypophorus* from a soil sample found in Japan. The antibiotic is isolated via extraction with ethyl acetate at pH 8 followed by precipitation with hexane or ether–petroleum ether to yield a crude powder. Purification is achieved by chromatography on silica gel or carbon to yield tolypomycin Y as yellow needles. *S. tolypophorus* also produces rifamycin B. The addition of small amounts of iron salts to the fermentation medium increases the production of tolypomycin Y (6,109–110).

The structure of tolypomycin Y (**14**) was arrived at by chemical degradation (111–112) and confirmed by x-ray crystallographic analysis (113). Mild acid hydrolysis of tolypomycin Y yields tolypomycinone [22356-23-6] and tolyposamine [23267-34-7] (**15**).

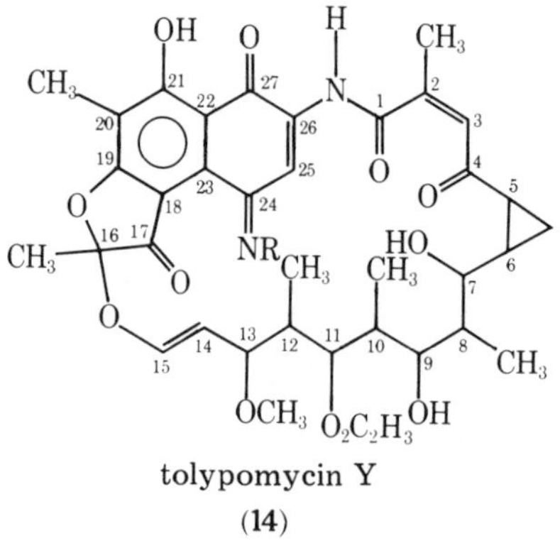

tolypomycin Y

(**14**)

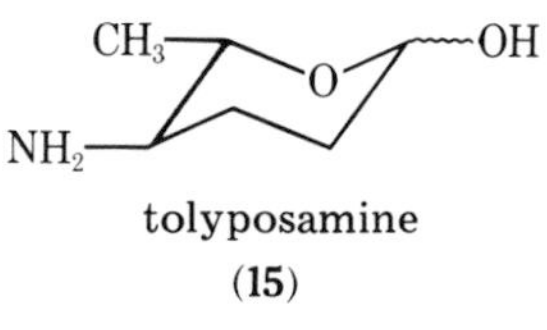

tolyposamine

(**15**)

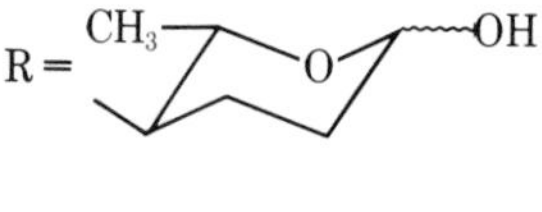

$R =$

Further hydrolysis of tolypomycinone with acid yields tolyponone [*24317-12-2*], which is also formed upon mild acid hydrolysis of rifamycin S. The structure of the *ansa*-bridge was determined by further chemical degradation and spectral studies. Reduction of tolypomycin Y produces tolypomycin R [*33889-22-4*] (**16**) (114).

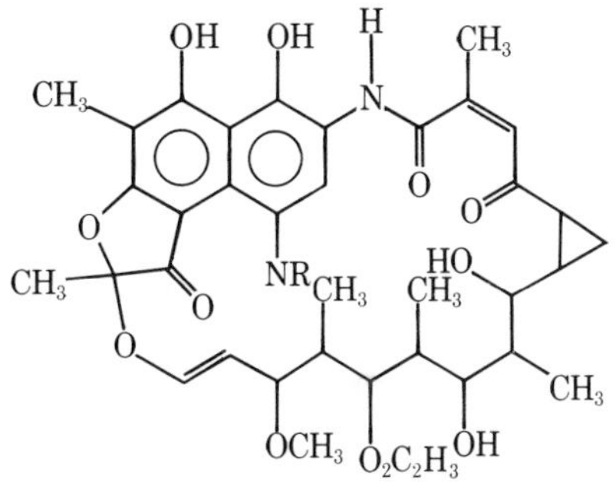

tolypomycin R
(**16**)

Tolypomycin Y shows strong antibacterial activity against gram-positive bacteria and *Neisseria gonorrheae*. When administered by subcutaneous, intraperitoneal, and intravenous routes, tolypomycin Y is effective in experimental infections in mice caused by *Staphylococcus aureus, Streptococcus pyrogenes*, and *Diplococcus pneumoniae*. Cross-resistance is observed with rifampicin but not with other antibiotics. Resistance to tolypomycin Y develops rapidly. The bioactivity of tolypomycin R is very similar to that of tolypomycin Y (114).

A differential bioassay was developed to distinguish tolypomycin Y from rifamycin B. The assay uses *Streptococcus alcalophilus* IFO 3531 as the test organism. This organism is inhibited by tolypomycin Y but not by rifamycin B (115).

Halomicins

The halomicins are a group of four antibiotics (A, B, C, D) produced by *Micromonospora halophytica*, an organism found in a soil sample from Syracuse, New York. The complex was isolated by extracting the filtered beer with ethyl acetate or chloroform followed by precipitation with ethyl ether–petroleum ether. The halomicins were separated by partition chromatography on Chromosorb W coated with formamide (14).

Halomicin B (**17**) is the only halomicin whose structure has been determined. Treatment of halomicin B with nitrous acid yields rifamycin S and the pyrrolidine (**18**). The structure of halomicin B was confirmed by heating rifamycin O and (**18**) in tetrahydrofuran to yield halomicin B (15). Halomicin B can also be converted to rifamycin S by electrochemical oxidation (116).

The halomicins are active against gram-positive bacteria. The halomicin complex exhibited high activity against bacterial strains resistant to penicillin G. Halomicin C appeared to be the most active component of the complex (14).

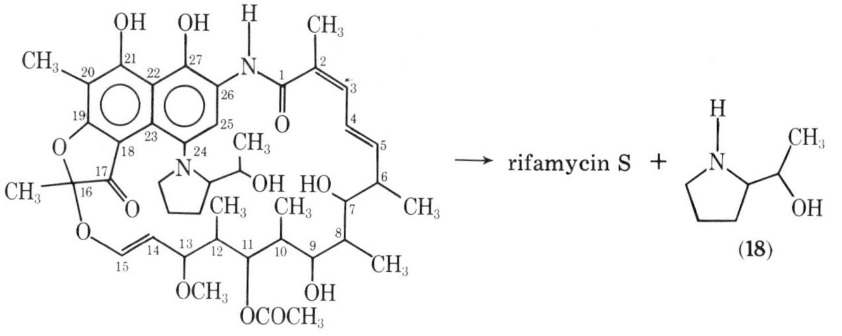

halomicin B

(17)

Naphthomycin

Naphthomycin (**19**) is isolated from the fermentation beer of *Streptomyces collinus* by extraction with ethyl acetate. It is separated from other components by extraction with base followed by acidification and reextraction with ethyl acetate. Purification is achieved by chromatography over silica gel followed by crystallization (16).

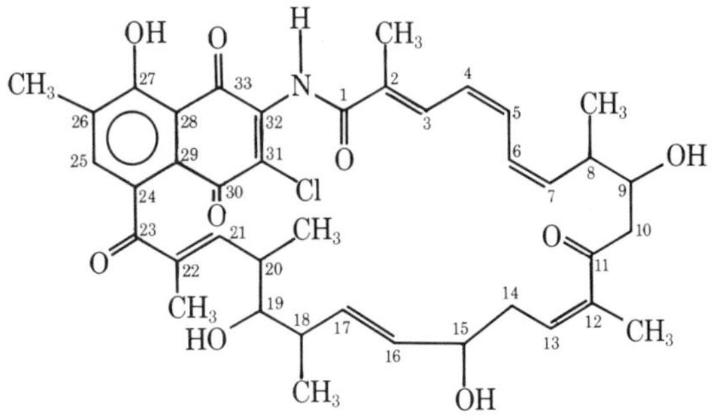

naphthomycin

(19)

The structure of naphthomycin was arrived at solely on the basis of nmr studies using lanthanide shift reagents (117). The position of the phenolic group has recently been disputed. Based on spectral data obtained for streptovaricin precursors, it has been proposed that the phenolic group of naphthomycin is at C-25 rather than at C-27 (118). The antibiotic is active against gram-positive bacteria, but this activity is reversed by the addition of cysteine. Naphthomycin is also a vitamin K antagonist.

BENZOQUINOIDS

Geldanamycin

Geldanamycin (**20**) is isolated from the filtered beer of *Streptomyces hygroscopicus* var. *geldanus* var. *nova*, an organism isolated from a soil sample from Michigan, by extraction with butanol. Upon concentration, crude crystals are obtained which are recrystallized from chloroform–ethyl ether to yield yellow crystals (17). The structure of geldanamycin was assigned in great part on the basis of nmr studies on geldanamycin and on its derivatives (4,119). Unlike the other ansamacrolides, geldanamycin has very little antibacterial activity, being primarily active against protozoa and fungi, especially *Tetrahymena pyriformis* and *Crithidia fasciculata* (17).

Geldanamycin undergoes reaction with *o*-phenylenediamines and *o*-aminophenols to give compounds similar to rifazine. The corresponding geldanazines and geldanoxazines are active against reverse transcriptase. Geldanamycin also yields compounds similar to rifaldehyde and rifampicin by reaction with formaldehyde and *tert*-butylamine followed by oxidation. Oxime and hydrazone derivatives of the generated aldehyde have been prepared and found to inhibit reverse transcriptase (4,120).

Maytansinoids and Maytansides

Unlike the other ansamacrolides, which are obtained from microorganisms, the maytansinoids are isolated after repeated column chromatography and preparative thin layer chromatography, from ethanol extracts of plants obtained in Ethiopia and Kenya. Maytansinoids are those compounds similar to maytansine; maytansides are maytansinoids possessing the macrocyclic ring system but lacking the ester moiety (20). The structure of maytansine was established by x-ray crystallographic analysis (18,121) and the structures of the other maytansinoids were arrived at by comparative nmr studies with maytansine (19–22) (Fig. 3). The absolute configuration of maytansine is 3*S*, 4*S*, 5*S*, 6*R*, 7*S*, 9*S*, 10*R*, and 2′*S*. Maytanvaline is converted to maysine and *N*-isovaleryl-*N*-methyl-L-alanine by basic methanolysis. Basic methanolysis of maytansine also yields maysine along with *N*-acetyl-*N*-methyl-L-alanine. Normaysine is converted to maysenine by treatment with chromous chloride in acetic acid. Maytanbutine and maytanacine are converted to maytansinol upon reduction with LiAlH$_4$. Maytansinol can be converted to maytanacine by treatment with acetic anhydride–pyridine.

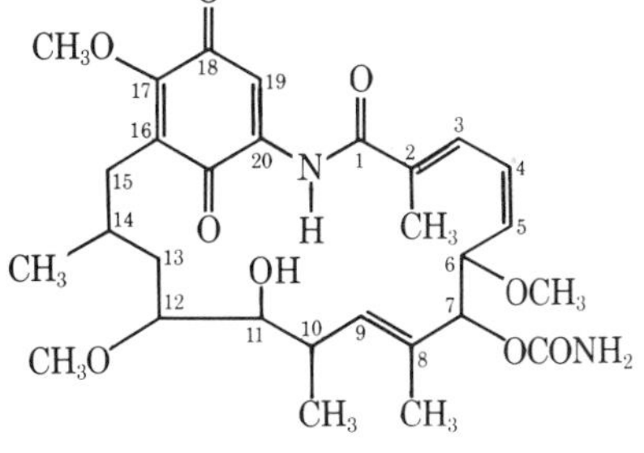

geldanamycin

(20)

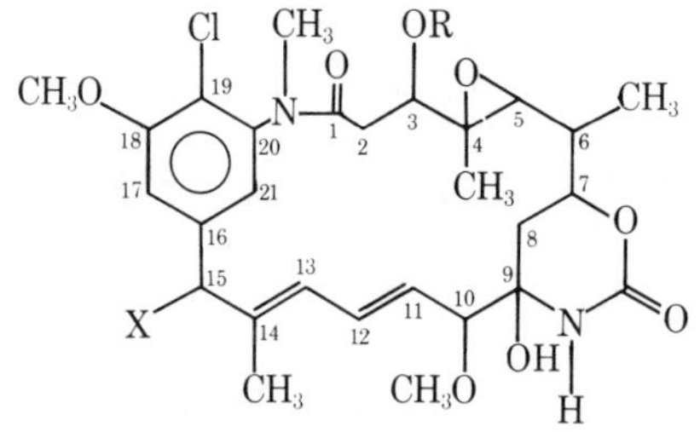

maytanvaline X = H; R = COCHCH$_3$NCH$_3$COCH$_2$CH(CH$_3$)$_2$
maytansine X = H; R = COCHCH$_3$NCH$_3$COCH$_3$
maytanprine X = H; R = COCHCH$_3$NCH$_3$COCH$_2$CH$_3$
maytanbutine X = H; R = COCHCH$_3$NCH$_3$COCH(CH$_3$)$_2$
maytanacine X = H; R = COCH$_3$
maytansinol X = R = H
colubrinol X = OH; R = COCHCH$_3$HCH$_3$COCH(CH$_3$)$_2$
colubrinol acetate X = OCOCH$_3$; R = COCHCH$_3$NCH$_3$COCH(CH$_3$)$_2$

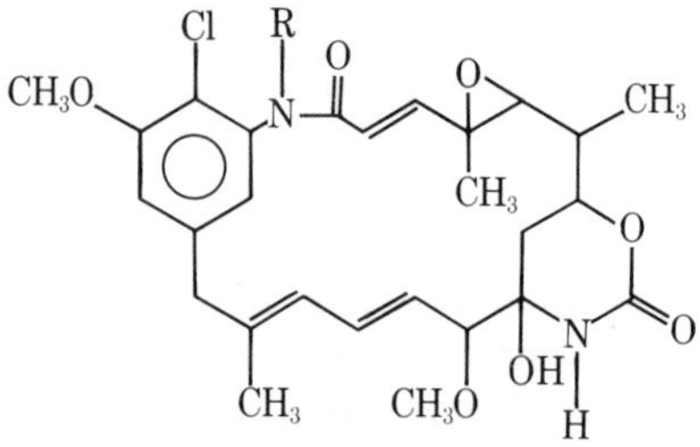

maysine R = CH$_3$
normaysine R = H

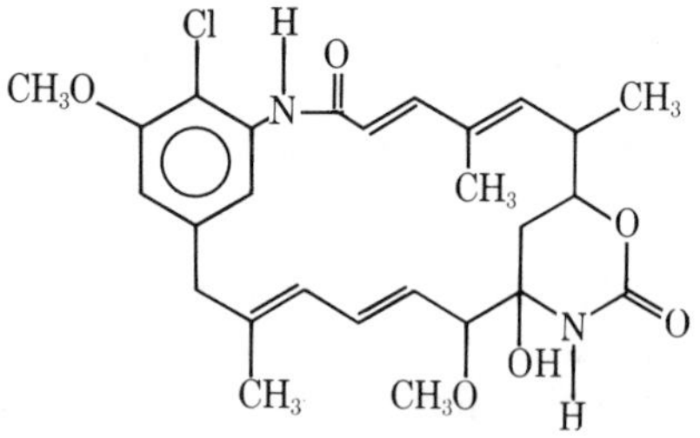

maysenine

Figure 3. Structures of the maytansinoids and maytansides.

The maytansinoids possess antitumor activity, particularly against P388 lymphocytic leukemia, B16 melanocarcinoma, and Lewis lung carcinoma. The maytansinoids act by inhibiting DNA synthesis by an as yet unknown mechanism (122). A number of semisynthetic esters of maytansinol have been prepared and exhibit good antileukemic activity (22). The maytansides (maysine, normaysine, maysenine, and maytansinol) lack antitumor activity, indicating that the ester side chain is a requirement for activity (20,22). The maytansinoids do not inhibit bacterial RNA polymerase as do the other ansamacrolides.

Mode of Action

The mode of action of the ansamacrolides was established through studies with the rifamycins and streptovaricins (36,94,123–124). The ansamacrolides inhibit bacterial growth by inhibiting RNA synthesis. This is accomplished by forming a tight complex with DNA-dependent RNA polymerase. This complex is between the ansamacrolide and the β-unit of RNA polymerase. The formation of the complex inhibits the initiation step of RNA synthesis. Apparently the complex does not prevent the formation of the first phosphodiester bond but inhibits formation of the second phosphodiester bond (125–126). The ansamacrolides form no such complex with

mammalian RNA polymerase, thus accounting for the low toxicity of the ansamacrolides.

The antiviral activity of the ansamacrolides is not due to inhibition of RNA
polymerase but due to the inhibition of the assembly of virus particles (94,124).

Commercially Available Ansamacrolides

The ansamacrolides commercially available in 1977 are shown below.

Compound	Trade name	Manufacturer
Rifamide	Rifocin M	Lepetit
Rifamysin SV	Rifocin	Lepetit
Rifampicin	Rimactane	Ciba-Geigy
	Rifadine	Dow; Lepetit

BIBLIOGRAPHY

1. V. Prelog, *Pure Appl. Chem.* **7,** 551 (1963).
2. A. Lüttringhaus and H. Gralheer, *Justus Liebigs Ann. Chem.* **550,** 67 (1942).
3. K. L. Rinehart, Jr., F. J. Antosz, K. Sasaki, P. K. Martin, M. L. Maheshwari, F. Reusser, L. H. Li, D. Moran, and P. F. Wiley, *Biochemistry* **13,** 186 (1974).
4. K. L. Rinehart, Jr., and L. S. Shield, *Fortschr. Chem. Org. Naturst.* **33,** 231 (1976).
5. P. Sensi, *Prog. Org. Biol. Med. Chem.* **1,** 337 (1964).
6. T. Kishi, H. Yamana, M. Muroi, S. Harada, M. Asai, T. Hasegawa, and K. Mizuno, *J. Antibiot.* **25,** 11 (1972).
7. S. Sugawara, K. Karasawa, M. Watanabe, and T. Hidaka, *J. Antibiot. Ser. A* **17,** 29 (1964).
8. W. Kump and H. Bickel, *Helv. Chim. Acta* **56,** 2323 (1973).
9. G. Lancini and C. Hengeller, *J. Antibiot.* **22,** 637 (1969).
10. J. Leitich, V. Prelog, and P. Sensi, *Experientia* **23,** 505 (1967).
11. G. C. Lancini, G. G. Gallo, G. Sartori, and P. Sensi, *J. Antibiot.* **22,** 369 (1969).
12. E. Martinelli, G. G. Gallo, P. Antonini, and R. J. White, *Tetrahedron* **30,** 3087 (1974).
13. R. J. White, E. Martinelli, and G. Lancini, *Proc. Nat. Acad. Sci. U.S.A.* **71,** 3260 (1974).
14. M. J. Weinstein, G. M. Luedeman, E. M. Oden, and G. H. Wagman, *Antimicrob. Agents Chemother.* 435 (1968).
15. A. K. Ganguly, S. Szmulewicz, O. Z. Sarre, D. Greeves, J. Morton, and J. McGlotten, *J. Chem. Soc. Chem. Commun.* 395 (1974).
16. M. Balerna, W. Keller-Schierlein, C. Martius, H. Wolf, and H. Zähner, *Arch. Mikrobiol.* **65,** 303 (1969).
17. C. DeBoer, P. A. Meulman, R. J. Wnuk, and D. H. Peterson, *J. Antibiot.* **23,** 442 (1970).
18. S. M. Kupchan, Y. Komoda, W. A. Court, G. J. Thomas, R. M. Smith, A. Karim, C. J. Gilmore, R. C. Haltiwanger, and R. F. Bryan, *J. Am. Chem. Soc.* **94,** 1354 (1972).
19. S. M. Kupchan, Y. Komoda, G. J. Thomas, and H. P. J. Hintz, *J. Chem. Soc. Chem. Commun.* 1065 (1972)
20. S. M. Kupchan, Y. Komoda, A. R. Branfman, R. G. Dailey, Jr., and V. A. Zimmerly, *J. Am. Chem. Soc.* **96,** 3706 (1974).
21. M. C. Wani, H. L. Taylor, and M. E. Wall, *J. Chem. Soc. Chem. Commun.* 390 (1973).
22. S. M. Kupchan, A. R. Branfman, A. T. Sneden, A. K. Verma, R. G. Dailey, Jr., Y. Komoda, and Y. Nagao, *J. Am. Chem. Soc.* **97,** 5294 (1975).
23. P. Siminoff, R. M. Smith, W. T. Sokolski, and G. M. Savage, *Am. Rev. Tuber. Pulm. Dis.* **75,** 576 (1957).
24. U.S. Pat. 3,116,202 (Dec. 31, 1963), A. Dietz, C. DeBoer, R. M. Smith, P. Siminoff, G. A. Boyack, and G. B. Whitfield (to The Upjohn Company).
25. G. B. Whitfield, E. C. Olson, R. R. Herr, J. A. Fox, M. E. Bergy, and G. A. Boyack, *Am. Rev. Tuber. Pulm. Dis.* **75,** 584 (1957).
26. H. Yamazaki, *J. Antibiot.* **21,** 204 (1968).
27. K. L. Rinehart, Jr., *Acc. Chem. Res.* **5,** 57 (1972).

28. K. Sasaki, K. L. Rinehart, Jr., and F. J. Antosz, *J. Antibiot.* **25,** 68 (1972).
29. A. H.-J. Wang, I. C. Paul, K. L. Rinehart, Jr., and F. J. Antosz, *J. Am. Chem. Soc.* **93,** 6275 (1971).
30. A. H.-J. Wang and I. C. Paul, *J. Am. Chem. Soc.* **98,** 4612 (1976).
31. R. S. Cohn, C. Ingold, V. Prelog, *Angew. Chem. Int. Ed. Eng.* **5,** 385 (1966).
32. K. L. Rinehart, Jr., and J. C. Cook, Jr., *J. Antibiot.* **27,** 1 (1974).
33. K. Kakinuma, B. I. Milavetz, and K. L. Rinehart, Jr., *J. Org. Chem.* **41,** 1358 (1976).
34. K. L. Rinehart, Jr., W. M. J. Knöll, K. Kakinuma, F. J. Antosz, I. C. Paul, A. H.-J. Wang, F. Reusser, L. H. Li, and W. C. Krueger, *J. Am. Chem. Soc.* **97,** 196 (1975).
35. K. L. Rinehart, Jr., F. J. Antosz, P. V. Deshmukh, K. Kakinuma, P. K. Martin, B. I. Milavetz, K. Sasaki, T. R. Witty, L. H. Li, and F. Reusser, *J. Antibiot.* **29,** 201 (1976).
36. D. M. Byrd and W. A. Carter in W. A. Carter, ed., *Selective Inhibitors of Viral Function,* Chemical Rubber Co. Press, Cleveland, Ohio, 1973, p. 329.
37. K. Sasaki, T. Naito, T. Satomi, and K. Onodera, *J. Antibiot.* **29,** 147 (1976).
38. K. Onodera, Y. Aoi, and K. Sasaki, *Agric. Biol. Chem.* **40,** 1381 (1976).
39. K. L. Rinehart, Jr., P. K. Martin, and C. E. Coverdale, *J. Am. Chem. Soc.* **88,** 3149 (1966).
40. P. Sensi, A. M. Greco, and R. Ballotta, *Antibiot. Annu.* **1959–1960,** 262 (1960).
41. Ger. Pat. 1,089,513 (Sept. 22, 1960), P. Sensi and P. Margalith (to Lepetit S.p.A.).
42. P. Margalith and H. Pagani, *Appl. Microbiol.* **9,** 320 (1961).
43. Ref. 42, p. 325.
44. D. Kluepfel, G. C. Lancini, and G. Sartori, *Appl. Microbiol.* **13,** 600 (1965).
45. P. Sensi, R. Ballota, and A. M. Greco, *Farmaco Ed. Sci.* **15,** 228 (1960).
46. P. Sensi, R. Ballota, A. M. Greco, and G. G. Gallo, *Farmaco Ed. Sci.* **16,** 165 (1961).
47. W. Oppolzer and V. Prelog, *Helv. Chim. Acta* **56,** 2287 (1973).
48. W. Oppolzer, V. Prelog, and P. Sensi, *Experientia* **20,** 336 (1964).
49. M. Brufani, W. Fedeli, G. Giacomello, and A. Vaciago, *Experientia* **20,** 339 (1964).
50. M. Brufani, W. Fedeli, G. Giacomello, and A. Vaciago, *Experientia* **23,** 508 (1967).
51. M. Brufani, S. Cerrini, W. Fedeli, and A. Vaciago, *Mol. Biology* **87,** 409 (1974).
52. J. Leitich, W. Oppolzer, and V. Prelog, *Experientia* **20,** 343 (1964).
53. H. Fuhrer, *Helv. Chim. Acta* **56,** 2377 (1973).
54. E. Martinelli, R. J. White, G. G. Gallo, and P. J. Beynon, *Tetrahedron Lett.* 1367 (1974).
55. E. Martinelli, R. J. White, and G. G. Gallo, *Tetrahedron* **29,** 3441 (1973).
56. P. Ferrari and G. G. Gallo, *Farmaco Ed. Sci.* **30,** 676 (1975).
57. M. T. Timbal, *Antibiot. Annu.* **1959–1960,** 271 (1960).
58. N. Bergamini and G. Fowst, *Arzneim. Forsch.* **15,** 951 (1965).
59. W. Wehrli and M. Staehelin, *Bacteriol. Rev.* **35,** 290 (1971).
60. S. Riva and L. G. Silvestri, *Ann. Rev. Microbiol.* **26,** 199 (1972).
61. E. A. C. Follett and T. H. Pennington in M. A. Lauffer, F. B. Bang, K. Maramorosch, and K. M. Smith, eds., *Advances in Virus Research,* Vol. 18, Academic Press, Inc., New York, 1973, p. 105.
62. B. Moss in W. A. Carter, ed., *Selective Inhibitors of Viral Functions,* Chemical Rubber Co. Press, Cleveland, Ohio, 1973, p. 313.
63. R. C. Ting, S. S. Yang, and R. C. Gallo, *Nature (London) New Biol.* **236,** 163 (1972).
64. R. G. Smith, J. Whang-Peng, R. C. Gallo, P. Levine, R. C. Ting, *Nature (London) New Biol.* **236,** 166 (1972).
65. R. G. Smith and R. C. Gallo, *Life Sci.* **15,** 1711 (1974).
66. P. Sensi, N. Maggi, R. Ballotta, S. Füresz, R. Pallarza, and V. Arioli, *J. Med. Chem.* **7,** 596 (1964).
67. F. R. Quinn, J. S. Driscoll, and C. Hansch, *J. Med. Chem.* **18,** 332 (1975).
68. N. Maggi, G. G. Gallo, and P. Sensi, *Farmaco Ed. Prat.* **20,** 147 (1965).
69. R. Pallanza, S. Füresz, M. T. Timbal, and G. Carniti, *Arzneim. Forsch.* **15,** 800 (1965).
70. S. Füresz, V. Arioli, and R. Scotti, *Arzneim. Forsch.* **15,** 802 (1965).
71. V. Dezulian, M. G. Serralunga, and G. Maffii, *Toxicol. Appl. Pharmacol.* **8,** 126 (1966).
72. P. Sensi, M. T. Timbal, and A. M. Greco, *Antibot. Chemother.* **12,** 488 (1962).
73. P. Sensi, N. Maggi, S. Füresz, and G. Maffii, *Antimicrob. Agents Chemother.* 699 (1966).
74. H. Bickel, F. Knüsel, W. Kump, and L. Neipp, *Antimicrob. Agents Chemother.* 352 (1966).
75. Neth. Pat. 6,411,694 (Apr. 12, 1965), (to CIBA Ltd.); *Chem. Abstr.* **65,** 12216f (1966).
76. G. G. Gallo, C. R. Pasqualucci, N. Maggi, R. Ballotta, and P. Sensi, *Farmaco Ed. Sci.* **21,** 68 (1966).
77. W. Kump and H. Bickel, *Helv. Chim. Acta* **56,** 2348 (1973).
78. U.S. Pat. 3,923,791 (Dec. 2, 1975), W. D. Celmer (to Pfizer Inc.).
79. F. Kradolfer, L. Neipp, and W. Sackmann, *Antimicrob. Agents Chemother.* 359 (1966).

80. M. Green, J. Bragdon, and A. Rankin, *Proc. Nat. Acad. Sci. U.S.A.* **69**, 1294 (1972).
81. M. F. Dampier and H. W. Whitlock, Jr., *J. Am. Chem. Soc.* **97**, 6254 (1975).
82. N. Maggi, V. Arioli, and P. Sensi, *J. Med. Chem.* **8**, 790 (1965).
83. N. Maggi, R. Pallanza, and P. Sensi, *Antimicrob. Agents Chemother.* **1965**, 765.
84. S. Füresz, V. Arioli, and R. Pallanza, *Antimicrob. Agents Chemother.* **1965**, 770.
85. Neth. Pat. 6,509,961 (Feb. 1, 1966), (to Lepetit S.p.A.).
86. N. Maggi, C. R. Pasqualucci, R. Ballotta, and P. Sensi, *Chemotherapy (Basel)* **11**, 285 (1966).
87. H. D. Cohn, *J. Clin. Pharmacol. J. New Drugs* **9**, 118 (1969).
88. G. Binda, E. Domenichini, A. Gottardi, B. Orlandi, E. Ortelli, B. Pacini, and G. Fowst, *Arzneim. Forsch.* **21**, 1907 (1971).
89. A. Vall-Spinosa, W. Lester, T. Moulding, P. T. Davidson, and J. K. McClatchy, *N. Eng. J. Med.* **283**, 616 (1970).
90. G. S. Avery, ed., *Drugs* **1**, 354 (1971).
91. W. Lester, *Ann. Rev. Microbiol.* **26**, 85 (1972).
92. D. B. Radner, *Chest* **64**, 213 (1973).
93. R. J. Clark, *N. Eng. J. Med.* **284**, 675 (1971).
94. P. Sensi, *Pure Appl. Chem.* **35**, 383 (1973).
95. A. N. Tischler, U. R. Joss, F. M. Thompson, and M. Calvin, *J. Med. Chem.* **16**, 1071 (1973).
96. F. M. Thompson, A. N. Tischler, J. Adams, and M. Calvin, *Proc. Nat. Acad. Sci. U.S.A.* **71**, 107 (1974).
97. A. N. Tischler, F. M. Thompson, L. J. Libertini, and M. Calvin, *J. Med. Chem.* **17**, 948 (1974).
98. A. M. Fietta and L. G. Silvestri, *Eur. J. Biochem.* **52**, 391 (1975).
99. R. Cricchio, G. Lancini, G. Tamborini, and P. Sensi, *J. Med. Chem.* **17**, 396 (1974).
100. G. Pelizza, G. C. Allievi, and G. G. Gallo, *Farmaco Ed. Sci.* **31**, 31 (1976).
101. J. M. Finkel, R. F. Pittillo, and L. B. Melleit, *Chemotherapy (Basel)* **16**, 380 (1971).
102. J. W. Lightbrown and P. deRossi, *Analyst* **90**, 89 (1965).
103. G. G. Gallo, P. Sensi, and P. Radaelli, *Farmaco Ed. Prat.* **15**, 283 (1960).
104. C. R. Pasqualucci, A. Vigevani, P. Radaelli, and G. G. Gallo, *J. Pharm. Sci.* **59**, 685 (1970).
105. G. G. Gallo, L. Chiesa, and P. Sensi, *Anal. Chem.* **34**, 423 (1962).
106. G. G. Gallo, L. Chiesa, and P. Sensi, *Farmaco Ed. Sci.* **17**, 668 (1962).
107. P. Sensi, C. Coronelli, and B. J. R. Nicolaus, *J. Chromatogr.* **5**, 519 (1961).
108. P. Sensi, C. Coronelli, and A. Binaghi, *Farmaco Ed. Prat.* **15**, 283 (1960).
109. M. Shibata, T. Hasegawa, and E. Higashide, *J. Antibiot.* **24**, 810 (1971).
110. T. Hasegawa, E. Higashide, and M. Shibata, *J. Antibiot.* **24**, 817 (1971).
111. T. Kishi, M. Asai, M. Muroi, S. Harada, E. Mizuta, S. Terao, T. Miki, and K. Mizuno, *Tetrahedron Lett.* **1969**, 91.
112. T. Kishi, S. Harada, M. Asai, M. Muroi, and K. Mizuno, *Tetrahedron Lett.* **1969**, 97.
113. K. Kamiya, T. Sugino, Y. Wada, M. Nishikawa, and T. Kishi, *Experientia* **25**, 901 (1969).
114. M. Kondo, T. Oishi, and K. Tsuchiya, *J. Antibiot.* **25**, 16 (1972).
115. T. Hasegawa, *J. Antibiot.* **25**, 25 (1972).
116. A. K. Ganguly, P. Kabasakalian, S. Kalliney, O. Sarre, S. Szmulewicz, and A. Westcott, *J. Org. Chem.* **41**, 1258 (1976).
117. T. H. Williams, *J. Antibiot.* **28**, 85 (1975).
118. P. V. Deshmukh, K. Kakinuma, J. J. Ameel, K. L. Rinehart, Jr., P. F. Wiley, and L. H. Li, *J. Am. Chem. Soc.* **98**, 870 (1976).
119. K. Sasaki, K. L. Rinehart, Jr., G. Slomp, M. F. Grostic, and E. C. Olson, *J. Am. Chem. Soc.* **92**, 7591 (1970).
120. L. H. Li, T. D. Clark, C. H. Cowie, and K. L. Rinehart, Jr., *Cancer Treatment Rep.* **61**, (1977).
121. R. F. Bryan, C. J. Gilmore, and R. C. Haltiwanger, *J. Chem. Soc. Perkin Trans.* 2 **1973**, 897.
122. M. K. Wolpert-Defilippes, R. H. Adamson, R. L. Cysyk, and D. G. Johns, *Biochem. Pharmacol.* **24**, 751 (1975).
123. W. Wehrli and M. Staehelin, *Bacteriol. Rev.* **35**, 290 (1971).
124. W. Wehrli and M. Staehelin in J. W. Corcoran and F. E. Hahn, eds., *Antibiotics,* Vol. 3, Springer-Verlag New York, Inc., New York, 1975, p. 252.
125. W. Stender and K. H. Scheit, *Eur. J. Biochem.* **65**, 333 (1976).
126. L. R. Yarbrough, F. Y.-H. Wu, and C.-W. Wu, *Biochem.* **15**, 2669 (1976).

FREDERICK J. ANTOSZ
The Upjohn Company

β-LACTAMS

The β-lactam antibiotics comprise two groups of therapeutic agents of considerable clinical importance—the penicillins and cephalosporins—and several recently discovered fermentation products of unestablished utility (in 1977), including the cephamycins, nocardicins, thienamycins, and clavulanic acid. Figure 1 illustrates the essential structural features of these antibiotics (**1–6**). As their name implies, these substances have in their chemical structures a 4-membered lactam. With the exception of the nocardicins, the β-lactam is fused through the nitrogen and the adjacent tetrahedral carbon atom to a second heterocycle—a 5-membered thiazolidine, pyrroline, or oxazolidine for the penicillins, thienamycin, and clavulanic acid, respectively, or a 6-membered dihydrothiazine for the cephalosporins and cephamycins. These antibiotics carry a variety of substituents which contribute to their biological properties. A structural feature common to virtually all of the β-lactam antibiotics is the carboxyl group on the carbon adjacent to the lactam nitrogen, although this group has now been chemically converted to a tetrazole with retention of biological activity (see (**26**)). Another feature shared by the penicillins, cephalosporins, and cephamycins is the functionalized amino group on the carbon atom opposite the nitrogen of the β-lactam. The cephalosporins (**2**) and cephamycins (**3**) have the same basic structure except that the cephamycins have a methoxy group instead of a hydrogen on the amide-bearing carbon atom (C-7).

The β-lactam antibiotics inhibit bacteria, exhibiting activities that differ in

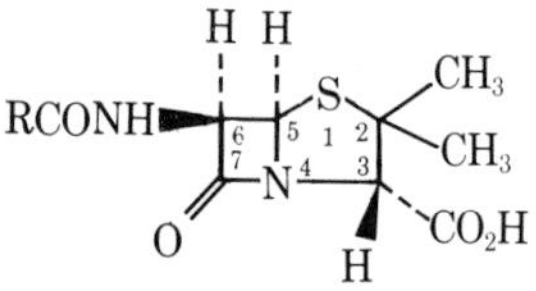

Penicillins
(**1**)

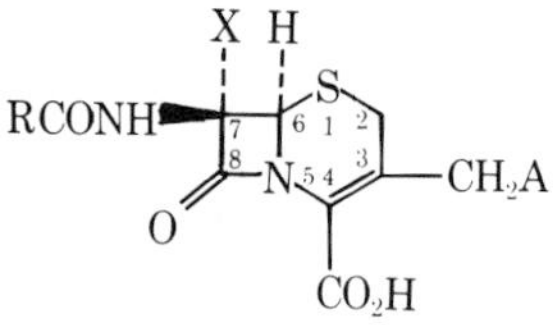

Cephalosporins (X = H) (**2**)
Cephamycins (X = OCH_3) (**3**)

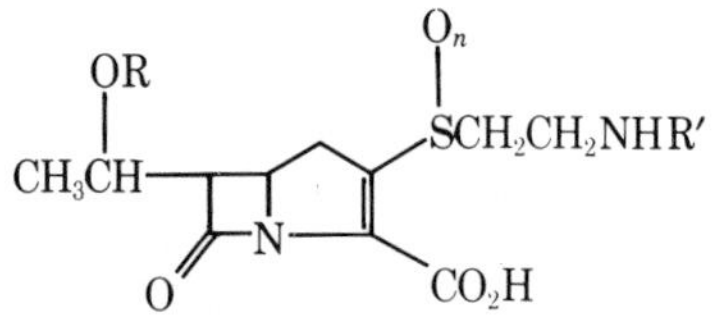

R = H, SO_3H; R′ = H, $COCH_3$; n = 0, 1
(Epi) thienamycins
(**4**)

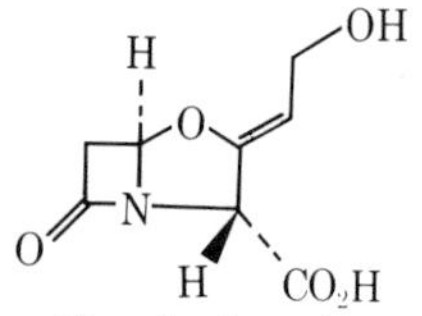

Clavulanic acid
(**5**)

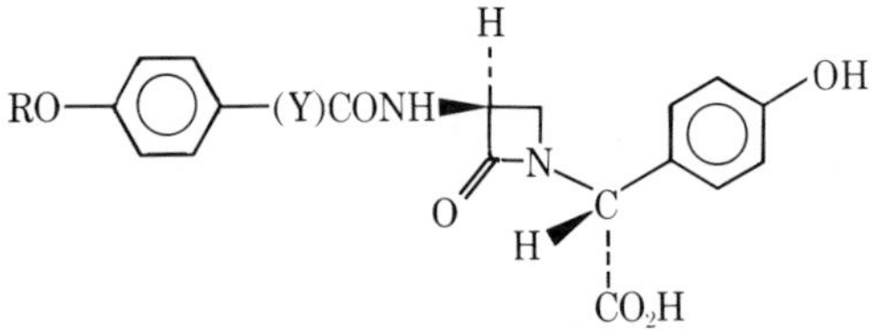

R′ = H, D-$HO_2CCH(NH_2)CH_2CH_2$—;
Y = C=NOH(syn, anti), $CHNH_2$, C=O
Nocardicins A–G
(**6**)

Figure 1. β-Lactam antibiotics.

pattern and intensity. In general, they exert their biological effect by interfering with the synthesis of essential structural components of the bacterial cell wall. These components are absent in mammalian cells so that synthesis of bacterial cell-wall structure can be inhibited with little or no effect on mammalian cell metabolism. In addition, these antibiotics tend to be irreversible inhibitors of cell wall synthesis and they are usually bactericidal at concentrations close to their bacteriostatic levels. As a consequence, the penicillins and cephalosporins are used widely for treating bacterial infections, and are regarded as highly effective antibiotics with low toxicity.

Since the thienamycins, nocardicins, cephamycins and clavulanic acid, were discovered more recently than the penicillins and the cephalosporins, nearly all of the present knowledge of the β-lactam antibiotics relates to the latter two antibiotic classes. This article deals with the information concerning the penicillins and cephalosporins; references to the other members of the group are included where appropriate.

Nomenclature. *Chemical Abstracts* indexes most penicillins as 4-thia-1-azabicyclo[3.2.0]heptanes, and cephalosporins and cephamycins as 5-thia-1-azabicyclo[4.2.0]oct-2-enes (Fig. 2). Using this system, penicillin G [(1) R = $C_6H_5CH_2$] is 6-(2-phenylacetamido)-3,3-dimethyl-7-oxo-4-thia-1-azabicyclo[3.2.0]heptane-2-carboxylic acid and cephalosporin C [(2) R = $HO_2CCH(NH_2)(CH_2)_3$—, A = — $OCOCH_3$] is 3-(acetoxymethyl)-7-(D-5-amino-5-carboxyvaleramido)-8-oxo-5-thia-1-azabicyclo[4.2.0]oct-2-ene-2-carboxylic acid. Obviously, the chemical substance names derived from this nomenclature system are too cumbersome for general use. One simplification designates the unsubstituted bicyclic ring systems of the penicillins and cephalosporins as penam (7) (1) and cepham (8) (2), respectively. Thus the penicillins are generally 6-acylamino-2,2-dimethylpenam-3-carboxylic acids and the cephalosporins are 3-acetoxymethyl-7-acylamino-3-cephem-4-carboxylic acids. This nomenclature is widely used, especially in the chemically oriented literature dealing with the cephalosporins and cephamycins. A further simplification with narrower structural latitude is the use of the terms penicillanic acid (1) and cephalosporanic acid (3) to designate the penicillin and cephalosporin ring systems with the substituents indicated in structures (9) and (10). In this case the penicillins and cephalosporins are named as the appropriate acylaminopenicillanic and cephalosporanic acids. Although convenient, this naming becomes restrictive for the cephalosporins in which the 3-acetoxymethyl grouping has been replaced by other substituents. For the penicillins a straightforward naming system is widely used that relies on the fact that nearly all of the variations of the penicillin structure are on the acyl group; in this case the carbonyl of the acyl group is included in the basic moiety name penicillin (11); here penicillin G is named benzylpenicillin (Table 1).

The discovery of penicillin in 1929 by Sir Alexander Fleming (4) and the subsequent recognition in 1940 by Florey, Chain, Abraham, and their colleagues of the potential utility of penicillin for controlling infections in animals (5), and shortly afterward in man (6), has been recounted many times (7), including the autobiographical writings of the principals in a review of the penicillins (8). The realization that penicillin was a useful drug occurred during World War II and an immediate attempt was made to produce the antibiotic on a large scale in the United States and later in Britain. Accompanying the scale-up of production were widespread studies on the chemical properties and structure of the antibiotic involving many industrial concerns, universities, and hospitals on both sides of the Atlantic. The results of this research were kept secret until after the war when the chronological account and the details of the chemical studies were published in 1949 (9).

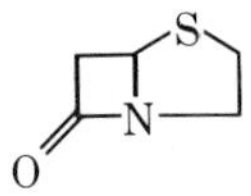

Penam
7-Oxo-4-thia-1-azabicyclo[3.2.0]heptane
[53908-04-6]
(7)

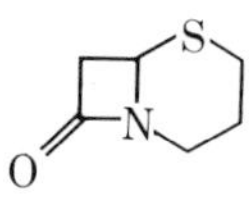

Cepham
8-Oxo-5-thia-1-azabicyclo[4.2.0]octane
[25795-42-0]
(8)

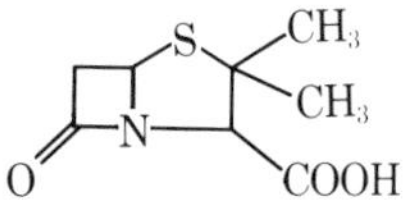

Penicillanic acid
[87-53-6]
(9)

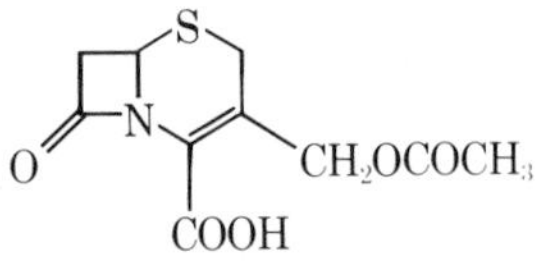

Cephalosporanic acid
[4704-60-3]
(10)

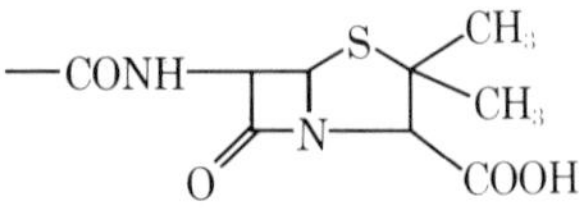

Penicillin
(11)
(see Table 1)

Figure 2. Nomenclature systems.

Table 1. Biosynthetic Penicillins

Name	CAS Registry Number[a]	United States designation	British designation	Side chain (11)
2-pentenylpenicillin	[118-53-6]	F	I	$CH_3CH_2CH=CHCH_2—$
pentylpenicillin	[4493-18-9]	dihydro F	dihydro I	$CH_3(CH_2)_4—$
heptylpenicillin	[525-97-3]	K	IV	$CH_3(CH_2)_6—$
benzylpenicillin	[61-33-6]	G	II	$C_6H_5CH_2—$
p-hydroxybenzylpenicillin	[525-91-7]	X	III	$p\text{-}HO—C_6H_4CH_2—$
D-4-amino-4-carboxybutyl-penicillin	[525-94-0]	N[b]		$D\text{-}HO_2CCH(NH_2)(CH_2)_3—$
L-4-amino-4-carboxybutyl-penicillin	[525-94-0]	iso-N		$L\text{-}HO_2CCH(NH_2)(CH_2)_3—$
phenoxymethylpenicillin	[87-08-1]	V		$C_6H_5OCH_2—$
butylthiomethylpenicillin	[525-87-1]		BT	$C_4H_9SCH_2—$
allylthiomethylpenicillin	[87-09-2]	O	AT	$CH_2=CHCH_2SCH_2—$
4-carboxybutylpenicillin	[18991-52-1]			$HO_2C(CH_2)_4—$
p-aminobenzylpenicillin	[2510-42-1]	T		$p\text{-}NH_2—C_6H_4CH_2—$
p-nitrobenzylpenicillin	[36143-18-7]			$p\text{-}NO_2—C_6H_4CH_2—$

[a] Salts of these acids with cations other than hydrogen have different registry numbers.
[b] Also known as cephalosporin N and synnematin B.

Penicillin was first obtained as a product of the fungus *Penicillium notatum*. Its early manufacture utilized this organism on surface cultures that were cumbersome and not amenable to large-scale handling. The American workers, notably Coghill and colleagues, quickly introduced modifications which included replacing the surface cultures with deep fermentations, adopting high-yielding strains of *Penicillium chrysogenum* and substituting corn steep liquor for the less readily available yeast extract (10). As soon as reasonably pure samples of the penicillins were obtained it became obvious that the penicillin initially crystallized by workers in the United States was different from the one under study by the British investigators. Strong hydrolysis of the penicillins yielded phenylacetic acid in the case of the American preparations and 2-hexenoic acid from the British penicillin. It was soon recognized that penicillins with different acyl side chains could be obtained from unaided fermentations depending on the strain of the mold used and the composition of the fermentation medium (eg, corn steep liquor vs yeast extract). Subsequently it was found that various modified penicillins could be obtained by adding appropriate side-chain precursors to the fermentation mixture (Table 1) (11). For example, benzylpenicillin was obtained by adding phenylacetic acid or various benzenoid precursors of this acid to the fermentations. About 50 biosynthetic penicillins were investigated; three (penicillin G, V, and O) were produced commercially. Only penicillins with an unsubstituted methylene adjacent to the amide carbonyl (monosubstituted acetamides) could be generated by this approach.

Although there was an intense effort to purify the antibiotic and determine its structure from 1940 onward, it was 1945 before the combined results of chemical degradations and x-ray crystallography made it possible to be certain that the penicillin structure contained the β-lactam-thiazolidine ring system (12). This was partly due to the extreme lability of the molecule, making it difficult to obtain pure samples, and to the unexpectedness of the β-lactam ring in a natural substance.

In 1959, Bachelor and his colleagues reported the isolation of the penicillin nucleus, 6-aminopenicillanic acid (1) (6-APA; RCO = H) from fermentations deficient in side-chain precursors (13). It was soon found that 6-APA could be produced more efficiently by enzymatically removing the acyl group from various penicillins using penicillin acylases. Subsequently this intermediate has been made for manufacturing purposes by chemically removing the 6-acyl group after first protecting the carboxyl group. The availability of 6-aminopenicillanic acid has resulted in the preparation and testing of literally thousands of penicillin analogues derived by acylation of the 6-amino group. The amino group has also been converted to a variety of other substituents. From this vast chemical investment only a dozen or so semisynthetic penicillins have found wide use in clinical medicine (see Table 2).

The discovery and development of the cephalosporins began with the finding by Brotzu that a *Cephalosporium* species produced antibiotic material that was active against certain gram-negative as well as gram-positive organisms (14). This fungus was later found by the Oxford workers to produce at least six antibiotic substances. Five were steroidal (cephalosporin P_1–P_5) and active only against gram-positive bacteria. A major hydrophilic component, active against gram-positive and gram-negative organisms and originally called cephalosporin N, was found to be D-4-amino-4-carboxybutyl penicillin (Table 1), identical to synnematin B which had been described earlier (15). It has been renamed penicillin N. In the process of studying the ion-exchange chromatography of the products from the acid degradation of penicillin N, Abraham and Newton discovered a second hydrophilic antibiotic that had survived the degradation (16). This material was apparently present only in minute amounts in the original fermentation mixture. They named the new product cephalosporin C (Table 3).

Chemical studies demonstrated a similarity between penicillin N and cephalosporin C; both contained an α-aminoadipamido substituent and a fused β-lactam ring system. Additional studies led Abraham and Newton to suggest the correct structure for cephalosporin C which was confirmed by x-ray crystallographic studies (17). This work has been described in detail (18). In contrast to the penicillins where many an-

Table 2. Penicillins in Clinical Use

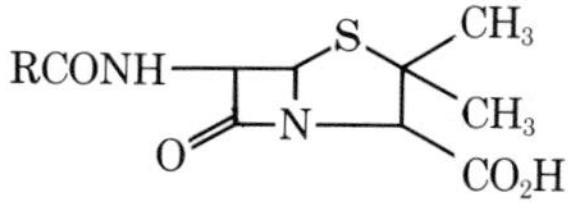

Generic name	CAS Registry Number	R	Route[a]	Av daily dose, g
Narrow spectrum				
benzylpenicillin (penicillin G)	[61-33-6]		iv im po	3–12[b] 1–7[c] 0.6–6[d]
phenoxymethylpenicillin (penicillin V)	[87-08-1]		po	0.3–6
phenethicillin	[132-93-4]	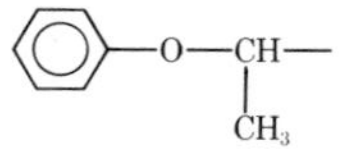	po	0.5–1
β-Lactamase resistant				
methicillin	[132-92-3]		im iv	6–12 4–6
oxacillin, X = H, Y = H	[66-79-5]	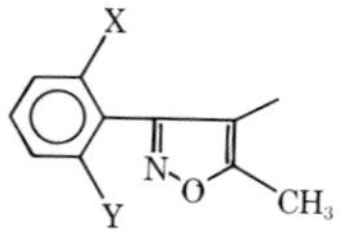	po, im, iv	1–6
cloxacillin, X = H, Y = Cl	[61-72-3]		po	1–6
dicloxacillin, X = Cl, Y = Cl	[3116-76-5]		po	1–6

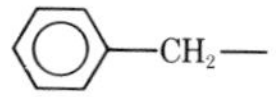

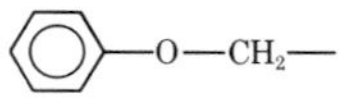

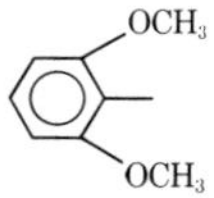

	CAS No.	Structure	Route[a]	Dose
nafcillin	[985-16-0]	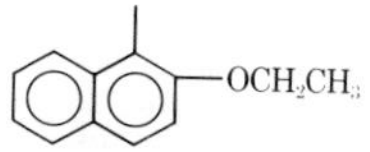 methylnaphthalene–OCH$_2$CH$_3$	po	1–2
Broad spectrum				
ampicillin	[69-53-4]	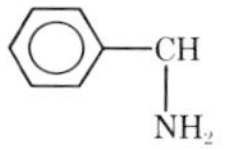 phenyl–CH–NH$_2$	po	1–4
hetacillin	[3511-16-8]	(acetonide)	iv/im	2–4
amoxicillin	[26787-78-0]	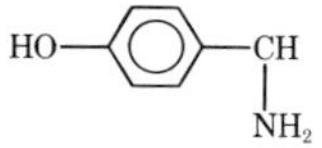 HO–phenyl–CH–NH$_2$	po	0.75–1.5
Broad spectrum–narrow use				
carbenicillin	[4697-36-3]	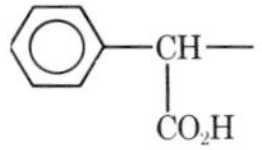 phenyl–CH–CO$_2$H	iv	to 40
– indanyl ester	[26605-69-6]			
ticarcillin	[34787-01-4]	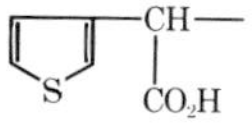 thiophene–CH–CO$_2$H		
sulbenicillin	[41744-40-5]	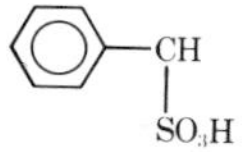 phenyl–CH–SO$_3$H		
acylated ampicillins		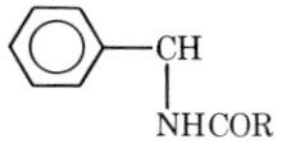 phenyl–CH–NHCOR		

[a] iv, intravenously; im, intramuscularly; po, orally.
[b] 5–20 million units.
[c] 2–12 million units.
[d] 1–10 million units.

Table 3. Naturally Occurring Cephalosporins and Cephamycins

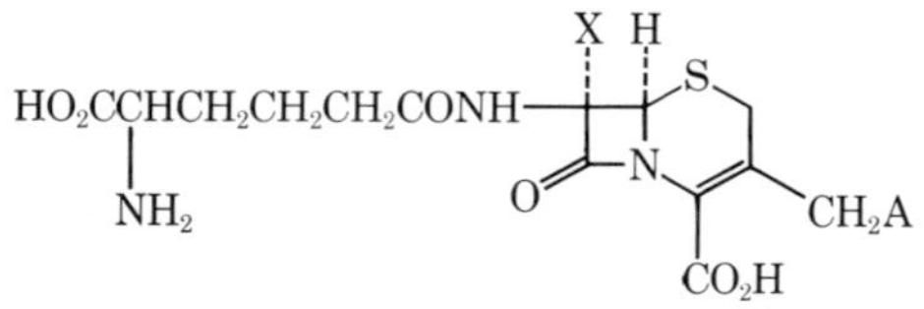

Name	CAS Registry Number	X	A
cephalosporin C	[61-24-5]	H	$OCOCH_3$
deacetylcephalosporin C	[1476-46-6]	H	OH
deacetoxycephalosporin C	[26924-74-3]	H	H
carbamyldeacetylcephalosporin C	[32178-83-9]	H	$OCONH_2$
3'-methylthiodeacetoxycephalosporin C	[60890-86-0]	H	SCH_3
cephamycin A	[34279-78-2]	OCH_3	$OCOC(OCH_3)=CHC_6H_4OSO_2OH$ (p)
cephamycin B	[34279-77-1]	OCH_3	$OCOC(OCH_3)=CHC_6H_4OH$ (p)
Takeda C2801X	[62851-50-7]	OCH_3	$OCOC(OCH_3)=CHC_6H_3(OH)_2$ (m, p)
cephamycin C	[34279-51-1]	OCH_3	$OCONH_2$
7α-methoxycephalosporin C	[32178-82-8]	OCH_3	$OCOCH_3$

alogues were obtained depending on the precursors present in the fermentation mixture, all cephalosporins found in nature have the same 7-acyl side chain, D-α-aminoadipic acid. Initial attempts to improve cephalosporin C paralleled the earlier penicillin experiences. A substantial amount of work was directed toward replacing the aminoadipic acid side chain or modifying it appropriately. However, modified cephalosporins could not be produced by precursor-fed fermentation or by enzymatic transfer of acyl groups using cephalosporin C as a substrate. Similarly, attempts to produce 7-aminocephalosporanic acid (7-ACA) by splitting off the aminoadipoyl side chain with the enzymes that readily removed the acyl group from penicillins were uniformly unsuccessful. A practical chemical process to remove this side chain by using nitrosyl chloride in anhydrous formic acid was reported by Morin and his co-workers in 1962 (2). Several related processes were subsequently developed centering around carboxyl-protected imino ether intermediates.

Like 6-APA, 7-aminocephalosporanic acid has given rise to thousands of new semisynthetic cephalosporins. The cephalosporin structure offers more opportunities for chemical modification than the penicillins (Table 3). In addition to the sulfur, double bond, carboxyl group, and unsubstituted positions, there are two side chains that especially lend themselves to chemical manipulation: the 7-acylamino and the 3-acetoxymethyl substituents. Nearly all possible modifications have been tried through a huge investment in research on this chemical system by the academic and pharmaceutical communities.

The cephamycins were described almost simultaneously by workers at Lilly and at Merck in 1971 (19). These antibiotics are produced by *Streptomyces* species. They have the basic cephalosporin ring system with differences in the substituents at the 7α- and 3-positions (Table 3) (20). Again, the natural products from the fermentation have the D-α-aminoadipamido substituent at the 7-position. The chemical experiences with the cephalosporins and penicillins were applied to the cephamycins to produce semisynthetic analogues (21). These have been obtained by chemically introducing a methoxy group at the 7α-position of the cephalosporin ring system and by manipulating the 3- and 7-substituents of the natural cephamycins. One derivative is now under intensive clinical evaluation (22).

Thienamycin was first described by workers at Merck in 1976 (23). Like the cephalosporins and cephamycins, it was discovered as a fermentation product with broad antibacterial activity, in this case from *Streptomyces cattleya*. The nocardicins, first described in 1976 by workers at Fujisawa, were discovered in a screen using a mutant of *Escherichia coli* specifically supersensitive to β-lactams, and confirmed to be a β-lactam-containing substance by inactivation with β-lactamases (24). Clavulanic acid, also reported first in 1976 by Beecham Laboratories, was discovered by still another approach, a program of screening for novel β-lactamase inhibitors. This material is only weakly active against bacteria and is produced along with penicillin N and two cephalosporins by *Streptomyces clavuligerus* (25). Other than structure determination and initial biological studies, very little chemical work has yet been reported for these three new β-lactam systems.

Physical Properties

There are several properties that are shared by a sufficient number of the structurally divergent β-lactam antibiotics to allow them to be cited as characteristic

(26). For the most part, these antibiotics when obtained in reasonably pure form are white, off-white, tan, or yellow solids that are usually amorphous, sometimes crystalline. They do not usually have sharp melting points, but decompose upon heating to elevated temperatures. Most natural members have a free carboxyl group; as their salts, they are soluble in polar solvents, especially water. When other ionizable substituents are absent they are soluble in organic solvents as their free acids. For example, benzylpenicillin and other biosynthetic penicillins are routinely extracted from acidified fermentation broths into organic solvents as a part of the isolation process. Obviously, the presence of other polar substituents, especially an amino group (eg, cephalosporin C, penicillin N, ampicillin, cephalexin) will appropriately modify this behavior. The acid strength (pK_a) of the carboxyl group indigenously attached to the central ring system varies, depending on its environment. The pK_a values extrapolated to the pK_a in water if determined in mixed solvents are included in Table 4.

One of the most distinguishing physical characteristics of these substances is the infrared stretching frequency of the β-lactam carbonyl group. Values for this property, along with the carbonyl stretching frequencies for the amide groupings, when present in the molecule, are included in Table 4. The β-lactam-carbonyl stretching occurs at characteristically high frequencies (1770–1815 cm^{-1} in the penicillins and cephalosporins) compared to the absorptions for secondary amide (1504–1695 cm^{-1}) and ester (1720–1780 cm^{-1}) carbonyl groups. Its absorption frequency provides information about the integrity of the β-lactam, the nature of rings fused thereto, and the oxidation state of the sulfur atom of the fused ring in the penicillins and cephalosporins.

Similarly, the nuclear magnetic resonance signals derived from the protons attached to the two tetrahedral carbon atoms of the β-lactam ring (eg, C-5 and C-6 of the penicillins, C-6 and C-7 of the cephalosporins) provide information about the integrity of the ring, attachments to the ring and the stereochemistry of the attachments. In the penicillins and cephalosporins these protons form an ABX system with the vicinal proton on the side-chain amide nitrogen atom. Thus the proton on the amide-bearing carbon atom gives rise to a quartet (or a doublet in solvents providing NH–deuterium exchange) (δ_{PEN} = 5.42–6.15, δ_{CPH} = 5.23–6.21; J_{AB} (cis) = 4–5 Hz, J_{AB} (trans) = 1.5–2 Hz, J_{AX} = 8–11 Hz) and the proton on the bridgehead carbon gives rise to a doublet (δ_{PEN} = 4.66–5.60, δ_{CPH} = 4.24–5.46; J_{AB} = as above). More detailed information on the influence of structure and adjacent groupings on spectral behavior (ir and nmr) is in the references cited in Table 4.

The penicillin and clavulanic acid rings do not absorb ultraviolet light. However, the natural (Δ-3) cephalosporins display absorption maxima (Table 4) at about 260 nm. The fact that this occurs at a longer wavelength than expected for an α,β-unsaturated amide acid (α-acetamide-β,β-dimethylacrylic acid absorbs at 223 nm) has been explained in terms of participation of the d-orbital of the sulfur atom with the nitrogen atom and the double bond of the dihydrothiazine ring (31). Saturation of the double bond results in loss of the ultraviolet absorption. Thienamycin has an ultraviolet absorption maximum at 296 nm (23).

Chemical Properties

In the past thirty-five years, there have been many determinations of basic chemical properties, degradations and structure elucidations of the β-lactam antibiotics (8–9,19,23–25,32), as well as total syntheses of penicillins and cephalosporins (33),

Table 4. Physical Properties of Some β-Lactam Antibiotics[a]

Name	CAS Registry Number	Melting point	pKa[b]	β-Lactam ir stretching frequency, cm⁻¹ [c]	Ring system uv absorbance, nm [d]	Nmr resonance[e] δ(HA)	δ(HB)	JAB	Optical rotation[f] Temp, °C	[α]D[b]
6-APA	[551-16-6]	209–210 (dec)	2.29, 4.90	1775		4.64d	5.54d	4.0	31	+273 (c, 1.2)[g]
benzylpenicillin sodium salt	[69-57-8]	215 (dec)	2.76	1775		5.56d	5.44d	4.0	24.8	+301 (c, 2.0)
ampicillin	[69-53-4]	199–202 (dec)	2.53, 7.24	1770		5.51s	5.51s		23	+287.9
7-ACA	[957-68-6]	>200 (dec)	1.75, 4.63	1806	261 (ε8500)	50% 5.53d 50% 4.83d	5.13d	4.5	20	+114 (c, 1)
cephalosporin C	[61-24-5]		<2.6, 3.1, 9.8	1780	260 ($E_{1cm}^{1\%}$ 200)	5.66d	5.75d	4.7	20	+103[h]
cephalothin sodium	[58-71-9]			1760	265 ($E_{1cm}^{1\%}$ 204)	5.70d	5.14d	4.5		+130 (c, 5)
cephalexin	[15686-71-2]		5.2, 7.3	1775	260 (ε7750)	6.10d	5.45d	4.201-01.153 (c, 1)		+153 (c, 1)
cephamycin C	[34279-51-1]		4.2, 5.6, 10.4[i]	1770	264, 242 (ε6900, 5700)		5.19s			
thienamycin	[59995-64-1]		3.08[j]	1765[k]	296.5 (ε7900)	3.39dd	4.25m	2.9	27	+82.7 (c, 0.1)
nocardicin A	[39391-39-4]	234–235 (dec)	3.2, 4.5, 10.0, 11.6, 12.7[m]	1730	270 (ε14900)	4.96m[n]	3.83t (4α)			−135 (c, 1)
clavulanic acid	[58001-44-8]		2.4–2.7			3.54dd (6α)[o]	5.72dd (5α)	2.8	20	+47[o]
methyl ester	[57943-82-5]			1800					22	+38.0[p]

[a] Refs. 9, 19, 23–25, and 27–30.
[b] Except where noted pKa values are for aqueous solutions, determined directly or extrapolated from mixed solvents.
[c] In most cases from Nujol mull or natural film.
[d] In aqueous solution except nocardicin A (ethanol–water).
[e] In D2O except where noted: s, singlet; d, doublet; m, multiplet; δ, ppm relative to TMS; J, coupling constant in Hz; HA, α proton on penultimate carbon from β-lactam nitrogen; HB; α proton on carbon adjacent to β-lactam nitrogen.
[f] In water unless indicated.
[g] In 0.1 N HCl.
[h] For dihydrate.
[i] In 66% DMF.
[j] In phosphate buffer.
[k] Methyl ester 1779 cm⁻¹.
[l] In phosphate buffer at pH 6.95.
[m] In 50% DMSO.
[n] In DMSO-d6.
[o] Solvent unreported.
[p] Amine salt of tetrahydrate.

interconversions of penicillins and cephalosporins, modifications of the substituents and the basic chemical structures of these antibiotics, and, most recently, semisynthesis and total synthesis of new β-lactam-containing compounds that resemble the fermentation-derived antibiotics in structure and biological activity. Described below are the chemical properties that pertain to the manufacture and use of these antibiotics and to those manipulations that have been carried out to create new derivatives and analogues of the natural antibiotics with improved biological characteristics (9,26,34).

Stereochemistry. The stereochemical configurations of the penicillins, cephalosporins, and cephamycins are indicated in the structures in Figure 1. The stereochemistry around the β-lactam is the same in these three series, ie, the asymmetric centers at C-5 and C-6 in the penicillins correspond to those at C-6 and C-7 in the cephalosporins and cephamycins. The amide-bearing carbon atom (C-6 of the penicillins and C-7 of the cephalosporins) has the R-configuration. The fused rings are, of course, not coplanar but are folded along the C-5 to N-4 axis of the penicillins and the C-6 to N-5 bond of the cephalosporins and cephamycins. The configuration of the fused rings is such that the hydrogen on the carbon atom at the ring junction is cis to the hydrogen (or methoxy group) on the amide-bearing carbon atom. In the penicillins the carbon atom carrying the carboxyl group (C-3) has the S-configuration, thus placing the carboxyl group on the opposite side of the ring system from the amide group at C-6. This asymmetric center does not exist in the cephalosporins and cephamycins because of the endocyclic double bond in the dihydrothiazine ring. In summary, the absolute stereochemistry of the penicillins is $3S:5R:6R$, and for the cephalosporins it is $6R:7R$. The stereochemistry of the substituents attached to the rings is designated by the α and β notations. Accordingly, the β-lactam hydrogens are α, the acylamino groups are β, the penicillin carboxyl is α, and the 17-methoxy group of the cephamycins is α.

β-Lactam. The β-lactam antibiotics are generally reactive substances. The level of reactivity ranges from the nocardicins (24), which are stable over a fairly wide pH range, through the penicillins, which are only moderately stable in solutions that are near to neutrality (pH 5–8), to thienamycin (23), which is extremely unstable outside of a very narrow pH range (pH 6–7), requires the presence of phosphate buffer or its equivalent for reasonable stability even within this pH range, and rapidly undergoes self-condensation at concentrations above 1.0 mg/mL.

Much of the chemical reactivity of these molecules is associated with the β-lactam. The simple β-lactam (eg, in nocardicin) has little amide-resonance stabilization, indicated by its relatively high carbonyl stretching frequency (1730 cm^{-1}). In the fused ring systems the geometry and the accompanying increased ring strain results in even less resonance stabilization (carbonyl stretching frequency: penicillins, 1770–1790 cm^{-1}; cephalosporins, 1760–1800 cm^{-1}) and greater reactivity. In many situations the reactivity of the lactam carbonyl group is analogous to that of a carboxylic acid anhydride (9). Thus the fused-β-lactam antibiotics are readily attacked by nucleophiles and by electrophiles with resultant opening of the lactam ring and loss of biological activity (9). The penicillins are rapidly hydrolyzed by aqueous alkali to the corresponding penicilloic acids (12) which are stable as their salts, but which decarboxylate on acidification to yield penilloic acids (13).

$$(12) \qquad (13)$$

This ring-opening sequence serves as a basis for the chemical assay of penicillins and, to a lesser extent, cephalosporins. The alkali required for the initial hydrolysis is determined by back titration with acid, or the penicilloic acid is assayed by titration with iodine. Hydroxylamine reacts with the β-lactam to give the corresponding hydroxamic acid which can be assayed colorimetrically as its ferric complex. Alkoxides, ammonia, amines, and other nucleophiles will react analogously with the penicillins to give penicilloic acid esters and amides.

Penicillins are also destroyed by aqueous acids. This degradation proceeds via initial interaction of the side-chain carbonyl group with the lactam, probably after protonation of the lactam nitrogen, to give penicillenic acids (14) when the hydrolysis is carried out at pH 4 and penillic acids (15) at pH 2.

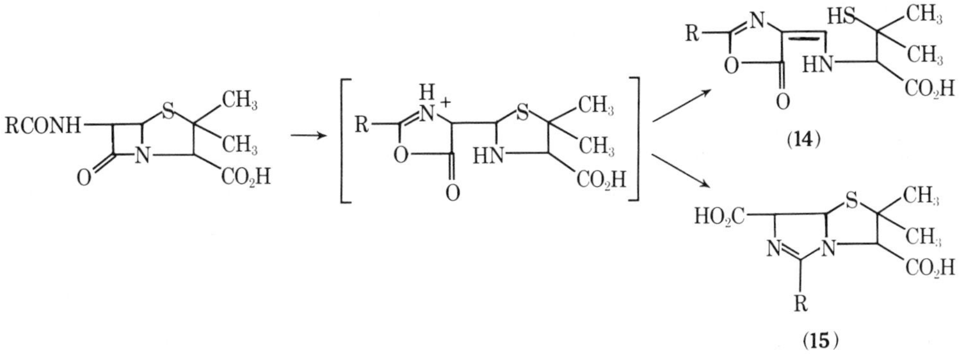

Electron withdrawing groups at the α-position of the 6-acyl substituent influence this attack by the side-chain carbonyl. Thus penicillins, such as phenoxymethylpenicillin and ampicillin, are more stable to acids, and are absorbed more efficiently than benzylpenicillin by the oral route. Neutral solutions of penicillins are fairly stable but trace impurities can catalyze decomposition. The reaction of penicillins with alcohols is catalyzed by mercury and other heavy metal ions and hydrolysis in neutral aqueous solution is speeded up by traces of sulfite or thiols such as cysteine. Surprisingly, 6-aminopenicillanic acid undergoes decomposition to a penillic acid-like structure in solutions containing sodium bicarbonate even though it has no assisting 6-acyl group. In this case, carbon dioxide adds to the amino group to form a carbamic acid which rearranges to the penillic acid structure (15) shown above where, in the enol form, R equals hydroxyl (35). 7-ACA also forms the analogous carbamic acid since the 7-methyl carbamate can be obtained on treatment with methyl iodide, but in contrast to 6-APA it does not undergo the succeeding rearrangement (36).

The cephalosporins are more resistant to ring-opening than the penicillins. For example, although alcohols readily attack the penicillin lactam, cephalosporins are sufficiently stable to permit the use of methanol as a recrystallization solvent. The cephalosporins are also more resistant to acids. They are attacked by nucleophiles, such as alkoxide or hydroxylamine, but because of the nature of the dihydrothiazine ring, products equivalent to penicilloic and penilloic acids are not obtained. Rather, studies by Abraham and others indicate involvement of the 3-substituent analogously to the formation of (16) (37).

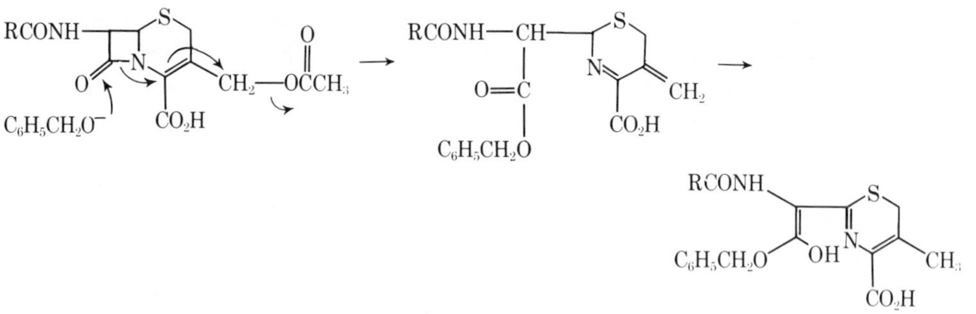

(16)

In harmony with this, 3-deacetoxycephalosporins are found to be more stable to these degradation conditions than cephalosporins with 3-substituents that can be readily lost. These relationships appear to correlate with biological activity, which can be influenced by substituents on the 3-position of the cephalosporin ring, the deacetoxy analogues generally showing lower levels of *in vitro* activities than their 3-functionalized analogues.

   Penicillin to Cephalosporin Conversions. The penicillin sulfoxides have provided a means for chemically correlating the penicillin and cephalosporin structures, and a commercial process for obtaining cephalosporins from the less expensive penicillins. In 1963, Morin and co-workers reported that penicillin V sulfoxide methyl ester, when heated with acetic anhydride gave a mixture of penicillin acetate (17) and cepham acetate (18) (38). When heated in toluene with a trace of acid, the sulfoxide gave the deacetoxycephalosporanic acid (19) (R = $C_6H_5OCH_2$, R′ = CH_3 [10209-06-0]). The identical compound (19) was obtained by hydrogenolysis of 7-phenoxyacetamido-cephalosporanic acid methyl ester [57943-82-5], thus establishing the correlation between the penicillin and cephalosporin structures (39). This conversion has been studied intensively and improved so that it is now the primary industrial route to 7-ADCA and the deacetoxycephalosporins cephalexin and cephradine. Reaction conditions and the choice of protective groups are discussed on page 122. The free sulfenic acid intermediates (20) are unstable and rapidly cyclize to the penicillin sulfoxide (21) and cephalosporin (19) structures. The ring-opened form can be trapped by electrophiles to give, eg, the trimethylsilyl esters, or by nucleophiles (dihydropyran, thiols) which produce sulfides, disulfides, and the like. The myriad reactions and mechanism studies which this work has generated have been extensively reviewed (40).

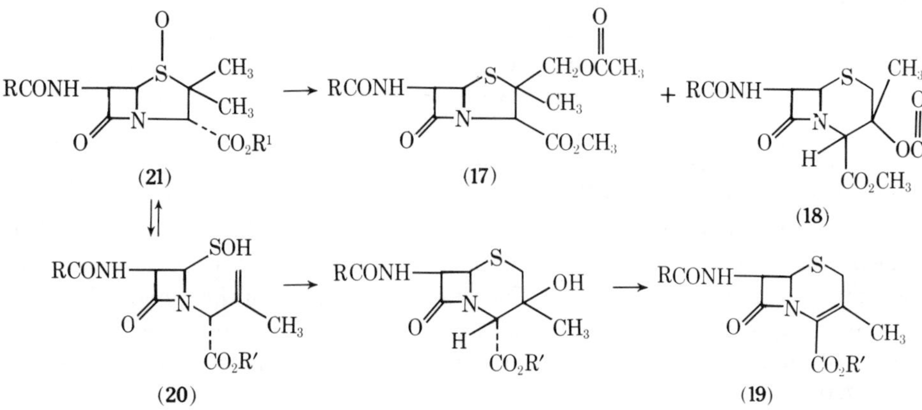

New β-Lactam-Containing Structures.   Both the penicillin and cephalosporin structures have been constructed by total synthesis for academic purposes (32–33). The penicillin ring system was obtained by forming the thiazolidine ring first and then annelating the β-lactam via attached substituents. Cephalosporin C was synthesized by constructing the β-lactam first and annelating the dihydrothiazine to it. More recently, a large number of unnatural β-lactam-containing structures have been synthesized, and several have been found to possess significant antibacterial activities. Many of these new structures have been obtained through the β-lactam sulfenic acids formed from the thiazolidine-ring openings of penicillin sulfoxides ($21 \rightarrow 20$). Others were made by constructing the β-lactam chemically, and attaching entirely new rings. Reviews of this rapidly expanding area of chemistry are starting to appear (40–41).

Biological Properties

Structure–Activity Relationships.   Much of the chemical work that has been done on the β-lactam antibiotics has been directed toward modifying and improving the antibacterial and pharmacokinetic properties of these substances. These chemical studies are closely coupled with extensive biological evaluations which examine properties, such as *in vitro* and *in vivo* antibacterial activities (minimum inhibitory concentrations (MIC), minimum bactericidal concentrations (MBC), and protective effectiveness in laboratory animals (PD_{50})), and pharmacokinetic characteristics (including: efficiency of absorption by oral and parenteral routes, serum levels, tissue distribution, urinary excretion, metabolism, serum binding, serum and tissue inactivation, biliary excretion and recycling, etc). The modified antibiotics are also tested for their abilities to resist inactivation by enzymes, specifically β-lactamases (penicillinases, cephalosporinases) produced by both gram-positive and gram-negative bacteria. Although many of these data are retained within the research organizations that generated them, many structure–activity studies have been published. Only a few correlations are considered here (for additional information, see Ref. 42).

Until recently, the data on structure–activity relationships of the β-lactam antibiotics suggested that the minimal structural characteristics required for significant antibacterial activity could be summarized by structure (**22**); these data suggested the need for a fused ring to confer a degree of strain on the β-lactam; the requirement of the sulfur atom was assumed, but untested. The penicillins and cephalosporins (3-cephems) appear to be optimal in this respect, equipping the β-lactam with a high level of chemical reactivity, but retaining sufficient stability to survive in the biological environment of the host. The isomeric 2-cephems were found to have a low level of antibacterial activity. This has been attributed to the lower degree of strain on the β-lactam. An exception to the assumed structural requirements indicated by (**22**) were penicillins in which the acylamino side chain is replaced by an amidine structure, eg, in structure (**23**) (43). These derivatives are significantly less active than benzylpenicillin or ampicillin against gram-positive bacteria, but more active against most of the gram-negative bacteria tested. They interfere with cell wall synthesis, but appear to have a mechanism of inhibition different from that of the 6-acylaminopenams (44). Some β-lactam-containing structures described recently further restrict (**22**) as the synoptic structure associated with antibacterial activity. Semisynthetic and totally synthetic structures with new rings fused to the β-lactam, which display good antibacterial activities, indicate a lack of necessity for sulfur at the 1-position (**24**) (45), or carbon at the 2-position (25) (46). The broad antibacterial activity of thienamycin violates the assumed requirement of the functionalized amino group in (22), but it-supports the assumption that ring strain contributes to the level of biological activity observed.

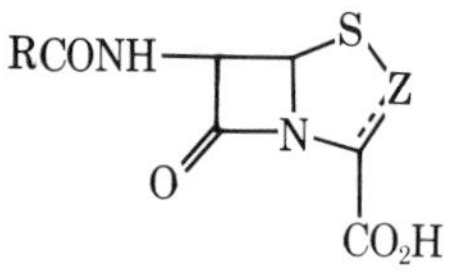

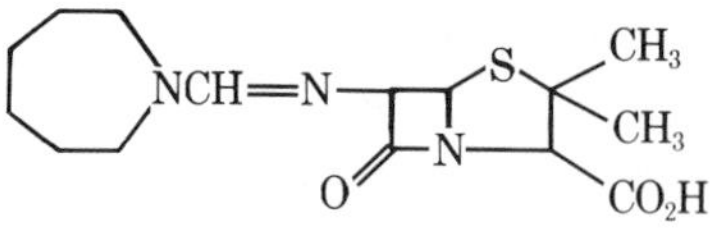

6-(1-*H*-hexahydroazapin-1-yl-methylene)-aminopenicillanic acid
[32887-01-7]
(23)

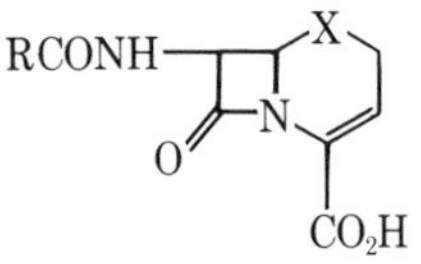

X = CH₂, O

(24)

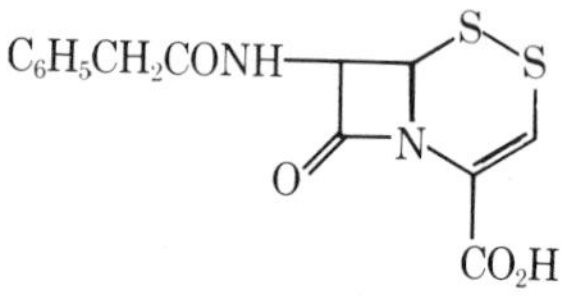

7-phenylacetamido-2-thia-3-*H*-cephalosporanic acid
[38287-60-4]
(25)

Conversely, the nocardicins would seem to negate the ring-strain requirement for activity, but while the activity of the nocardicins again seems to be directed at the cell wall, the level and type of activity observed differs from that exhibited by the bicyclic structures, and the specific location and mechanism of action are likely different.

Important structure–activity relationships within the scope of the penicillins and cephalosporins (cephamycins) can be inferred from comparison of the properties of the clinical agents (see pages 129, 130, and 133). It should be kept in mind that desired characteristics include pharmacokinetic as well as antibacterial properties. As mentioned already, changes on the penicillin structure other than those involving the 6-acyl group have been generally unprofitable. The exceptions to this are the derivatives in which the 3-carboxyl group has been converted to a tetrazole ring (26).

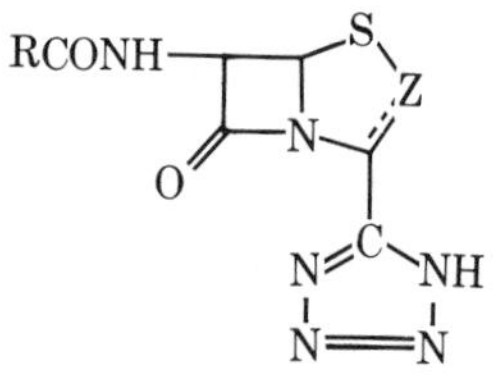

(26)

Acyl groups that tend to confer the highest gram-positive activity on the penicillin structure are acetic acids substituted by an aromatic moiety—usually a phenyl group or a simple heterocycle such as thiophene—attached directly, or through a hetero atom (oxygen, sulfur). Homologation of the acetic acid moiety lowers activity. The effect of benzene-ring substitution on activity is variable. Introduction of a *p*-amino group slightly broadens the gram-negative activity. A *p*-hydroxy group has little effect on antibacterial activity but can improve the pharmacokinetic properties (eg, amoxicillin). Introduction of a second substituent on the α-carbon atom of the acyl side-chain has a profound effect on activity. Bulky, neutral groups (eg, aryl or alkyl) lower the gram-positive activity but increase penicillinase resistance. Amino (ampicillin), acylamino, carboxyl (carbenicillin), and sulfonic acid (sulbenicillin) groups broaden the *in vitro* activity against gram-negative bacteria with retention of gram-positive activity. Penicillinase susceptibility is essentially unaffected. The importance of the D-phenylglycine side chain in both penicillins and cephalosporins should be noted. The L-phenylglycine analogues display much lower activities. Direct attachment of the aromatic ring to the side-chain amide carbonyl (6-aroylamino substituents) lowers the *in vitro* activity significantly. However, aroyl derivatives with ortho substituents which provide sufficient steric blocking, while of low antibacterial activity, have good penicillinase resistance and provide a group of valuable agents for treating infections caused by benzylpenicillin-resistant staphylococci (methicillin, oxacillin).

For the cephalosporins too, the highest antibacterial activities are observed when the acyl side chains are substituted acetic acids. However, in this series there is more latitude for the type of substituent attached to the α-carbon of the side chain. The phenyl and phenoxyacetyl side chains are less effective in conferring activity on the cephalosporins than the penicillins. More effective are acetic acid side chains carrying heterocyclic rings, notably: thiophene, pyridine, tetrazole, furan, and sydnone. Instead of the aromatic ring, much smaller and nonaromatic substituents can confer high levels of *in vitro* activity on the structures. These include the cyano, methylthio, methylsulfonyl, and trifluoromethylthio groupings. The effect of a second substituent on the α-carbon of the acyl group differs from the effect on activity in the penicillins. Since the cephalosporins inherently have a broader spectrum of activity than the penicillins, the carboxyl and sulfonic acid groups do not particularly improve activity. On the other hand, the 7-D-mandelamido derivatives (α-hydroxy) display good broad-spectrum activities. As with the phenylglycine analogues, derivatives with the L-mandelamido side chain are less active. The nature of the 3-substituent also influences the pharmacokinetic properties as well as the activity of the cephalosporins. Analogues with a 3-methyl substituent generally have a low level of antibacterial activity except when the 7-acyl group is D-mandelic acid or D-phenylglycine (or its 1,3-cyclohexadiene analogue). Thus an α-hydroxyl or amino group on the side chain compensates, at least in part, for the lack of a nucleophilic leaving group on the 3-methylene. The 7-phenylglycine analogues are the only known cephalosporins that combine good *in vitro* activity and efficient oral absorption. The 3′-acetoxy group has been displaced by many nucleophiles. Most of these displacements do not result in improved antibacterial activity, but improvement is seen with pyridinium (mostly gram-positive) and certain heterocyclic thio groups, notably the 5-methyl-1,2,4-thiadiazole, 1-methyltetrazole- and 2-pyridine-N-oxide-thiomethyl groups. The primary effect of these heterocyclethiomethyl substituents is to increase the level of *in vitro* activity against gram-negative bacteria. The 1-methyltetrazolethiomethyl group is generally the most efficient of the heterocyclethiomethyl substituents in improving the level of *in vitro* activity against already susceptible gram-negative bacteria. Many other 5- and 6-membered heterocyclethiomethyl substituents have little effect on *in vitro* activity, or lower it. The effect of the 3-substituent on pharmacokinetic properties is variable. The 3′-acetoxy group is metabolized in the body to the less active 3′-alcohol. The other substituents discussed, and the 3′-carbamate, are metabolically stable. The complete removal of the 3-substituent (3-deacetoxymethylcephalosporanic acid analogues (**27**), W = H) results in derivatives that behave biologically very much like the 3-methyl analogues (cephalexin, cephradine). The 3-chloro or 3-methyl analogues ((**27**), W = OCH$_3$, Cl) are more active than the 3-methyl cephalosporins. The introduction of a methoxy substituent on the 7α-position of the cephalosporins, and the resulting effect on biological activity including resistance to β-lactamases, are discussed below.

(**27**)

Many other changes on the penicillin and cephalosporin structures give products with reduced antibacterial activities. Examples include: sulfoxides, sulfones, 6α-alkyl-penicillins, 2-substituted cephalosporins, 2-cephems, etc.

Resistance.   Bacterial resistance to β-lactam antibiotics can be natural or acquired. In many cases, resistance results from the production of a β-lactamase enzyme which opens the β-lactam (47). Bacteria produce chromosomally and R plasmid (resistance factor) mediated β-lactamases. The nature of the β-lactamases and the physiological factors controlling their production contribute to the role these enzymes play in the resistance of bacteria to penicillins and cephalosporins. β-Lactamases are commonly distinguished from one another by substrate profile, sensitivity to inhibitors, analytical isoelectric focusing, immunological studies, and molecular weight determination. Individual enzymes may inactivate primarily penicillins, cephalosporins, or both. The substrate specificity predetermines the antibiotic resistance of the producing strain. The level of the β-lactamase produced is controlled by mutation, induction, and the acquisition of R plasmids. Some β-lactamases are produced only in the presence of a β-lactam antibiotic (inducible) and others are produced continuously (constitutive). The transfer of resistance due to the production of β-lactamases between strains and even species has enhanced the problems of β-lactam antibiotic resistance. Species previously easily controlled by β-lactam antibiotics are now becoming significant medical problems.

Gram-positive organisms produce extracellular enzymes but gram-negative organisms commonly produce cell-bound β-lactamases. In the former, the extracellular β-lactamases act on the antibiotic before it enters the cell. The cell wall structure of gram-negative microorganisms provides a natural defense against many penicillins and cephalosporins. In these bacteria the β-lactam antibiotic must penetrate the outer cell membrane before coming in contact with the β-lactamase. Thus the inherent permeability of the antibiotic determines the amount of antibiotic which reaches the β-lactamase.

Mode of Action.   The penicillins and cephalosporins inhibit the biosynthesis of bacterial cell walls. The cell wall contains a matrix of complex macromolecules that provide rigidity and mechanical stability by way of cross-linked latticework-like structures. One such structure is the peptidoglycan layer, apparently present in both gram-positive and gram-negative bacteria. This is made up of glycan strands (alternating N-acetylglucosamine and N-acetylmuramic acid units) and, forming the second dimension, peptide chains which cross-link the glycan strands. In some models (*S. aureus*) the N-acetylmuramic acid units carry, initially, pentapeptide side chains that become cross-linked by pentaglycine bridges. The final step in the construction of the peptidoglycan cross-link involves a transpeptidase catalyzed reaction in which the terminal glycine unit of the pentaglycine bridge is linked to the fourth unit (D-alanine) of the muramic acid pentapeptide, with the loss of the fifth (terminal) unit, which is also D-alanine. Although various cell-wall active antibiotics inhibit other stages in the biosynthesis of the peptidoglycan components and their assembly into the macro-molecular units, the β-lactam antibiotics have been found to inhibit the transpeptidase and carboxypeptidase enzymes involved in the final cross-linking of the peptidoglycan chains. The transpeptidase is irreversibly inhibited; the carboxypeptidase, although more sensitive to these antibiotics, is reversibly inhibited. Strominger (48) has ex-tensively reviewed the specific mechanism of cell wall inhibition and has proposed that the penicillins are structural analogues of the terminal D-alanyl-D-alanine residue of the peptidoglycan strands that is operated on by these enzymes. However, the sensitivity of the enzymes to the penicillins and cephalosporins does not seem to fully explain the killing of the bacterial cell since bactericidal activities of different β-lactam antibiotics do not correlate well with the enzyme inhibition data. In addition, ra-dioactively labeled β-lactam antibiotics bind to multiple sites on the cell wall and different antibiotics display different reactivities toward these binding sites (49). The nature and specific relationship to the killing of the cell of these other binding sites have not been completely resolved.

Biosynthesis. The β-lactam antibiotics which contain an α-aminoadipic acid side chain are structurally bicyclic tripeptides composed of α-aminoadipic acid, cysteine and valine (50–51). Labeling studies with carbon-14, and more recently with carbon-13, indicate that penicillins and cephalosporins are formed from these primary metabo-lites. Mutations that affect the synthesis of α-aminoadipic acid, cysteine and valine correspondingly influence the synthesis of β-lactam antibiotics. Structural elucidation and labeling studies of cephamycins from *Streptomyces* species also indicate that α-aminoadipic acid, cysteine, and valine are precursors of the antibiotic.

Microbial synthesis of β-lactam antibiotics from *P. chrysogenum* and *C. acre-monium* has been extensively reviewed (51). The tripeptide theory has dominated the theme of β-lactam biosynthesis since the isolation of δ-(α-aminoadipyl)cys-teinylvaline from *P. chrysogenum*. Recently, three sulfur-containing peptides, in-cluding δ-(L-α-aminoadipyl)-L-cysteinyl-D-valine, have been isolated from *P. acre-monium*. This tripeptide has also been synthesized in broken cells. Labeled isomers of δ-(L-α-aminoadipyl)-L-cysteinylvaline have been incorporated into penicillin N by cell extracts. The involvement of tripeptide in penicillin and cephalosporin bio-synthesis has been further supported by the accumulation of peptides in mutants blocked in antibiotic synthesis.

The biosynthetic penicillins are believed to be derived from isopenicillin N which contains an L-α-aminoadipic acid side chain. Lysine-requiring mutants of *P. chryso-genum,* blocked prior to α-aminoadipic acid, produce penicillins only when supple-mented with α-aminoadipic acid. Mutants blocked between α-aminoadipic acid and lysine, on the other hand, produce antibiotic without supplementation. The biosyn-thetic penicillins are synthesized by the exchange of a monosubstituted acetic acid moiety for the L-α-aminoadipic acid of isopenicillin N. The acyl transferase enzyme which catalyzes the reaction has been detected in cell-extracts from *P. chrysogenum* but not *C. acremonium*.

The terminal steps in the biosynthesis of cephalosporin C have been partially elucidated with the aid of antibiotic negative mutants and the use of cell-free synthesis (52). These studies support a biosynthetic scheme in which deacetoxycephalosporin

C is converted to deacetylcephalosporin C, followed by acetylation to form cephalosporin C. Many questions remain unsolved in the biosynthesis of both penicillin and cephalosporin antibiotics.

Manufacture and Processing

At present all of the β-lactam antibiotics are derived from fermentation processes. Penicillins G and V are obtained by direct fermentation; the other penicillins in Table 2 and all of the cephalosporins (Table 5) are produced by a combination of fermentation and subsequent chemical manipulation of the fermentation product. The manufacturing process consists of four stages: fermentation, isolation, chemical modification, and finishing.

Fermentation. The β-lactam antibiotics are produced by submerged fermentation under optimal physical and nutritional conditions to provide the desired microbial product. The specific characteristics of the industrial microbial strains, media, and fermentation conditions cannot be described in detail since these facts are considered

Table 5. Clinically Important Cephalosporins

Name	CAS Registry Number	R	A	Route[a]	Av daily dose, g
Injectable					
cephalothin	[153-61-7]	(thiophene)CH$_2$—	—OCOCH$_3$	im/iv	4–6
cephapirin	[21593-23-7]	N(pyridyl)—SCH$_2$—	—OCOCH$_3$	im/iv	2–6
cephacetrile	[23239-41-0]	N≡CCH$_2$	—OCOCH$_3$		
cephaloridine	[50-59-9]	(thiophene)CH$_2$—	±N(pyridinium)	im	1–3
cefazolin	[25953-19-9]	(tetrazole)—CH$_2$—	—S—(thiadiazole)CH$_3$	im/iv	0.75–4(6)
Oral					
cephaloglycin	[3577-01-3]	D(phenyl)—CH(NH$_2$)—	—OCOCH$_3$	po	1–2
cephalexin	[15686-71-2]	D(phenyl)—CH(NH$_2$)—	—H	po	1–4
cephradine	[3882-53-3]	D(cyclohexadienyl)—CH(NH$_2$)—	—H	po[b]	1–2

[a] iv, intravenously; im, intramuscularly; po, orally.
[b] Also iv and im.

trade secrets. The origin of strains, and general principles of culture maintenance, fermentation equipment, innoculum preparation, media, and fermentation conditions for penicillin and cephalosporin production, are public knowledge and are reviewed here (see Fermentation).

Microorganisms.   The organisms used for the commercial production of the penicillins and cephalosporins are mutants of *Penicillium chrysogenum* and *Cephalosporium acremonium,* respectively (51). Both are true fungi (eucaroytes). In contrast, the cephamycins (7α-methoxycephalosporins) are produced by certain species of procaryotic *Streptomyces.*

Fleming's original strain of *P. notatum* provided only low yields of penicillin and responded poorly to submerged fermentation techniques. However, a specific strain of *P. chrysogenum* designated NRRL 1951 was found to respond well under conditions of submerged fermentation and provided greater yields of penicillins. Superior penicillin-producing strains of *P. chrysogenum* have since been obtained by random screening of variant strains following mutation induction. All of the present-day high-yielding industrial strains are descendants of the NRRL 1951 strain. The physiological characteristics, such as nutritional requirements, sensitivity to precursors, pigment production, and sporulation, differ markedly from the original isolate. The mutant strains used for manufacturing cephalosporin C have been derived from *Cephalosporium acremonium* (CMI 49,137) isolated by Brotzu (53). The first high-yielding strain, culture 8650, was obtained from CMI 49,137 following mutagenesis with ultraviolet light. Markedly divergent lines have since been developed from the 8650 mutant. These strains generally grow poorly, produce almost no pigment, and appear to be impaired in some facet of sporulation. The cephamycins are produced by several species of *Streptomycetes* including *S. lipmania* and *S. clavuligerus.* Although no cephamycin has yet been marketed, considerable research is being devoted to the isolation of high-yielding strains.

Strain Maintenance.   Once a high-yielding strain has been isolated, it is essential that the organism be maintained so that it remains viable and capable of producing the antibiotic at its original rate (54). Such mutant strains are frequently unstable, a factor that must be considered in maintaining the stock cultures. The best method for maintenance depends on the particular organism and the characteristic being preserved. The high-yielding strains of both *P. chrysogenum* and *C. acremonium* are commonly stored in liquid nitrogen at −196°C, or the spores are lyophilized. The success of either of these methods is dependent upon the inherent genetic stability of the culture, the method of preparing the cell suspension, the suspending menstrum, and the specific storage procedures used. Under suitable conditions high-yielding strains can be preserved for many years without loss of viability or antibiotic-producing ability. Working cultures of *P. chrysogenum* and *C. acremonium* are generally prepared by transferring preserved cells to agar media. Several sporulation media have been developed for mutants of both species. Frequent transfers of these fungi on agar media tend to select for natural variants which sporulate profusely, but good sporulation is not necessarily associated with high yields; in fact, the reverse frequently applies. It is therefore common practice to limit the transfers of cultures on agar slants to as few as possible.

Equipment.   The penicillins and cephalosporins are both produced by large-scale submerged fermentation processes in tanks providing high levels of aeration and agitation. These fermenters vary in size from 38,000 to 380,000 L and have been designed to provide conditions that are optimal for the specific strains used, and to fit the needs of the individual company. Obviously, these fermenters must be capable of being sterilized and operated under aseptic conditions; they are usually equipped with facilities for adding sterile nutrients during the fermentation and for removing the broth for processing either continuously or by the batch method. Other design factors include the ability to handle the liquid broth and associated gases under pressure, to monitor and control the environmental conditions of pH, temperature, and foam, and to provide high levels of agitation and effective exchange of air and carbon dioxide between the liquid and gaseous phases. In order to effectively control these conditions, the fermenters have become highly instrumented and in some modern facilities they are computer controlled. The methods and equipment design for achieving the fermentation conditions listed here have been extensively reviewed (55–57). A fermentation facility for manufacturing β-lactam antibiotics must be equipped with culture laboratories, fermenters for growing the inoculum, production scale fermenters, and, of course, all of the necessary services including steam, cooling water, sterile air, power, etc.

Inoculum Development. For every fermentation set up in the manufacturing plant, inoculum must be developed from the original spore suspension in sufficient quantity to provide a proper rate of growth and antibiotic production in the final tank. The size of the production fermenters usually requires that the inoculum be developed in several stages of increasing volume. For *C. acremonium* and *P. chrysogenum*, spores are developed at 24°C for 5–10 d on solid agar media. The spores from these heavily sporulated cultures are suspended in sterile water with a wetting agent and a specific quantity is used as inoculum for the first of several vegetative stages. These stages are designed to provide 5–10% inoculum to the succeeding stage. The early stages are usually grown in shake flasks or bottles, the later stages in small replicas of the production fermenters. The conditions used (typically 28°C, 48–96 h for *C. acremonium*, 48–72 h for *P. chrysogenum,* with high aeration and agitation) provide heavy mycelial growth.

Media. The antibiotic products are commonly produced by metabolic reactions that differ from those responsible for the growth and reproduction of the microorganism. In order to enhance antibiotic synthesis, nutrients must be diverted from the primary to the antibiotic biosynthetic sequences. Although most media for production of penicillins and cephalosporins are similar, they are individually designed for the specific requirements of the high-yielding strains and the fermentation equipment used. The development of these media has been largely empirical.

A typical fermentation medium for penicillin production contains lactose, corn steep liquor, and calcium carbonate (51). In most industrial processes the carbohydrate source (glucose, beet molasses, or lactose) is continuously added to the fermentation. Maintenance of growth-limiting amounts of glucose in the fermentation has led to longer periods of penicillin production. If excess glucose is added inadvertently, synthesis of the penicillin can be markedly reduced. The rate of glucose addition is commonly determined by following the pH or the rate of oxygen utilization. Alternative sources of nitrogen, such as cottonseed, peanut, linseed, or soybean meal, have been substituted for corn steep liquor. During the later phases of the penicillin fermentation the available nitrogen may become limited and additional nitrogenous material must then be added. Other ingredients that have been added to the medium to provide maximum penicillin production are monopotassium phosphate (for additional phosphorus and pH control) and sodium or magnesium sulfate (for additional sulfur). Some ingredients, such as excess iron or copper, can reduce penicillin synthesis. Several synthetic fermentation media for penicillin production have been developed, but none have proven to be superior to the complex organic media (58).

As mentioned earlier, the penicillin fermentations are usually supplemented with appropriate monosubstituted acetic acid precursors in order to direct the fermentation to the production of specific penicillins (benzylpenicillin, phenoxymethylpenicillin). Precursors, such as phenylacetic acid, are toxic to *P. chrysogenum* and therefore must be added in many small portions over the course of the fermentation. Recently high-yielding strains of *P. chrysogenum* have been developed that are more resistant to the precursors.

Media for large-scale fermentation of cephalosporin C generally contain fish meal, peanut meal or soybean meal, corn steep liquor, beet molasses, lard oil or methyl oleate, glucose, and methionine (59). In the cephalosporin medium lipids rather than glucose provide the main source of carbon and energy. The sulfur for the cephalosporin C molecule is derived more efficiently from methionine than from sulfate. Cephalosporin C yields are potentiated by both methionine and methyl oleate. The molecular basis for this potentiation has not yet been established.

Procedures. The commercial penicillin and cephalosporin fermentations can be divided into three interrelated phases. Rapid growth occurs during the first phase which lasts approximately 30 h (penicillins) and 48 h (cephalosporins). This phase produces most of the mycelia for the fermentation. The antibiotic is produced at a rapid rate during the second phase which lasts 5–7 d. The growth rate is markedly reduced during this period. The third phase is characterized by depletion of the carbon and nitrogen sources, followed by a termination of antibiotic synthesis. The cells lyse, releasing ammonia, and the pH rises.

The optimum temperatures for penicillin and cephalosporin C fermentations are 25° and 28°C, respectively. Slight variations (2–4°C) can drastically lower antibiotic yield. Recent studies suggest that better yields can be achieved by adjusting the temperature to the phase of the fermentation, eg, 30–32°C for optimal cell growth, then 24°C for the antibiotic-production phase (60). In a batch fermentation process the pH changes as specific medium ingredients are used up and metabolites are released (61). The pH of the fermentation mixture can be maintained constant by including in the initial medium ingredients which function as internal buffers (eg, calcium carbonate) or by adding acid or alkali to the fermentation as it progresses. The pH of the penicillin fermentation is commonly controlled by the rate of addition of glucose. On the other hand, the medium for cephalosporin C production is highly buffered. Both the penicillin and cephalosporin C fermentation media contain large amounts of particulate ingredients which must be kept in suspension. This is achieved by using high aeration and agitation rates. The formation of foam which results from these conditions is controlled by adding nontoxic defoamers such as animal or vegetable oils or synthetic derivatives from petroleum. The efficient exchange of metabolic carbon dioxide from the liquid mixture and in oxygen to it is controlled by the air flow, back pressure, agitation speed, and fermentor design (62). Generally, these parameters are adjusted to produce maximum gas exchange while controlling foam. The available oxygen is commonly monitored using dissolved oxygen probes and gas analyzers. During the course of the fermentation the concentration of the antibiotic is monitored using various standard assay methods. These include procedures based on high pressure liquid chromatography, chemical reactions of the β-lactam and microbiological assay.

Isolation.   The isolation procedures rely primarily on solubility, adsorption, and ionic characteristics of the antibiotic to separate it from the large number of other substances present in the fermentation mixture. The penicillins are monobasic carboxylic acids which lend themselves to solvent extraction techniques. The separation process of amphoteric cephalosporin C is more complex. In general, the recovery process is greatly simplified when the antibiotic in the fermentation broth is present in high concentration. If the penicillin, or cephalosporin C, is to be used as a manufacturing intermediate it is frequently carried into the chemical processing stage with a relatively low degree of purity.

Penicillins.   At the completion of the fermentation the mixture is usually transferred to a holding tank. The penicillins are relatively unstable chemically, and if the broth is contaminated they are subject to inactivation by penicillinases. To decrease penicillin loss the mixture (usually at pH 7.5–8.0) is cooled rapidly to 5–10°C and/or adjusted with mineral acids to pH 6.0. These conditions retard both the enzymatic and chemical destruction of the antibiotic. The fermentation mixture is filtered to remove the mycelia and other solids. The filtered broth is adjusted to pH 2–2.5 using, eg, phosphoric acid, and it is then extracted with a smaller volume of an organic solvent such as amyl acetate, butyl acetate, methyl isobutyl ketone, or the like. It is important that the extraction be carried out in such a way that the time that the broth is held at an acid pH is minimized. In some cases this extraction is carried out using an in-line high-speed homogenizer followed by a continuous-flow centrifuge to separate the emulsified phases (63). The Podbielniak centrifugal countercurrent separator accomplishes the emulsification and centrifugation functions in essentially one step (see Centrifugal separation).

In a typical isolation sequence (64) the initial penicillin-containing solvent (amyl acetate) is treated with charcoal to remove colored impurities and then is back extracted with a 2% phosphate buffer solution at pH 7.5. This transfers the penicillin to the aqueous phase as its salt. The buffer solution is then acidified with phosphoric acid and the penicillin is again extracted into amyl acetate or its equivalent. By transferring the product into progressively smaller volumes of solvent with each extraction, concentration factors of up to 80–100-fold can be realized. At this stage the penicillin, in organic solution, can be converted into a stable salt form in a number of ways. It can be extracted into a calcium carbonate slurry which is filtered and lyophilized or spray-dried; it can be extracted into other buffers and freeze- or spray-dried to give the sodium or potassium salt; or it can be precipitated from the dried organic phase using organic bases such as triethylamine or N-ethylpiperidine.

Crystalline sodium or potassium penicillin can be obtained by dissolving the crude material in water and adding an excess of n-butyl alcohol. The water is then completely removed by distillation and upon further concentration the penicillin crystallizes. In a second procedure a saturated solution of the crude alkali metal salt in a cold polar solvent, such as methanol, is warmed to 20–30°C to induce crystallization. The addition of a nonpolar solvent facilitates the process. A third technique is based on the salting out of penicillin from a saturated aqueous solution of crude penicillin by the addition of a neutral, highly water-soluble salt, such as potassium chloride or sodium chloride at pH 5.5–7.0, until turbidity appears. After standing, the crystals are filtered. The crystalline salt of penicillin which is produced is generally a salt of the same metal as the salt used for salting out. Salts can also be formed in solutions of penicillins in organic solvents such as butyl alchol. A typical process for the preparation of crystalline procaine penicillin involves dissolving the crude sodium or potassium salt to a concentration of 20–30% in a 40–60% aqueous solution of procaine hydrochloride. Procaine penicillin crystallizes upon standing.

Cephalosporin C. The amphoteric nature of cephalosporin C precludes its direct extraction into organic solvents. Methods for converting cephalosporin C into an organic solvent-extractable product by acylating the side-chain amino group have been described. However, it has been a more common practice to isolate this antibiotic through the use of a combination of ion exchange and precipitation procedures originally outlined by Abraham (65). More recently techniques using adsorption on neutral macroporous resins (XAD resins) and precipitations as sparingly soluble metal ion complexes have been combined with the ion exchange process. The isolation of cephalosporin C is complicated by the presence in the fermentation broth of several other antibiotics having an α-aminoadipic acid side chain: penicillin N, deacetylcephalosporin C, deacetylcephalosporin C lactone [2429-86-9], and deacetoxycephalosporin C. The first three are effectively separated from the desired product by an acid treatment step followed by adsorption on an ion-exchange resin.

As with the penicillin fermentations, the cells are removed by filtration at the completion of the fermentation cycle. The clarification of the cephalosporin C fermentation broth is more difficult than for the penicillin fermentation. To facilitate the removal of the cells 2% filter aid is commonly added directly to the broth which is then filtered through a rotary vacuum unit precoated with filter aid. The broth is acidified to pH 2.5–3.0 before or after the filtration and held at pH 2–3 until any penicillin N present is destroyed. This procedure also lactonizes any deacetylacephalosporin C present in the broth. If the pH is adjusted after the mycelia are removed, the resulting proteinaceous precipitate must be removed before the subsequent separations are carried out.

In a typical procedure (65) the cephalosporin C is removed from the filtered and acid-treated broth by adsorption on a weakly basic ion-exchange resin such as IR-4B or IRA-68. However, if the broth contains high concentrations of inorganic anions (chloride, sulfate) these ions will also adsorb on the resin, seriously reducing its capacity for retaining the cephalosporin C. In this case, the competing ions are eliminated by first passing the broth through a column filled with a strong base ion exchange resin such as IRA-400 or Dowex-50. This resin adsorbs the cephalosporin and the inorganic ions, but it binds the latter more strongly. If the column is loaded to the point of chloride-ion breakthrough, the cephalosporin C will be completely eluted, having been displaced by the more strongly bound inorganic anions. The cephalosporin C is commonly eluted from the IRA-68 column (or its equivalent) by relatively small volumes of pyridine acetate buffer. If care is exercised in the elution the lactonized deacetylcephalosporin C can be separated from the product. The pyridine acetate buffer is removed by vacuum distillation (<30°C) and, if necessary, the adsorption and elution steps are repeated until the cephalosporin C is sufficiently concentrated and pure to allow its precipitation from aqueous solution by the addition of water-miscible organic solvents such as alcohols or acetone.

The use of neutral macroporous resins (XAD-2, XAD-4) allows a more rapid elimination of impurities from the cephalosporin C in the initial steps of the isolation (66). These polymers will readily adsorb the cephalosporin C while rejecting inorganic ions and other impurities in the cephalosporin fermentation broth. The cephalosporin

C is commonly loaded on the XAD resin at pH 2.5–3.0 and, after the resin is washed with water, it can be eluted with aqueous alcohols, eg, 50% methanol or 10% isopropyl alcohol. Subsequent to the XAD cycle, the cephalosporin C can be further purified by adsorption on and elution from a weak base ion-exchange resin as already described.

Once the cephalosporin C has been partially purified (20–40%), it can be obtained as a solid in reasonably good purity by precipitating it from water–alcohol mixtures as a complex with metal ions such as Zn^{2+} or Cd^{2+} (67). This process appears to be most suitable for the later stages of cephalosporin C recovery. Although the yields are often moderate in this step the purification factor is relatively good, and the complexes can be used directly in the chemical modification steps.

Several processes have been described in which the amino group on the aminoadipic acid side chain of cephalosporin C is acylated (benzoyl, chloroacetyl, i-butoxycarbonyl, acetoacetyl) (68) or otherwise converted to a neutral substituent (hydantoin, dihydropyridines) (69). The chemical conversion can be carried out in the fermentation broth, where competing hydrolysis requires the use of relatively large amounts of the acylating agent, or on partially purified concentrates. The cephalosporin C so modified can then be extracted from the acidified broth using immiscible organic solvents and purified by procedures similar to those used with the penicillins. Reported recovery yields are relatively poor. These cephalosporin C derivatives can usually be used in the subsequent chemical modification (side chain removal) reactions.

Chemical Modification.   Only benzylpenicillin and phenoxymethylpenicillin are used in their original chemical form. The rest of the penicillins, and all of the cephalosporins are chemically modified derivatives of the natural fermentation products. The semisynthetic penicillins are derived from 6-aminopenicillanic acid which is obtained, in turn, by removal of the 6-acyl group from a fermentation-produced penicillin. Likewise 7-aminocephalosporanic acid, obtained by removal of the α-aminoadipic acid side chain of cephalosporin C, is a key intermediate for the cephalosporins that have a 3-acetoxymethyl group, or a functionalized 3-substituent derived therefrom. On the other hand, the cephalosporins with a 3-methyl substituent (deacetoxycephalosporanic acids) are derived from the penicillins. These interrelationships are summarized in Figure 3. As with the fermentation processes, specific information on the reaction and processing conditions and yields for actual manufacturing processes are considered proprietary and are seldom disclosed.

In addition to all of the other chemical work carried out on the penicillins and cephalosporins, a considerable amount of effort has been directed toward modifications that may change the biological properties of these substances. As a result, each position on the penicillin and cephalosporin rings has been subjected to chemical alteration, with the exception of the 4(5)-bridgehead nitrogen atom. Table 6 is partial listing of modifications that have been described in the patent or published literature. Most are single substituent changes; in some cases two or more substituents were changed simultaneously. Most of the modifications were accomplished without major disruption to the essential ring systems. Some entailed migration of, or addition to, the dihydrothiazine double bond, and a very important group of reactions has involved opening of the ring fused to the β-lactam and reclosure to new structures. Especially important has been the opening of the thiazolidine and recyclization to dihydrothiazine allowing the conversion of penicillins to cephalosporins. Of the chemistry implied in Table 6 only a few of the more significant reactions are discussed here. Several reviews (9,26,34) give more thorough discussions of the specific chemical topics and access to publications of the original studies.

6(7)β-Substituents.   7-Aminocephalosporanic acid cannot be made by direct fermentation, nor can it be obtained by enzymatic removal of the aminoadipic acid side chain from cephalosporin C. Therefore two chemical methods have been developed for converting cephalosporin C to 7-ACA. One method is based on a peculiar property of the 7α-aminoadipamido group. Diazotization of the α-amino group results in loss of nitrogen and intramolecular reaction of the α-carbon with the amide carbonyl group of the side chain. This produces the cyclic imino ether (**28**). In aqueous solution this imino ether hydrolyzes and the resulting 7-ACA is destroyed by diazotization of the 7-amino group and loss of nitrogen. When formic acid is used as the solvent instead of water, and nitrosyl chloride is substituted for nitrous acid, hydrolysis of the imino ether can be delayed until the excess nitrosating agent is removed. This reduces the secondary diazotization of the 7-amino group allowing yields of 7-ACA to be obtained (2,70). The second method is more general and can be used to remove the acyl side chains from the penicillins or cephalosporin C. It is based on the conversion of the secondary amide grouping to an imino chloride (**29a**) using phosphorus pentachloride. This intermediate reacts readily with an alcohol to form the corresponding imino ether (**29b**) which hydrolyzes on contact with water to the amine and the side-chain acid ester (30). It is necessary to protect the carboxyl group(s) before this reaction sequence, is carried out eg, with silyl esters (71).

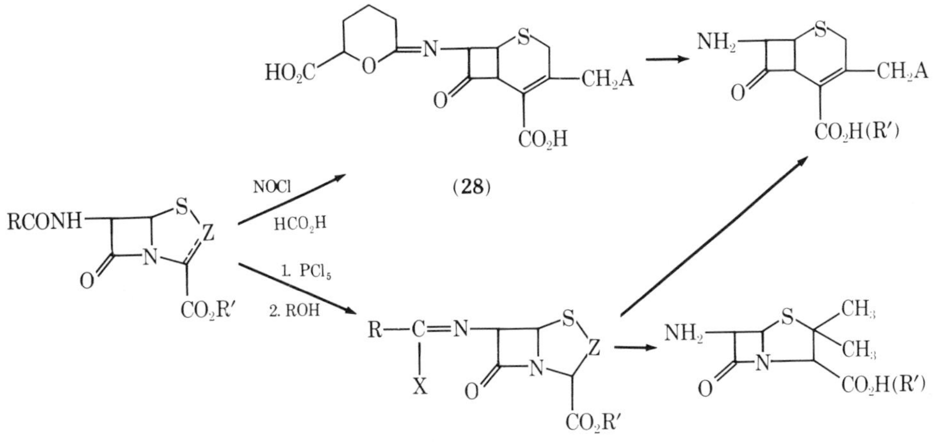

(28)

(29a, b)

penicillins: R = $C_6H_5CH_2$, $C_6H_5OCH_2$; Z = $-\overset{|}{C}(CH_3)_2$
cephalosporins: R = $R'O_2CCH(NH_2)(CH_2)_3$; Z = $=C(CH_2A)CH_2$
R' = $Si(CH_3)_3$, $CH_2C_6H_4NO_2$, CH_2CCl_3; A = H, $OCOCH_3$, S-heterocyle, etc
(**29a**), X = Cl;   (**29b**), X = OCH_3

They have sufficient chemical stability to allow the chemical manipulation described to be carried out in their presence, and they hydrolyze under conditions that are sufficiently mild to avoid opening of the β-lactam ring, in this case during the reaction work-up which hydrolyzes the imino ether. This process when used to convert cephalosporin C to 7-ACA is complicated by the presence of an amino group and two

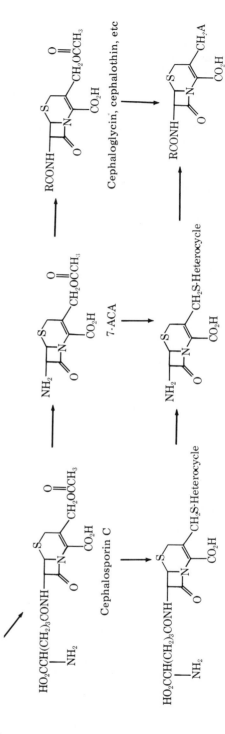

Figure 3. Manufacture of penicillins and cephalosporins.

116

Table 6.   Chemical Modifications of Penicillins and Cephalosporins

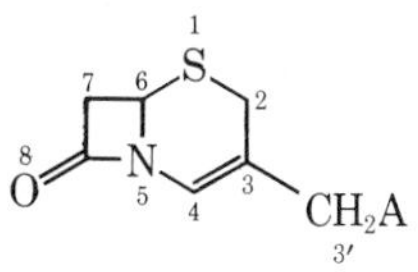

Position	From	To
1	S	SO, SO_2, $\overset{+}{S}CH_3$
2-Pen	$(CH_3)_2$	H_2, cycloalkyl
2-Cep	H_2	$=CHSAr$; H, OAc; H, CH_3; CH_3, H; $=CH_2$; Br, CH_2Br; H, CH_2SR; CH_2SR, H; $=CHSR$; $=O$
$2\alpha, \beta$	H	$OCOCH_3$, Br, OCH_3
3-Cep	CH_2OCOCH_3	CHO, CO_2H, ($=CH_2$), OH, OR, Cl, F, NH_2, NHCOOR
3'	$OCOCH_3$	H, OH, OCOR, OR, SR, $\overset{+}{N}C_5H_4X$, S_2O_3Na, N_3, NH_2, CN, SO_nCH_3, $S(C=NH)NR_2$, $S(C=S)NR_2$, $S(CS)OR$, SCOR, SO_2Ar, Br, $OCONH_2$, OCONHR, S-heterocycle, NCS, Ar, heterocycle, $CH=CHAr$, $CH=CHCO_2H$
3-Pen, 4-Cep	CO_2H	H, CO_2R, CO_2CH_2OCOR, $CONH_2$, CO_2OCOR, $CONHCH(R)CO_2H$, CO_2SiR_3, CON_3, CH_2OH, CH_2CO_2H, $COCHN_2$, $COCH_2Cl$, CN, tetrazole
5-Pen, 6-Cep	H	C_6H_5
6β-Pen, 7β-Cep	RCONH	H, NH_2, R^1CONH, $R^2N=C=N$, $ArC=N$, R_2N, RNH
6α-Pen, 7α-Cep	H	CH_3, OCH_3, RCONH, NH_2, Cl, OH, OCOR, CH_2OH, CH_2Cl, CH_2F, CH_2NH_2, CH_2CH_2CN, SCH_3, CH_2COOCH_3, CH_2Ar, CO_2H, CH_2COAr, $C(OH)(CH_3)_2$, $NHCOOC_2H_5$
7-Pen, 8-Cep	$=O$	$=S$

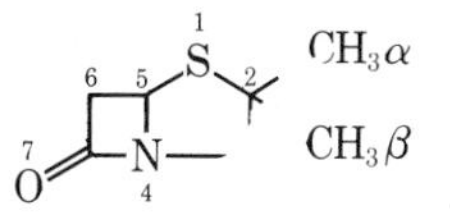

carboxyl groups in the molecule. Fortunately, the use of silylation to protect the carboxyl groups allows the reaction with phosphorus pentachloride to be carried out without further protection of the amino group. These reactions are important to the manufacture of semisynthetic pencillins and cephalosporins (see page 120).

The primary amino groups of 6-APA, 7-ACA, and their related analogues have reacted with a large number of chemical reagents. The most thoroughly studied reaction, and the most profitable one in terms of biological results, is the acylation of the amino group with carboxylic acids. The acylations have been accomplished using a large variety of agents. In addition to the acid chlorides and mixed anhydrides discussed on page 123, acylations have been carried out using carboxylic acids with N,N'-dicyclohexylcarbodiimide and similar condensing agents, activated esters with N-hydroxysuccinimide, N-hydroxyphthalimide and nitrophenols, cyclic anhydrides of amino acids, and other acylating agents commonly used in peptide synthesis. Side-chain acids with polar or reactive groupings require the prior attachment of protective groupings capable of being removed without destruction of the penicillin or cephalosporin β-lactam. The acylations can be carried out in aqueous or nonaqueous media. Recently, several less conventional methods for introducing desired acyl groups on the 6(7)-positions have been described. These include direct acylation of benzylpenicillin iminochloride esters (**29a**) to the diacyl derivative (**30**), followed by selective removal of the phenylacetyl group with thiophenolate (72). A route to α-carboxyphenylacetaminocephalosporins utilizes the reaction of isocyanate (**31**) derived from 7-aminodeacetylcephalosporanic acid (7-ADCA) with the anion of *tert*-butyl phenylacetate (73).

(30)

(31)

The amino group has been alkylated with trityl chloride, and mono- and di-methylations have been reported. Diazotization of 6-APA produces various 6α-substituted penicillanic acids (configuration inverted at the 6-carbon atom) depending on the anion present. Derivatives include 6α-chloro, bromo, acetoxy, and hydroxy-penicillanic acids. Although the halo derivatives can be hydrogenated to penicillanic acid, they cannot be displaced by nucleophiles such as azide without loss of the β-lactam.

For epimerization of the 6(7)-substituents and introduction of groupings at the 6α- and 7α-positions of 6-APA, 7-ACA, and related analogues, it is desirable in some cases to have derivatives in which the 6(7)-nitrogen atom carries no hydrogens. The 6(7)-phthalimido derivatives have been made by reaction of 6-APA or 7-ACA with N-carbethoxyphthalamic acid and a condensing agent, or with N-carbethoxy phthalimide. Various Schiff bases have been prepared in aqueous or alcoholic solvents including those from 6-APA and benzaldehyde (90% yield) or salicylaldehyde (78% yield) and 7-ACA with 4-hydroxy-3,5-di-*tert*-butyl benzaldehyde. Epimerization at the 6-carbon atom of the penicillins, and the 7-carbon atom of the cephalosporins, has been accomplished in several ways. For example, hetacillin, 6-phthalimidopeni-cillanic acid, and 6-(p-nitrobenzylidenimino)penicillanic acid have been epimerized under conditions that lead to formation of the 6-anion (sodium hydride in THF, tri-ethylamine in methylene chloride, etc) and cephalothin sulfoxide esters were epim-erized in DMS, triethylamine. The epipenicillins and cephalosporins are essentially devoid of antibacterial activity.

6(7)α-Substituents. A prediction that alkylation at the 6α-position of penicillins might enhance antibacterial activity (74) led to the synthesis of 6α-methyl penicillins and cephalosporins with reduced antibacterial activities. The alkylation step was accomplished by treating methyl 6-(N-benzylidenimino)penicillanate and *tert*-butyl 7-(N-benzylidenimino)deacetylcephalosporanate [64265-54-9] with sodium hydride followed by an excess of methyl iodide (75). This has been followed by the preparation of a large number of penicillins and some cephalosporins with other 6α- and 7α-sub-stituents (CH_2OH, $CH_2OSO_2C_6H_4CH_3$, CH_2NH_2, CH_2Cl, CH_2F, CH_2CH_2CN, $COOCH_3$, COOH, CHO, $COCH_3$) by a similar synthetic route using p-nitrobenzylidene derivatives and phenyl lithium (**32–34**) (76–77).

Of the various 6α-substituted penicillins and cephalosporins now known, only the cephalosporins with a 7α-methoxy group (cephamycins) have interesting biological characteristics. Interest in these structures has resulted in the development of several methods for preparing 7α-methoxycephalosporins: (*1*) The anion from (**32**) reacts with methyl methylthiosulfonate ($CH_3SSO_2CH_3$) to give the 7-methylthio derivative ((**33**) X = SCH_3). Hydrolysis of the imine and treatment of the amine with mercuric chloride in methanol gives the 7β-amino-7α-methoxy derivative (78). (*2*) Benzyl 7-diazo-cephalosporanate (**35**) and bromine azide gives the 7-azido-7-bromo adduct (**36**) which reacts with silver fluoroborate in methanol to form the 7β-azido-7α-methoxyce-phalosporanate (**37**). Reduction of the azide, acylation and deblocking of the acid group

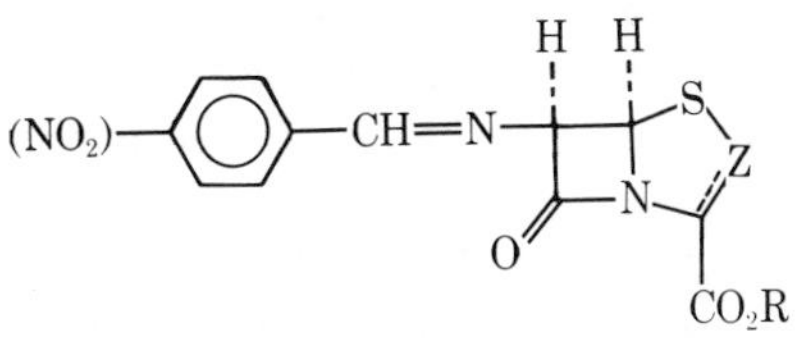

(32) 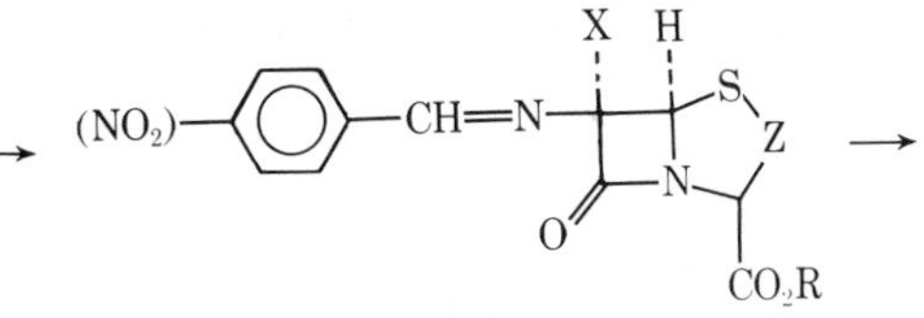   (33)

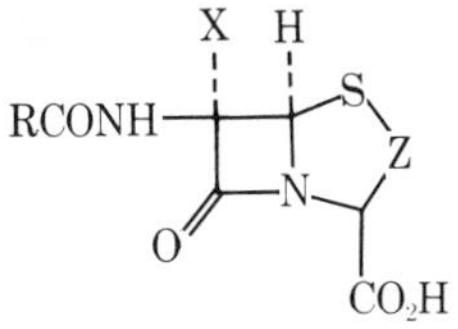

(34)

gives the desired 7α-methoxycephalosporins (79). (3) A more direct method employs the oxidation of a 7-amide function to an acylimine (38) using *tert*-butylhypochlorite in methanol containing lithium methoxide with immediate capture of the solvent (80). (4) Methanol is added to the quinoidal compound (40) prepared by lead dioxide oxidation of Schiff base (39) (81).

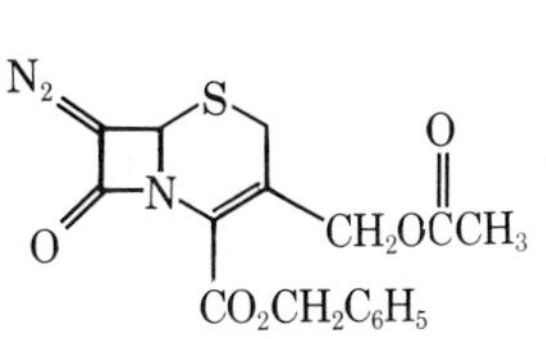

(35) 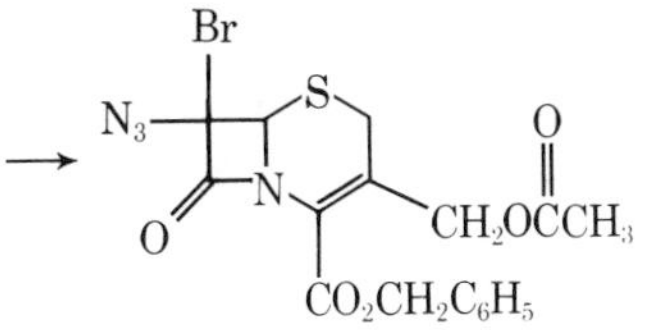   (36) 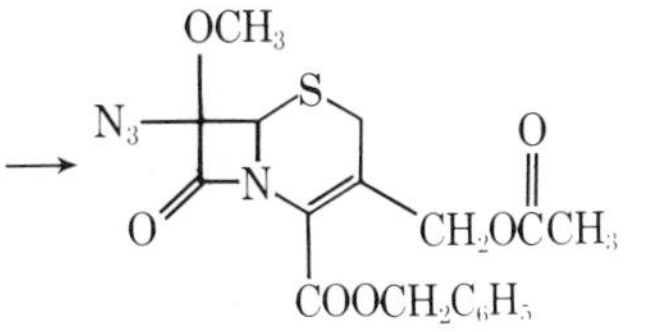   (37)

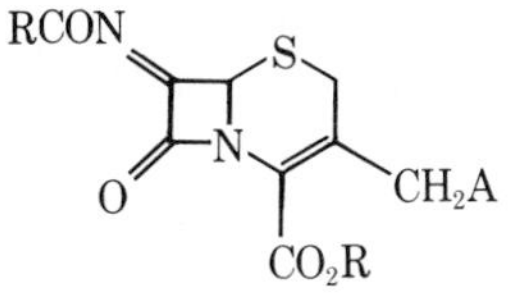

(38) 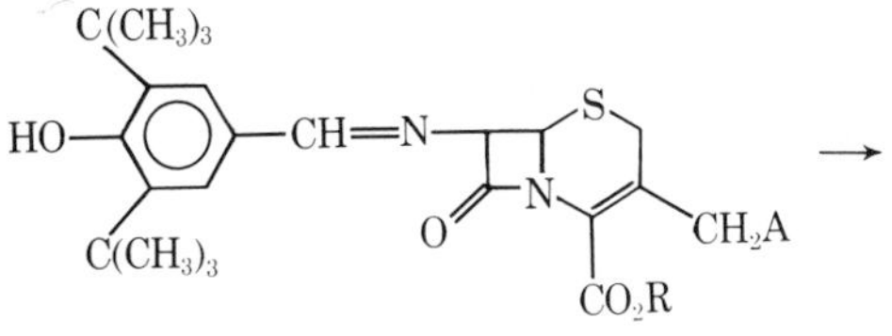   (39)

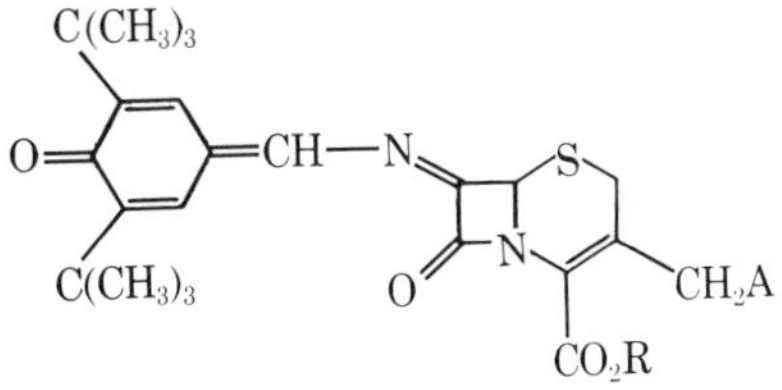

(40)

6-Aminopenicillanic Acid. The direct fermentation of 6-APA in media deficient in side-chain precursors was hampered by poor yields and difficult isolation procedures. It has been replaced by processes based on the chemical or enzymatic removal of the acyl group from a penicillin, usually benzylpenicillin. Penicillin acylases are produced by many living organisms including bacteria, fungi, and mammals (hog kidney acylase). They differ in the type of penicillin that can serve as substrate. Those derived from actinomycetes and filamentous fungi generally hydrolyze aliphatic and phenoxymethyl penicillins, but they split benzylpenicillin only slowly. Those of bacterial origin, eg, from the genera *Escherichia* and *Alcaligenes,* readily remove the phenylacetic acid side chain from benzylpenicillin, but they hydrolyze phenoxymethylpenicillin poorly. Some of these enzymes are bound to the cellular material, others are found mainly in the culture broths. Whole cell systems, as well as extracellular enzyme preparations in various stages of purification, have been used. This includes enzymes adsorbed or bound to insoluble substances, such as bentonite, or (diethylamino)ethyl cellulose. Used as slurries, or in columns, these bound enzyme preparations are reported to be stable for long periods of time allowing the conversion of large amounts of penicillin per unit of enzyme. Optimal pH and temperature depend on the enzyme preparation used. Reported working temperatures range from 28° to 50°C, pH ranges from 5.5 to 9. The preparation and use of penicillin acylases, including source organisms, isolation procedures, operating conditions, substrate specificity, and investigators, has been reviewed (82).

The chemical route to 6-APA based on the conversion of the secondary amide grouping to its imino chloride (**29a**) followed by conversion to an imino ether (**29b**) and hydrolytic removal of the side chain is discussed on page 115. In a typical procedure, penicillin G or V reacts at room temperature with trimethylchlorosilane or dimethyldichlorosilane in methylene chloride in the presence of pyridine or triethyl amine and then treated with phosphorus pentachloride at −59°C. Cold methanol is added at −70°C followed by water. The mixture is adjusted to pH 4 and the precipitated 6-APA is removed and washed with aqueous acetone. Yields of 85–95% and purities of 95% have been reported.

7-Aminocephalosporanic Acid.   The conversion of cephalosporin C to 7-ACA can be accomplished by the two discrete chemical sequences discussed earlier. The reaction using nitrosyl chloride in formic acid gave 7-ACA in approximately 40% yield. Addition of co-solvents, such as acetonitrile or nitroparaffins, results in slightly higher yields. The excess nitrosyl chloride can be destroyed by adding a large volume of methanol to the reaction mixture eliminating the need to distill the solvent.

The process for converting cephalosporin C to 7-ACA via the imino chloride–imino ether intermediates provides yields in excess of 90%. The several reaction steps can be carried out in one vessel. The zinc complexes described earlier for isolating cephalosporin C from fermentation broths can be used in place of the sodium salt. Likewise, *N*-chloroacetylcephalosporin C extracted from acylated fermentation broths and obtained in solid form as its quinoline salt, can be substituted for the cephalosporin C sodium salt normally used in this process.

A considerable number of other groups for protecting the carboxyl and amino functions were investigated before and after the development of the silylation-based process just described. One appears promising (83); the *N*-chloroacetylcephalosporin C quinoline salt is converted to the bis-mixed anhydride using acetyl chloride, dimethylaniline, and a catalytic amount of dimethylformamide. This protected derivative is then carried through the imino chloride–imino ether sequence at −20°C followed by hydrolysis and pH adjustment to give 7-ACA in yields and purity comparable to those obtained in the silylation processes.

3-Substituent Modifications.   The 3′-acetoxy group of the cephalosporins is easily displaced by many nitrogen, sulfur, and carbon nucleophiles (84). The displacements tend to follow S_N1 kinetics. Oxygen nucleophiles do not readily displace the acetoxy group. The displacement reactions cannot utilize the cephalosporin sulfoxides or esters. The carboxylate group does not attack the 3-methylene during the displacements by nucleophiles to give the lactone, although the latter is obtained by treating cephalosporins, especially deacetylcephalosporins, with acids. These characteristics and the surprising ease with which the displacement reactions occur have been explained in terms of resonance stabilization through the dihydrothiazine ring and the carboxylate ion (41) (85).

Nitrogen nucleophiles used to displace the 3'-acetoxy group include many substituted pyridines, quinolines, pyrimidines, triazoles, pyrazoles, azide, and even aniline and methylaniline if the pH is controlled at 7.5. The azide grouping has been reduced to a primary amine and cyclized to 1,2,3-triazole and tetrazole structures. Sulfur nucleophiles used in the displacement are legion, including alkyl thiols (—SR), thiosulfate (—S_2O_3Na), thio and dithio acids, carbamates and carbonates, thioureas, thioamides, and most important biologically, heterocyclic thiols.

Early manipulation of this substituent included hydrogenolysis of the 3'-acetoxy group to give 3-methyl derivatives ((42) A = H) and the inadvertent generation of the 3-pyridiniummethyl substituent ((42) A = $C_5H_5N^+$) through contact with warm pyridine acetate buffer used to elute cephalosporin C from ion-exchange columns. The 3-hydroxymethyl derivatives ((42) A = OH) cannot be obtained in any practical yield by acid or alkaline hydrolysis of the ester group because of the lability of the cephalosporin molecule and the ready lactonization of the alcohol and carboxyl in the presence of acids. The acetyl grouping has been removed enzymatically by esterases obtained from orange peel or from various microorganisms. It has been replaced by other aliphatic and aromatic acid groups by acylation of this alcohol. Similarly, the hydroxymethyl derivatives have been allowed to react with isocyanates to prepare 3-carbamyloxymethyl analogues. The primary carbamate ((42) A = $OCONH_2$) occurs naturally on some cephamycins and has been introduced synthetically on the cefuroxime structure. The 3-halomethyl substituent ((42) A = Cl, Br) has been obtained by treating deacetylcephalosporanic acid esters (eg, benzhydryl) with thionyl chloride or its equivalent. These 3-substituents can also be generated by treating deacetoxycephalosporanic acid ester sulfoxides with N-bromosuccinimide using photochemical induction or by the reaction of NBS with 3-methyl-2-cephem-4-carboxylate esters followed by isomerization of the double bond to the Δ^3-position. These halides undergo allylic displacements with the carboxyl group esterified and provide 3'-derivatives not obtainable by the nucleophilic displacements of the acetoxy group, eg, 3-cyanomethyl and 3-methoxymethyl analogues.

The 3-hydroxymethyl substituent has been oxidized with chromium oxide or its equivalent to the 3-aldehyde ((27) W = CHO) and various aldehyde derivatives have been prepared. Both Δ^3- and Δ^2-aldehydes (see structure (45), W = CHO) are known. The latter, on treatment with decarbonylation catalysts, such as tris(triphenylphosphine) rhodiumtrichloride, lose carbon monoxide and undergo double bond rearrangement to deacetoxymethylcephalosporanic acids ((27) W = H) (86). Several new reduction methods (electrochemical, chromium (II) salts) have been used to convert the 3-acetoxymethyl substituent to an exomethylene group (43) (87). This isomer of deacetoxycephalosporanic acid is also obtained by Raney nickel desulfurization of 3-heterocyclethiomethyl derivatives, eg, (42) A = 2-thio(pyridine-1-oxide) (88). The 3-exomethylene analogues can be isomerized to deacetoxycephalosporanic acid ((42) A = H) or ozonized to give the 3-ketone which exists largely as the enol (44). The enol function has been converted to the methyl ether, and to halo derivatives such as the chloride (cefachlor) and fluoride ((27) W = OCH_3, Cl, F) (89).

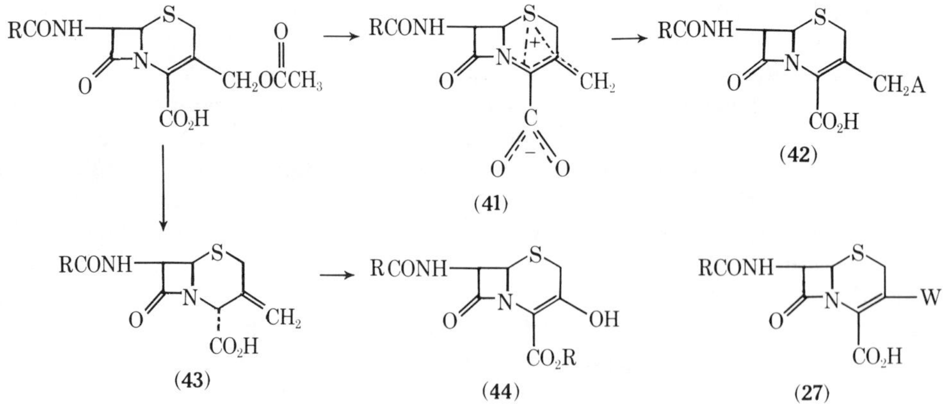

7-Aminodeacetoxycephalosporanic Acid. The original preparation of 7-ADCA [26395-99-3] was accomplished by catalytic hydrogenolysis of the acetoxy group from 7-ACA (90). The reaction gave moderate yields (62%) of 7-ADCA and required relatively large amounts of noble metal catalyst (palladium). Hydrogenation conditions were modified to achieve better yields (86%) of 7-ADCA by this route. However, this intermediate and its carboxylic acid esters are now more economically derived from penicillins via the ring expansion reaction discovered by Morin and co-workers (17–21) (39).

Several synthetic alternatives exist depending on the starting penicillin and the carboxylic acid protecting group selected. The protecting group, required to prevent decarboxylation during the ring expansion, must be removable in high yield at the end of the reaction sequence using conditions that will not destroy the final cephalosporin product. Groupings that have been used in this way include, among others, 2,2,2-trichloroethyl, *p*-nitrobenzyl, and trimethylsilyl. The penicillin ester is oxidized to the sulfoxide using sodium metaperiodate or organic peracids (the esterification–oxidation sequence can be reversed) and the ring expansion is carried out using one of a number of reaction conditions now on record, eg, benzene-trimethylphosphite, dimethylacetamide-*p*-toluenesulfonic acid, dimethyl formamide–acetic anhydride or acetonitrile–pyridine–dimethyldichlorosilane. Removal of the acyl (phenylacetyl, phenoxyacetyl) side chain via the imino chloride–imino ether intermediates, and the carboxyl protecting group, gives 7-ADCA. A process of special merit uses excess silylating agent in the presence of organic amines to protect the carboxyl group of the penicillin sulfoxide, and to accomplish the ring expansion as well (91). 7-ADCA is an item of commerce and is used in the manufacture of cephradine. For the manufacture of cephalexin, it has been found convenient to use the intermediate 7-ADCA esters, eg, starting with phenoxymethylpenicillin, the 2,2,2-trichloroethyl ester is obtained by reaction with 2,2,2-trichloroethyl chloroformate followed by thermal decarbonylation of the mixed anhydride. The oxidation, ring expansion, and acyl side-chain removal closely parallel procedures just described. The resulting product is the 2,2,2-trichloroethyl ester of 7-ADCA which can be isolated as its *p*-toluenesulfonate salt. The ester is acylated in high yield with an *N*-protected D-phenylglycine using a carboxyl-activating agent. Removal of the two protective groups gives cephalexin.

7-Amino-3-Heterocyclethiomethyl-3-Cephem-4-Carboxylic Acids.   In cefazolin and cefamandole the 3-acetoxymethyl grouping of the cephalosporanic acid structure has been replaced by a heterocyclethiomethyl moiety. These substituents are constructed by the 3′-acetoxy displacement reactions discussed earlier. The displacement reaction can be carried out on cephalosporin C, 7-aminocephalosporanic acid, or the appropriate 7-acylaminocephalosporanic acid (Fig. 3). Present manufacturing procedures appear to use one of the first two alternatives; although not yet marketed, the production of cefatrizine is now accomplished most efficiently using the third. The displacement of the acetoxy group on 7-ACA by 2-mercapto-5-methyl-1,3,4-thiadiazole or 5-mercapto-1-methyltetrazole is readily accomplished in refluxing aqueous-acetone solution using an excess of the heterocyclic thiol. The reaction mixture is maintained at about pH 7–8 by adding sodium bicarbonate as required. Yields are 40–60%.

Semisynthetic Penicillins.   The semisynthetic penicillins are obtained from 6-APA by techniques commonly used in peptide synthesis. Acylation of the 6-APA is accomplished by reaction with a suitably activated derivative of a carboxylic acid, most frequently an acid chloride or a mixed anhydride. The coupling reaction can be carried out in organic solvents under anhydrous conditions or in aqueous solution. Organic amines, such as triethyl amine, are added to the anhydrous reactions; the aqueous reactions are frequently carried out in acetone–water mixtures in the presence of sodium bicarbonate. The resulting penicillins are usually isolated by distributing the product as its free acid into a water-immiscible organic solvent and the salts and other impurities into water. This can be followed by one or more transfers from organic to aqueous solvents and back, with charcoal treatment and the like as required. The penicillins can be precipitated from organic solution as amine salts, or as alkali metal salts. Potassium or sodium ethylhexanoate dissolved in lower aliphatic alcohols has been used for this purpose. For parenteral preparations, the penicillin in organic solution can be extracted with a stoichiometric amount of cold aqueous alkali and the resulting aqueous solution of the salt concentrated *in vacuo,* filtered sterile, and lyophilized; or the penicillin can be crystallized and finished by procedures similar to those described earlier for benzylpenicillin and phenoxymethylpenicillin.

For the neutral side chains, the acid chlorides serve as efficient acylating agents. Ampicillin presents a more complicated synthetic problem. Early procedures used *N*-benzyloxycarbonyl phenylglycine as its mixed anhydride with lower alkyl chloroformates, or phenylazidoacetyl chloride. Both required hydrogenation procedures to generate the unblocked phenylglycine side chain. Improvements include the use of D-phenylglycyl chloride hydrochloride (in the presence of acetone this gives the cyclic acetone adduct hetacillin), or D-phenylglycine *N*-protected by the enamine adduct ($-C(CH_3)=CHCOOC_2H_5$) obtained from its reaction with ethyl acetoacetate in the presence of base. This adduct, called the Dane salt, is activated for coupling by forming the mixed anhydride with isobutyl chloroformate. After the acylation, the *N*-protecting group is removed under acidic conditions sufficiently mild (CO_2–water) to avoid destruction of the penicillin. The *tert*-butoxycarbonyl protecting group used frequently in cephalosporin syntheses cannot be used here since the acid conditions required for its removal also open the β-lactam. For carbenicillin, the bis-acid chloride obtained initially by treating phenylmalonic acid with phosphorous pentachloride is quickly transformed into its half-ketene-half-acid chloride. This intermediate reacts smoothly with 6-APA to give carbenicillin. Care must be exercised in the reaction workup to minimize the decarboxylation of this material to benzylpenicillin. In the nonaqueous acylations, the low solubility of the 6-APA in organic solvents is a problem. The reaction conditions, and yields, can be improved considerably by first converting the 6-APA to soluble trialkylsilyl esters through reaction with hexamethyldisilazane. The silyl group is, of course, lost upon contact with water in the reaction workup.

   Semisynthetic Cephalosporins.   The general procedures used for the acylation of 6-APA are also used for the acylations of 7-ACA, 7-ADCA, and the 7-amino-3-heterocyclethiomethyl-3-cephem-4-carboxylic acids. Thus cephalothin can be made by reaction of 7-ACA with thiophene acetyl chloride in aqueous acetone and cephapirin by reaction of 7-ACA with pyridine-4(thioacetyl chloride) hydrochloride and triethylamine in methylene chloride. Cephacetrile is obtained in nearly quantitative yield by acylating 7-ACA in THF with a mixed anhydride obtained from cyanoacetic acid and trichloracetyl or phthaloyl chloride, or in methylene chloride with cyanoacetyl chloride. The acylations of 7-ADCA and its 2,2,2-trichloroethyl ester to give cephradine and cephalexin were mentioned earlier. Cefazolin can be efficiently obtained by first displacing the acetoxy group from cephalosporin C followed by removal of the α-aminoadipic acid side chain and acylation of the 7-amino-3-(2-methyl-1,3,4-thiadiazole-5-thiomethyl)-3-cephem-4-carboxylic acid [30246-33-4] in either aqueous acetone or methylene chloride with the mixed anhydride obtained from 1-(1H)-tetrazoleacetic acid and pivaloyl or benzoyl chloride. Purification of the cephalosporins parallel the methods used to purify the penicillins.

   Other Modifications.   The carboxyl groups of penicillins and cephalosporins have been modified in the expected ways. Penicillin esters are readily obtained by reaction of the alkali metal salts in DMF with appropriate halides, by activation of the carboxyl group (acid chlorides, mixed anhydrides) and treatment with alcohols, by decarbonylation of mixed anhydrides with carbonic acids (2,2,2-trichloroethyl), or by other conventional methods. The preparation of cephalosporin esters is complicated by the predisposition of the 3-cephem double bond to isomerize to the 2-cephem position (**45**). This occurs in the presence of base (amines, etc) when the carboxyl group is blocked (ester, amide, chloride, anhydride). The isomerization process is reversible and equilibrium mixtures are usually encountered. The nature of the 3-substituent influences the composition of the mixture. Cephalosporanic acid derivatives (**42**) give mixtures rich in the 2-cephem isomers; deacetoxymethylcephalosporanic acid derivatives ((**27**) W = H) give mixtures that are rich in the 3-cephem isomers. Because of the double bond isomerization under these conditions, cephalosporin esters are more easily obtained by reaction of the acid group with diazoalkanes (diazomethane, phenyldiazomethane, diphenyldiazomethane). The *tert*-butyl esters of the cephalosporins are convenient chemical intermediates. The *tert*-butyl esters of 7-ACA, 7-ADCA, and other 3-substituted-7-amino-3-cephem-4-carboxylic acids can be obtained by treatment with isobutylene in dioxane–sulfuric acid. Amides of penicillins and cephalosporins have been described. For cephalosporin amide synthesis, the double bond isomerization problems parallel those of the ester preparations. Cephalosporin sulfoxides readily undergo decarboxylation when warmed with tertiary amines (**46**). In an interesting series of reactions, the penicillin carboxyl group has been replaced by a tetrazole ring through a multiple-step reaction sequence (carboxyl, amide, nitrile, tetrazole). This penicillin analogue ((**26**) Z = $=$C(CH$_3$)$_2$) has been converted to its analogous cephalosporin ((**26**) Z = $=$C(CH$_3$)CH$_2$—). Both display surprisingly good antibacterial activities (92).

   An early reaction of the sulfur atom was the desulfurization of benzylpenicillin

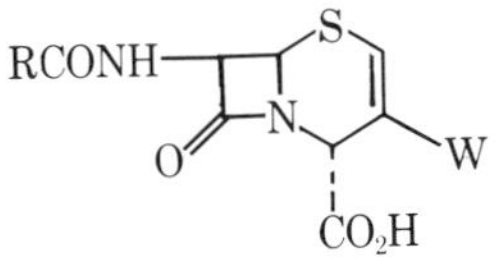

(45) 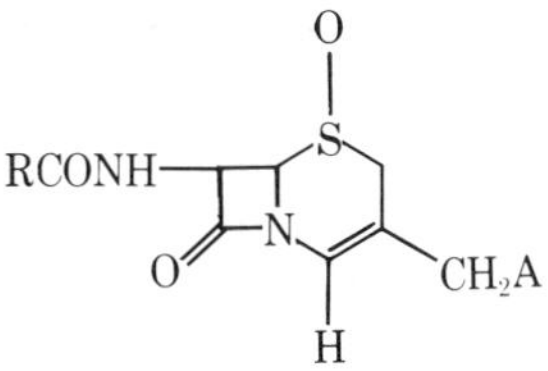   (46)

by Raney nickel to give desthiobenzylpenicillin [4425-26-7]. This reaction played a role in the original determination of the penicillin structure (9). The sulfur atom in both the penicillins and the cephalosporins is readily oxidized by various reagents (sodium metaperiodate, hydrogen peroxide, organic peracids) to the sulfoxide. The penicillins oxidize somewhat more easily than the cephalosporins, and stronger oxidation conditions (potassium permanganate) produce penicillin sulfones. Sulfoxides obtained from penicillins having an N–H grouping in the side chain have the (S)- or β-configuration (cis to the 6-side chain). Oxidation (peracid) of methyl 6-phthalimidopenicillanate gives the epimeric (R)-sulfoxide. Under certain oxidation conditions, mixtures of the two epimeric oxides can be obtained. A thorough analysis of the course of these oxidations and interconversions of the epimers has been published (93). Normally when 2-cephem structures are oxidized, the 3-cephem sulfoxide is obtained. This is a valuable method for converting 2-cephems to 3-cephems. The 3-cephem sulfoxides, so obtained, can be converted in good yield to the 3-cephems (sulfide) by reaction with reducing agents such as iodide, stannous or cuprous ions, or thiosulfate in the presence of acyl halides.

Finishing. As antibiotics, the penicillins and cephalosporins used in medicine are subject to production and testing controls under federal regulation including batch certification prior to distribution. Standards for potency and purity are established by the FDA in the form of regulations published from time to time in the *Federal Register*. Required labeling data include the lot number or an identifying mark, the number of antibiotic units (biosynthetic penicillins) or the weight of the product in the container or dosage unit (tablet, capsule) and the expiration date. When the material complies only with the standards for oral or nonparenteral use, the label must indicate this. Data required for certification include moisture content, pH, identification, specific rotation, pyrogenicity, sterility, safety, and potency.

The final isolation and purification of these antibiotics to give bulk chemicals suitable for incorporation into clinical dosage forms is controlled by the nature of the chemical substance and the federal certification controls indicated. The other products are carried through similar final purification steps which are followed by procedures for sterilization and removal of pyrogens and particulate matter for the parenteral dosage forms. These individual processes as well as those used to incorporate the bulk chemical into tablet, capsule, and vial dosage forms, are largely proprietary in nature and depend on the procedures adopted by the individual manufacturer.

Economic Aspects

Of the many substances, both natural and synthetic, that fall within the definition of the β-lactam antibiotics, only about fourteen penicillins (Table 2) and eight cephalosporins (Table 5) are important items of commerce. One semisynthetic cephamycin and several additional penicillins and cephalosporins (see pages 131 and 132) are now under development, and a few of these may be added to this group of commercially available drugs. It is estimated that worldwide retail antibiotic sales in 1975 were 4.5 billion dollars, with sales of 700 million dollars (15%) in the United States (94). The penicillins and the cephalosporins accounted for 37% and 12%, respectively, of the approximately 430 million dollars of United States sales which were made to outpatients, primarily through retail pharmacies. The remaining 270 million dollars of sales of antibiotics were used in hospitals, where the β-lactams accounted for 71% (penicillins, 30%; cephalosporins, 41%) of the antibiotics administered orally and 64% (penicillins, 22%; cephalosporins, 42%) of those given by injection.

The retail use of the penicillins and cephalosporins is controlled by prescription. Many of these drugs are covered by patents in the United States and elsewhere. Those still under patent protection may be distributed by one or more suppliers. The older antibiotics, such as benzylpenicillin and phenoxymethylpenicillin, on which patent coverage no longer exists are frequently distributed by many suppliers, and are sold under both brand and generic names. The retail price varies considerably depending on the brand of drug and the dispensing pharmacy (retail or hospital). Contract sales to large volume users also influence the cost per dose. Three annual publications afford specific information on the sources and prices of these antibiotics for retail use (95–96).

The manufacture of penicillins since the mid 1940s and of cephalosporins since the early 1960s has undergone rapid and continuous growth. For example, production of biosynthetic penicillins in the United States was 4000 kg in 1945, 195,000 kg in 1951 (97), and in excess of 3 million kg in 1974 (98). With increasing production the cost has declined, progressing from $20 to $1 to less than 2¢ to less than 1¢ per 100,000 units in 1943, 1945, 1951 and 1974, respectively (97–98). The production of cephalosporin C has followed a similar growth pattern but the decline in cost has been less spectacular. In 1976 the cost of cephalosporin C in bulk quantities was in the range of $150–200/kg; the cost of benzylpenicillin was approximately $25/kg. Plants for the production of penicillins are distributed widely throughout the world; those for making cephalosporins are less broadly distributed. Table 7 lists the primary manufacturers of penicillins in the United States and of cephalosporins in the United States and other parts of the world. The list is derived in part from data reported annually by the United States International Trade Commission (98). This organization also reports annually on the United States production and sales of bulk medicinal chemicals. Their data on the production of bulk penicillins are summarized in Table 8. Similar data on the cephalosporins are not available since the production and sales of bulk cephalosporins are included with those of all antibiotics produced or sold in the United States other than the penicillins, tetracyclines, neomycin, and antifungal and antitubercular antibiotics.

Health and Safety Factors

The toxicity characteristics relating to the clinical use of the penicillins and cephalosporins are discussed below. The large-scale handling of these agents associated with their manufacture and formulation entails some risk. Certain manufacturing intermediates, eg, 7-aminocephalosporanic acid, have been found to produce contact dermatitis in operators chronically exposed to the chemical. In rare cases, individuals

Table 7. Primary Manufacturers and Bulk Suppliers of Penicillins in the United States and Cephalosporins in the United States and Elsewhere

Chemical	Company	Chemical	Company
penicillin G	Wyeth Laboratories	amoxicillin	Beecham, Inc.
	E. R. Squibb & Sons		Bristol Laboratories
	Pfizer, Inc.		Roche Laboratories
	Bristol Laboratories	carbenicillin	Beecham, Inc.
	Eli Lilly & Co.		Roerig Laboratories
penicillin V	Eli Lilly & Co.	cephalothin	Eli Lilly & Co.
	E. R. Squibb & Sons		Glaxo Laboratories, Ltd. (UK)
	Bristol Laboratories	cephapirin	Bristol Laboratories
	Wyeth Laboratories	cephacetrile	Ciba-Geigy, Ltd. (Switz.)
	Abbott Laboratories	cephaloridine	Glaxo Laboratories, Ltd. (UK)
phenethicillin	Bristol Laboratories		Eli Lilly & Co.
	Pfizer, Inc.	cefazolin	Fujisawa Pharmaceutical Corp. (Jpn.)
methicillin	Beecham, Inc.		Eli Lilly & Co.
	Bristol Laboratories		Smith Kline & French Laboratories
oxacillin	Beecham Laboratories	cephaloglycin	Eli Lilly & Co.
	Bristol Laboratories	cephalexin	Eli Lilly & Co.
cloxacillin	Beecham Laboratories		Glaxo Laboratories, Ltd. (UK)
	Bristol Laboratories	cephradine	Smith Kline & French Laboratories
dicloxacillin	Beecham Laboratories		E. R. Squibb & Sons
	Bristol Laboratories	cephalosporin C	Glaxo Laboratories, Ltd. (UK)
	Ayerst Laboratories		Eli Lilly & Co.
	Wyeth Laboratories		Fujisawa Pharmaceutical Corp. (Jpn.)
nafcillin	Wyeth Laboratories		Montedison Pharmaceutical Div. (Italy)
ampicillin	Beecham Laboratories		Antibioticos S.A. (Spain)
	Biocraft Laboratories, Inc.	7-ADCA	Gist-Brocades N.V. (Neth.)
	Bristol Laboratories		Glaxo Laboratories, Ltd. (UK)
	E. R. Squibb & Sons		Eli Lilly & Co.
	Wyeth Laboratories		Montedison Pharmaceutical Div. (Italy)
	Ayerst Laboratories		Antibioticos S.A. (Spain)
hetacillin	Bristol Laboratories		

sensitized to penicillins when exposed to minute amounts of the substances may exhibit hypersensitivity reactions that range from mild to severe skin rashes and life-threatening anaphylaxes.

Specifications and Analytical Methods

The extensive production and clinical use of the penicillins and cephalosporins have produced an array of specifications and procedures for characterizing and analyzing these antibiotics. The tests required in each case are tailored to the particular antibiotic and dosage form and have to do with identity (high pressure liquid chromatography, color reactions, optical and magnetic spectra, etc), quality and purity (water content, pH, specific rotation), safety (pyrogens, histamine, sterility), and strength (microbiological or chemical assay). The listings of required tests, and detailed

Table 8.   United States Production and Sales of Bulk Antibiotics[a]

Antibiotics	Production, t	Sales		
		t	$ $\times 10^3$	$/kg
antibiotics total	9340	3750	254,477	67.86
biosynthetic penicillins	3550	1886	47,656	25.27
benzylpenicillin for medicinal use only	1422			
all other biosynthetic for all uses	2128	1886	47,656	25.27
semisynthetic penicillins	661	142	27,461	193.39
ampicillin	502	117	23,070	197.18
all other semisynthetic	159	25	4,391	175.64
cephalosporins and all other antibiotics for medicinal use except tetracyclines, neomycin, antifungal, and antitubercular antibiotics[b]	1030	400	109,954	274.88

[a] Ref. 98.
[b] Production and sales data are reported separately for the excepted antibiotics, Ref. 98.

procedures for carrying them out, are published in the *Federal Register* and summarized annually in the *Code of Federal Regulations* (99).

The dosage and antibacterial potency of the penicillins and the cephalosporins are usually expressed in terms of weight. For penicillin G these values are frequently expressed in penicillin units. An international unit of penicillin was established by the International Conference on the Standardization of Penicillin held in London in 1944; it represents the penicillin activity contained in 0.6 μg of a master standard of the crystalline sodium salt of penicillin G. Thus 1 mg of pure penicillin G sodium salt equals 1667 units.

The β-lactam antibiotics have been characterized qualitatively in a variety of ways. These substances can be detected in screening programs for new antibiotics by the use of test bacteria that have been made supersensitive to the β-lactam structure and by the loss of antibacterial activity in the presence of added β-lactamases (24). Principal quantitative assay methods rely on microbiological determinations (plate assay and turbidometric assay) and chemical procedures (titrametric, iodometric, colorimetric) based on the hydrolytic opening of the β-lactam by dilute alkali or β-lactamases (12), or ring opening with hydroxylamine. More recently, high pressure liquid chromatography has been found effective for the quantitative determination of cephalosporins (100). This technique is especially useful for quantitative determination of individual cephalosporins in fermentation broths and isolates containing mixtures of several analogues, eg, cephalosporin C, deacetylcephalosporin C, and deacetoxycephalosporin C. Other separation systems adapted to quantitative methods have been used with cephalosporin and penicillin mixtures including paper chromatography, thin layer chromatography, and paper electrophoresis. Additional chemical assay procedures based on structural features other than the β-lactam have been used. These include ninhydrin determinations of 6-APA, 7-ACA, and amino-substituted penicillins and cephalosporins, and the displacement of the 3'-acetoxy group of cephalosporanic acids with nicotinamide, followed by conversion of the pyridinium moiety to a chromophore by reaction with 1,3-dihydroxyacetone. Details of these detection and assay procedures are available from a number of sources (101).

Uses and Applications

The penicillins and cephalosporins are used for treating infectious diseases of bacterial origin in man and animals. In fact, the clinical technique of treating bacterial infections by the systemic administration of fermentation-derived substances known as antibiotics began with the first use of penicillins in humans in 1941 (7–8); and the penicillins and cephalosporins have dominated this therapeutic field since that time (102). In spite of the subsequent discovery and development of many new classes of antibiotics, the biosynthetic penicillins (benzylpenicillin, phenoxymethylpenicillin) continue to be the drugs of choice for treating most infections caused by gram-positive bacteria. The cephalosporins, ampicillin, and more recently the carbenicillin-type penicillins and the cephamycins, have extended the applicability of the β-lactam antibiotics to include the treatment of infections caused by many gram-negative bacteria as well (7,102–103).

The clinical effectiveness of the penicillins and cephalosporins, depends on a number of properties associated with the individual antibiotic. It must inhibit or preferably kill bacteria at acceptable concentrations of the drug (*in vitro* activity). Its toxicity properties must allow it to be administered safely to the host. It must be capable of achieving concentrations in the host (serum and tissue levels) greater than those required to inhibit the pathogenic organism. This capability is controlled by such pharmacokinetic properties as efficiency and rate of absorption, rate of metabolism and excretion, tissue distribution, serum binding, serum and tissue inactivation, and the like. These properties form the basis for the comparison and selection of the various penicillins and cephalosporins for therapeutic use (7).

In Vitro Activities.   The *in vitro* antibacterial activities of six representative β-lactam antibiotics, three penicillins, and three cephalosporins, are presented in Table 9 (103). These activities are expressed in terms of minimum inhibitory concentrations (MIC), the minimum concentration (µg/mL) of antibiotic required to inhibit the bacterium (105). A studied comparison of these MIC values for the six antibiotics should supply the reader with a feel for the relative potency and spectrum of antibacterial activity that the various penicillins and cephalosporins possess.

Toxicity.   The penicillins are striking in their general lack of toxicity. For example, carbenicillin is recommended in parenteral doses of up to 40 g/d for treating certain severe systemic infections (106). The lack of toxicity is impressive in normal individuals, but the wide use of these substances is accompanied by a sufficient incidence of unpredictable adverse reactions to necessitate caution in their prescription. The most common adverse effect from the use of penicillins is an allergic reaction which can range from a mild rash to fatal anaphylactic shock in rare cases. The cephalosporins are also considered to be particularly safe antibiotics, but they cannot be used with the level of inattention to potential toxicity applied to the penicillins. Of the cephalosporins that have been used extensively in humans, cephaloridine has the highest incidence of toxic reactions, producing significant renal tubular damage in a small number of patients when given in high and prolonged doses. The cephalosporins have a lower incidence of allergic reactions than the penicillins. Cross allergenicity between the cephalosporins and penicillins has occurred, but its incidence is also low, and cephalosporins have been used to treat patients with known allergy to penicillins. Because of their broad-spectrum activity, overgrowth by fungi or resistant bacteria can occur with prolonged use.

Table 9. *In Vitro* **Antibacterial Activities of Representative Penicillins and Cephalosporins**[a,b]

Bacterial species	Penicillin G MIC mode (range), μg/mL	Penicillin G Proportion resistant[c], %	Ampicillin MIC mode (range), μg/mL	Ampicillin Proportion resistant[c], %	Carbenicillin MIC mode (range), μg/mL	Carbenicillin Proportion resistant[c], %	Cephalothin MIC mode (range), μg/mL	Cephalothin Proportion resistant[c], %	Cefazolin MIC mode (range), μg/mL	Cefazolin Proportion resistant[c], %	Cephalexin MIC mode (range), μg/mL	Cephalexin Proportion resistant[c], %
Strep. pneumoniae	0.01 (<0.01–0.02)	(0)	0.02 (<0.01–0.1)	(0)	0.4 (0.1–1)	(1)[d]	0.1 (0.02–0.4)	(0)	0.1 (0.1–0.3)	(0)	2 (0.1–12)	(1)[d]
Strep. pyogenes (A)	<0.01 (<0.01–0.02)	(0)	0.01 (<0.01–0.2)	(0)	0.2 (0.1–1)	(1)	0.12 (0.05–0.5)	(0)	0.1 (0.1–0.3)	(0)	0.6 (0.2–6)	(1)
Staph. aureus nonpenicillinase	0.06 (0.02–0.2)	(0)	0.1 (0.04–0.3)	(0)	5 (1–10)	(1)	0.1 (0.08–0.8)	(0)	0.1 (0.06–2)	(0)	2.6 (0.5–16)	(1)
Enterococci	3 (2–5)	(1)	1.25 (0.5–5)	(1)	50	(100)	0.2 (0.06–2)	(0)	0.3 (0.06–8)	(0)	2.9 (0.5–16)	(1)
N. gonorrhoeae	0.05 (<0.01–2.5)	(v)[e]	0.02 (0.01–1.0)	(v)			24 (8–32)	(100)	32 (15–50)	(100)	100 (32–256)	(100)
N. meningitidis	0.06	(0)	0.03	(0)	0.1		(0.25–3)	(1)	1 (0.1–>50)	(1)	3 (0.1–6.3)	(1)
H. influenzae	0.6 (0.1–3)	(1)	0.2 (0.05–1.0)	(5)	(0.5–125c)		(2–8)	(1)	(2–12)	(1)	>100 (125–>100)	(100)
E. coli	16–>125 (2–64)	(30c)	3 (<1–>125)	(20c)	5 (2–>125)	(20c)	4 (2–128)	(15c)	2 (1–256)	(5c)	4 (1–32)	
Salmonella			1 (0.4–>125)	(10c)	(4–16)		(1.5–12)		2 (1–6.25)		5 (4–50)	(20c)
Proteus mirabilis	8 (2–>125)		1 (0.5–>125)	(10c)	1 (0.5–>125)	(10c)	2 (0.5–12)	(10)	1 (0.5–5)	(5)	8 (4–50)	
Proteus (other)	16–>250	(90c)	125 (32–>125)	(90c)	2 (0.5–>125)	(15c)	(32–>256)	(100)	50 (2.5–100)	(60c)	>100 (25–>100)	(100)
K. pneumoniae	>250		12 (4–>125)	(80c)	>125 (50–>125)	(100)	4 (1.8–>256)	(15c)	2 (1.8–>256)	(15c)	12 (1–>100)	(30c)
Enterobacter	>250		50 (25–>125)	(85c)	12 (6–>125)	(25c)	>100 (2–>256)	(90c)	>100 (2–>256)	(80c)	>100 (50–>100)	(100c)
Pseudomonas	>250		>250		32 (8–>250)	(20+c)	>256		>256		>256	

[a] Reproduced with permission from *Annual Review of Pharmacology*, Vol. 14 (103). Copyright 1974 by Annual Reviews Inc.
[b] MIC, minimum inhibitory concentration.
[c] Resistant to serum concentrations of drug achieved with normal dosage. Proportion may vary markedly depending on strain selection, nosocomial origin, and testing methodology including inoculum size.
[d] 1 = Many strains intermediate in susceptibility.
[e] v = Variable proportion of strains (approximately 5–30%) with MICs at high end of range, depending on population studied.

Penicillins. *Biosynthetic Penicillins.* The penicillins available for clinical use in the United States are included in Table 2. Benzylpenicillin is the most widely used member of the group, primarily for therapy in infections caused by gram-positive bacteria (Table 9). It is rapidly destroyed by gastric acid so that oral absorption is erratic, therefore, it is usually administered by the parenteral route. Alkali metal salts of benzylpenicillin produce transient high blood levels especially when given intravenously. Salts with procaine or dibenzylethylenediamine give low, but sustained blood levels on intramuscular injection. Phenoxymethylpenicillin and phenethicillin have antibacterial activities similar to those of benzylpenicillin, but they are more resistant to destruction by gastric acid. When given orally, especially in a fasting state, they produce blood levels higher than those obtained by an equal dose of benzylpenicillin.

Penicillinase-Resistant Penicillins. At one time the usefulness of the penicillins as therapeutic agents was threatened by the emergence of pathogenic staphylococci which are resistant to these drugs. These organisms produce penicillin-specific β-lactamases (penicillinases) that rapidly destroy those penicillins already described, and others such as ampicillin and carbenicillin. Table 2 lists five semisynthetic penicillins—methicillin, oxacillin, cloxacillin, dicloxacillin, and nafcillin—that were developed in response to this problem. These agents have antibacterial spectra similar to that of benzylpenicillin although they are significantly less active *in vitro.* They are highly resistant to staphylococcal penicillinase and, therefore, they are specifically indicated for treating infections caused by benzylpenicillin-resistant staphylococci. Methicillin requires parenteral dosing, but nafcillin and the oxacillins are more resistant to acids and can be given orally.

Broad-Spectrum Penicillins. Ampicillin closely resembles benzylpenicillin in its activity against the gram-positive bacteria, but it is more active than the latter against some gram-negative bacteria. Thus, in addition to *Haemophilis influenzae, Neisseriae,* and gram-positive cocci susceptible to benzylpenicillin, it is active against *Proteus mirabilis* and some *Escherichia coli, Shigella, Salmonella,* and *Klebsiella* strains (Table 9). Ampicillin is destroyed by penicillinase at about the same rate as benzylpenicillin. It is acid stable, readily absorbed when given orally, and water soluble so that it can be given by the intravenous and intramuscular routes as well. Hetacillin is an acetone adduct of ampicillin, and amoxicillin is the *p*-hydroxy analogue. Both have *in vitro* activities virtually identical to ampicillin. The pharmokinetic properties of hetacillin are also essentially those of ampicillin; amoxicillin shows improved absorption on oral administration giving higher serum levels and better urinary recovery than ampicillin.

Broad-Spectrum–Narrow-Use Penicillins. For the most part, the penicillins, and the cephalosporins, are ineffective against *Pseudomonas aeruginosa.* Exceptions are carbenicillin and its related analogues. Carbenicillin's antibacterial spectrum includes activity against *Pseudomonas aeruginosa,* strains of indole-positive *Proteus,* some strains of *Escherichia coli, Serratia, Providentia, Citrobacter,* and a few other newly emerging highly resistant pathogenic strains of enteric bacteria. Because of its effectiveness against *Pseudomonas aeruginosa,* indole-positive *Proteus* and the other resistant bacteria named above, carbenicillin is indicated primarily for use in serious infections caused by this relatively narrow group of organisms. It must be administered parenterally since it has poor acid stability, undergoing decarboxylation to benzylpenicillin. Frequently, impressively high amounts are given by intravenous infusion to achieve serum peak concentrations of several hundred micrograms per milliliter since its MICs against *Pseudomonas aeruginosa* often range from 50 to 250 µg/mL. Its chemical stability is improved by conversion to its indanyl ester (side-chain carboxyl). This ester is absorbed orally (about 40%) and is rapidly hydrolyzed by esterases to carbenicillin, but the relatively low serum levels of carbenicillin attained restrict its use. Two closely related analogues of carbenicillin—ticarcillin and sulbenicillin—have been marketed overseas. Both show slightly better chemical stability, *in vitro* activities and serum levels than carbenicillin. A growing number of *N*-acyl derivatives of ampicillin have been found to display significantly better *in vitro* activities against *Pseudomonas aeruginosa* and other gram-negative bacteria than carbenicillin. Although several of these penicillins have undergone clinical trials, none have yet been cleared for marketing. Some of the acyl groups that confer this activity are listed below.

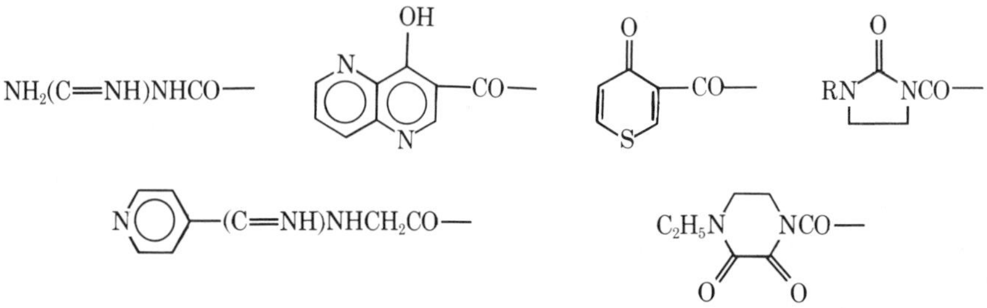

Cephalosporins.   Tables 5 and 10 list the cephalosporins that are available for clinical use and those that have been subjected to extensive premarketing clinical evaluation. The antibacterial spectra of the commercially available cephalosporins (Table 5) are practically identical, although there are quantitative differences in potency. All are characterized by high activity against a large number of gram-positive and gram-negative organisms (Table 9) including penicillin-resistant staphylococci. Several of the cephalosporins in Table 10 extend the range of activity against the gram-negative bacteria beyond that obtained with the antibiotics listed in Table 5. The cephalosporins in both tables differ in pharmacokinetic properties that relate to parenteral and oral absorption, serum levels, biliary excretion, serum protein binding, and the like.

Injectable Cephalosporins.   Cephalothin occupies a position among the cephalosporins similar to that of benzylpenicillin among the penicillins. Although marketed first and followed by analogues with improved properties, it continues to account for a significant part of cephalosporin use. It possesses broad-spectrum activity with important exceptions in the gram-negative group (eg, indole-positive *Proteus, Enterobacter, Pseudomonas,* etc). It has good resistance to staphylococcal penicillinase which contributes to its broad use. Only about 2% of cephalothin is absorbed when it is given orally. Therefore it is administered intravenously or intramuscularly where pain on injection is moderately high. Cephalothin is partially metabolized to the less active deacetylcephalothin [30200-18-1]. Cephapirin and cephacetrile are remarkably like cephalothin in their antimicrobial activities, pharmacokinetic behavior, and clinical indications. Cephaloridine displays better activity than cephalothin against the gram-positive cocci, it produces higher serum levels with equivalent doses, and it causes less pain on injection. These advantages are offset by a somewhat lower re-

Table 10. Cephalosporins and Cephamycins with Clinical Evaluation

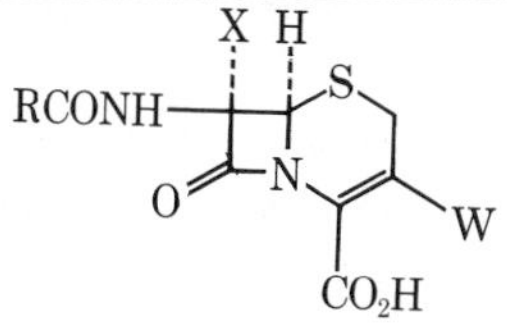

Name	CAS Registry Number	R	X	W
Injectable cephalosporins				
cefamandole (nafate)	[34444-01-4]	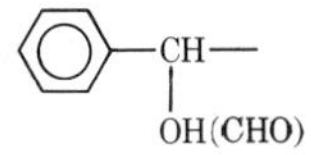	H	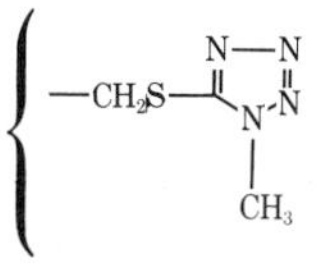
cefazaflur	[58665-96-6]	CF₃SCH₂	H	
cefuroxime	[55268-75-2]	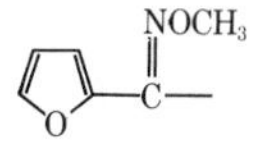	H	$-CH_2OCONH_2$
cephanone	[24209-51-6]	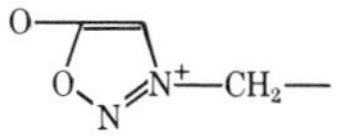	H	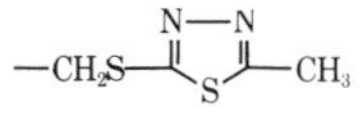
Oral cephalosporins				
cefatrizine	[51627-14-6]	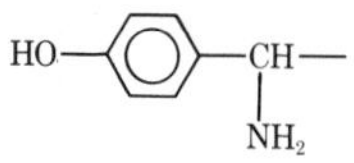	H	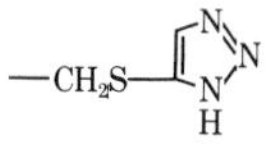
cefachlor	[53994-73-3]	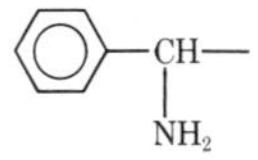	H	$-Cl$
cefadroxil	[50370-12-2]	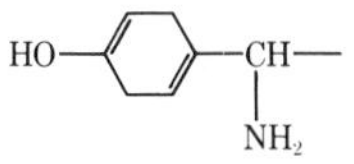	H	$-CH_3$
Injectable cephamycin				
cefoxitin	[35607-66-0]	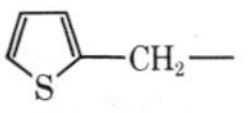	OCH₃	$-CH_2OCONH_2$

sistance to penicillinase and a renal toxicity liability that restricts its dosage to less than 4 g/d. Cefazolin is active against the gram-positive cocci at about the same level as cephalothin, but its activity against susceptible gram-negative pathogens is usually better. As with the other cephalosporins in this group, it is not appreciably absorbed when given orally. However, on intramuscular administration it gives serum levels that are four times the levels obtained with an equal dose of cephalothin. It has low renal toxicity in animals. Like cephaloridine, the 3-substituent is of a type that resists metabolic removal.

Oral Cephalosporins. Unlike the penicillins, which are absorbed orally except when limited by instability to gastric acid, the relatively acid-stable cephalosporins described so far are exceedingly poorly absorbed by the oral route. It is surprising therefore that cephalexin and cephradine (Table 5) are absorbed orally with efficiencies (80% or better) greater than for the penicillins. These agents are very similar in their antimicrobial and pharmacokinetic properties. They are generally less active *in vitro* than the injectable cephalosporins. Both are efficiently excreted through the kidney, giving high urine titers. They are indicated for treatment of mild to moderate infections, including infections of the urinary tract. Cephaloglycin is a less stable member of this group that is rather poorly absorbed orally (10–25%). It produces relatively low serum levels but adequate urinary concentrations for treatment of some urinary tract infections.

New Cephalosporins. Four injectable cephalosporins that have undergone clinical evaluations are listed in Table 10. Cefamandole (107) has about the same activity as cefazolin against normally susceptible gram-negative bacteria, such as *E. coli* and *Klebsiella,* but its activity extends to a somewhat broader group of gram-negative organisms, including some strains of *Enterobacter* and indole-positive *Proteus.* Its activity against gram-positive cocci is significantly lower than, eg, cephalothin's, but is still sufficient for effective therapy. Serum levels are between those obtained with cephalothin and cefazolin. Cefuroxime (108) extends the gram-negative spectrum less broadly than cefamandole but retains more gram-positive activity. Cefazaflur (109) exhibits exceptionally high *in vitro* activities against gram-positive and gram-negative organisms and also extends the spectrum of activity against the latter but less broadly than cephamandole. Cephanone (110) displayed good *in vitro* activities and high serum levels on intramuscular injection, but it has been withdrawn from clinical trials.

Two of the oral cephalosporins listed in Table 10 (cefatrizine (111), cefachlor (112)) have higher *in vitro* activities than cephalexin, giving serum levels on oral dosing equal to or somewhat lower than those obtained with an equivalent dose of the latter. Cefadroxil (113) with essentially the activity of cephalexin, is reported to produce serum levels of longer duration.

Cephamycins. Cefoxitin (22) is the first cephamycin to undergo clinical trials. Like cefamandole, it is more active than cephalothin against many of the gram-negative organisms susceptible to the latter, and its antibacterial spectrum is broader, including activity against indole-positive *Proteus* and some strains of *Serratia.* Its gram-positive activity is poorer than that of cephalothin, but still adequate. This antibiotic has been shown to be resistant to most β-lactamases produced by gram-negative bacteria, including organisms that are not susceptible to it. Cefoxitin must be given intravenously; it produces serum levels in the same range as cefamandole.

BIBLIOGRAPHY

"Penicillin" in *ECT* 1st ed., Vol. 9, pp. 922–943, by W. E. Brown, Squibb Institute for Medical Research; "Penicillins" in *ECT* 2nd ed., Vol. 14, pp. 652–707, by Kenneth Butler, Chas. Pfizer & Co., Inc.

In many cases reviews rather than individual original articles are cited.

1. J. C. Sheehan, K. R. Henery-Logan, and D. A. Johnson, *J. Am. Chem. Soc.* **75,** 3292 (1953).
2. R. B. Morin, B. G. Jackson, E. H. Flynn, and R. W. Roeske, *J. Am. Chem. Soc.* **84,** 3400 (1962).
3. B. Loder, G. G. F. Newton, and E. P. Abraham, *Biochem. J.* **79,** 408 (1961).
4. A. Fleming, *Br. J. Exp. Pathol.* **10,** 226 (1929).
5. E. Chain, H. W. Florey, A. D. Gardner, N. G. Heatley, M. A. Jennings, J. Orr-Ewing, and A. G. Sanders, *Lancet* **1940**(ii), 226.
6 E. P. Abraham, E. Chain, C. M. Fletcher, A. D. Gardner, N. G. Heatley, M. A. Jennings, and H. W. Florey, *Lancet* **1941**(ii), 177.
7. L. Weinstein in L. S. Goodman and A. Gilman, eds., *The Pharmacological Basis of Therapeutics,* 5th ed., Macmillan Publishing Co., New York, 1975, Chapt. 57.
8. H. W. Florey, E. Chain, N. G. Heatley, M. A. Jennings, A. G. Sanders, E. P. Abraham, and M. E. Florey, *Antibiotics,* Vol. II, Oxford University Press, London, New York, Toronto, 1949.
9. H. T. Clarke, J. R. Johnson, and R. Robinson, eds., *The Chemistry of Penicillin,* Princeton University Press, Princeton, N. J., 1949.
10. A. J. Moyer and R. D. Coghill, *J. Bacteriol.* **53,** 329 (1947).

11. Q. F. Soper, C. W. Whitehead, O. K. Behrens, J. J. Corse, and R. G. Jones, *J. Am. Chem. Soc.* **70,** 2849 (1948).

12. D. Crowfoot, C. W. Bunn, B. W. Rogers-Low, and A. Turner-Jones in Ref. 9, p. 310; H. T. Clarke, J. R. Johnson, and Sir R. Robinson in Ref. 9, p. 5; Ref. 8, p. 667.

13. F. R. Batchelor, F. P. Doyle, J. H. C. Nayler, and G. N. Rolinson, *Nature (London)* **183,** 257 (1959); F. R. Batchelor, E. B. Chain, T. L. Hardy, K. R. L. Mansford, and G. N. Rolinson, *Proc. Roy. Soc. London Ser. B.* **154,** 498 (1961).

14. G. Brotzu, *Richerche su di Nuovo Antibiotico,* Lav. Ist. Igiene Cagliari, 1948.

15. E. P. Abraham, G. G. F. Newton, J. R. Schenck, M. P. Hargie, B. H. Olson, D. M. Shuurmans, M. W. Fisher, and S. A. Fusari, *Nature (London)* **176,** 551 (1955).

16. G. G. F. Newton and E. P. Abraham, *Nature (London)* **175,** 548 (1955); G. G. F. Newton and E. P. Abraham, *Biochem. J.* **62,** 651 (1956).

17. E. P. Abraham and G. G. F. Newton, *Biochem. J.* **79,** 377 (1961); D. C. Hodgkin and E. N. Maslen, *Biochem. J.* **79,** 393 (1961).

18. E. P. Abraham, *Pharm. Rev.* **14,** 473 (1962); E. P. Abraham, *Q. Rev. Chem. Soc.* **21,** 231 (1967); R. B. Morin and B. E. Jackson, *Fortschr. Chem. Org. Naturst.* **28,** 343 (1970).

19. R. Nagarajan, L. D. Boeck, M. Gorman, R. L. Hamill, C. E. Higgens, M. M. Hoehn, W. M. Stark, and J. G. Whitney, *J. Am. Chem. Soc.* **93,** 2308 (1971); E. O. Stapley, D. Hendlin, S. Hernandez, M. Jackson, J. H. Mater, A. K. Miller, H. B. Woodruff, T. W. Miller, G. Albers-Schönberg, B. H. Arison, and J. L. Smith, *Abstr. 15, 11th Interscience Conference on Antimicrobial Agents and Chemotherapy,* Atlantic City, N. J., 1971.

20. A. K. Miller and co-workers, *Antimicrob. Agents Chemother.* **2,** 287 (1972) and prior articles in this series; H. Fukase and co-workers, *J. Antibiot.* **29,** 113 (1976) and related articles.

21. H. R. Onishi and co-workers, *Antimicrob. Agents Chemother.* **5,** 38 (1974) and prior articles in this series; H. Nakao and co-workers, *J. Antibiot.* **29,** 554 (1976).

22. W. Brumfitt, J. Kosmidis, J. M. T. Hamilton-Miller, and J. N. G. Gilchrist, *Antimicrob. Agents Chemother.* **6,** 290 (1974); S. Schwartz and co-workers, *Abstr. 77, 16th Interscience Conference on Antimicrobial Agents and Chemotherapy,* Chicago, Ill., 1976.

23. F. M. Kahan and co-workers, *Abstr. No. 227;* H. Kropp and co-workers, *Abstr. No. 228;* G. Albers-Schönberg and co-workers, *Abstr. No. 229; 16th Interscience Conference on Antimicrobial Agents and Chemotherapy,* Chicago, Ill., 1976; U.S. Pat. 3,950,357 (Apr. 13, 1976), J. S. Kaham, F. M. Kahan, E. O. Stapley, R. T. Goegelman, and S. Hernandaz (to Merck & Co., Inc.).

24. M. Hashimoto, T. Komori and T. Kamiya, *J. Am. Chem. Soc.* **98,** 3023 (1976); H. Aoki and co-workers, *J. Antibiot.* **29,** 492 (1976); M. Hashimoto, T. Komori, and T. Kamiya, *J. Antibiot.* **29,** 890 (1976).

25. P. A. Hunter and C. Reading, *Abstr. No. 211, 16th Interscience Conference on Antimicrobial Agents and Chemotherapy,* Chicago, Ill., 1976; T. T. Howarth, A. G. Brown, and T. J. King, *J. Chem. Soc. Chem. Commun.* 266 (1976); A. G. Brown, T. T. Howarth, I. Stirling, and T. J. King, *Tetrahedron Lett.* **1976,** 4203.

26. E. H. Flynn, ed., *Cephalosporins and Penicillins, Chemistry and Biology,* Academic Press, Inc., New York, 1972.

27. M. Windholz, ed., *The Merck Index,* 9th ed., Merck & Co., Inc., Rahway, N. J., 1976.

28. J. P. Hou and J. W. Poole, *J. Pharm. Sci.* **60,** 503 (1971).

29. P. V. Demarco and R. Nagarajan in Ref. 26, Chapt. 8; G. F. H. Green, J. E. Page, and S. E. Staniforth, *J. Chem. Soc.* **1965,** 1595.

30. B. Fechtig, H. Peter, H. Bickel, and E. Vischer, *Helv. Chim. Acta* **51,** 1108 (1968); U.S. Pat. 3,697,515 (Oct. 10, 1972), B. Fechtig and co-workers (Ciba-Geigy Corp.).

31. D. M. Green, A. G. Long, P. J. May, and A. F. Turner, *J. Chem. Soc.* **1964,** 766.

32. E. P. Abraham and G. G. F. Newton in A. Goldin, F. Hawking, and R. J. Schnitzer, eds., *Advances in Chemotherapy,* Vol. II, Academic Press, Inc., New York, 1965, p. 23; E. Van Heyningen in N. J. Harper and A. B. Simmonds, eds., *Advances in Drug Research,* Vol. IV, Academic Press, Inc., New York, 1967, p. 1.

33. J. C. Sheehan and K. R. Henery-Logan, *J. Am. Chem. Soc.* **79,** 1262 (1957); **81,** 3089 (1959); **81,** 5838 (1959); J. C. Sheehan and J. P. Ferris, *J. Am. Chem. Soc.* **81,** 2912 (1959); R. B. Woodward, K. Heusler, J. Gosteli, P. Naegeli, W. Oppolzer, R. Ramage, S. Ranganathan, and H. Vorbrüggen, *J. Am. Chem. Soc.* **88,** 852 (1966); R. B. Woodward, *Science* **153,** 487 (1966); R. Heymès, G. Amiard, and G. Nominé, *C. R. Acad. Sci. Ser. C.* **263,** 170 (1966); R. Heymès, G. Amiard, and G. Nominé, *Bull. Soc. Chim. Fr.* 2343 (1973); 563 (1974); B. G. Christensen and R. W. Ratcliffe, *Tetrahedron Lett.* 4649 (1973); N. G. Sternberg, R. W. Ratcliffe, and B. G. Christensen, *Tetrahedron Lett.* 3567 (1974); J. A. Edwards,

A. Guzman, R. Johnson, P. J. Beeby, and J. H. Fried, *Tetrahedron Lett.* 2031 (1974); K. Heusler in Ref. 26, Chapt. 6.

34. R. B. Morin and B. E. Jackson, *Fortschr. Chem. Org. Naturst.* **28,** 343 (1970); R. J. Stoodley, *Tetrahedron* **31,** 2321 (1975); P. G. Sammes, *Chem. Rev.* **76,** 113 (1976); R. D. G. Cooper in D. H. Hey and D. I. John, eds., *MTP International Review of Science, Organic Chemistry Series One,* Vol. 6, University Park Press, Baltimore, Md., 1973, pp. 247–281; J. G. Gleason and G. L. Dunn in *Organic Compounds of Sulfur, Selenium and Tellurium,* Vol. 4, The Chemical Society, London, 1977, p. 466.

35. F. R. Batchelor, D. Gazzard, and J. H. C. Nayler, *Nature (London)* **191,** 910 (1961); D. A. Johnson and G. A. Hardcastle, Jr., *J. Am. Chem. Soc.* **83,** 3534 (1961).

36. R. A. Archer and B. S. Kitchell, *J. Org. Chem.* **31,** 3409 (1966).

37. G. G. F. Newton, E. P. Abraham, and S. Kawabara, *Antimicrob. Agents Chemother-1967,* 449 (1968); S. H. Eggers, V. V. Kane, and G. Lowe, *J. Chem. Soc.* 1262 (1965).

38. R. B. Morin, B. G. Jackson, R. A. Mueller, E. R. Lavagnino, W. B. Scanlon, and S. L. Andrews, *J. Am. Chem. Soc.* **85,** 1896 (1963).

39. R. B. Morin, B. G. Jackson, R. A. Mueller, E. R. Lavagnino, W. B. Scanlon, and S. L. Andrews, *J. Am. Chem. Soc.* **91,** 1401 (1969).

40. R. D. G. Cooper and D. O. Spry in Ref. 26, p. 181; P. G. Sammes in Ref. 34; R. J. Stoodley in Ref. 34; J. G. Gleason and G. L. Dunn in Ref. 34.

41. G. Lowe, *Chem. Ind. (London)* 459 (1975); A. K. Mukerjee and R. C. Srivastava, *Synthesis* 327 (1973); N. S. Isaacs, *Chem. Soc. Rev.* **5,** 181 (1976).

42. M. Gorman and C. W. Ryan in Ref. 26, Chapt. 12; J. P. Hou and J. W. Poole, *J. Pharm. Sci.* **60,** 503 (1971); A. E. Bird and J. H. C. Nayler in E. J. Ariens, ed., *Drug Design,* Vol. 2, Academic Press, Inc., New York, 1971, p. 277; J. R. E. Hoover and R. J. Stedman in A. Burger, ed., *Medicinal Chemistry,* 3rd ed., Interscience Publishers, a division of John Wiley & Sons, Inc., New York, 1970, p. 371; E. Van Heyningen in Ref. 31; F. P. Doyle and J. H. C. Nayler in N. J. Harper and A. B. Simonds, eds., *Advances in Drug Research,* Vol. I, Academic Press, Inc., New York, 1964, p. 1.

43. L. Tybring, *Antimicrob. Agents Chemother.* **8,** 266 (1975).

44. J. T. Park and L. Burman, *Biochem. Biophys. Res. Commun.* **51,** 863 (1973).

45. L. D. Cama and B. G. Christensen, *J. Am. Chem. Soc.* **96,** 7582 (1974).

46. K. Heusler in Ref. 26, p. 275.

47. R. B. Sykes and M. Matthew, *J. Antimicrob. Chemother.* **2,** 115 (1976).

48. J. L. Strominger, *Johns Hopkins Med. J.* **133,** 63 (1973); P. M. Blumberg and J. L. Strominger, *Bact. Rev.* **38,** 291 (1974).

49. M. R. J. Salton and A. Tomasz, eds., *Ann. N. Y. Acad. Sci.* **235,** 1 (1974).

50. C. H. Nash, N. DeLaHiguera, N. Neuss, and P. A. Lemke, *Dev. Ind. Microbiol.* **15,** 114 (1974); P. Fawcett and E. P. Abraham, *Biosynthesis* **4,** 248 (1976).

51. P. A. Lemke and D. R. Brannon in Ref. 26, Chapt. 9; A. L. Demain, *Lloydia* **37,** 147 (1974); T. Kanzaki and Y. Fujisawa, *J. Takeda Res. Lab.* **34,** 324 (1975).

52. M. Lieisch, J. Nuesch, and H. J. Treichler in K. O. Macdonald, ed., *Second International Symposium on Genetics of Industrial Microorganisms,* Academic Press, Inc., New York, 1976, p. 179; Lemke and Nash, *Can. J. Microbial.* **18,** 255 (1972); M. Kohsaka and A. L. Demain, *Biochem. and Biophys. Res. Commun.* **70,** 465 (1976).

53. R. P. Elander, C. J. Corum, H. DeValeria, and R. M. Wilgus in K. O. Macdonald, ed., *Second International Symposium on the Genetics of Industrial Microorganisms,* Academic Press, Inc., New York, 1976, p. 253.

54. G. Germonti, *Genetics of Antibiotic-Producing Microorganisms,* Interscience Publishers, a division of John Wiley & Sons, Inc., New York, 1969, p. 39.

55. G. L. Solomons, *Materials and Methods in Fermentation,* Academic Press, Inc., New York, 1969.

56. S. Aiba, A. E. Humphey, and N. F. Mills, *Biochemical Engineering,* Academic Press, Inc., New York, 1965.

57. R. Steel and T. L. Miller, *Adv. Appl. Microbiol.* **12,** 153 (1970).

58. D. Perlman, *Ann. N. Y. Acad. Sci.* **139,** 258 (1966).

59. J. L. Ott, C. W. Godzeski, D. Pavey, J. D. Farran, and D. R. Horton, *Appl. Microbiol.* **10,** 515 (1962).

60. A. Constantinides, J. Spencer, and E. Gaden, *Biotechnol. Bioeng.* **12,** 803 (1970).

61. Brit. Pat. 1,109,362 (Apr. 10, 1968), D. S. Callow.

62. C. J. Feren and R. W. Squires, *Biotechnol. Bioeng.* **11,** 583 (1969); J. A. Auden, J. Gruner, M. Lieisch, and J. Neusch, *Pathol. Microbiol.* **34,** 240 (1969).

63. J. W. Foster, *Chemical Activities of Fungi*, Academic Press, Inc., New York, 1949.
64. J. J. Gordon, E. Grenfell, E. Knowles, B. J. Legge, R. C. A. McAllister, and T. J. White, *J. Gen. Microbiol.* **1**, 187 (1947).
65. U.S. Pat. 3,184,454 (May 18, 1965), E. P. Abraham, G. G. F. Newton, and C. W. Hale (to National Research Development Corporation).
66. U.S. Pat. 3,725,400 (Apr. 3, 1973), W. Voser (to CIBA, Ltd.).
67. U.S. Pat. 3,661,901 (May 9, 1972), H. Bickel and co-workers (to CIBA, Ltd.).
68. U.S. Pat. 3,227,709 (Jan. 4, 1966), A. A. Patchett (to Merck & Co., Inc.); U.S. Pat. 3,641,018 (Feb. 8, 1972), H. B. Hayes and G. L. Huff (to Eli Lilly & Co.); U.S. Pats. 3,573,295; 3,573,296 (Mar. 30, 1971), D. A. Johnson and co-workers (to Bristol-Myers Co.); U.S. Pat. 3,825,473 (July 23, 1974), F. Garginolo (to Alfa Farmaceutici S.p.A.).
69. U.S. Pats. 3,296,258 (Jan. 3, 1967), 3,454,564 (July 8, 1969), E. Vischer (to CIBA, Ltd.); U.S. Pat. 3,821,208 (June 28, 1974), H. C. Stables and co-workers (to Glaxo Laboratories, Ltd.).
70. R. B. Morin, B. G. Jackson, E. H. Flynn, R. W. Roeske, and S. L. Andrews, *J. Am. Chem. Soc.* **91**, 1396 (1969).
71. U.S. Pats. 3,499,909 (Mar. 10, 1970), 3,575,970 (Apr. 20, 1971), H. W. O. Weissenburger and M. G. van der Hoeven (to Koninklijke Ned Gistern Spiritusfab.); Belg. Pat. 719,712 (Feb. 20, 1969), (to Glaxo Laboratories, Ltd.); Neth. Pat. 6,812,413 (Mar. 3, 1969), (to CIBA, Ltd.); Ref. 26, p. 37.
72. I. Buskooszczapowicz, J. Kazimierczak, and J. Cieslak, *Rocz. Chem.* **48**, 253 (1974).
73. G. A. Koppel, *Tetrahedron Lett.* 2427 (1974).
74. J. L. Strominger and D. J. Tipper, *Am. J. Med.* **39**, 708 (1965).
75. E. H. W. Böhme, H. E. Applegate, B. Toeplitz, J. E. Dolfini, and J. Z. Gongoulos, *J. Am. Chem. Soc.* **93**, 4324 (1971).
76. R. A. Firestone, N. Schelechow, D. B. R. Johnston, and B. G. Christensen, *Tetrahedron Lett.* 375 (1972); D. B. R. Johnston, S. M. Schmitt, R. A. Firestone, and B. G. Christensen, *Tetrahedron Lett.* 4917 (1972); G. H. Rassamussen, G. F. Reynolds, and G. E. Arth, *Tetrahedron Lett.* 145 (1973).
77. W. A. Spitzer, T. Goodson, R. J. Smithey, and I. G. Wright, *J. Chem. Soc. Chem. Commun.* 1138 (1972).
78. T. Jen, J. Frazee, and J. R. E. Hoover, *J. Org. Chem.* **38**, 2857 (1973); W. A. Slusarchyk, H. E. Applegate, P. Funke, W. Koster, M. S. Puar, M. Young, and J. E. Dolfini, *J. Org. Chem.* **38**, 943 (1973); H. E. Applegate and co-workers, *J. Org. Chem.* **39**, 2794 (1974).
79. L. D. Cama, W. J. Leanza, T. R. Beattie, and B. G. Christensen, *J. Am. Chem. Soc.* **94**, 1408 (1972).
80. G. A. Koppel and R. E. Koehler, *J. Am. Chem. Soc.* **95**, 2403 (1973); R. A. Firestone and B. G. Christensen, *J. Org. Chem.* **38**, 1436 (1973); W. H. W. Lunn and E. V. Mason, *Tetrahedron Lett.* 1311 (1974).
81. H. Yanagisawa, M. Fukushima, A. Ando, and H. Nakoa, *Tetrahedron Lett.* 2705 (1975).
82. Ref. 26, p. 29.
83. Belg. Pat. 758,800 (May 12, 1971), R. R. Chauvette (to Eli Lilly & Co.).
84. Ref. 26, p. 151.
85. J. D. Cocker, B. R. Cowley, J. S. G. Cox, S. Eardley, G. I. Gregory, J. K. Lazenby, A. G. Long, J. C. P. Sly, and G. A. Somerfield, *J. Chem. Soc.* 5015 (1965).
86. H. Peter and H. Bickel, *Helv. Chim. Acta* **57**, 2044 (1974); R. Scartazzini and H. Bickel, *Helv. Chim. Acta* **55**, 423 (1972).
87. M. Ochiai, O. Aki, A. Morimoto, T. Okada, K. Shinozaki, and Y. Asaki, *Tetrahedron Lett.* 2341 (1972); M. Ochiai, O. Aki, A. Morimoto, T. Okada, K. Shinozaki, and Y. Asaki, *J. Chem. Soc. Perkin Trans. 1* 258 (1974); M. Ochiai, O. Aki, A. Morimoto, T. Okada, and K. Morita, *Tetrahedron* **31**, 115 (1975).
88. R. R. Chauvette and P. A. Pennington, *J. Org. Chem.* **38**, 2994 (1973).
89. R. R. Chauvette and P. A. Pennington, *J. Am. Chem. Soc.* **96**, 4986 (1974); R. R. Chauvette and P. A. Pennington, *J. Med. Chem.* **18**, 403 (1975); R. Scartazzini and H. Bickel, *Helv. Chim. Acta* **57**, 1919 (1974); B. Müller, H. Peter, P. Schneider, and H. Bickel, *Helv. Chim. Acta* **58**, 2469 (1975).
90. R. J. Stedman, K. Swered, and J. R. E. Hoover, *J. Med. Chem.* **7**, 117 (1964).
91. Neth. Pat. 7,211,213 (Feb. 20, 1973), (to Gist-Brocades N.V.).
92. A. R. English and co-workers, *Antimicrob. Agents Chemother.* **10**, 132 (1976); A. R. English and co-workers, *Abstr. No. 224, 225, 16th Interscience Conference on Antimicrobial Agents and Chemotherapy*, Chicago, Ill., 1976.
93. Ref. 26, p. 185.
94. *FDC Reports* **38**(12), 12 (Mar. 22, 1976).

95. *Physicians' Desk Reference,* 30th ed., Medical Economics Co., Oradell, N.J., 1976. Published annually.

96. *Drug Topics Red Book,* E. Prinz and co-eds., Medical Economics Co., Oradell, N.J., 1977; *American Druggist Blue Book,* S. Siegelman and co-eds., Hearst Corp., New York, 1976.

97. S. B. Lee, *Ind. Eng. Chem.* **41,** 1868 (1949); **42,** 1672 (1950); **43,** 1948 (1951).

98. *Synthetic Organic Chemicals, United States Production and Sales 1974, U.S. International Trade Commission Publication 776,* U.S. Government Printing Office, Washington, D.C., 1976.

99. *Code of Federal Regulations,* Vol. 21, Parts 300 to 499, U.S. Government Printing Office, Washington, D.C., 1976.

100. R. E. White, M. A. Carroll, J. E. Zarembo, and A. D. Bender, *J. Antibiot.* **28,** 205 (1975); R. D. Miller and N. Neuss, *J. Antibiot.* **29,** 902 (1976).

101. F. Kavanagh, ed., *Analytical Microbiology,* Vol. 1, 1963; Vol. 2, 1972, Academic Press, Inc., New York; D. W. Hughes and W. L. Wilson, *Can. J. Pharm. Sci.* **8,** 67 (1973); D. W. Hughes, A. Vilim, and W. L. Wilson, *Can. J. Pharm. Sci.* **11,** 97 (1976); L. P. Marrelli in Ref. 26, Chapt. 14.

102. P. Dineen in W. Modell, ed., *Drugs of Choice (1976–1977),* C. V. Mosby Co., St. Louis, Mo., 1976, Chapt. 9; *AMA Drug Evaluations,* 2nd ed., Publishing Sciences Group, Inc., Acton, Mass., 1973, Chapts. 48, 49; *Medical Letter* **18,** 9 (1976).

103. L. D. Thrupp, *Ann. Rev. Pharmacol.* **14,** 435 (1974); J. H. Thompson in J. H. Bevan, ed., *Essentials of Pharmacology,* 2nd ed., Harper & Row, Publishers, New York, 1976, p. 429; G. N. Rolinson and R. Sutherland, *Adv. Pharmacol. Chemother.* **11,** 151 (1973); C. H. Nightingale, D. S. Greene, and R. Quintiliani, *J. Pharm. Sci.* **64,** 1899 (1975); D. W. Owens, D. K. Luscombe, A. D. Russell, and P. J. Nicholls, *Adv. Pharmacol. Chemother.* **13,** 83 (1975).

104. J. A. Washington, Jr., *Mayo Clin. Proc.* **51,** 237 (1976).

105. F. Kavanagh in Ref. 101, Vol. 1, pp. 58, 126.

106. Ref. 95, p. 1315; W. J. Martin, *Lancet* **87,** 79 (1967).

107. I. W. Fong, E. D. Ralph, E. R. Engelkin, and W. M. Kirby, *Antimicrob. Agents Chemother.* **9,** 65 (1976).

108. C. H. O'Callaghan, R. B. Sykes, A. Griffiths, and J. E. Thornton, *Antimicrob. Agents Chemother.* **9,** 511 (1976).

109. P. Actor, J. V. Uri, J. R. Guarini, I. Zajac, L. Phillips, C. S. Sacks, R. M. DeMarinis, J. R. E. Hoover, and J. A. Weisbach, *J. Antibiot.* **28,** 471 (1975).

110. E. R. Noriega, E. Rubinstein, M. S. Simberkoff, and J. J. Rahal, Jr., *Am. J. Med. Sci.* **267,** 353 (1974).

111. R. DelBusto, E. Haas, T. Madhavan, K. Burch, F. Cox, E. Fisher, E. Quinn, and D. Pohlod, *Antimicrob. Agents Chemother.* **9,** 397 (1976).

112. H. R. Black, K. S. Israel, G. L. Brier, and J. D. Wolny, *Abstr. No. 354, 16th Interscience Conference on Antimicrobial Agents and Chemotherapy,* Chicago, Ill., 1976.

113. A. Cordero, *J. Int. Med. Res.* **4,** 176 (1976).

JOHN R. E. HOOVER
CLAUDE H. NASH
Smith Kline & French Laboratories

CHLORAMPHENICOL AND ITS ANALOGUES

Chloramphenicol (1) is the first of the so-called broad-spectrum medicinal antibiotics. It was originally isolated from aerobic broth cultures of an actinomycete, *Streptomyces venezuelae* (1), in 1947. The antibiotic is a neutral, crystalline substance with a bitter taste and is moderately soluble (4.4 mg/mL at 28°C) in water and freely soluble in many organic solvents. It is manufactured by chemical synthesis and is commercially available as the free compound and its esters (Table 1).

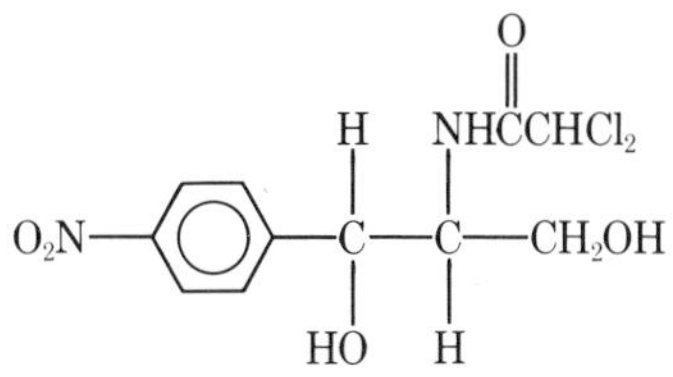

$$O_2N-\langle\bigcirc\rangle-\overset{\overset{\displaystyle H}{|}}{\underset{\underset{\displaystyle HO}{|}}{C}}-\overset{\overset{\displaystyle NH\overset{O}{\overset{||}{C}}CHCl_2}{|}}{\underset{\underset{\displaystyle H}{|}}{C}}-CH_2OH$$

(1)

Chloramphenicol is antimicrobially active against a wide range of gram-positive and gram-negative bacteria, rickettsiae, the lymphogranuloma-psittacosis group, and *Vibrio cholerae* (1–2). It is particularly active against *Salmonella typhi* and *Hemophilus influenzae*. The chloramphenicol esters, such as the palmitate or succinate, are essentially inactive microbiologically until hydrolyzed *in vivo* to the free antibiotic.

Physical and Chemical Properties

A list of properties of chloramphenicol is shown in Table 2. The molecule may be considered as comprising two parts, the 2-acylamidopropanediol side chain containing two asymmetric carbon atoms, and the *p*-nitrophenyl group. Of the four possible stereoisomers, the D-threo is by far the most active against microorganisms. The stereochemical configuration of the side chain is thus rather specific in conferring antimicrobial properties. The aromatic part of the molecule is less specific for antimicrobial activity, as shown by the moderate activity of analogues in which the nitro group is replaced by iodine or by the methylsulfonyl group.

Table 1. Alphabetical List of Chloramphenicol Derivatives Referred to in the Text

Compound	CAS Registry No.	Formula
chloramphenicol glycinate	[2980-74-7]	$C_{13}H_{15}Cl_2N_3O_6$
chloramphenicol palmitate	[530-43-8]	$C_{27}H_{42}Cl_2N_2O_6$
chloramphenicol palmitoylglycolate	[60595-52-0]	$C_{29}H_{44}Cl_2N_2O_8$
chloramphenicol stearate	[16255-48-4]	$C_{29}H_{46}Cl_2N_2O_6$
chloramphenicol stearoylglycolate	[24292-47-5]	$C_{31}H_{48}Cl_2N_2O_8$
chloramphenicol succinate monoacid	[3544-94-3]	$C_{15}H_{15}Cl_2N_2NaO_8$
chloramphenicol succinate sodium salt	[982-57-0]	$C_{15}H_{15}Cl_2N_2NaO_8$

Table 2.   Properties of Chloramphenicol

Property	Value	Refs.
CAS Registry No.	[56-75-7]	
mol formula	$C_{11}H_{12}Cl_2N_2O_5$	
mol wt	323	
mp, °C	150.5–151.5	
$[\alpha]_D^{25}$	+19° (5% in C_2H_5OH)	
	−25.0° (5% in $C_2H_5OOCCH_3$)	
specific	589 +18.5 ± 1.5°	
rotation	578 +19.8°	
(5% in	546 +23.8°	
C_2H_5OH),	436 +59.7°	
nm		
solubility at	2.5 mg/mL H_2O	
25°C	150.8 mg/mL $HOCH_2CH_2CH_2OH$	
	very sol in CH_3OH, C_2H_5OH, BuOH^n,	
	CH_3COCH_3, ethyl and amyl	
	acetate, and DMAC	
	fairly sol in $C_2H_5OC_2H_5$	
	insol in C_6H_6 and pet. ether	
	solubilities at 28°C	3
uv	ϵ max 278 nm, min at 237 nm	
	$E_{1\,cm}^{1\%} = 298_{H_2O}$ at 278 nm	
	$= 312_{C_2H_5OH}$ at 274 nm	
ir	3340, 3260, 1697, 1568, 1530, 1358, and	
	1068 cm^{-1}	
nmr		4
tlc		5–7
summary of physical		8
properties		

Esterification of the primary alcohol group of the propanediol side chain with palmitic acid readily yields chloramphenicol palmitate: $[\alpha]_D^{26}$ +24.6° (5% in absolute ethyl alcohol); $E_{1\,cm}^{1\%}$ 179 at 271 nm in ethyl alcohol. This white crystalline substance is only slightly soluble in water and petroleum ether but freely soluble in ethyl alcohol, chloroform, ether, and benzene. The monopalmitate shows no significant antimicrobial activity *in vitro* but is hydrolyzed in the duodenum to active chloramphenicol. The ester is tasteless and in suspension provides an oral-dosage form of the antibiotic acceptable to those unable to take capsules (9–12).

Esterification of the primary alcohol of the propanediol side chain with succinic acid yields chloramphenicol acid succinate: $[\alpha]_D^{20}$ +25° (5% in absolute ethyl alcohol); $E_{1\,cm}^{1\%}$ 231 at 276 nm in water (13). The free acid ester is converted to chloramphenicol succinate sodium salt, anhydrous: $[\alpha]_D^{23}$ +5.7° (4.91% in water); $E_{1\,cm}^{1\%}$ 215 at 276 nm in water; this is a faintly yellow crystalline substance, freely soluble in water. The salt is essentially inactive *in vitro* but upon parenteral injection is hydrolyzed by tissue enzymes, liberating chloramphenicol within the body. Thus the sodium salt of the monosuccinate ester provides a product form for intramuscular, intravenous, or subcutaneous administration when oral therapy is not feasible, when it is important to achieve a high blood level quickly (11–12, 14).

Preparation and Manufacture

Chloramphenicol, now produced by synthesis, was originally prepared and later manufactured by a fermentation process.

Fermentation Process. Complex media are subjected to submerged, aerobic fermentation by various strains of the actinomycete *Streptomyces venezuelae* (15–20). The fermented broth is extracted with amyl acetate and the acetate is concentrated, washed, and concentrated further. Crude crystals obtained upon cooling are filtered, dried, and dissolved in hot water. The hot solution is decolorized, clarified, and cooled to induce crystallization. The purified crystals are filtered, washed, dried, pulverized, and sieved. This process yields a single optical entity having the D-threo configuration (21–23) (see Fermentation).

Synthesis. Four synthetic procedures account for most worldwide production.

The first synthesis involved the addition of benzaldehyde (**2**) to β-nitroethanol to yield 2-nitro-1-phenyl-1,3-propanediol (**3**) in an uneconomical D,L-erythro–D,L-threo isomer ratio of about 2:1 (24). Chemists at Boehringer Mannheim G.m.b.H. devised a technique for obtaining exclusively the D,L-threo racemate. Reduction to the aminodiol (**4**), *swing* resolution, subsequent nitration, and dichloroacetylation have made Figure 1 the process of choice throughout the 1960s and 1970s.

In Figure 2, acetophenone or, preferably, *p*-nitroacetophenone may be used as starting material (25). The bromination of structure (**7**) to (**8**) may be carried out in a variety of inert solvents, yield >90%. The formation of a hexamethylenetetramine complex (**9**) is usually carried out in a chlorinated solvent and followed by an alcoholic mineral acid hydrolysis to obtain the corresponding mineral acid salt, (**10**). Acetylation of (**10**) is carried out in cold water with acetic anhydride and mild alkali, overall yield, (**8**) to (**11**), 67%. The addition of formaldehyde to (**11**) occurs in the presence of sodium bicarbonate, yield 86%. The Meerwein-Pondorf reduction of structure (**12**) to (**13**) yields almost exclusively the D,L-threo racemate in 41% yield. (If acetophenone is used as a starting material, the hydroxyl groups of the compound analogous to structure

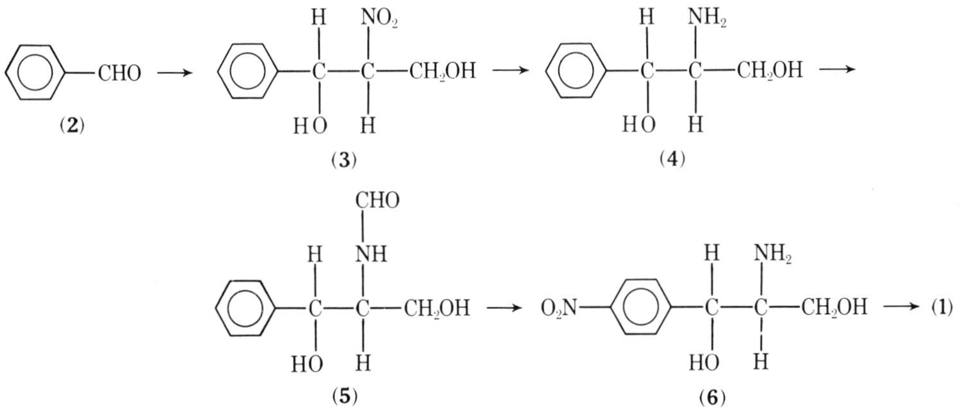

Figure 1. The preferred process of chloramphenicol synthesis.

(13) are protected by acetylation and the triacetyl derivative (15) is nitrated with fuming nitric acid to give (16).) Acid hydrolysis of either (13) or (16) yields the racemic base (14), which is resolved into its optical antipodes by crystallization of its salt with an optically active acid, eg, tartaric acid in methanol. After recovery of the optically active D-base by precipitation with alkali, 30% yield, main crop, the dried base may be acylated by a variety of agents, the most commonly used being methyl dichloroacetate, to give chloramphenicol (1). The overall yield is about 6%.

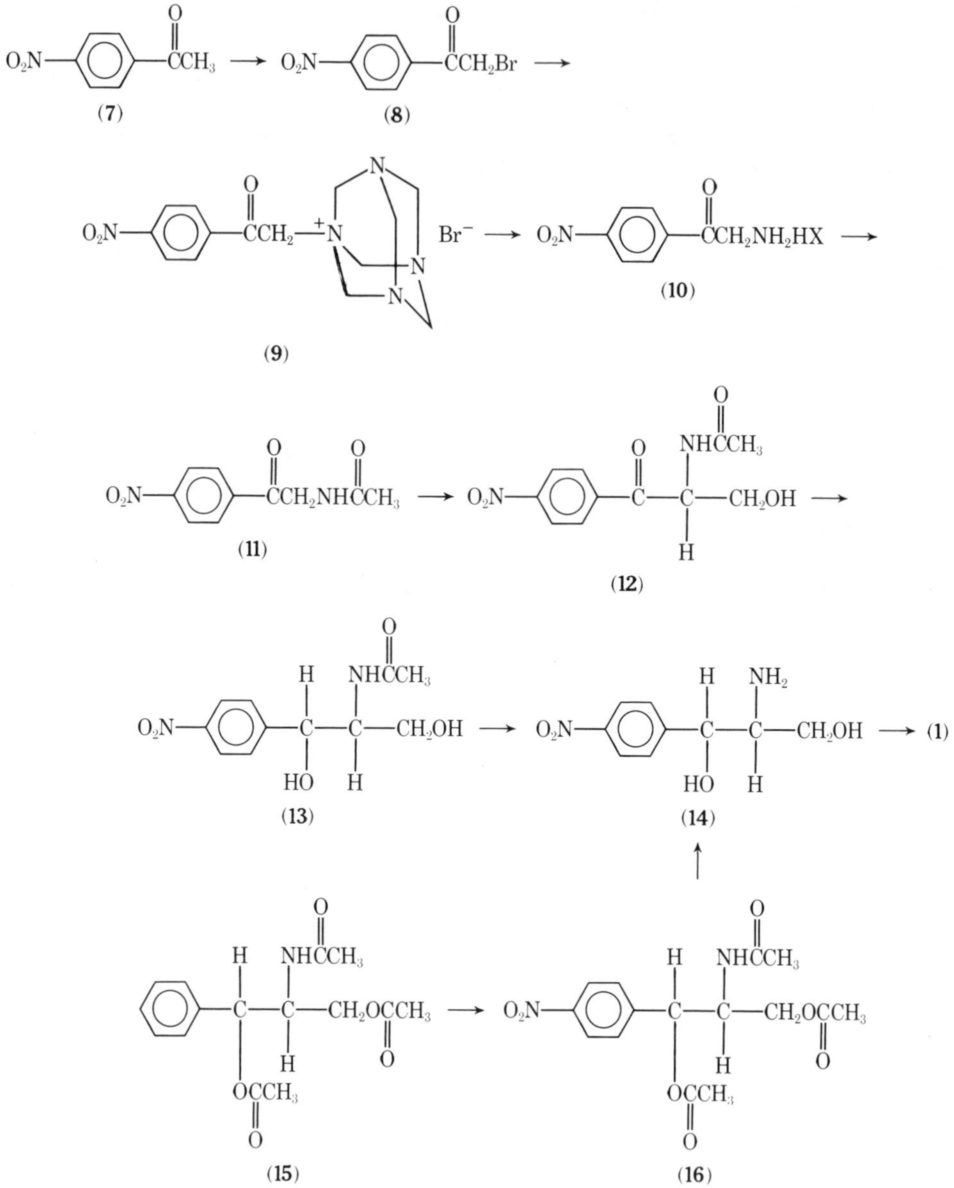

Figure 2. A process of chloramphenicol synthesis.

A process (Fig. 3) used for a considerable time in Western Europe involved cinnamyl alcohol (17) which is converted to its bromohydrin (18) and in turn to the bromodioxane (19). Reaction with ammonia gives the aminodioxane (20) which is resolved, acylated to the dichloroacetamido compound (21), nitrated, and gently hydrolysed to (1) (26).

A further procedure, which is understood to have been utilized in Eastern Europe, involves use of phenyl serine derivatives (Fig. 4). p-Nitrobenzaldehyde (22) is condensed with glycine to obtain the Schiff's base of D,L-*threo-p*-nitrophenyl serine (23). Cleavage of the Schiff's base followed by esterification gives D,L-*p*-nitrophenyl serine methyl ester (24) which may be resolved with D-tartaric acid and the ester of the correct configuration (corresponding to L-*p*-nitrophenyl serine) reduced by sodium or calcium borohydride to the desired p-nitrophenyl serinol (6).

Market Forms

Chloramphenicol is marketed for use in human and veterinary medicine in product forms suitable for oral, parenteral, and topical administration (see Table 3). Some rectal formulations are marketed overseas. Oral product forms include capsules and tablets of chloramphenicol and flavored syrups and suspensions of the esters such as the palmitate, palmitoylglycolate, stearate, and stearoylglycolate. Parenteral product forms include sterile solutions and powders for suspension, and solutions of salts of chloramphenicol succinic acid and glycine esters. Topical product forms include powders, solutions, creams, and ointments for use on or in the eye, ear, nose, skin, vagina, and bovine udder. Product combinations of chloramphenicol with other antibiotics are available outside the United States.

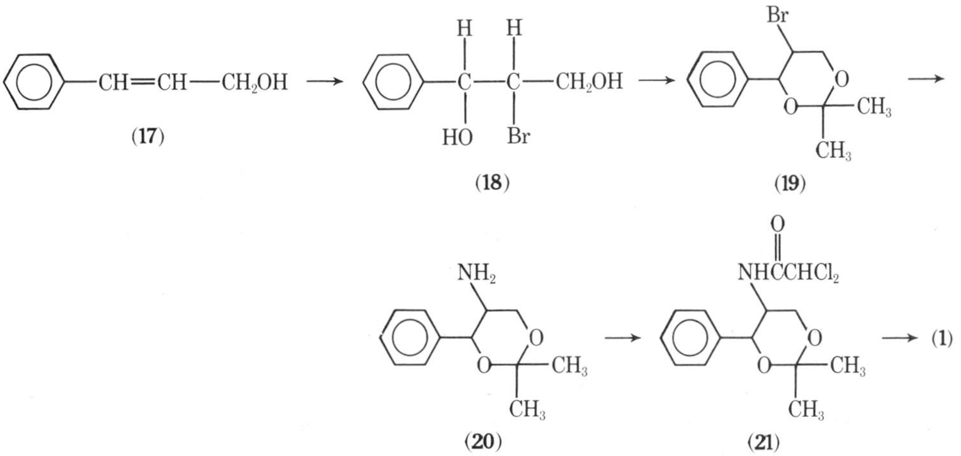

Figure 3. A process of chloramphenicol synthesis used in Western Europe.

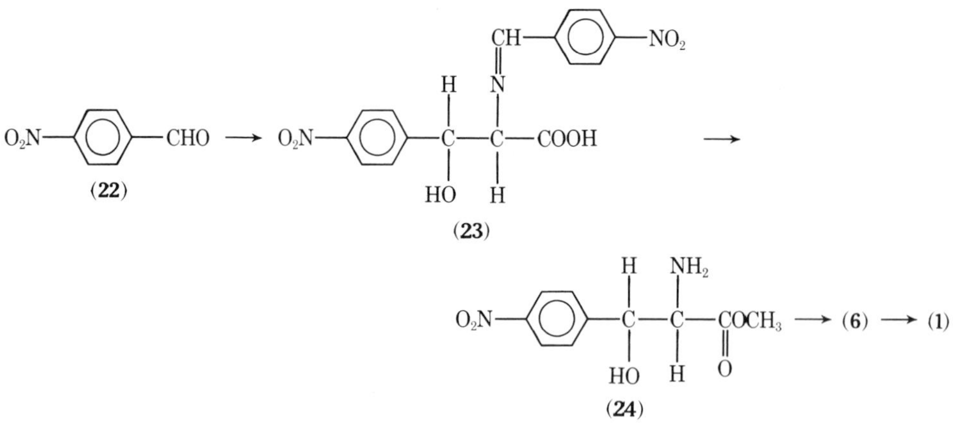

Figure 4. A process of chloramphenicol synthesis used in Eastern Europe.

Table 3.   Chloramphenicol Producers and Trade Names

Company	Trade name
Boehringer, Ger.	Paraxin
Carlo Erba, Italy	Chemicetina
Farmitalia, Italy	Farmicetina
Lepetit, Italy	Sintomycetina
Parke, Davis and Co. (a division of Warner-Lambert), U.S.A.	Chloromycetin
Rachelle Laboratories, U.S.A.	
Roussel, Fr.	Tifomycine (in France)
	Chloranfetina (in Italy)
Zambon, Italy	Micoclorina

Stability

Chloramphenicol solutions, when exposed to a uv source (sunlight) or to high temperature, decompose with the formation of hydrochloric and dichloroacetic acids. The two primary routes of decomposition have been determined (27–30) to be amide hydrolysis with the formation of 1-(p-nitrophenyl)-2-amino-1,3-propanediol and hydrolysis of the covalent chlorine of the dichloroacetamide moiety. The dry solid is stable at room temperature in ordinary diffuse light for at least five years. Sterile aqueous solutions held at 100°C retain their antimicrobial activity >5 h but lose approximately half their activity if heated at 100°C for approximately 16 h. At 37°C, activity remains practically unimpaired for a month but deteriorates slowly thereafter, dropping to approximately half after six months. At room temperature (about 25°C) sterile aqueous solutions protected from light are stable for three to six months and lose approximately half their activity over a two-year period. At 5°C there is little or no loss in activity of aqueous solutions for at least two years. Chloramphenicol is also relatively pH stable; aqueous solutions adjusted to levels between pH 4.0 and pH 9.5 retain their activity at 25°C for at least 24 h but those above pH 10 do not.

Specifications

Chloramphenicol is certified as an antibiotic by the FDA which specifies test methods and standards for the antibiotic itself and for the various certified market forms (31). The USP monograph on chloramphenicol specifies conformity to FDA regulations and gives data on solubility, identification, melting range, specific rotation, absorptivity, pH, assay, content variation, packaging, and storage (32).

For FDA certification, chloramphenicol batches must pass the following standards of identity, strength, quality, and purity dependent on the clinical use of the formulated product: (1) crystallinity; (2) a potency of not less than 900 μg/mg; (3) sterility; (4) nontoxic; (5) nonpyrogenic; (6) free of histamine and histamine-like substances; (7) exhibit a pH of 4.5–7.5 (saturated solution in water); (8) a rotation of $[\alpha]_D^{20}$ +20 ± 1.5° and $[\alpha]_D^{25}$ + 18.5 ± 1.5° (5% in absolute ethyl alcohol); (9) 151 ± 2°C; and (10) absorptivity at 278 nm (20 μg/mL in H$_2$O), varying no more than ±3% of the chloramphenicol working standard, similarly treated. Specifications (3), (5), and (6) are not required of batches to be used in manufacture of capsules and tablets, or ointment and creams not intended for ophthalmic use (31).

Chloramphenicol palmitate must be crystalline, have a potency of 555–595 μg/mg, be nontoxic, have a melting point of 91 ± 4°C, a specific rotation $[\alpha]_D^{25}$ +23 ± 2° (5% absolute ethyl alcohol), and must pass the safety test (31).

Chloramphenicol sodium succinate must have a potency of not less than 650 and not more than 765 μg/mg; be sterile, nonpyrogenic, pass the safety test, contain no histamine nor histamine-like substances, and have a moisture content of not more than 5%. An aqueous solution of the succinate (250 mg/mL) should exhibit a pH of not less than 6.4 and not more than 7.0, and a specific rotation $[\alpha]_D^{25}$ +6.5 ± 2.5° (5% in water) (31).

Assay

Chloramphenicol may be assayed by various techniques. These include microbiological as well as physical and chemical test methods. Solutions of chloramphenicol in water or body fluids can be assayed by two microbiological methods, turbidimetrically (31), or by agar diffusion (33–34). An enzymatic assay based on acetyl transferase has been reported (35). Physical methods include uv spectrophotometry, titrimetry (36–38), and polarography (39–45). A colorimetric procedure based on reduction of the nitro group can be made specific for chloramphenicol (46). Other chemical tests are available (47–48) including a hydroxamic acid colorimetric method (49–50) and an isonicotinic acid hydrazide method (51–53).

Microbiological Properties

Antimicrobial Spectrum. Chloramphenicol is classed as a broad-spectrum antibiotic because it exerts marked inhibitory activity toward many gram-positive and gram-negative cocci and bacilli, some mycobacteria, spirochetes and actinomycetes, a wide range of anaerobic bacteria, several rickettsias, the lymphogranuloma-psitta-cosis group, and *Vibrio cholerae* (54–56). In acute infections caused by *Salmonella typhi,* it is a drug of choice and it is particularly useful in the treatment of *Hemophilus influenzae* meningitis since the recent clinical appearance of ampicillin-resistant strains. Chloramphenicol is generally inactive, however, against protozoa and other animal parasites, fungi, and viruses.

Development of Resistance. As with most antimicrobial drugs, populations of some strains of bacteria exposed for many generations to chloramphenicol *in vitro* exhibit a gradually increasing resistance to its inhibitory action. With chloramphenicol, this tendency is particularly true of gram-negative bacilli. Such resistant populations usually retain their original degree of susceptibility to other medicinal antibiotics. Increased resistance to chloramphenicol is often reversible in whole or in part when the organism grows in the absence of the antibiotic (57).

Mode of Action. Chloramphenicol is typically bacteriostatic at low concentrations. It inhibits protein synthesis in bacteria and in cell-free systems (58). It acts primarily on the smaller, the 50S ribosomal subunit. The enzyme, peptidyl transferase, which catalyzes peptide bond formation, is suppressed although ribosomes may still bind to and move along strands of mRNA (messenger RNA). It is not known whether chloramphenicol binds directly to the transferase enzyme, or inactivates it, or prevents the interaction of other ribosome-bound components with the enzyme.

Toxicity. Chloramphenicol is a relatively nontoxic substance in animals. The maximum tolerated single intravenous dose (LD) in mg/kg is 75 (in propylene glycol) for rabbits, 125 (in water) for albino mice, 150 (in propylene glycol) for dogs, and 200–225 (in dimethylacetamide) for albino rats. Considerably higher doses are tolerated orally: >300 mg/kg by dogs; 1500 by albino mice, and 3000 by rabbits. No cumulative toxic effect has been observed in dogs on oral daily divided dosage of 200 mg/kg, five days a week, for over eighteen months. Albino mice tolerate 425 mg/(kg·d) orally for four weeks. Rabbits have tolerated 1 g/(kg·d), five days a week, for twelve weeks, and albino rats have been found to tolerate 1% in the diet for over a year without evidence of cumulative toxic effects (59–60).

In humans, therapeutic doses of chloramphenicol are generally well tolerated. Aplastic anemia, hypoplastic anemia, thrombocytopenia, and granulocytopenia have been associated with the administration of chloramphenicol. There is some evidence that the most serious toxicity associated with chloramphenicol, ie, aplastic anemia, may not occur after exclusively parenteral use. Glossitis and stomatitis may occur after several days of oral therapy. On rare occasions superimposed infection by *Candida albicans* may produce widespread oral lesions of the thrush type. Diarrhea and irritation of perianal tissues have been reported. Angioneurotic edema, urticaria, and various types of dermatitis have been reported in patients sensitive to chloramphenicol. Headache, mild depression, mental confusion, and delirium have been described in patients receiving the drug for a variety of infectious diseases. Optic and peripheral neuritis, as probable effects of prolonged therapy, have been reported. The use of this antibiotic, as with other antibiotics, may result in an overgrowth of nonsusceptible organisms, particularly *Candida* (55).

Uses

In Medicine. Chloramphenicol is used for treating a wide range of infectious diseases of humans (55, 61). Notably responsive are the rickettsial diseases, including epidemic and murine typhus fevers, Brill's disease, scrub typhus fever, and rickettsial pox; typhoid fever, for which chloramphenicol is a drug of choice; meningeal infections caused by *Hemophilus influenzae*; anaerobic bacterial infections including *Bacillus fragilis* (62); brain abscesses caused by intracranial pathogens (63). Chloramphenicol is also used for susceptible nontyphoidal salmonelloses; urinary, severe respiratory, surgical, and dermatologic infections; and diverse infections including brucellosis, bartonellosis, relapsing fever, granuloma inguinale, plague, ornithosis, and susceptible staphylococcal infections of various organs and tissues.

In Veterinary Medicine. Chloramphenicol is used to treat many infections of both large and small animals (64–69). Responsive diseases (caused by susceptible microorganisms) include bacterial pulmonary infections (64–65), infections of the urinary tract (64,66), enteritis (64), and infections associated with canine distemper (64). Regulations vary in different countries concerning administration to meat-, milk-, or egg-producers for human consumption because of inadequate data on the persistance of residues. Where permitted, chloramphenicol has been successfully used in the treatment of colibacillosis of calves (67–68) and piglets (68–69), salmonellosis in piglets (69), and fowl cholera and *E. tenella* in poultry (68). Topically, it is useful in treating bacterial conjunctivitis (66,68).

BIBLIOGRAPHY

"Chloromycetin" in *ECT* 1st ed., Vol. 3, p. 870, by H. B. Woodruff, Merck & Co., Inc.; "Chloramphenicol" under "Streptomyces Antibiotics," Vol. 13, pp. 81–89, by John Ehrlich, Parke, Davis & Company; "Chloramphenicol" in *ECT* 2nd ed., Vol. 4, pp. 928–937, by John Ehrlich, Parke, Davis & Company.

1. J. Ehrlich, Q. R. Bartz, R. M. Smith, D. A. Joslyn, and P. R. Burkholder, *Science* **106**, 417 (1947).
2. J. E. Smadel and E. B. Jackson, *Science* **106**, 418 (1947).
3. P. J. Weiss, M. L. Andrew, and W. W. Wright, *Antibiot. Chemother.* **7**, 374 (1957).
4. O. Jardetzky, *J. Biol. Chem.* **238**, 2498 (1963).
5. Y. T. Lin and K. T. Wang, *J. Chromatogr.* **21**, 158 (1966).
6. E. Schlederer, *Cosm. Pharma.* **3**, 17 (1966).
7. J. Lacharme and D. Netien, *Bull. Trav. Soc. Pharm. Lyon* **8**, 122 (1964).
8. D. Szulczewski and F. Eng, *Anal. Profiles Drug Subst.* **4**, 48 (1975).
9. A. J. Glazko, W. H. Edgerton, W. A. Dill, and W. R. Lenz, *Antibiot. Chemother.* **2**, 234 (1952).
10. W. H. Edgerton, V. H. Maddox, and J. Controulis, *J. Am. Chem. Soc.* **77**, 27 (1955).
11. *New and Nonofficial Drugs 1962*, J. B. Lippincott Co., Philadelphia, Pa., 1964, pp. 49–52.
12. *The Pharmacopeia of the United States of America, U.S.P. XVI*, Washington, D.C., 1960, pp. 139–145; First Suppl., 1962, pp. 9–11.
13. G. Ceriotti, A. Defrancheschi, I. De Carneri, and V. Zamboni, *Il Farmaco Ed. Sci.* **9**, 21 (1954).
14. A. J. Glazko, H. E. Carnes, A. Kazenko, L. M. Wolf, and T. F. Reutner in H. Welch and F. Marti-Ibañez, eds., *Antibiotics Annual 1957–1958*, Medical Encyclopedia, Inc., New York, 1958, pp. 792–802.
15. D. Gottlieb, P. K. Bhattacharyya, H. W. Anderson, and H. E. Carter, *J. Bacteriol.* **55**, 409 (1948).
16. J. Ehrlich, D. Gottlieb, P. R. Burkholder, L. E. Anderson, and T. G. Pridham, *J. Bacteriol.* **56**, 467 (1948).
17. R. M. Smith, D. A. Joslyn, O. M. Gruhzit, I. W. McLean, Jr., M. A. Penner, and J. Ehrlich, *J. Bacteriol.* **55**, 425 (1948).
18. H. Umezawa, T. Tazaki, H. Kanari, Y. Okami, and S. Fukuyama, *Jpn. Med. J.* **1**, 358 (1948).
19. H. Umezawa and K. Maeda, *J. Antibiot.* **3**, 41 (1949).
20. K. Ogata, M. Shibata, T. Ueno, and K. Nakazawa, *J. Antibiot.* **4** (Suppl. A), 44 (1951).
21. W. H. Mohrhoff and W. D. Mogerman, *Proc. Ind. Quart.* **12**(1), 1 (1949).

22. T. R. Olive, *Chem. Eng. N.Y.* **56,** 107, 172 (1949).
23. D. W. Anderson and E. F. Lau, *Chem. Eng. Progr.* **51,** 507 (1955).
24. J. Controulis, M. C. Rebstock, and H. M. Crooks, Jr., *J. Am. Chem. Soc.* **71,** 2458 (1949).
25. L. M. Long and H. D. Troutman, *J. Am. Chem. Soc.* **71,** 2473 (1949).
26. Brit. Pats. 735,454 (Aug. 24, 1955), 741,711 (Dec. 7, 1955), C. F. Boehringer u. Soehne (to G.m.b.H., Mannheim).
27. T. Higuchi and C. D. Bias, *J. Am. Pharm. Assoc. Sci. Ed.* **42,** 707 (1953).
28. T. Higuchi and A. Marcus, *J. Am. Pharm. Assoc. Sci. Ed.* **43,** 530 (1954).
29. T. Higuchi, A. Marcus, and C. Bias, *J. Am. Pharm. Assoc. Sci. Ed.* **43,** 135 (1954).
30. C. Trolle-Lassen, *Arch. Pharm. Chemi* **60,** 689 (1953).
31. *Title 21, Code of Federal Regulations,* Washington, D.C., S 436.102, 436.106, 455.10, 455.10b, 455.11, 455.12a.
32. *United States Pharmacopeia, U.S.P. XIX, July 1, 1975, United States Pharmacopeial Convention, Inc., Rockville, Md,* pp. 77–79.
33. D. G. Smith, C. B. Landers, and J. Forgacs, *J. Lab. Clin. Med.* **36,** 154 (1950).
34. R. Hans, M. Galbraith, and W. C. Alegnani in F. Kavanagh, ed., *Analytical Microbiology,* Academic Press, Inc., New York, 1963, pp. 271–281.
35. R. Daigneault and M. Grutard, *J. Infect. Dis.* **133,** 515 (1976).
36. W. Awe and H. Stohlman, *Arch. Pharm. (Weinheim, Ger.)* **289,** 61, 276 (1956).
37. M. Hadicke and G. Schmid, *Pharm. Zentralhalle* **95,** 387 (1956).
38. W. Awe and H. Stohlman, *Arzneim. Forsch.* **7**(8), 495 (1959).
39. K. Fossdal and E. Jackson, *Anal. Chim. Acta* **56,** 105 (1971).
40. G. B. Hess, *Anal. Chem.* **22,** 649 (1950).
41. C. G. Macros, *Chem. Chron. A.* **32,** 104 (1967).
42. C. Russo, I. Cruceanu, D. Monciu, and V. Barcaru, *Il. Farmaco* **20,** 22 (1965).
43. C. Russo, I. Cruceanu, and V. Barcaru, *Pharmazie* **18,** 799 (1963).
44. A. F. Summa, *J. Pharm. Sci.* **54,** 442 (1963).
45. P. Zuman, *Organic Polarographic Analysis,* MacMillan Co., New York, 1964, pp. 186.
46. A. J. Glazko, L. M. Wolf, and W. A. Dill, *Arch. Biochem.* **23,** 411 (1949).
47. C. F. Weiss, A. J. Glazko, and J. K. Weston, *New Engl. J. Med.* **262,** 787 (1960).
48. D. W. O'G. Hughes and L. K. Diamond, *Science* **144,** 296 (1964).
49. T. H. Aihara, H. Machida, and Y. Yoneda, *J. Pharm. Soc. Jpn.* **77,** 1318 (1957).
50. M. S. Karawya and M. G. Ghourab, *J. Pharm. Sci.* **59,** 1331 (1970).
51. K. Kakemi, T. Arito, and S. Ohasaki, *Yakugaku Zasshi* **82,** 342 (1962).
52. G. L. Resnick, D. Corbin, and D. H. Sandberg, *Anal. Chem.* **38,** 582 (1966).
53. R. C. Shah, P. V. Raman, and P. V. Sheth, *Indian J. Pharm.* **30,** 68 (1968).
54. I. W. McLean, Jr., J. L. Schwab, A. B. Hillegas, and A. S. Schlingman, *J. Clin. Invest.* **28,** 953 (1949).
55. T. E. Woodward and C. L. Wisseman, *Chloromycetin (Chloramphenicol) Antibiotics Monographs No. 8,* Medical Encyclopedia Inc., New York, 1958.
56. H. Welch, *A Guide to Antibiotic Therapy,* Medical Encyclopedia Inc., New York, 1959, pp. 18–19.
57. G. L. Coffey, J. L. Schwab, and J. Ehrlich, *J. Infect. Dis.* **87,** 142 (1950).
58. E. F. Gale, E. Cundliffe, P. E. Reynolds, M. H. Richmond, M. J. Waring, *The Molecular Basis for Antibiotic Action,* John Wiley & Sons, Inc., New York, 1972, pp. 325–331.
59. O. M. Gruzhit, R. A. Fisken, T. F. Reutner, and E. Martino, *J. Clin. Invest.* **28,** 943 (1949).
60. T. F. Reutner, R. E. Maxwell, K. E. Weston, and J. K. Weston, *Antibiot. Chemother.* **5,** 679 (1955).
61. A. M. Walter and L. Heilmeyer, *Antibiotika-Fibel,* Georg Thieme Verlag, Stuttgart, Ger., 1954.
62. S. J. Bodner, M. G. Koenig, J. S. Goodman, *Ann. Intern. Med.* **73,** 537 (1970).
63. P. Kramer, R. S. Griffith, and R. L. Campbell, *J. Neurosurg.* **31,** 295 (1969).
64. R. W. Kirk, *Current Veterinary Therapy V. Small Animal Practice,* W. B. Saunders Co., Philadelphia, Pa., 1974, pp.17–21.
65. Ref. 64, pp. 215–218.
66. *The Merck Veterinary Manual,* 4th ed., Merck & Co., Inc., Rahway, N. J., 1973, pp. 850–851.
67. W. J. Gibbons, E. J. Catcott, and J. F. Smithcors, *Bovine Medicine and Surgery,* American Veterinary Publications, Inc., Wheaton, Ill., 1970, pp. 689–695.
68. I. S. Rossoff, *Handbook of Veterinary Drugs,* Springer Publishing Co., New York, 1974, pp. 96–99.
69. G. C. Brander and D. M. Pugh, *Veterinary Applied Pharmacology and Therapeutics,* 2nd ed., Baillere Tindall, London, 1971, pp. 362–363.

General References

M. E. Florey, *Clinical Applications of Antibiotics*, vol. VIII, Oxford University Press, New York, 1957, pp. 1–381.

V. S. Malik, *Advance in Applied Microbiology: Chloramphenicol*, Academic Press, Inc., New York, 1972, pp. 297–336.

M. J. Snyder and T. E. Woodward, "The Clinical Use of Chloramphenicol," *Med. Clin. North Am.* 54(5); 1187 (1970).

JOHN EHRLICH
Detroit Institute of Technology

LINCOSAMINIDES

The lincosaminide antibiotics are characterized by an alkyl 6-amino-6,8-dide-oxy-1-thio-α-D-*galacto*-octopyranoside joined with a proline moiety by an amide linkage. An alphabetical list of lincosaminides is shown in Table 1.

Lincomycin

The discovery and biological properties of lincomycin (1) were described in 1962 (1). It is active *in vitro* and *in vivo* against clinical isolates of gram-positive organisms (streptococci, pneumococci, staphylococci). It does not show cross-resistance with any

Table 1. Lincosaminides

Compound	CAS Registry No.	Formula
celesticetin (2)	[2520-21-0]	$C_{24}H_{36}N_2O_9S$
clindamycin (10)	[18323-44-9]	$C_{18}H_{33}ClN_2O_5S$
clindamycin hydrochloride	[17431-55-9]	$C_{18}H_{34}Cl_2N_2O_5S$
clindamycin palmitate	[36688-78-5]	$C_{34}H_{63}ClN_2O_6S$
clindamycin phosphate	[24729-96-2]	$C_{18}H_{34}ClN_2O_8PS$
1'-demethyllincomycin (6)	[16843-70-2]	$C_{17}H_{32}N_2O_6S$
1-demethylthio-1-ethylthiolincomycin (5)	[14042-43-4]	$C_{19}H_{36}N_2O_6S$
1-demethylthio-1-ethylthio-1'-demethythio-1'-ethylthiolinco-mycin (7)	[21085-65-4]	$C_{20}H_{38}N_2O_6S$
1-demethylthio-1-hydroxylincomycin (9)	[22099-01-0]	$C_{17}H_{32}N_2O_7$
4'-depropyl-4'-ethyllincomycin (4)	[2520-24-3]	$C_{17}H_{32}N_2O_6S$
desalicetin (3)	[19246-70-9]	$C_{17}H_{32}N_2O_7S$
lincomycin (1)	[154-21-2]	$C_{18}H_{34}N_2O_6S$
lincomycin hydrochloride	[17017-16-2]	$C_{18}H_{35}ClN_2O_6S$
lincomycin sulfoxide (8)	[23444-78-2]	$C_{18}H_{34}N_2O_7S$

major known antibiotic; resistance to lincomycin develops at a relatively slow rate and its activity is not influenced by body fluids at concentrations up to 50% (2).

Lincomycin was produced originally by the actinomycete *Streptomyces lincolnensis* var. *lincolnensis*, NRRL 2936. Subsequently, it was produced by *Streptomyces umbrinus* var. *cyaneoniger*, var. *nova.* (3); by *Streptomyces espinosus* Dietz, sp. *nova.* (4–5); by *Streptomyces pseudogriseolus chemovar. linmyceticus* Dietz var. *nova.* (6); by *Streptomyces variabalis chemovar. liniabilis* Dietz var. *nova.* (7); by strain no. 1146 *Actinomyces roseolus* (8) and by *Streptomyces vellosus* sp *nova.* (9).

Properties.   Lincomycin isolated from a 1-butanol extract is a white colorless, fluffy, needlelike, crystalline hydrochloride salt, having the empirical formula $C_{18}H_{34}N_2O_6S.HCl.\frac{1}{2}H_2O$ (10).

A second form of small, dense crystals exists as the monohydrate (11). This is the commercially available form of lincomycin hydrochloride (Lincocin, Upjohn).

The extraction was followed by standard bioassay procedures against *Sarcina lutea* on agar trays (12).

The structure of lincomycin was elucidated from classical chemical degradation studies and interpretation of proton magnetic resonance spectra (13–18). Lincomycin hydrochloride is readily soluble in water, moderately soluble in methanol and ethanol, and relatively insoluble in less polar organic solvents. It contains one basic function, pK_a' 7.5, and shows a specific rotation $[\alpha]_D^{25} + 137°$ (c = 1, H_2O).

Biosynthesis.   *Origin of methyl groups.*   The methyl groups attached to sulfur at C-1, to nitrogen at N-1′ and the terminal methyl group of the propyl moiety attached to C-4′ are derived from methionine (19). The methyl group attached at C-7 and the methylene groups of the propyl moiety at C-4′ are not derived from methionine.

Origin of the aminoacid portion.   Several logical precursors of the propylhygric acid moiety of lincomycin, eg, L-proline [U-^{14}C] (uniformly labeled), hydroxy-L-proline [2-^{14}C], L-glutamic acid [U-^{14}C] and 5-amino-levulinic acid [4-^{14}C] were not incorporated (20).

4-Propylproline accumulates when *Streptomyces lincolnensis* is grown in sulfur deficient media (21). Addition of L-tyrosine or L-dihydroxyphenylalanine stimulated propylproline production. By the use of radioactive L-tyrosine it was found that all of the carbon atoms, except for the methyl group on nitrogen and the terminal methyl group of the propyl side chain were derived from tyrosine.

In complex media excellent incorporation of radioactive L-tyrosine into lincomycin was demonstrated: all of the label was found in the propylhygric acid portion of the antibiotic.

Mechanism of Action.   The earliest studies on the mechanism of action of lincomycin showed that lincomycin had the immediate effect on *Staphylococcus aureus* of complete inhibition of protein synthesis (22). Little effect on DNA and RNA synthesis was observed.

The site of lincomycin action is on the 50S (svedberg unit) subunit of the ribosome where it inhibits the binding of phenylalanine–t-RNA (transfer-RNA) to the ribosome–messenger complex (23).

Lincomycin causes a breakdown of polyribosomes into 30S and 50S subunits (24). These results suggested that lincomycin either causes premature detachment of ribosomes from m-RNA (messenger-RNA) or that it inhibits the initiation of polypeptide synthesis.

Lincomycin exerts its effect on protein synthesis inhibition by acting on 70S complexes, thus inhibiting the process of peptide chain initiation (25).

Pharmacology and Uses. Lincomycin hydrochloride is available in oral dosage forms and as a sterile solution for injection.

After oral administration to adults mean peak serum levels were achieved within 2 and 6 h. Single 500 and 1000 mg doses gave peak levels of 1.8–5.3 and 2.5–6.7 μg/mL, respectively (26–30). The half-life is 4.2–5.4 h (31).

Intramuscular administration gave peak levels at 0.5–2 h. After 300 and 600 mg doses, mean peak levels were 11.7–15 and 9.3–18.5 μg/mL, respectively, (26–27,30,32).

Lincomycin activity is widely distributed in human body tissues and fluids. Significant concentrations were found in bile, peritoneal fluid, pleural fluid, eye, bone, and brain (30,33–36). It is excreted both in the urine and in the feces (26–30).

Lincomycin has found use in the treatment of diseases of the ear, throat, nose, skin, respiratory, skin and soft tissue, bone, joint, dental, and septicemic infections caused by staphylococci, pneumonococci, and streptococci (other than enterococci). It has also been used in the treatment of diphtheria and a variety of anaerobic infections, including actinomycosis (37).

Celesticetin

Although the structural assignment of lincomycin was completed first, the production of a related antibiotic, celesticetin, by the actinomycete *Streptomyces caelestis* sp *nova*. NRRL 2418, was reported earlier (38). Its isolation was described by Hoeksema and co-workers (39).

The structure of celesticetin (**2**) was assigned by Hoeksema in 1968 (40). Desalicetin (**3**), the antibacterially active alkaline hydrolysis product from celesticetin, and celesticetin itself, were deemed lacking in clinical potential and were not developed past laboratory studies.

4′-Depropyl-4′-ethyllincomycin

Argoudelis and co-workers (41–43) reported the isolation, properties and structure of an antibiotic, 4′-depropyl-4′-ethyllincomycin (**4**), which was co-produced with lincomycin in fermentations of *S. lincolnensis*. It is a homologue of lincomycin and possesses about one-tenth the activity of lincomycin.

Others

A series of modified lincomycins was obtained by manipulating fermentation conditions, and adding presumed precursors, biochemical antagonists and fragments of the lincomycin molecule to the parent *Streptomyces lincolnensis* and mutants of it. None of these possessed properties superior to those of lincomycin itself.

The addition of ethionine to the lincomycin-producing organisms resulted in the formation of 1-demethylthio-1-ethylthiolincomycin (**5**) (3,41,44–46).

Addition of the sugar moiety of lincomycin to *S. lincolnensis* fermentations resulted in the formation of 1′-demethyllincomycin (**6**) (47). The production of (**6**) occurs under the influence of methylation inhibitors (48–49).

The 1-demethylthio-1-ethylthio-1′-demethylthio-1′-ethylthio analogue (**7**) was formed by the addition of ethionine to *S. lincolnensis* growing in synthetic media (50–51).

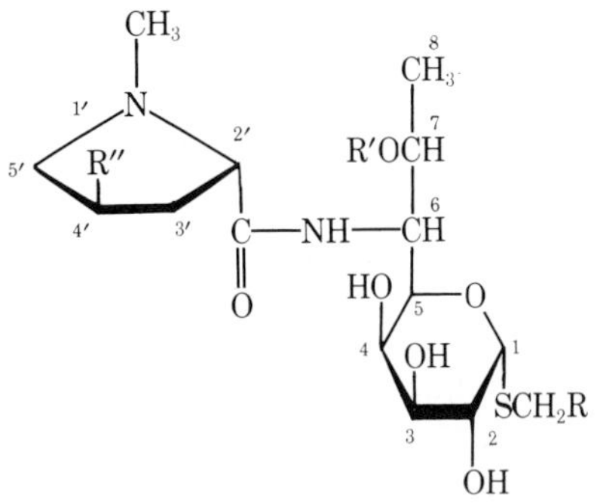

	R	R'	R''
(1) lincomycin	H	H	$CH_2CH_2CH_3$
(2) celesticetin	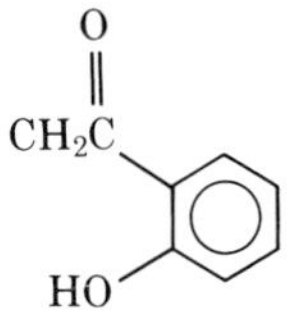 (see structure below)	CH_3	H
(3) desalicetin	CH_2OH	CH_3	H
(4) 4'-depropyl- 4'- ethyllincomycin	H	H	CH_2CH_3

Extension of normal fermentation (6 d) of *S. lincolnensis* to 12 d resulted in the formation of lincomycin sulfoxide **(8)** and 1-demethylthio-1-hydroxylincomycin **(9)**.

Clindamycin

The successful reaction of lincomycin with thionyl chloride (52) resulted in the replacement of the 7*R*-hydroxyl group to form 7*S*-chloro-7-deoxylincomycin in **(10)**, whose structure was confirmed by x-ray crystallography (53).

Preparation. Birkenmeyer and Kagan (54) described three procedures for the conversion of lincomycin to clindamycin (Cleocin, Upjohn).

In the first procedure, lincomycin reacted with thionyl chloride at reflux temperatures to give clindamycin as a 3,4-cyclic sulfite and a 3,4-cyclic sulfite-2-linear sulfite. Treatment of the reaction mixture with methanol and strong base afforded clindamycin.

In the second procedure, lincomycin reacted with triphenylphosphine dichloride; in the third procedure, it reacted with triphenylphosphine in carbon tetrachloride. In all three cases, clindamycin was isolated as the crystalline hydrochloride–hydrate.

Clindamycin Palmitate and Clindamycin Phosphate. The 2-palmitate ester of clindamycin is tasteless and is readily hydrolysed *in vivo* to active clindamycin (55). It has been developed as the pediatric formulation of clindamycin (Cleocin Pediatric, Upjohn).

When given intramuscularly, clindamycin hydrochloride causes pain at the in-

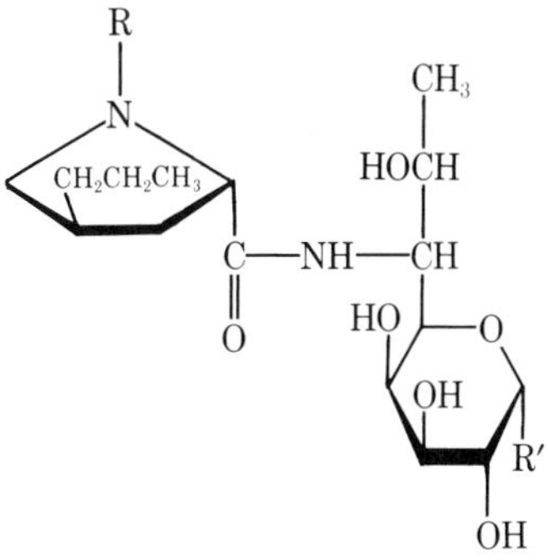

	R	R'
(5) 1-demethyl-1-ethylthiolincomycin	CH$_3$	SCH$_2$CH$_3$
(6) 1'-demethyllincomycin	H	SCH$_3$
(7) 1-demethylthio-1-ethylthio-1'-demethylthio-1'-ethylthiolincomycin	CH$_2$CH$_3$	SCH$_2$CH$_3$
(8) lincomycin sulfoxide	CH$_3$	$\overset{\text{O}}{\overset{\uparrow}{\text{S}}}CH_3$
(9) 1-demethylthio-1-hydroxylincomycin	CH$_3$	⁓OH

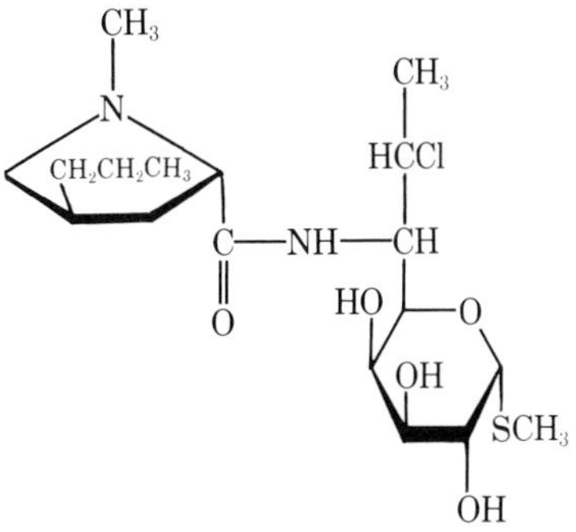

(10)

clindamycin

jection site. A modification program to alter this undesirable characteristic resulted in the preparation of clindamycin 2-phosphate (56) (Cleocin Phosphate, Upjohn). Clindamycin 2-phosphate, although antibacterially inactive per se, is rapidly hydrolysed after injection to the active clindamycin.

Pharmacology and Uses.   Oral administration of clindamycin hydrochloride gave peak serum levels of 1.9–2.7, 3.6, and 5.6 µg/mL one hour after single doses of 150, 300, and 450 mg, respectively. The half-life is 2.0–3.8 h (57–60).

Clindamycin palmitate was also absorbed rapidly, following oral administration, but serum concentrations were lower than after clindamycin hydrochloride (58).

Intramuscular injection of single 300, 450, and 600 mg doses of clindamycin phosphate gave mean peak serum levels of 3.8–4.9, 5.3, and 6.2–6.3 µg/mL respectively, 2–4 h after administration (58,61–62).

Clindamycin, like lincomycin, is distributed widely in human body tissues except that no significant levels are found in the brain or eye (37).

Antibacterial activity is found both in urine and feces after administration of clindamycin. Some of this activity is due to clindamycin. The N-demethyl analogue of clindamycin has been isolated from the urine of human subjects who had received clindamycin, and tlc bioautographic analysis which detected the presence of N-demethylclindamycin in serum has been described (63).

Clindamycin has found use in the treatment of common infections caused by gram-positive cocci. It is also highly efficacious in treating anaerobic infections, including actinomycosis (37).

BIBLIOGRAPHY

1 D. J. Mason, A. Dietz, and C. DeBoer, *Antimicrob. Agents Chemother.* (*1962*) 544 (1963).
2. C. Lewis, H. W. Clapp, and J. E. Grady, *Antimicrob. Agents Chemother.* (*1962*) 570 (1963).
3. E. L. Patterson, J. H. Hash, M. Lincks, P. A. Miller, and N. Bohonos, *Science* 146, 1691 (1964).
4. U.S. Pat. 3,697,380 (Oct. 10, 1972), A. D. Argoudelis, J. H. Coats, and T. R. Pyke (to The Upjohn Company).
5. U.S. Pat. 3,833,475 (Sept. 3, 1974), F. Reusser and A. D. Argoudelis (to The Upjohn Company).
6. U.S. Pat. 3,726,766 (Apr. 10, 1973), A. D. Argoudelis and J. H. Coats (to The Upjohn Company).
7. U.S. Pat. 3,812,014 (May 21, 1974), A. D. Argoudelis and J. H. Coats (to The Upjohn Company).
8. U.S.S.R. Pat. 287,743 (Feb. 18, 1975), G. F. Gause, O. A. Lapchinskaya, M. A. Sveshnikova, T. P. Preobrazhenskaya, R. S. Ukholina, N. P. Nechaeva, V. V. Pogozheva, T. P. Korobkova, and G. A. Trenina (to The University of Moscow).
9. Belg. Pat. 830,068 (Dec. 10, 1975), M. E. Bergy, J. H. Coats, and V. S. Malik (to The Upjohn Company).
10. R. R. Herr and M. E. Bergy, *Antimicrob. Agents Chemother.* (*1962*) 560 (1963).
11. U.S. Pat. 3,313,695 (Apr. 11, 1967), D. VanOverloop (to The Upjohn Company).
12. L. J. Hanka, D. J. Mason, M. R. Burch, and R. W. Treick, *Antimicrob. Agents Chemother.* (*1962*) 565 (1963).
13. H. Hoeksema, *Abstr. Papers, 149th Meeting of the American Chemical Society,* Detroit, Mich., 1965, p. 9-C.
14. H. Hoeksema, B. Bannister, R. D. Birkenmeyer, F. Kagan, B. J. Magerlein, F. A. MacKellar, W. Schroeder, G. Slomp, and R. R. Herr, *J. Am. Chem. Soc.* 86, 4223 (1964).
15. R. R. Herr and G. Slomp, *J. Am. Chem. Soc.* 89, 2444 (1967).
16. W. Schroeder, B. Bannister, and H. Hoeksema, *J. Am. Chem. Soc.,* 89, 2448 (1967).
17. G. Slomp and F. A. MacKellar, *J. Am. Chem. Soc.* 89, 2454 (1967).
18. B. J. Magerlein, R. D. Birkenmeyer, R. R. Herr, and F. Kagan, *J. Am. Chem. Soc.,* 89, 2459 (1967).
19. A. D. Argoudelis, T. E. Eble, J. A. Fox, and D. J. Mason, *Biochemistry* 8, 3408 (1969).
20. T. E. Eble, "Lincomycin," in D. Gottlieb and P. D. Shaw, eds., *Antibiotics II, Biosynthesis,* Springer-Verlag New York, Inc., New York, 1967, p. 353.
21. D. F. Witz, E. J. Hessler, and T. L. Miller, *Biochemistry* 10, 1128 (1971).
22. J. J. Josten and P. M. Allen, *Biochem. Biophys. Res. Commun.* 14, 241 (1964).
23. F. N. Chang, D. J. Sih, and B. Weisblum, *Proc. Nat. Acad. Sci. U.S.A.* 55, 431 (1966).
24. E. Cundliffe, *Biochemistry* 8, 2063 (1969).
25. F. Reusser, *Antimicrob. Agents Chemother.* 7, 32 (1975).
26. J. J. Vavra, W. T. Sokolski, and J. B. Lawson, *Antimicrob. Agents Chemother.* (*1963*) 176 (1964).
27. K. Kaplan, W. H. Chew, and L. Weinstein, *Am. J. Med. Sci.* 250, 137 (1965).
28. C. E. McCall, N. H. Steigbigel, and M. Finland, *Am. J. Med. Sci.* 254, 144 (1967).
29. R. F. McGehee, Jr., C. B. Smith, C. Wilcox, and M. Finland, *Am. J. Med. Sci.* 256, 279 (1968).
30. A. Medina, N. Fiske, I. Hjelt-Harvey, C. D. Brown, and A. Prigot, *Antimicrob. Agents Chemother.* (*1963*), 189 (1964).
31. J. G. Wagner, J. I. Northam, and W. T. Sokolski, *Nature (London)* 207, 201 (1965).
32. P. Ma, M. Lim, and J. H. Nodine, *Antimicrob. Agents Chemother.* (*1963*) 183 (1964).
33. P. A. Thomas and P. C. Jolly, *Am. Rev. Respir. Dis.* 96, 1044 (1967).
34. E. F. Becker, *Am. J. Ophthalmol.* 67, 963 (1969).
35. W. McL. Davis, Jr., *Oral Surg.* 27, 688 (1969).
36. V. J. Nemecek, M. Hejzlar, and V. Vacek, *Arzneim. Forsch.* 19, 1760 (1969).
37. R. J. Fass, "Lincomycin and Clindamycin," in E. M. Kagan, ed., *Antimicrobial Therapy,* 2nd ed., W. B. Saunders Company, Philadelphia, Pa., 1974, p. 83.
38. C. DeBoer, A. Dietz, J. R. Wilkins, C. Lewis, and G. M. Savage, *Antibiot. Annu.,* 831 (1954–1955).

39. H. Hoeksema, G. F. Crum, and W. H. DeVries, *Antibiot. Annu.*, 837 (1954–1955).
40. H. Hoeksema, *J. Am. Chem. Soc.* **90,** 755 (1968).
41. A. D. Argoudelis, J. A. Fox, D. J. Mason, and T. E. Eble, *J. Am. Chem. Soc.* **86,** 5044 (1964).
42. U.S. Pat. 3,359,164 (Dec. 19, 1967), A. D. Argoudelis, J. A. Fox, and M. E. Bergy (to The Upjohn Company).
43. A. D. Argoudelis, J. A. Fox, and T. E. Eble, *Biochemistry* **4,** 698 (1965).
44. A. D. Argoudelis and D. J. Mason, *Antimicrob. Agents Chemother., Abstr.* 15 (1964).
45. U.S. Pat. 3,359,163 (Dec. 19, 1967), A. D. Argoudelis and D. J. Mason (to The Upjohn Company).
46. A. D. Argoudelis and D. J. Mason, *Biochemistry* **4,** 704 (1965).
47. A. D. Argoudelis, J. A. Fox, and D. J. Mason, *Biochemistry* **4,** 710 (1965).
48. U.S. Pat. 3,313,801 (Apr. 11, 1967), A. D. Argoudelis, L. E. Johnson, and T. R. Pyke (to The Upjohn Company).
49. A. D. Argoudelis, L. E. Johnson, and T. R. Pyke, *J. Antibiot.* **26,** 429 (1973).
50. U.S. Pat. 3,395,139 (July 30, 1968), D. J. Mason and A. D. Argoudelis (to The Upjohn Company).
51. A. D. Argoudelis, T. E. Eble, and D. J. Mason, *J. Antibiot.* **23,** 1 (1970).
52. R. D. Birkenmeyer, B. J. Magerlein, and F. Kagan, *Abstr. 5th Intersci. Conf. Antimicrob. Agents and Chemother., 1965,* p. 18.
53. D. J. Duchamp, *Abstracts American Crystallography Association Summer Meeting D5, 1967.*
54. R. D. Birkenmeyer and F. Kagan, *J. Med. Chem.* **13,** 616 (1970).
55. A. A. Sinkula, W. Morozowich, and E. L. Rowe, *J. Pharm. Sci.* **62,** 1106 (1973).
56. W. A. Morozowich, D. J. Lamb, R. M. DeHaan, and J. E. Gray, *Abstracts, Papers, American Pharmaceutical Association Meeting, Washington, D.C., 1970,* p. 63.
57. R. M. DeHaan, C. M. Metzler, D. Schellenberg, W. D. VandenBosch, and E. L. Masson, *Int. J. Clin. Pharmacol.* **62,** 105 (1972).
58. C. M. Metzler, R. M. DeHaan, D. Schellenberg, W. D. VandenBosch, *J. Pharm. Sci.* **62,** 591 (1973).
59. B. R. Meyers, K. Kaplan, and L. Weinstein, *Appl. Microbiol.* **17,** 653 (1969).
60. J. G. Wagner, E. Novak, N. C. Patel, C. G. Chidester, and W. L. Lummis, *Am. J. Med. Sci.* **256,** 25 (1968).
61. R. M. DeHaan, C. M. Metzler, D. Schellenberg, and W. D. VandenBosch, *J. Clin. Pharmacol.* **13,** 190 (1973).
62. R. J. Fass and S. Saslaw, *Am. J. Med. Sci.* **263,** 369 (1972).
63. T. F. Brodasky, A. D. Argoudelis, and T. E. Eble, *J. Antibiot.* **21,** 327 (1968).

THOMAS E. EBLE
The Upjohn Company

MACROLIDES

Picromycin (1) was the first of a large number of macrolide antibiotics to be isolated from soil actinomycetes mainly of the genus *Streptomyces*. As a class they are characterized by having excellent antibacterial activity particulary against gram-positive bacteria. Macrolide antibiotics are classified according to the size of the macrocyclic lactone ring forming the aglycone, either as 12-, 14-, or 16-membered ring macrolides (see Table 1). They are polyfunctional molecules and the majority of macrolides contain at least one aminosugar moiety and are basic compounds. However, neutral macrolides containing only neutral sugar moieties attached to the aglycone are also known. There are a number of reviews dealing with the chemistry (2–14), the biosynthesis (2–4,15–18), the biological activity (11,19,20), the development of resistance (21–26), and the mechanism of action (27–30).

Table 1.   Alphabetical List of Macrolides

Compound	CAS Registry Number	Structure number	Molecular formula
acumycin	[25999-30-8]	(74)	$C_{37}H_{59}NO_{12}$
albocycline	[25129-91-3]	(25)	$C_{18}H_{28}O_4$
albomycetin	[19721-56-3]	(15)	$C_{28}H_{47}NO_8$
aldgamycin D	[20283-48-1]	(83)	$C_{35}H_{56}O_{14}$
aldgamycin E	[11011-06-6]	(86) partial structure	$C_{37}H_{58}O_{15}$
aldgamycin F	[55141-41-8]	(85)	$C_{37}H_{56}O_{16}$
amaromycin	[19721-56-3]	(15)	$C_{28}H_{47}NO_8$
angolamycin	[1402-83-1]	(72)	$C_{46}H_{77}NO_{17}$
antibiotic B-5050 A	[35908-44-2]	(31)	$C_{43}H_{71}NO_{16}$
antibiotic B-5050 B	[35908-45-3]	(32)	$C_{42}H_{69}NO_{16}$
antibiotic B-5050 C	[35775-82-7]	(33)	$C_{41}H_{67}NO_{16}$
antibiotic B-5050 D	[35942-56-4]	(34)	$C_{40}H_{65}NO_{16}$
antibiotic B-5050 E	[35942-57-5]	(35)	$C_{40}H_{65}NO_{16}$
antibiotic B-5050 F	[35775-66-7]	(36)	$C_{39}H_{63}NO_{16}$
antibiotic B-5050 G	[56078-81-0]	(37)	$C_{42}H_{69}NO_{16}$
antibiotic B-58941	[25999-30-8]	(74)	$C_{37}H_{59}NO_{12}$
antibiotic M-4209	[4564-87-8]	(27)	$C_{42}H_{67}NO_{16}$
antibiotic M-4365 A$_1$	[59227-84-8]	(78)	$C_{31}H_{53}NO_8$
antibiotic M-4365 A$_2$	[35834-26-5]	(75)	$C_{31}H_{51}NO_9$
antibiotic M-4365 A$_3$	[61475-37-4]	(77)	$C_{31}H_{53}NO_9$
antibiotic M-4365 G$_1$	[59227-83-7]	(81)	$C_{31}H_{53}NO_7$
antibiotic M-4365 G$_2$	[56689-42-0]	(82)	$C_{31}H_{51}NO_8$
antibiotic M-4365 G$_3$	[58947-83-4]	(79)	$C_{31}H_{53}NO_8$
antibiotic PA-148	[1402-83-1]	(72)	$C_{46}H_{77}NO_{17}$
antibiotic SF-837	[35457-80-8]	(57)	$C_{41}H_{67}NO_{15}$
antibiotic SF-837 A$_2$	[35457-81-9]	(58)	$C_{42}H_{69}NO_{15}$
antibiotic SF-837 A$_3$	[36025-69-1]	(40)	$C_{41}H_{65}NO_{15}$
antibiotic SF-837 A$_4$	[36083-82-6]	(41)	$C_{42}H_{67}NO_{15}$
antibiotic XK-41 A$_1$	[49669-77-4]	(11)	$C_{49}H_{86}N_2O_{17}$
antibiotic XK-41 A$_2$	[49669-76-3]	(10)	$C_{48}H_{84}N_2O_{17}$
antibiotic XK-41 B$_1$	[49669-75-2]	(9)	$C_{46}H_{82}N_2O_{16}$
antibiotic XK-41 C	[28022-11-9]	(8)	$C_{44}H_{80}N_2O_{15}$
antibiotic XK-41 B$_2$	[50692-34-7]	(12)	$C_{47}H_{84}NO_{16}$
antibiotic YC-17	[11091-33-1]	(3)	$C_{25}H_{43}NO_6$
antibiotic YL-704 A$_0$	[52310-62-0]	(62)	$C_{44}H_{73}NO_{15}$
antibiotic YL-704 A$_1$	[40615-47-2]	(63)	$C_{43}H_{71}NO_{15}$
antibiotic YL-704 A$_3$	[16846-24-5]	(48)	$C_{42}H_{69}NO_{15}$
antibiotic YL-704 B$_1$	[35457-80-8]	(57)	$C_{41}H_{67}NO_{15}$

Table 1 (*continued*)

Compound	CAS Registry Number	Structure number	Molecular formula
antibiotic YL-704 B$_3$	[18361-48-3]	(51)	C$_{40}$H$_{65}$NO$_{15}$
antibiotic YL-704 C$_1$	[35775-82-7]	(33)	C$_{41}$H$_{67}$NO$_{16}$
antibiotic YL-704 C$_2$	[35867-32-4]	(61)	C$_{40}$H$_{65}$NO$_{15}$
antibiotic YL-704 C$_3$	[35908-44-2]	(31)	C$_{43}$H$_{71}$NO$_{16}$
antibiotic YL-704 C$_4$	[35908-45-3]	(32)	C$_{42}$H$_{69}$NO$_{16}$
antibiotic YL-704 W$_1$	[35867-31-3]	(42)	C$_{43}$H$_{69}$NO$_{15}$
antibiotic YL-704 W$_2$	[52310-61-9]	(43)	C$_{44}$H$_{71}$NO$_{15}$
carbomycin A	[4564-87-8]	(27)	C$_{42}$H$_{67}$NO$_{16}$
carbomycin B	[21238-30-2]	(38)	C$_{42}$H$_{67}$NO$_{15}$
chalcomycin	[20283-48-1]	(83)	C$_{35}$H$_{56}$O$_{14}$
cineromycin B	[11033-23-1]	(26)	C$_{17}$H$_{26}$O$_4$
cirramycin A$_1$	[25339-90-6]	(73)	C$_{31}$H$_{51}$NO$_{10}$
cirramycin A$_2$	[65086-22-8]		
cirramycin A$_3$	[65086-23-9]		
cirramycin A$_4$	[65086-24-0]		
cirramycin A$_5$	[65086-25-1]		
cirramycin B$_1$	[25999-30-8]	(74)	C$_{37}$H$_{59}$NO$_{12}$
cirramycin B$_2$	[65086-26-2]		
cirramycin B$_3$	[65086-27-3]		
deltamycin A$_1$	[58880-22-1]	(28)	C$_{39}$H$_{61}$NO$_{16}$
deltamycin A$_2$	[58880-23-2]	(29)	C$_{40}$H$_{63}$NO$_{16}$
deltamycin A$_3$	[58880-24-3]	(30)	C$_{41}$H$_{65}$NO$_{16}$
deltamycin A$_4$	[4564-87-8]	(27)	C$_{42}$H$_{67}$NO$_{16}$
3″-de-*O*-methyl-2″,3″-anhydrolanka-mycin	[60462-94-4]	(24)	C$_{41}$H$_{68}$O$_{15}$
O-demethyloleandomycin	[64743-16-4]	(20)	C$_{34}$H$_{59}$NO$_{12}$
8,8a-deoxyoleandolide	[53428-54-9]	(21)	C$_{20}$H$_{36}$O$_6$
10,11-dihydropicromycin	[27656-56-0]	(18)	C$_{28}$H$_{49}$NO$_8$
erythromycin A	[114-07-8]	(4)	C$_{37}$H$_{67}$NO$_{13}$
erythromycin B	[527-75-3]	(5)	C$_{37}$H$_{67}$NO$_{12}$
erythromycin C	[1675-02-1]	(6)	C$_{36}$H$_{65}$NO$_{13}$
erythromycin D	[33442-56-7]	(7)	C$_{36}$H$_{65}$NO$_{12}$
erythromycin E	[41451-91-6]	(14)	C$_{37}$H$_{65}$NO$_{14}$
erythromycin estolate	[3521-62-8]		C$_{52}$H$_{97}$NO$_{18}$S
erythronolide B	[3225-82-9]	(13)	C$_{21}$H$_{38}$O$_7$
espinomycin A$_1$	[35457-80-8]	(57)	C$_{41}$H$_{67}$NO$_{15}$
espinomycin A$_2$	[40867-12-7]	(60)	C$_{42}$H$_{69}$NO$_{15}$
espinomycin A$_3$	[35867-32-4]	(61)	C$_{40}$H$_{65}$NO$_{15}$
josamycin	[16846-24-5]	(48)	C$_{42}$H$_{69}$NO$_{15}$
juvenimicin A$_1$	[63939-12-8]		
juvenimicin A$_2$	[61417-47-8]	(76)	C$_{30}$H$_{51}$NO$_8$
juvenimicin A$_3$	[35834-26-5]	(75)	C$_{31}$H$_{51}$NO$_9$
juvenimicin A$_4$	[61475-37-4]	(77)	C$_{31}$H$_{53}$NO$_9$
juvenimicin B$_1$	[58947-83-4]	(79)	C$_{31}$H$_{53}$NO$_8$
juvenimicin B$_2$	[63939-10-6]		
juvenimicin B$_3$	[61417-48-9]	(80)	C$_{31}$H$_{53}$NO$_9$
juvenimicin B$_4$	[63939-11-7]		
kitasamycin	[1392-21-8]		C$_{19}$H$_{25}$NO$_{10}$
kromin	[17681-07-1]		C$_{17}$H$_{28}$O$_5$
kromycin	[20509-23-3]	(17)	C$_{20}$H$_{30}$O$_5$
kujimycin A	[33955-27-0]	(23)	C$_{40}$H$_{70}$O$_{15}$
kujimycin B	[30042-37-6]	(22)	C$_{42}$H$_{72}$O$_{16}$
lankamycin	[30042-37-6]	(22)	C$_{42}$H$_{72}$O$_{16}$
leucomycin A$_1$	[16846-34-7]	(47)	C$_{40}$H$_{67}$NO$_{14}$
leucomycin A$_3$	[16846-24-5]	(48)	C$_{42}$H$_{69}$NO$_{15}$
leucomycin A$_4$	[18361-46-1]	(49)	C$_{41}$H$_{67}$NO$_{15}$
leucomycin A$_5$	[18361-45-0]	(50)	C$_{39}$H$_{65}$NO$_{14}$
leucomycin A$_6$	[18361-48-3]	(51)	C$_{40}$H$_{65}$NO$_{15}$

Table 1 (*continued*)

Compound	CAS Registry Number	Structure number	Molecular formula
leucomycin A_7	[18361-47-2]	(52)	$C_{38}H_{63}NO_{14}$
leucomycin A_8	[18361-50-7]	(53)	$C_{39}H_{62}NO_{15}$
leucomycin A_9	[18361-49-4]	(54)	$C_{37}H_{61}NO_{14}$
leucomycin U	[31642-61-2]	(55)	$C_{37}H_{61}NO_{14}$
leucomycin V	[22875-15-6]	(56)	$C_{35}H_{59}NO_{13}$
9-*epi*-leucomycin A_3	[54274-45-2]		$C_{42}H_{69}NO_{15}$
leucomycin complex	[1392-21-8]		
magnamycin	[4564-87-8]	(27)	$C_{42}H_{67}NO_{16}$
magnamycin B	[21238-30-2]	(38)	$C_{42}H_{67}NO_{15}$
maridomycin I	[35908-44-2]	(31)	$C_{43}H_{71}NO_{16}$
maridomycin II	[35908-45-3]	(32)	$C_{42}H_{69}NO_{16}$
maridomycin III	[35775-82-7]	(33)	$C_{41}H_{67}NO_{16}$
maridomycin IV	[35942-56-4]	(34)	$C_{40}H_{65}NO_{16}$
maridomycin V	[35942-57-5]	(35)	$C_{40}H_{65}NO_{16}$
maridomycin VI	[35775-66-7]	(36)	$C_{39}H_{63}NO_{16}$
maridomycin G	[56078-81-0]	(37)	$C_{42}H_{69}NO_{16}$
megalomicin A	[28022-11-9]	(8)	$C_{44}H_{80}N_2O_{15}$
megalomicin B	[49669-75-2]	(9)	$C_{46}H_{82}N_2O_{16}$
megalomicin C_1	[49669-76-3]	(10)	$C_{48}H_{84}N_2O_{17}$
megalomicin C_2	[49669-77-4]	(11)	$C_{49}H_{86}N_2O_{17}$
9-*O*-methylmidecamycin	[55648-53-8]		$C_{42}H_{69}NO_{15}$
methymycin	[497-72-3]	(1)	$C_{25}H_{43}NO_7$
methynolide	[534-32-7]	(64)	$C_{17}H_{28}O_5$
midecamycin	[35457-80-8]	(57)	$C_{41}H_{67}NO_{15}$
midecamycin metabolite M_1	[37906-56-0]	(59)	$C_{38}H_{63}NO_{14}$
midecamycin metabolite M_2	[38456-05-2]		$C_{38}H_{63}NO_{15}$
midecamycin A_2	[35457-81-9]	(58)	$C_{42}H_{69}NO_{15}$
midecamycin A_3	[36025-69-1]	(40)	$C_{41}H_{65}NO_{15}$
midecamycin A_4	[36083-82-6]	(41)	$C_{42}H_{67}NO_{15}$
mikonomycin	[20283-48-1]	(83)	$C_{35}H_{56}O_{14}$
narbomycin	[6036-25-5]	(16)	$C_{28}H_{47}NO_7$
narbonolide	[32885-75-9]		$C_{20}H_{32}O_5$
neomethymycin	[497-73-4]	(2)	$C_{25}H_{43}NO_7$
neutramycin	[1404-08-6]	(84)	$C_{34}H_{54}O_{14}$
niddamycin	[20283-69-6]	(39)	$C_{40}H_{65}NO_{14}$
oleandomycin	[3922-90-5]	(19)	$C_{35}H_{61}NO_{12}$
picromycin	[19721-56-3]	(15)	$C_{28}H_{47}NO_8$
picronolide	[51724-55-1]	(65)	$C_{20}H_{32}O_6$
platenomycin Ao	[52310-62-0]	(62)	$C_{44}H_{73}NO_{15}$
platenomycin A_1	[40615-47-2]	(63)	$C_{43}H_{71}NO_{15}$
platenomycin A_3	[16846-24-5]	(48)	$C_{42}H_{69}NO_{15}$
platenomycin B_1	[35457-80-8]	(57)	$C_{41}H_{67}NO_{15}$
platenomycin B_3	[18361-48-3]	(51)	$C_{40}H_{65}NO_{15}$
platenomycin C_1	[35775-82-7]	(33)	$C_{41}H_{67}NO_{16}$
platenomycin C_2	[35867-32-4]	(61)	$C_{40}H_{65}NO_{15}$
platenomycin C_3	[35908-44-2]	(31)	$C_{43}H_{71}NO_{16}$
platenomycin C_4	[35908-45-3]	(32)	$C_{42}H_{69}NO_{16}$
platenomycin W_1	[35867-31-3]	(42)	$C_{43}H_{69}NO_{15}$
platenomycin W_2	[52310-61-9]	(43)	$C_{44}H_{71}NO_{15}$
9-propionylmaridomycin III	[35775-84-9]		$C_{44}H_{71}NO_{17}$
relomycin	[62902-06-1]	(71)	$C_{46}H_{79}NO_{17}$
rosamicin	[35834-26-5]	(75)	$C_{31}H_{51}NO_9$
shincomycin A	[1402-83-1]	(72)	$C_{46}H_{77}NO_{17}$
spiramycin I	[24916-50-5]	(44)	$C_{43}H_{74}N_2O_{14}$
spiramycin II	[24916-51-6]	(45)	$C_{45}H_{76}N_2O_{15}$

Table 1 (*continued*)

Compound	CAS Registry Number	Structure number	Molecular formula
spiramycin III	[24916-52-7]	(46)	$C_{46}H_{78}N_2O_{15}$
triacetyloleandomycin	[2751-09-9]		$C_{41}H_{67}NO_{15}$
tylosin	[1401-69-0]	(70)	$C_{46}H_{77}NO_{17}$

Production and Isolation

Macrolide antibiotics are produced as secondary metabolites of soil microorganisms and the majority have been produced by various strains of *Streptomyces*. The macrolide antibiotics are invariably produced as a complex mixture of closely related components by submerged aerobic fermentation of suitable cultures at 20–40°C in an aqueous nutrient medium containing a variety of carbohydrate and nitrogen sources. The optimum yields of the antibiotic are usually obtained after 3 or 4 days. The antibiotic complex is then isolated by adjusting the whole broth to pH 9.5 and extracting with suitable solvents such as ethyl acetate, chloroform, or methylene chloride. Evaporation of the solvent extract affords the crude antibiotic complex (31) which may be further purified by passage over Sephadex LH20. The separation of the complex into its individual components has been effected by counter current distribution (32–36), column chromatography on alumina (36–38), silica gel (36,38–39), Amberlite IRC 50 (H^+) ion exchange resin (40), or by high-pressure liquid chromatography (41). Analytical separations of the components of the complex are usually carried out using paper chromatography or thin-layer chromatography (35,39,42).

12-Membered Ring Macrolides.   Methymycin (1), produced by *Streptomyces venezuelae* (43), has the distinction of being the first macrolide for which a structure was determined (44–47). Mild acidic hydrolysis gave the aglycone, methynolide (Fig. 1) (64), and D-desosamine (44) (see Table 2). The absolute stereochemistry of methymycin (1) has been established as 2*R*, 3*S*, 4*S*, 6*R*, 8,9-*trans;* 10*S*, 11*R* (100–104). The results of biosynthetic studies on the aglycone are shown in Figure 1 (105–106).

Neomethymycin (2) which is coproduced with (1) has the isomeric structure (2) (107–108). The partial absolute stereochemistry has been shown to be 2*R*, 3*S*, 4*S*, 6*R* (100–101,103,109).

Antibiotic YC-17 (3), isolated from the early culture filtrate of *Streptomyces venezuelae* MCRL 0376 along with (1) and (2), has been identified as being the 10-deoxy derivative of (1) (110). The absolute stereochemistry of YC-17 (3) has not been determined.

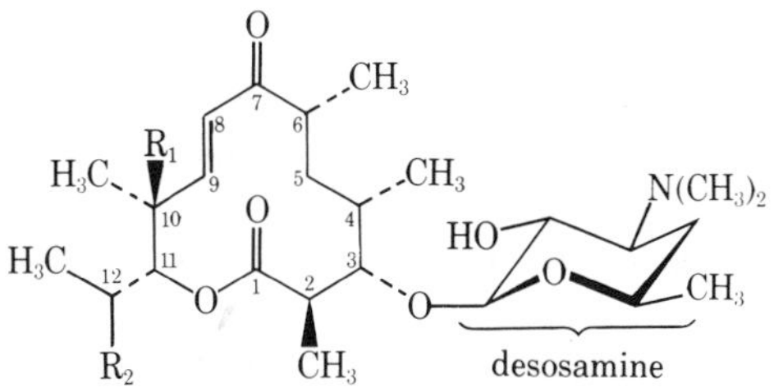

(1) R_1 = OH, R_2 = H   methymycin
(2) R_1 = H, R_2 = OH   neomethymycin
(3) R_1 = R_2 = H   antibiotic YC-17

Table 2. Alphabetical List of Macrolide Sugars Referred to in the Text

Compound	CAS Registry No.	References Structural studies	Synthesis
4-*O*-acetyl-L-arcanose[a]	[63887-63-8]	48	
D-aldgarose	[26428-87-5]	51,52	53–55
D-angolosamine	[14702-57-9]	56	
D-chalcose	[3150-28-5]	48	57
L-cinerulose	[33985-39-6]	58,59	
L-cladinose	[470-12-2]	60–63	
D-desosamine	[5779-39-5]	60,64–69	70–72
D-forosamine	[18423-27-3]	73	74,75
4-*O*-isovaleryl-L-mycarose	[63887-64-9]	76–78	
L-megosamine[b]	[65832-97-5]	79	79
D-mycaminose	[519-21-1]	77,78,82,83	84–86
L-mycarose	[6032-92-4]	62,63,76,87	63
D-mycinose	[21967-31-7]	88–92	93,94
L-oleandrose	[6786-76-1]	95–96	97–99
L-olivose	[25029-50-9]	9	

[a] D-Arcanose [26548-40-3] has been synthesized (49–50).

[b] Originally postulated to be D-rhodosamine [30636-50-1] (80–81).

14-Membered Ring Macrolides. The erythromycins are the most widely investigated members of this group and are produced by *Streptomyces erythreus* NRRL 2338 (32). Extensive chemical degradations on erythromycin A (4) established its structure (60,61,111–117). An x-ray crystallographic study on erythromycin A hydroiodide afforded the absolute stereochemistry of (4) (118). The structures of the coproduced minor components erythromycin B (5) (119–121), erythromycin C (6) (122), and erythromycin D (7) (123–124) have been determined.

A number of derivatives have been prepared with the objective of increasing blood and serum levels of the erythromycins and to improve their taste properties. These include esters (125–131), phosphates (132–133), *N*-alkylsuccinates (134), and fatty acid salts (135). Derivatives of erythromycin, modified in the cladinose ring (136–137), the desosamine ring (138–142), the aglycone (143–163), and at *C*-9 of the aglycone (114,163–176), have been described and have contributed greatly to the understanding of the chemistry and structure-activity relationships of the erythromycins. The mass spectral fragmentation patterns of the erythromycins under electron impact (177–178), chemical ionization (179) and field desorption (180) conditions have been described and extensive ¹H nmr and cd (circular dichroism) studies (7,181–189) have defined a single stable conformation for the aglycones, illustrated for erythronolide B (13). The ¹³C nmr spectral data (190–192) are in agreement with the conformations deduced earlier from the ¹H nmr studies.

Biosynthetic studies have shown that both propionate (193) and 2-methylmalonate (194) units are incorporated to form the aglycone, but the *C*-methyl, *O*-methyl and *N*-methyl groups of the sugars are derived from methionine (195–196). Some insight into the latter stages of the biosynthesis have been obtained by feeding various aglycone precursors to blocked mutants of *Streptomyces erythreus* (197–200), or to the oleandomycin producing strain, *Streptomyces antibioticus* ATCC 11891 (201). These results have been interpreted to indicate initial attachment of the mycarose unit to the aglycone followed by subsequent attachment of the desosamine unit in these antibiotics. A number of interesting shunt metabolites have been isolated from a blocked mutant (Abbott 4EB40) (187,202–203) and it has been demonstrated that (4) is slowly metabolized by the producing strain, to a novel ortho ester derivative, erythromycin E (14) (204).

The megalomicins represent novel members of this class produced by *Micromonospora megalomicea* (31,39) and the structures of megalomicin A (8), B (9), C_1 (10), and C_2 (11), have been elucidated (80–81,177,205–206) and revised following ^{13}C nmr and x-ray studies (79). A variety of acyl derivatives (206–209) and water soluble salts (210) have been prepared. *Micromonospora inositola* XK-41 (211–212) has been found to produce four components XK-41 A_1 (11), A_2 (10), B_1 (9), and C (8), that are identical to the natural megalomicins, as well as a fifth component B_2 (12), which is identical to a semisynthetic ester derivative of (8) (207).

Picromycin (albomycetin, amaromycin) (15), isolated from *Streptomyces felleus* (1,213), was originally thought to be an isomer of (1) (214–219) until mass spectral and ^1H nmr studies showed it to have the 14-membered lactone structure (15) (220). Hydrolysis at pH 6.5 afforded kromycin (17) (215–217,219–220), the structure and absolute stereochemistry of which was confirmed by x-ray analysis (221,222). From the above results and studies carried out on the acid degradation product kromin, the stereochemistry of (15) was defined as 2R, 4R, 5S, 6S, 8R, 12S, and 13R (97,223). The solution conformation of the aglycone of (15) has been determined (224) and the results of biosynthetic studies are illustrated in Figure 1 for picronolide (65) (225). The isolation of the aglycone, picronolide (65) has been reported from *Streptomyces venezuelae* MCRL 0376 (226), and a new metabolite of *Streptomyces venezuelae* ATCC 15068, namely 10,11-dihydropicromycin (18) (227), has been isolated. Reduction of (15) afforded the identical product (18) (227). Amaromycin, produced by *Streptomyces flavochromogenes* has been shown to be identical to picromycin (15) (228).

Narbomycin (16) produced by *Streptomyces narbonensis* has been shown to be the 12-deoxy analogue of picromycin (15) (229–231). The isolation of the aglycone, narbonolide, and its biological transformation into picromycin (15) via narbomycin (16) has been reported (232–234). The solution conformation of narbomycin (16) has also been determined (224).

Oleandomycin, produced by *Streptomyces antibioticus* (235) has the structure (19) (95,236–237) and the absolute stereochemistry of the aglycone has been shown to be 2R, 3S, 4S, 5S, 6S, 8R, 10R, 11S, 12R, 13R (238).

Triacetyloleandomycin has been prepared (239–240) and found to have improved taste and bioavailability relative to (19). A blocked mutant of the erythromycin producing strain, *Streptomyces erythreus* (Abbott 4EB40), has been found to produce 8,8a-deoxyoleandolide (21) (241). The biosynthesis of oleandomycin is shown in Figure 1 (66) (13,242) and the ^{13}C nmr spectrum has been reported (192). *O*-Demethyloleandomycin (20) has been isolated (9).

Several neutral 14-membered ring macrolides are known. Lankamycin (22), isolated from *Streptomyces violaceoniger*, has the structure (48,243–246) and stereochemistry (246–247) shown in (22). The ^{13}C nmr spectrum of (22) has been reported (192). *Streptomyces spinichromogenes* var. *kujimyceticus* has been found to produce kujimycin A (23) and kujimycin B (22) (245,248). A structure-activity relationship for some acetyl derivatives of (23) has been reported (249). A minor product isolated from the lankamycin fermentations has been found to be 3″-de-*O*-methyl-2″,3″-anhydrolankamycin (24) (250). The structures of two noncarbohydrate containing

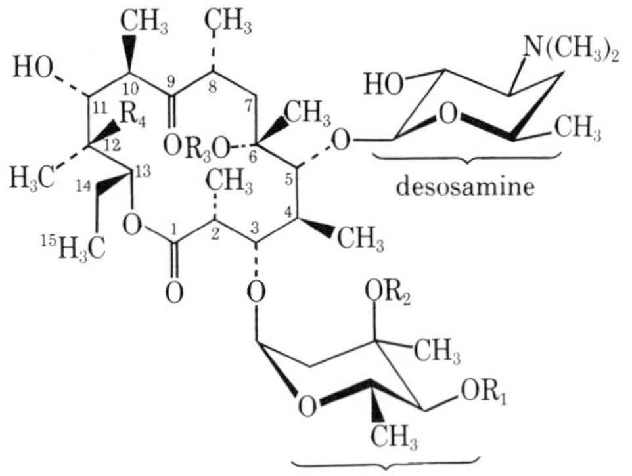

cladinose (R₁ = H, R₂ = CH₃)
mycarose (R₁ = R₂ = H)

(4) $R_1 = R_3 = H, R_2 = CH_3, R_4 = OH$ erythromycin A
(5) $R_1 = R_3 = R_4 = H, R_2 = CH_3$ erythromycin B
(6) $R_1 = R_2 = R_3 = H, R_4 = OH$ erythromycin C
(7) $R_1 = R_2 = R_3 = R_4 = H$ erythromycin D

(8) $R_1 = R_2 = H, R_3 =$ $, R_4 = OH$ megalomicin A

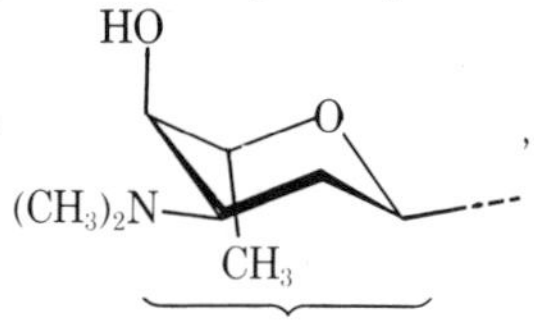

megosamine

(9) $R_1 = COCH_3, R_2 = H, R_3 =$ megosamine, $R_4 = OH$ megalomicin B
(10) $R_1 = R_2 = COCH_3, R_3 =$ megosamine, $R_4 = OH$ megalomicin C_1
(11) $R_1 = COCO_2CH_3, R_2 = COCH_3, R_3 =$ megosamine, $R_4 = OH$ megalomicin C_2
(12) $R_1 = COCH_2CH_3, R_2 = H, R_3 =$ megosamine, $R_4 = OH$ antibiotic XK-41 B_2

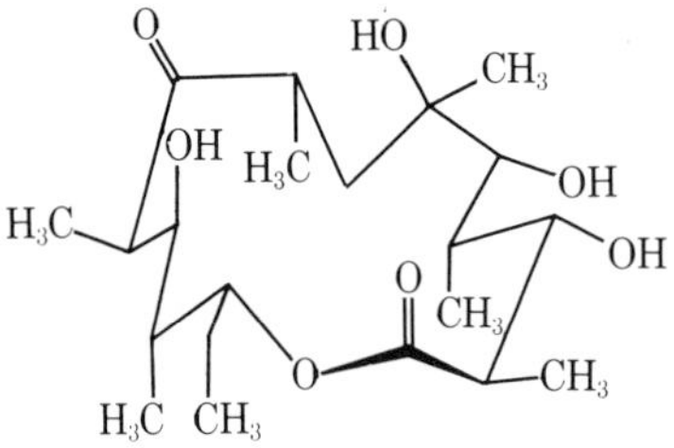

(13)
erythronolide B

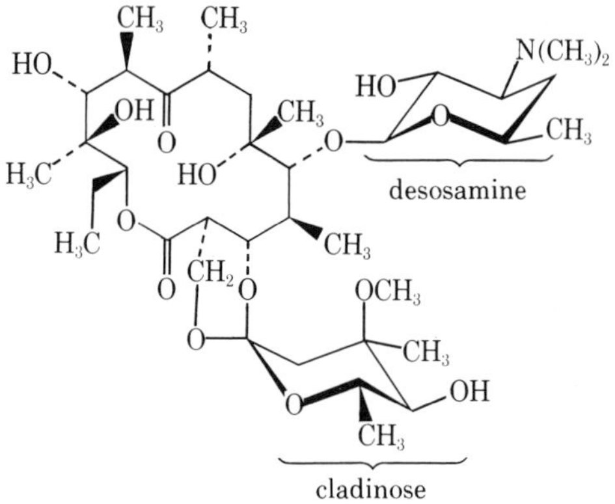

(14)
erythromycin E

macrolides, namely albocycline (25) from *Streptomyces brunneogriseus* (251–254) and cineromycin B (26) from *Streptomyces cinerochromogenes* (253–255), have been elucidated.

16-Membered Ring Macrolides. Extensive chemical studies on carbomycin A (magnamycin, M-4209, deltamycin A₄) (27) elaborated by *Streptomyces halstedii* (256,257), resulted in a structure (2,76–77,82,116,258) which was later revised to (27) (78,259). Biosynthetic studies have shown the incorporation of seven acetate units

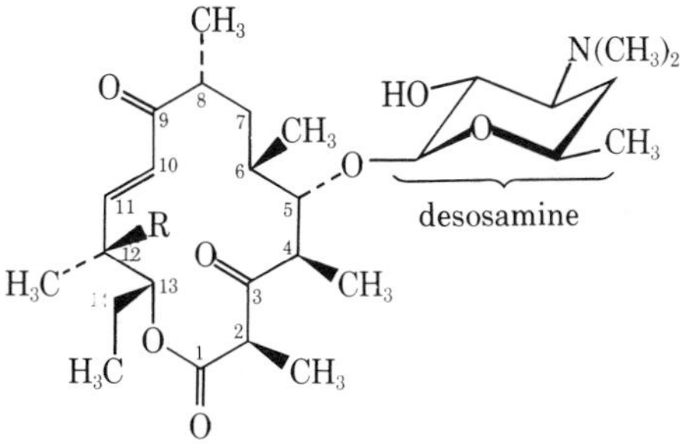

(15) R = OH   picromycin
(16) R = H   narbomycin

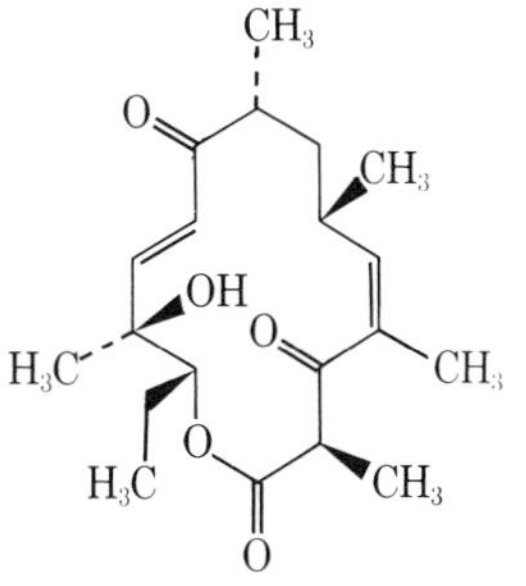

(17) kromycin

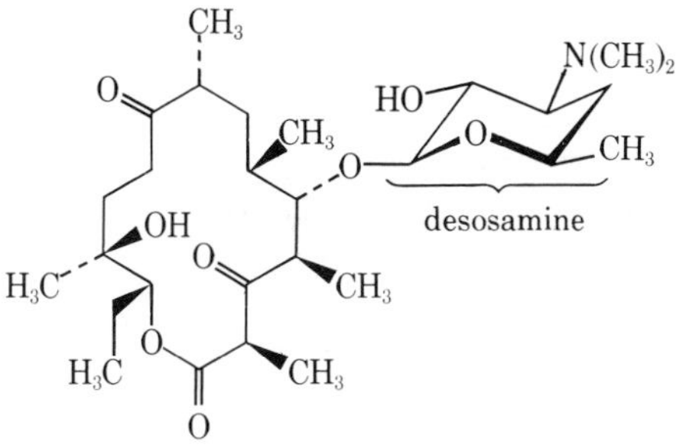

(18) 10, 11-dihydropicromycin

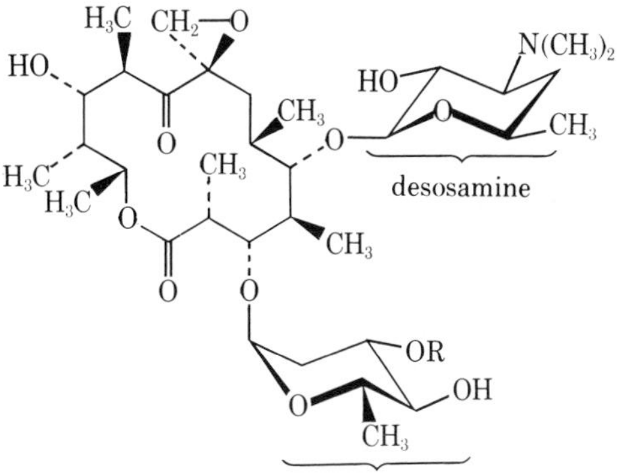

oleandrose (R = CH₃)
olivose (R = H)

(19) R = CH₃   oleandomycin
(20) R = H   O-demethyloleandomycin

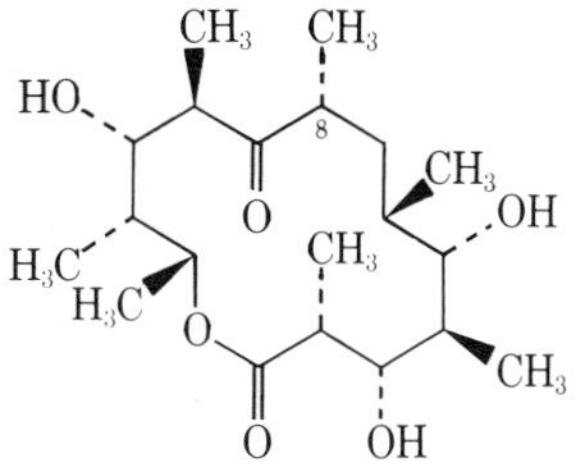

(21)
8,8a-deoxyoleandolide

(260) and one propionate unit (260–261) into the aglycone. The propionate unit was incorporated into C-7, C-8, and the 8-CH_3. The origin of C-5, C-6, and the aldehydic side chain remained in doubt although glucose was found to be incorporated (262). The absolute stereochemistry of (27) has been defined as 3R, 4S, 5S, 6R, 8R, 12S, 13S, 15R (238,263). The absolute stereochemistry at C-12 was originally assigned the R-configuration, but was subsequently shown to have the S-configuration as depicted in (27) (264).

Carbomycin B (magnamycin B) (38) is produced as a minor product of the fermentation (265). The ^{13}C nmr spectra of (27) and (38) have been reported (266). The

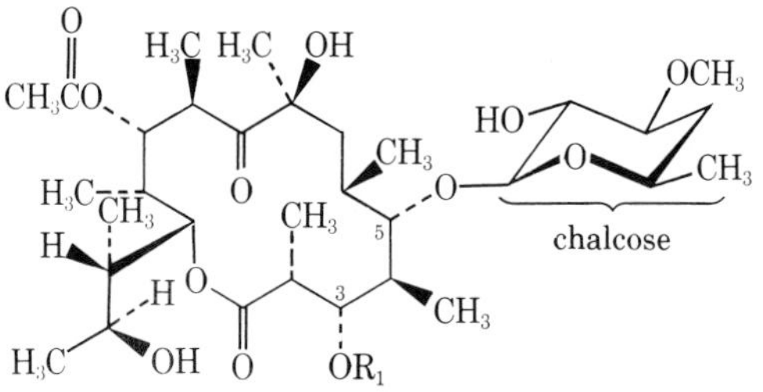

(**22**), $R_1 =$ 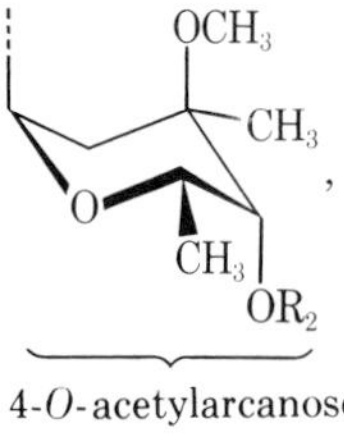 , $R_2 = COCH_3$ lankamycin

4-*O*-acetylarcanose

(**23**) R_1 = arcanose, R_2 = H   kujimycin A

(**24**), $R_1 =$ 3″-de-*O*-methyl-2″,3″-anhydrolankamycin

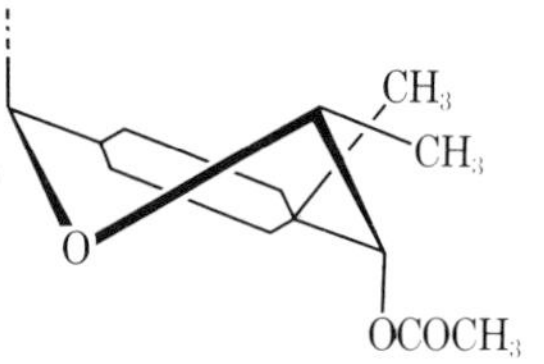

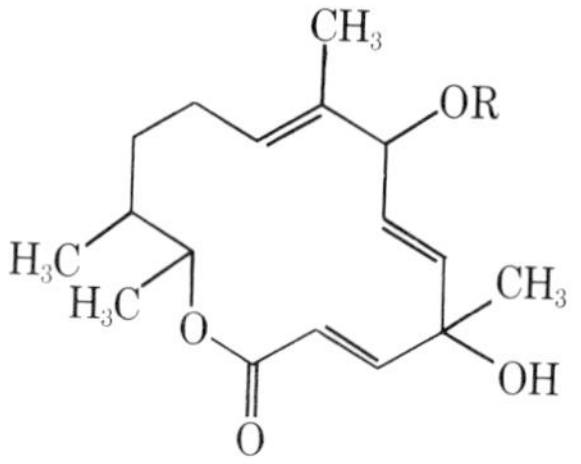

(**25**) R = CH$_3$ albocycline
(**26**) R = H   cineromycin B

deltamycins produced by *Streptomyces deltae*, have closely related structures and although their structures have not been published, a recent patent (267) describing microbial deacylation of the 4″-position has cited the gross structures of deltamycin A_1 (**28**), A_2 (**29**), A_3 (**30**), and A_4 (**27**). Niddamycin (**39**) produced by *Streptomyces djakartensis* was shown to be 3-desacetylcarbomycin B (268). The microbiological (269) and chemical (270) conversions of niddamycin (**39**) into the 9-dihydro derivatives have been reported. Microbiological deacylation of niddamycin has also been effected (271).

The spiramycins (foromacidines) produced by *Streptomyces ambofaciens* (34) have been separated into three components namely spiramycin I (**44**), spiramycin II (**45**), and spiramycin III (**46**) (272). Chemical studies led to proposed structures for the spiramycins (273–276) which were subsequently revised (78) and rerevised to (**44**), (**45**), and (**46**) (277). The ^{13}C nmr spectrum of (**46**) has been published (266). A number of acetyl derivatives of the spiramycins have been prepared (278), as well as Schiff base (279), and hydrazone (280) derivatives of the aldehyde group.

Detailed chemical studies have been carried out on the leucomycin complex (ki-

(27) R_1 = $COCH_3$, R_2 = $COCH_2CH(CH_3)_2$, R_3R_4 = =O   carbomycin A
(28) R_1 = R_2 = $COCH_3$, R_3R_4 = =O   deltamycin A_1
(29) R_1 = $COCH_3$, R_2 = $COCH_2CH_3$, R_3R_4 = =O   deltamycin A_2
(30) R_1 = $COCH_3$, R_2 = $COCH_2CH_2CH_,$, R_3R_4 = =O   deltamycin A_3
(31) R_1 = $COCH_2CH_3$, R_2 = $COCH_2CH(CH_3)_2$, R_3 = OH, R_4 = H   platenomycin C_3
(32) R_1 = $COCH_3$, R_2 = $COCH_2CH (CH_3)_2$, R_3 = OH, R_4 = H   platenomycin C_4
(33) R_1 = R_2 = $COCH_2CH_3$, R_3 = OH, R_4 = H   platenomycin C_1
(34) R_1 = $COCH_3$, R_2 = $COCH_2CH_3$, R_3 = OH, R_4 = H   maridomycin IV
(35) R_1 = $COCH_2CH_3$, R_2 = $COCH_3$, R_3 = OH, R_4 = H   maridomycin V
(36) R_1 = R_2 = $COCH_3$, R_3 = OH, R_4 = H   maridomycin VI
(37) R_1 = $COCH_2CH_3$, R_2 = $COCH_2CH_2CH_3$, R_3 = OH, R_4 = H   maridomycin G

tasamycin) which is elaborated by *Streptomyces kitasatoensis* (281). The complex has been separated into ten components namely leucomycin A_1 (47), A_3 (josamycin, YL-704 A_3, or platenomycin A_3) (48), A_4 (49), A_5 (50), A_6 (YL-704 B_3, or platenomycin B_3) (51), A_7 (52), A_8 (53), A_9 (54), U (55), and V (56) (35,40,41,282) which differ only in the nature of the acyl substituents at C-3 and C-4″.

The application of high pressure liquid chromatography to the separation of the leucomycins has recently been reported (41). Extensive chemical studies resulted in the elucidation of the structures of the leucomycins (282–292). The assignment of the R-configuration to C-9 in (48) (293–295) has made it necessary to revise the stereochemistry at C-9 in the spiramycins, midecamycins (SF-837), platenomycins (YL-704), and maridomycins (B-5050) as these compounds have all been shown to have the same basic aglycone as the leucomycins. The double bonds have been shown to have the *trans-trans* configuration and the solution conformation of the leucomycins has been deduced from cd and ^{1}H nmr studies (296). The cd studies suggest that the conformation of the 16-membered ring lactone, especially around the lactone region, is mobile and solvent dependent (296). There have been ^{13}C nmr studies on (48) and (50) (266). The biosynthesis of leucomycin A_3 is shown in Figure 1 (67) (297). The origin of C-3 and C-4 was not proved. A novel bicyclo lactone derivative prepared from leucomycin A_3 (48) by mild alkaline treatment has been reported (298,299). Deglycosylation of leucomycin A_3 (48) (300–301) and its derivatives (299), utilizing the Polonovsky reaction, has been studied. The preparation of acyl derivatives of the leucomycins has been reported (302–304). Deacylation of the 4″-acyl group may be effected with animal liver homogenate, or by means of microorganisms (305–306), but no microbial deacylation of C-3 has been observed. The 18-aldehyde function of (48) has been reduced to the primary alcohol (302,304) and also converted into the thiosemicarbazone, hydrazone, and bis-urea derivatives (302,304–305). Leucomycins modified in the mycaminose ring have been described (300,301,308), and a series of 17-halo derivatives of (48) have been prepared (309).

(38) $R_1 = COCH_3$, $R_2 = COCH_2CH(CH_3)_2$, $R_3R_4 = $ =O   carbomycin B
(39) $R_1 = H$, $R_2 = COCH_2CH(CH_3)_2$, $R_3R_4 = $ =O   niddamycin
(40) $R_1 = R_2 = COCH_2CH_3$, $R_3R_4 = $ =O   midecamycin A_3
(41) $R_1 = COCH_2CH_3$, $R_2 = COCH_2CH_2CH_3$, $R_3R_4 = $ =O   midecamycin A_4
(42) $R_1 = COCH_2CH_3$, $R_2 = COCH_2CH(CH_3)_2$, $R_3R_4 = $ =O   platenomycin W_1
(43) $R_1 = COCH_2CH_2CH_3$, $R_2 = COCH_2CH(CH_3)_2$, $R_3R_4 = $ =O   platenomycin W_2

(44) $R_1 = R_2 = R_4 = H$, $R_3 = (CH_3)_2N$ spiramycin I

forosamine

(45) $R_1 = COCH_3$, $R_2 = R_4 = H$, $R_3 = $ forosamine—O—   spiramycin II
(46) $R_1 = COCH_2CH_3$, $R_2 = R_4 = H$, $R_3 = $ forosamine—O—   spiramycin III
(47) $R_1 = R_4 = H$, $R_2 = COCH_2CH(CH_3)_2$, $R_3 = OH$ leucomycin A_1
(48) $R_1 = COCH_3$, $R_2 = COCH_2CH(CH_3)_2$, $R_3 = OH$, $R_4 = H$ leucomycin A_3
(49) $R_1 = COCH_3$, $R_2 = COCH_2CH_2CH_3$, $R_3 = OH$, $R_4 = H$ leucomycin A_4
(50) $R_1 = R_4 = H$, $R_2 = COCH_2CH_2CH_3$, $R_3 = OH$ leucomycin A_5
(51) $R_1 = COCH_3$, $R_2 = COCH_2CH_3$, $R_3 = OH$, $R_4 = H$ leucomycin A_6
(52) $R_1 = R_4 = H$, $R_2 = COCH_2CH_3$, $R_3 = OH$ leucomycin A_7
(53) $R_1 = R_2 = COCH_3$, $R_3 = OH$, $R_4 = H$ leucomycin A_8
(54) $R_1 = R_4 = H$, $R_2 = COCH_3$, $R_3 = OH$ leucomycin A_9
(55) $R_1 = COCH_3$, $R_2 = R_4 = H$, $R_3 = OH$ leucomycin U
(56) $R_1 = R_2 = R_4 = H$, $R_3 = OH$ leucomycin V
(57) $R_1 = R_2 = COCH_2CH_3$, $R_3 = OH$, $R_4 = H$ midecamycin
(58) $R_1 = COCH_2CH_3$, $R_2 = COCH_2CH_2CH_3$, $R_3 = OH$, $R_4 = H$ midecamycin A_2
(59) $R_1 = COCH_2CH_3$, $R_2 = R_4 = H$, $R_3 = OH$ midecamycin metabolite M_1
(60) $R_1 = COCH_2CH_3$, $R_2 = COCH(CH_3)_2$, $R_3 = OH$, $R_4 = H$ espinomycin A_3
(61) $R_1 = COCH_2CH_3$, $R_2 = COCH_3$, $R_3 = OH$, $R_4 = H$ espinomycin A_3
(62) $R_1 = COCH_2CH_2CH_3$, $R_2 = COCH_2CH(CH_3)_2$, $R_3 = OH$, $R_4 = H$ platenomycin A_0
(63) $R_1 = COCH_2CH_3$, $R_2 = COCH_2CH(CH_3)_2$, $R_3 = OH$, $R_4 = H$ platenomycin A_1

Streptomyces mycarofaciens produces two distinct groups of macrolides, namely midecamycin (SF-837, espinomycin A_1, YL-704 B_1, platenomycin B_1) (57), and midecamycin A_2 (SF-837 A_2) (58) of the leucomycin type, and midecamycins A_3 (SF-837 A_3) (40), and A_4 (SF-837 A_4) (41) of the carbomycin B (38) type (36,310–312). A variety of acyl derivatives of the midecamycins have been prepared (303,313–316) and 9-*O*-methylmidecamycin (317), as well as allylic rearrangement products from (57) and (58) (318) have been described. Two metabolites of midecamycin (57) namely M_1 (59) and M_2 (14-hydroxy analogue of (59) have been isolated and their structures have been determined (319).

Espinomycin A_1 (midecamycin, SF-837, YL-704 B_1, platenomycin B_1) (57), A_2 (60), and A_3 (YL-704 C_2, platenomycin C_2) (61) produced by *Streptomyces fungi-cidicus espinomyceticus* (320), are members of the leucomycin group. *Streptomyces*

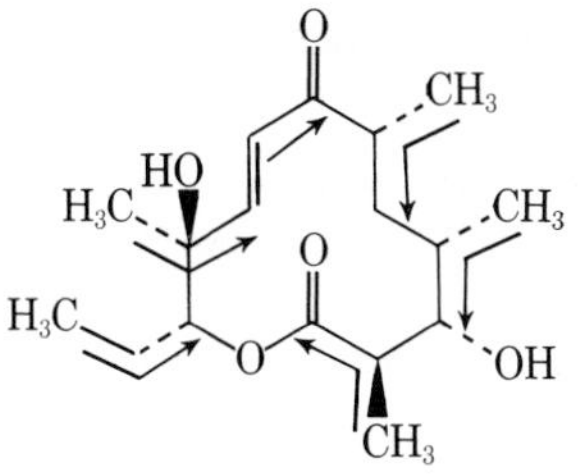

(64)
Methynolide

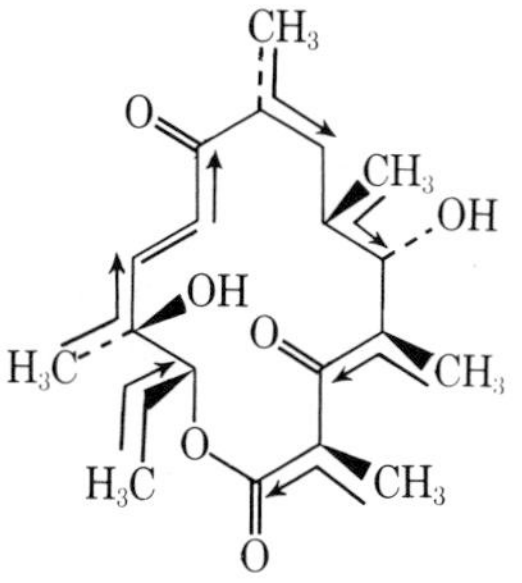

(65)
Picronolide

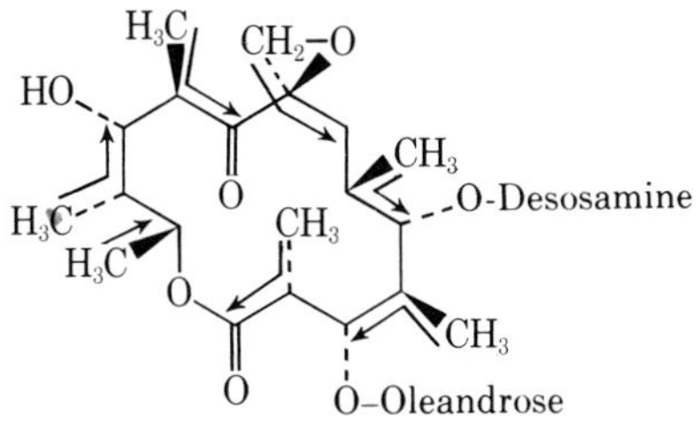

(66)
Oleandomycin

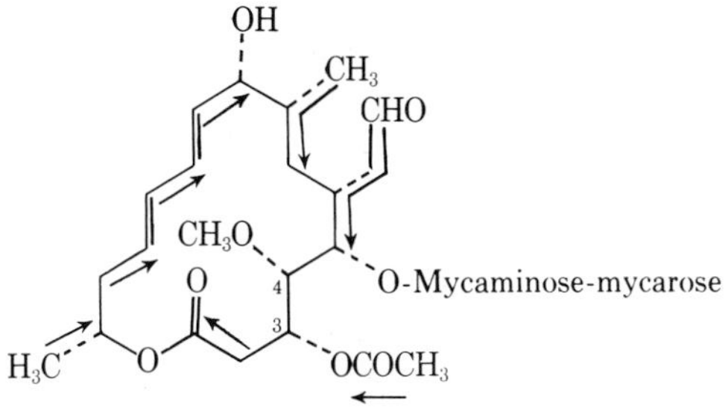

(67)
Leucomycin A₃

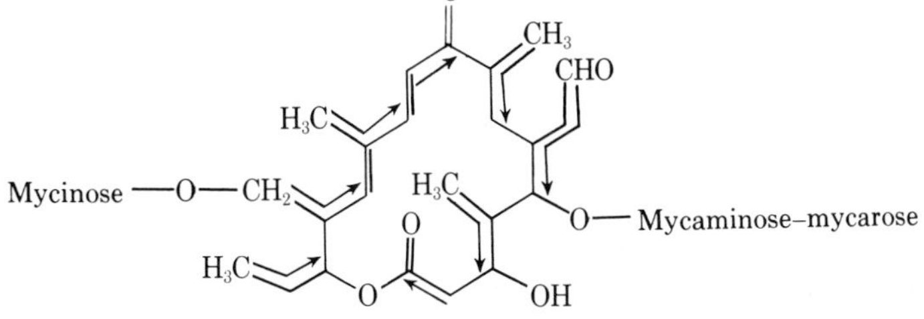

(68)
Tylosin

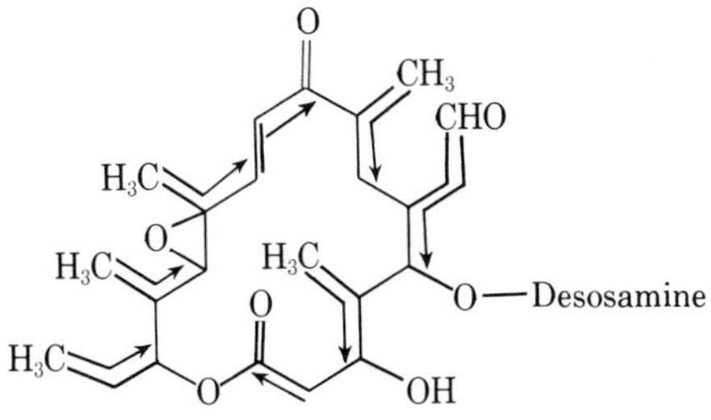

(69)
Rosamicin

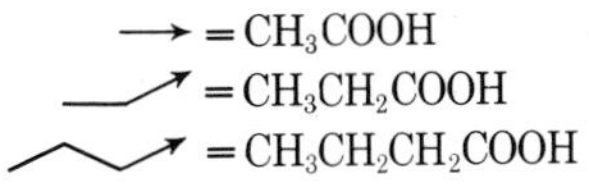

⟶ = CH₃COOH
↗ = CH₃CH₂COOH
↗ = CH₃CH₂CH₂COOH

Figure 1. Results of biosynthesis.

167

platensis produces macrolides of three structural types, namely platenomycin Ao (YL-704 Ao) (**62**), A$_1$ (YL-704 A$_1$) (**63**), A$_3$ (YL-704 A$_3$, josamycin, leucomycin A$_3$) (**48**), B$_1$ (YL-704 B$_1$, SF-837, midecamycin, espinomycin A$_1$) (**57**), B$_3$ (YL-704 B$_3$, leucomycin A$_6$) (**51**), and C$_2$ (YL-704 C$_2$, espinomycin A$_3$) (**61**) which are of the leucomycin type; platenomycin W$_1$ (YL-704 W$_1$) (**42**), and W$_2$ (YL-704 W$_2$) (**43**), which are of the carbomycin B type; and platenomycin C$_1$ (YL-704 C$_1$, maridomycin III, B-5050 C) (**33**), C$_3$ (YL-704 C$_3$, maridomycin I, B-5050 A) (**31**), and C$_4$ (YL-704 C$_4$, maridomycin II, B-5050 B) (**32**), which are of the maridomycin type (38,321–324). The absolute stereochemistry of the 12,13-epoxide has not been determined. Selective deacylation of the platenomycins using liver enzymes (325–326) and microbial acylation of the mycarose unit (327) have been reported. Blocked mutant strains of *Streptomyces platensis* have been used to study the biosynthesis of the platenomycins and it has been concluded that the mycaminose is attached to the aglycone, followed by the mycarose unit with the acylation of the latter as the final step in the biosynthesis (328–330).

The maridomycin complex produced by *Streptomyces hygroscopicus* no. B5050 has been shown to consist of maridomycin I (B-5050 A, YL-704 C$_3$, platenomycin C$_3$) (**31**), II (B-5050 B, YL-704 C$_4$, platenomycin C$_4$) (**32**), III (B-5050 C, YL-704 C$_1$, platenomycin C$_1$) (**33**), IV (B-5050 D) (**34**), V (B-5050 E) (**35**), VI (B-5050 F) (**36**), and G (B-5050 G) (**37**), the structures of which have been elucidated (264,331–335). Recent ^{1}H nmr, cd and x-ray crystallographic studies (264) on 9-propionylmaridomycin III have established the full absolute stereochemistry of these and many related macrolides. Microbial deacylation of the 4″-position and microbial reduction of the 18-aldehyde function of the maridomycins have been reported (336–340). Additional microbial transformation products (341) have been isolated, including 3‴-hydroxylated derivatives [(**31**) where R$_2$ = COCH$_2$C(OH)(CH$_3$)$_2$] (342). A number of ^{14}C-labeled precursors have been incorporated into maridomycin (343) and a variety of acyl derivatives have been prepared (344).

Tylosin (**70**), produced by *Streptomyces fradiae* has a different aglycone to the leucomycins and contains the neutral sugar D-mycinose (88–92). The biosynthesis of tylosin is shown in Figure 1 (**68**) (345). The gradual conversion of tylosin (**70**) into relomycin (**71**) (LL-AM 684β) by the producing strain has been demonstrated (346,347). Angolamycin (shincomycin A, PA 148) (**72**) elaborated by *Streptomyces eurythermus*, has a novel disaccharide unit containing D-angolosamine (56,348–349).

The cirramycin complex produced by *Streptomyces cirratus* has been separated into a number of components, namely cirramycin A$_1$ (**73**), A$_2$, A$_3$, A$_4$, A$_5$, B$_1$ (acumycin, B-58941) (**74**), B$_2$ and B$_3$ (350–352). The structure (**73**) has been determined (353) and the preparation of the desepoxy derivative, as well as a number of acyl derivatives, has been described (354). A closely related antibiotic B-58941 (cirramycin B$_1$, acumycin) (**74**) produced by *Streptomyces fradiae* var. *acinicolor* nov. var. B-58941 (58,355–358) has been converted to (**73**) by mild acidic hydrolysis (356). Cirramycin B$_1$ has also been converted to (**73**) by incubation with cane molasses (352). The neutral ketose, L-cinerulose has previously been found to occur in the anthracycline antibiotic cinerubin A (**59**) (Table 2). Acumycin which is produced by *Streptomyces griseoflavus* is thought to be identical to cirramycin B$_1$ and B-58941 (359). *Micromonospora rosaria* has been found to produce rosamicin (67-694, juvenimicin A$_3$, M-4365 A$_2$) (**75**), which has the same aglycone as cirramycin A$_1$ (**73**), and B-58941 (**74**), but has D-desosamine as the aminosugar component (360,361) (Table 2). The biosynthesis of rosamicin (**75**) is as shown in Figure 1, (69) (362). The juvenimicins (T-1124, jubenimycin) produced by *Micromonospora chalcea* var. *izumensis* consist of eight components, juvenimicin A_1, A_2 (76), A_3 (rosamicin, M-4365 A_2) (75), A_4 (77), B_1 M-4365 G_3) (79), B_2, B_3 (80), and B_4 (363–366). *Micromonospora capillata* sp. nov. (MCRL 0940) has been shown to produce the closely related antibiotics, M-4365 A_1 (78), A_2 (rosamicin, juvenimicin A_3) (75), A_3 (juvenimicin A_4) (77), G_1 (81), G_2 (82), and G_3 (juvenimicin B_1) (79) (367,368). The conversion of (78) into (81) has been reported (369).

The structures of several neutral 16-membered ring macrolides have been elucidated. Chalcomycin (aldgamycin D, mikonomycin) (83) produced by *Streptomyces bikiniensis* contains two neutral sugars, D-chalcose, and D-mycinose (Table 2), and has two *trans* double bonds in the aglycone (370–374). Both C-4 and C-6 have been shown to have the S-stereochemistry (373) and the x-ray crystallographic properties of (83) have been described (374). Neutramycin (84) from *Streptomyces rimosus* has a similar structure, but lacks the 6-methyl group (375–377). The aldgamycins produced by *Streptomyces lavendulae* (378) have been separated and aldgamycin E has been shown to have the partial structure (86) (379), while aldgamycin F (85) has the same aglycone as (83) (380). Mass spectral studies on the aldgamycins have been reported (381).

Activity

The macrolide antibiotics are considered to be medium or narrow spectrum antibiotics. Some possess activity against a wide range of gram-positive bacteria, but have only limited activity against gram-negative bacteria. Macrolides have also been shown to be active against *Rickettsia* strains, spirochetes, large viruses, protozoa, amoebae, schistosomes, and mycoplasma (11,30,257). Erythronolide B (13) has no antibacterial activity, but exhibits hypocholesterolemic activity as well as activity against schistosomes (150–151). With macrolide antibiotics there is often a considerable variation between the inhibitory concentrations measured *in vitro* and those observed *in vivo*. In general it has been observed that many macrolide-resistant clinical isolates of bacteria exhibit cross-resistance to other macrolides. Many are also resistant to lincomycin and chloramphenicol. Some macrolide-resistant mutant strains, however, are sensitive to other macrolides and most are sensitive to other classes of antibiotics (22,382–385). Clinical strains of *Staphylococcus aureus* show two types of resistance to macrolide antibiotics, namely induced and constitutive resistance (19,25,26,386–390). Several 14-membered macrolides such as (4), (8), (19), and (23) have been shown to be potent inducers of resistance in strains exposed to subinhibitory concentrations of the above macrolides. The strains then show resistance to all macrolides. No induction of resistance has been shown to occur with the 16-membered macrolides such as (27), (44), (47), and (48). The strains exhibiting constitutive resistance show a high degree of resistance to all macrolide antibiotics.

The mode of action of macrolide antibiotics has been shown to involve inhibition of protein synthesis (391) due to binding of the antibiotic to the 50S subunit of the ribosomes of the bacteria (23,392–394), although the specific step in the protein synthesis that is affected has not yet been identified. The effect of macrolides on metabolic processes other than protein synthesis has not been studied in detail and consequently inhibition of protein synthesis may not be the only mechanism by which these antibiotics inhibit bacterial growth. The ribosomal binding of a number of macrolides and

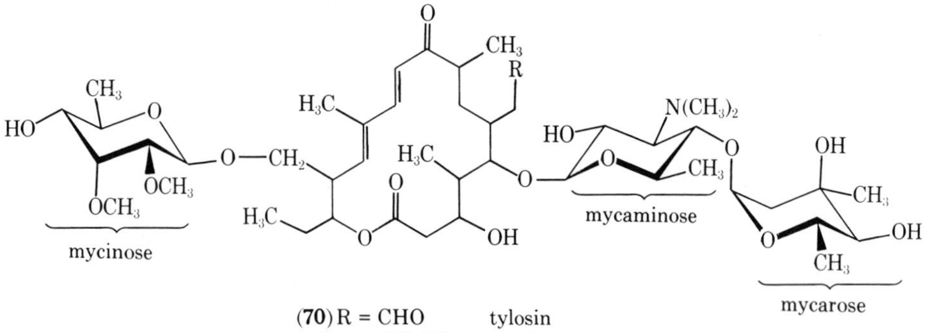
mycinose
mycaminose
mycarose

(**70**) R = CHO tylosin
(**71**) R = CH_2OH relomycin

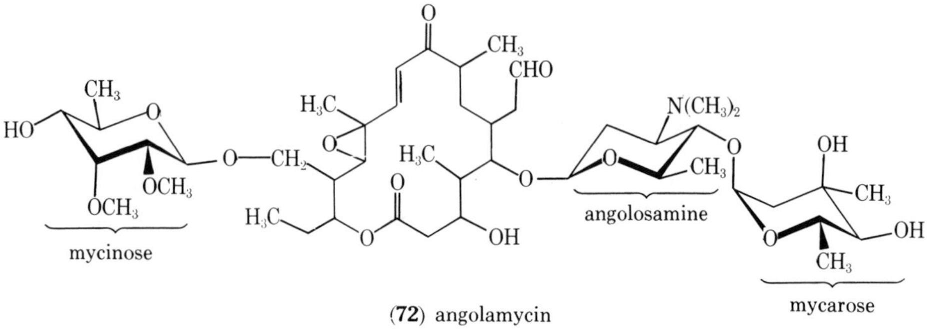
mycinose
angolosamine
mycarose

(**72**) angolamycin

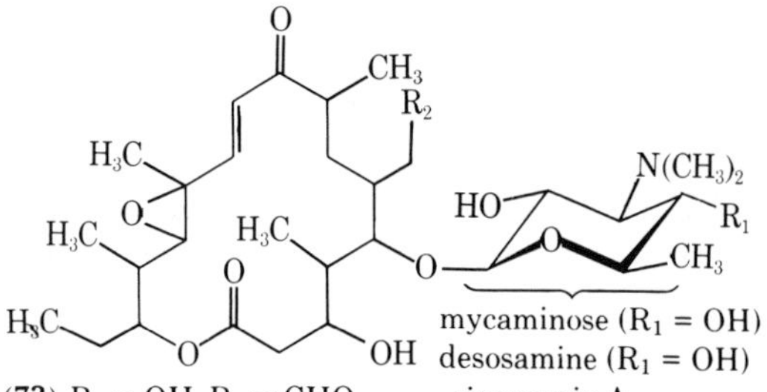
mycaminose (R_1 = OH)
desosamine (R_1 = OH)

(**73**) R_1 = OH, R_2 = CHO cirramycin A_1

(**74**) R_1 =

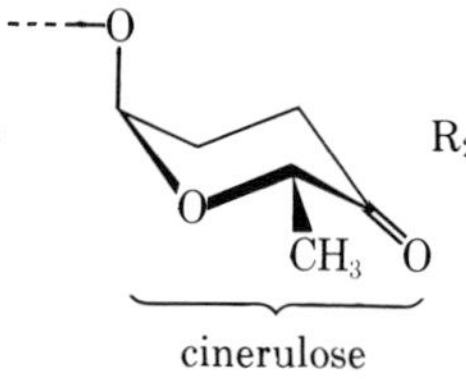
cinerulose

R_2 = CHO cirramycin B_1

(**75**) R_1 = H, R_2 = CHO rosamicin
(**76**) R_1 = R_2 = H juvenimicin A_2
(**77**) R_1 = H, R = CH_2OH juvenimicin A_4
(**78**) R_1 = H, R_2 = Ch_3 antibiotic M-4365 A_1

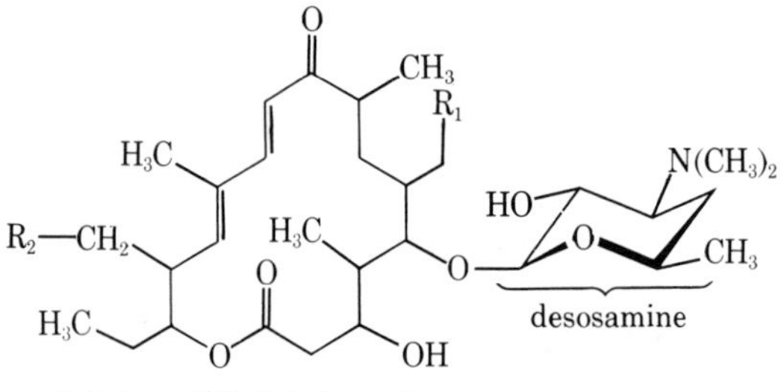
desosamine

(**79**) R_1 = CH_2OH, R_2 = H juvenimicin B_1
(**80**) R_1 = CH_2OH, R_2 = OH juvenimicin B_3
(**81**) R_1 = CH_3, R_2 = H antibiotic M-4365 G_1
(**82**) R_1 = CHO, R_2 = H antibiotic M-4365 G_2

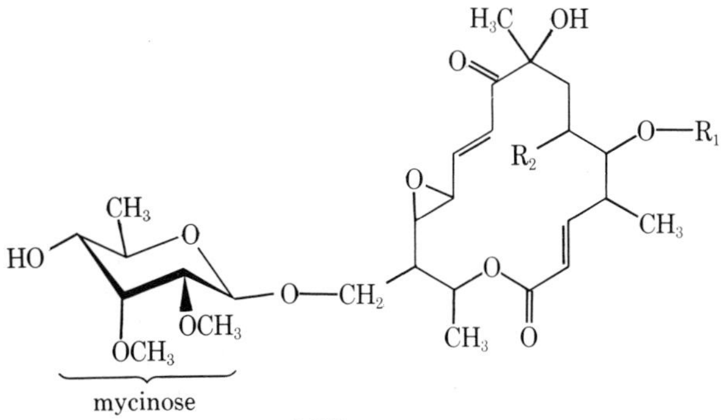

(83) R₁ = ... chalcose, R₂ = CH₃   chalcomycin

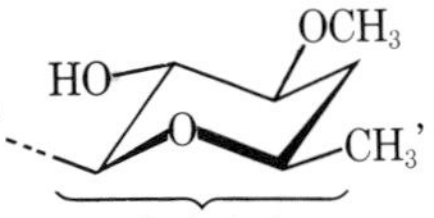

mycinose

chalcose

(84) R₁ = chalcose, R₂ = H   neutramycin

(85) R₁ = ... , R₂ = CH₃   aldgamycin F

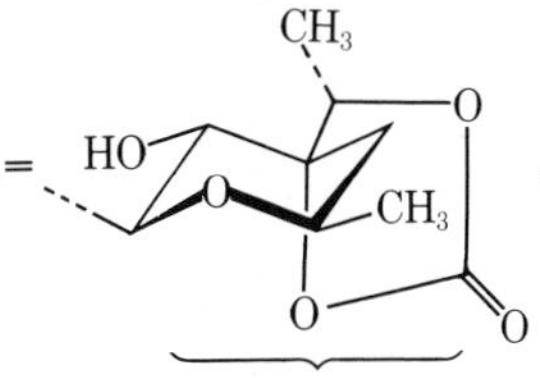

aldgarose

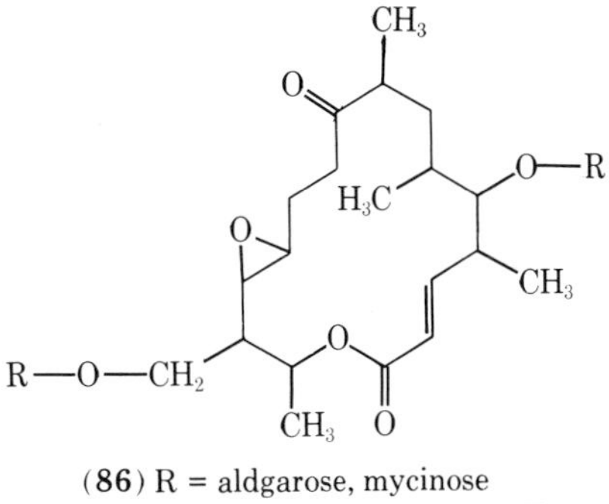

(86) R = aldgarose, mycinose
partial structure of aldgamycin E

various erythromycin derivatives has been studied and it has been demonstrated that macrolides having high antibacterial activities always have high ribosome-binding abilities, whereas, high binding activity does not necessarily correspond to high antibacterial activity (394–396).

A number of macrolide antibiotics have been used extensively in human medicine. Especially notable are erythromycin, oleandomycin, kitasamycin, and josamycin. Those marketed in the United States are shown in Table 3.

Tylosin has been used to treat mycoplasma in animals, as an animal feed supplement, and in the preservation of food. The major clinical use of the macrolides is against group A beta–hemolytic streptococcal infections as well as staphylococcal and pneumonococcal infections. Erythromycin has also been used to treat diphtheria,

Table 3.   Macrolide Antibiotics Marketed In The United States

Macrolide	Derivative	Trade name	Manufacturer
erythromycin[a]		Erythrocin	Abbott Laboratories
		E-Mycin	The UpJohn Company
			McKesson Laboratories (Div. of Foremost-McKesson, Inc.)
		Robimycin	A.H. Robins Company
		Ilotycin	Dista Products Company (Div. of Eli Lilly and Company)
	ethyl succinate[b]	Erythrocin Ethyl Succinate	Abbott Laboratories
	ethyl succinate[b]	Pediamycin	Ross Laboratories (Div. of Abbott Laboratories)
	lactobionate[b]	Erythrocin Lactobionate	Abbott Laboratories
	stearate[b]	Erythrocin Stearate	Abbott Laboratories
	stearate[b]	Bristamycin	Bristol Laboratories (Div. of Bristol-Myers Company)
	stearate[b]		Zenith Laboratories, Inc.
	stearate[b]	Ethril	E.R. Squibb and Sons
	stearate[b]	Erypar	Parke, Davis & Company (Div. of Warner Lambert Co.)
	stearate[b]	SK-Erythromycin	Smith, Kline and French Laboratories (Div. Smith Kline Corporation)
	stearate[b]	Pfizer-E	Pfipharmecs Div. (Pfizer, Inc.)
	stearate[b]		Wyeth Laboratories (Div. of American Home Product Corp.)
	estolate[b]	Ilosone	Dista Products Company (Div. of Eli Lilly and Co.)
	gluceptate[b]	Ilotycin Gluceptate	Dista Products Company (Div. of Eli Lilly and Co.)
oleandomycin[a]	triacetate[b]	TAO (Troleandomycin)	Roerig (Div. of Pfizer Pharmaceuticals)
tylosin[a,c]		Tylan	Elanco (Div. of Eli Lilly and Co.)

[a] Produced by fermentation.
[b] Produced by fermentation and chemical derivatization.
[c] Used exclusively for veterinary use.

erythrasma, and intestinal amebiasis (397). The toxicity of macrolide antibiotics is low (351). Serious adverse reactions are rare occurrences during macrolide therapy and are generally the result of patient hypersensitivity, the form of the drug used, or the use of unusually large doses of the drug (397). Higher blood levels and greater stability have been achieved by esterification of macrolides. Thus, erythromycin estolate (the lauryl sulfate salt of erythromycin 2′-propionate) is more stable and gives prolonged and higher blood levels than erythromycin. A very rare, but serious side effect produced by erythromycin estolate is cholestatic hepatitis (398). Other examples of esterified derivatives are triacetyl oleandomycin (399) and 9-propionylmaridomycin (400–401), both of which show enhanced biological properties relative to the parent antibiotics.

In view of the large number of structurally diverse naturally occurring macrolide antibiotics that are known, as well as their chemically modified derivatives, it is now possible to correlate some of the structural features governing biological activity (10–11,14,20,304,402–404). Future research on macrolide antibiotics will undoubtedly expand the structure-activity relationships and it is hoped that it will result in the synthesis of new clinically useful drugs.

BIBLIOGRAPHY

"Antibiotics" in *ECT* 1st ed., Vol. 2, pp. 7–37, by J. S. Kiser and H. B. Woodruff; "Antibiotics" in *ECT* 2nd ed., Vol. 2, pp. 533–540, by W. E. Brown, The Squibb Institute for Medical Research; "Macrolide Antibiotics" in *ECT* 2nd ed., Vol. 12, pp. 632–660, by Robert Morin and Marvin Gorman, Eli Lilly and Company.

1. H. Brockmann and W. Henkel, *Naturwissenschaften* **37,** 138 (1950).
2. R. B. Woodward, *Angew. Chem.* **69,** 50 (1957).
3. M. Berry, *Q. Rev.* **17,** 343 (1963).
4. H. Umezawa, *Recent Advances in Chemistry and Biochemistry of Antibiotics,* Microbial Chemistry Research Foundation, Tokyo, 1964, p. 44.
5. R. M. Evans, *The Chemistry of the Antibiotics Used in Medicine,* Pergammon Press, London, 1965, p. 135.
6. W. D. Celmer, in Z. Vanek and Z. Hostalek, eds., *Biogenesis of Antibiotic Substances,* Academic Press, New York, 1965, p. 99.
7. W. D. Celmer, *Antimicrob. Agents Chemother.* 144 (1966).
8. S. Masamune, G. S. Bates, and J. W. Corcoran, *Angew. Chem. Int. Ed. Engl.* **16,** 585 (1977).
9. W. D. Celmer, *Pure Appl. Chem.* **28,** 413 (1971).
10. T. J. Perun, in S. Mitsuhashi, ed., *Drug Action and Drug Resistance in Bacteria,* Vol. 1, *Macrolide Antibiotics and Lincomycin,* University Park Press, Tokyo, 1971, p. 123.
11. H. Toju and S. Omura, in S. Mitsuhashi, ed., *Drug Action and Drug Resistance in Bacteria,* Vol. 1, *Macrolide Antibiotics and Lincomycin,* University Park Press, Tokyo, 1971, p. 267.
12. K. L. Rinehart, Jr., and G. E. van Lear, in G. R. Waller, ed., *Antibiotics,* in *Biochemical Applications of Mass Spectrometry,* John Wiley & Sons, Inc., New York, 1972, p. 451.
13. W. Keller-Schierlein, *Progress in the Chemistry of Organic Natural Products,* Vol. 30, Springer-Verlag, Berl., 1973, p. 313.
14. S. Omura and A. Nakagawa, *J. Antibiot.* **28,** 401 (1975).
15. J. W. Corcoran, in Z. Vanek and Z. Hostalek, eds., *Biogenesis of Antibiotic Substances,* Academic Press, New York, 1965, p. 131.
16. H. Grisebach, *Beitr. Biochem. Physiol. Naturstoffen Fetschr.* 189 (1965).
17. J. W. Corcoran and M. Chick, in J. F. Snell, ed., *Biosynthesis of Antibiotics,* Vol. 1, Academic Press, New York, 1966, p. 159.
18. Z. Vanek and J. Majer, in D. Gottlieb and P. D. Shaw, eds., *Antibiotics,* Vol. 2, *Biosynthesis,* Springer-Verlag, New York, 1967, p. 154.
19. T. Osono and H. Umezawa, in S. Mitsuhashi, ed., *Drug Action and Drug Resistance in Bacteria,* Vol. 1, *Macrolide Antibiotics and Lincomycin,* University Park Press, Tokyo, 1971, p. 41.
20. K. Uzu and H. Takahira, in Ref. 19, p. 293.
21. H. Otaya, in ref. 19, p. 3.
22. S. Mitsuhashi and co-workers, ref. 19, p. 23.
23. J. W. Corcoran, ref. 19, p. 177.
24. K. Tanaka and co-workers, ref. 19, p. 201.
25. B. Weisblum, in ref. 19, p. 217.
26. T. Saito, M. Shimizu, and S. Mitsuhashi, ref. 19, p. 239.
27. D. Vazquez, in D. Gottlieb and P. D. Shaw, eds., *Antibiotics,* Vol. 1, *Mechanism of Action,* Springer-Verlag, New York, 1967, p. 366.
28. F. E. Hahn, in ref. 27, p. 378.
29. N. L. Oleinick, in J. W. Corcoran and F. E. Hahn, eds., *Antibiotics,* Vol. 3, *Mechanism of Action of Antimicrobial and Antitumor Agents,* Springer-Verlag, New York, 1975, p. 396.
30. D. Vazquez, in ref. 29, p. 459.
31. M. J. Weinstein and co-workers, *J. Antibiot.* **22,** 253 (1969).

32. J. M. McGuire and co-workers, *Antibiot. Chemother.* **2,** 281 (1952).
33. R. L. Sagner, F. A. Hochstein, and K. Murai, *J. Am. Chem. Soc.* **75,** 4684 (1953).
34. S. Pinnert-Sindico and co-workers, *Antibiot. Ann.* **2,** 274 (1954–1955).
35. T. Watanabe and co-workers, *Bull. Chem. Soc. Jpn.* **33,** 1104 (1960).
36. T. Tsuruoka and co-workers, *J. Antibiot.* **24,** 476 (1971).
37. Y. Sano, *J. Antibiot.* **7A,** 93 (1954).
38. A. Kinumaki and co-workers, *J. Antibiot.* **27,** 102 (1974).
39. J. Marquez and co-workers, *J. Antibiot.* **22,** 259 (1969).
40. T. Watanabe, *Bull. Chem. Soc. Jpn.* **33,** 1100 (1960).
41. S. Omura and co-workers, *J. Antibiot.* **26,** 794 (1973).
42. G. H. Wagman and M. J. Weinstein, *J. Chromatogr. Lib., Volume 1, Chromatography of Antibiotics,* Elsevier, New York, 1973.
43. M. N. Donin and co-workers, *Antibiotics Annual,* 179 (1953–1954).
44. C. Djerassi and J. A. Zderic, *J. Am. Chem. Soc.* **78,** 2907 (1956).
45. C. Djerassi, A. Bowers, and H. N. Khastgir, *J. Am. Chem. Soc.* **78,** 1729 (1956).
46. C. Djerassi and co-workers, *J. Am. Chem. Soc.* **78,** 1733 (1956).
47. C. Djerassi and J. A. Zderic, *J. Am. Chem. Soc.* **78,** 6390 (1956).
48. W. Keller-Schierlein and G. Roncari, *Helv. Chim. Acta* **45,** 138 (1962).
49. G. B. Howarth, W. A. Szarek, and J. K. N. Jones, *Chem. Comm.* 62 (1968).
50. G. B. Howarth, W. A. Szarek, and J. K. N. Jones, *Carbohydr. Res.* **7,** 284 (1968).
51. M. P. Kunstmann, L. A. Mitscher, and N. Bohonos, *Tetrahedron Lett.* 839 (1966).
52. G. A. Ellestad and co-workers, *Tetrahedron* **23,** 3893 (1967).
53. H. Paulsen and H. Redlich, *Angew. Chem.* **11,** 1021 (1972).
54. J. S. Brimacombe, C. W. Smith, and J. Minshall, *Tetrahedron Lett.* 2997 (1974).
55. J. S. Brimacombe, J. Minshall, and C. W. Smith, *J. Chem. Soc. Perkin I,* 682 (1975).
56. M. Brufani and W. Keller-Schierlein, *Helv. Chim. Acta* **49,** 1962 (1966).
57. B. T. Lawton and co-workers, *Can. J. Chem.* **47,** 2899 (1969).
58. T. Suzuki, N. Sugita, and M. Asai, *Chem. Lett.* 789 (1973).
59. W. Keller-Schierlein and W. Richle, *Antimicrob. Agents Chemother.* 68 (1970).
60. E. H. Flynn and co-workers, *J. Am. Chem. Soc.* **76,** 3121 (1954).
61. P. F. Wiley and O. Weaver, *J. Am. Chem. Soc.* **78,** 808 (1956).
62. W. Hofheinz, H. Grisebach, and H. Friebolin, *Tetrahedron* **18,** 1265 (1962).
63. D. M. Lemal, P. D. Pacht, and R. B. Woodward, *Tetrahedron* **18,** 1275 (1962).
64. R. K. Clark, Jr., *Antibiot. Chemother.* **3,** 663 (1953).
65. C. H. Bolton and co-workers, *J. Chem. Soc.* 4831 (1961).
66. C. H. Bolton and co-workers, *Chem. Ind. (London)* 1945 (1962).
67. A. B. Foster and co-workers, *Proc. Chem. Soc.* 279 (1963).
68. P. W. K. Woo and co-workers, *Tetrahedron Lett.* 735 (1962).
69. W. Hofheinz and H. Grisebach, *Tetrahedron Lett.* 377 (1962).
70. F. Korte, A. Bilow, and R. Heinz, *Tetrahedron* **18,** 657 (1962).
71. H. Newman, *Chem. Ind. (London),* 372 (1963).
72. A. C. Richardson, *Proc. Chem. Soc.* 131 (1963).
73. R. Paul and S. Tchelitcheff, *Bull. Soc. Chim. France* 734 (1957).
74. C. L. Stevens and co-workers, *Tetrahedron Lett.* 5717 (1966).
75. E. L. Albano and D. Horton, *Carbohydr. Res.* **11,** 485 (1969).
76. P. P. Regna and co-workers, *J. Am. Chem. Soc.* **75,** 4625 (1953).
77. R. L. Wagner and co-workers, *J. Am. Chem. Soc.* **75,** 4684 (1953).
78. M. E. Kuehne and B. W. Benson, *J. Am. Chem. Soc.* **87,** 4660 (1965).
79. T. T. Thang and co-workers, *J. Am. Chem. Soc.* **100,** 663 (1978).
80. A. K. Mallams, *J. Am. Chem. Soc.* **91,** 7505 (1969).
81. A. K. Mallams, *J. Chem. Soc. Perkin I,* 1369 (1973).
82. F. A. Hochstein and P. P. Regna, *J. Am. Chem. Soc.* **77,** 3353 (1955).
83. W. Hofheinz and H. Grisebach, *Z. Naturforsch.* **17b,** 355 (1962).
84. A. B. Foster and co-workers, *J. Chem. Soc.* 2116 (1962).
85. A. C. Richardson, *J. Chem. Soc.* 2758 (1962).
86. S. Yasuda and T. Matsumoto, *Tetrahedron Lett.* 4397 (1969).
87. A. B. Foster and co-workers, *Proc. Chem. Soc.* 254 (1962).
88. J. M. McGuire and co-workers, *Antibiot. Chemother.* **11,** 320 (1961).
89. R. L. Hamill and co-workers, *Antibiot. Chemother.* **11,** 328 (1961).

90. R. B. Morin and M. Gorman, *Tetrahedron Lett.* 2339 (1964).
91. H. W. Dion, P. W. K. Woo, and Q. R. Bartz, *J. Am. Chem. Soc.* **84,** 880 (1962).
92. R. B. Morin and co-workers, *Tetrahedron Lett.* 4737 (1970).
93. J. S. Brimacombe, M. Stacey, and L. C. N. Tucker, *J. Chem. Soc.* 5391 (1964).
94. J. S. Brimacombe, O. A. Ching, and M. Stacey, *J. Chem. Soc.* (C) 197 (1969).
95. H. Els, W. D. Celmer, and K. Murai, *J. Am. Chem. Soc.* **80,** 3777 (1958).
96. W. Neumann, *Ber.* **70,** 1547 (1937).
97. E. Vischer and T. Reichstein, *Helv. Chim. Acta* **27,** 1332 (1944).
98. F. Blindenbacher and T. Reichstein, *Helv. Chim. Acta* **31,** 2061 (1948).
99. S. Yasuda and T. Matsumoto, *Tetrahedron Lett.* 4393 (1969).
100. C. Djerassi and O. Halpern, *J. Am. Chem. Soc.* **79,** 3926 (1957).
101. C. Djerassi and co-workers, *Tetrahedron* **4,** 369 (1958).
102. L. D. Bergelson and S. G. Batrekov, *Bull. Acad. Sci. USSR Div. Chem. Sci.* 1982 (1966).
103. R. W. Rickards and R. M. Smith, *Tetrahedron Lett.* 1025 (1970).
104. D. G. Manwaring, R. W. Rickards, and R. M. Smith, *Tetrahedron Lett.* 1029 (1970).
105. A. J. Birch and co-workers, *Chem. and Ind.* (*London*), 1245 (1960).
106. A. J. Birch and co-workers, *J. Chem. Soc.* 5274 (1964).
107. C. Djerassi and O. Halpern, *J. Am. Chem. Soc.* **79,** 2022 (1957).
108. C. Djerassi and O. Halpern, *Tetrahedron* **3,** 255 (1958).
109. L. D. Bergelson and A. N. Grigoryan, *Izv. Akad. Nauk SSSR, Ser. Khim.* 282 (1966).
110. A. Kinumaki and M. Suzuki, *Chem. Comm.* 744 (1972).
111. P. F. Wiley and O. Weaver, *J. Am. Chem. Soc.* **77,** 3422 (1955).
112. P. F. Wiley and co-workers, *J. Am. Chem. Soc.* **77,** 3676 (1955).
113. P. F. Wiley and co-workers, *J. Am. Chem. Soc.* **77,** 3677 (1955).
114. M. V. Sigal, Jr. and co-workers, *J. Am. Chem. Soc.* **78,** 388 (1956).
115. K. Gerzon and co-workers, *J. Am. Chem. Soc.* **78,** 6396 (1956).
116. W. Hofheinz and H. Grisebach, *Chem. Ber.* **96,** 2867 (1963).
117. P. F. Wiley and co-workers, *J. Am. Chem. Soc.* **79,** 6062 (1957).
118. D. R. Harris, S. G. McGeachin, and H. H. Mills, *Tetrahedron Lett.* 679 (1965).
119. C. W. Pettinga, W. M. Stark, and F. R. van Abeele, *J. Am. Chem. Soc.* **76,** 570 (1954).
120. K. Gerzon and co-workers, *J. Am. Chem. Soc.* **78,** 6412 (1956).
121. P. F. Wiley and co-workers, *J. Am. Chem. Soc.* **79,** 6070 (1957).
122. P. F. Wiley and co-workers, *J. Am. Chem. Soc.* **79,** 6074 (1957).
123. J. Majer, J. R. Martin, and J. W. Corcoran, *14th Interscience Conference on Antimicrobial Agents and Chemotherapy,* San Francisco, California, Sept. 1974, Paper 200.
124. J. Majer and co-workers, *J. Am. Chem. Soc.* **99,** 1620 (1977).
125. V. C. Stephens and J. W. Conine, *Antibiot. Ann.* 346 (1958–1959).
126. A. Banaszek, J. St. Pyrek, and A. Zamojski, *Rocz. Chem.* **43,** 763 (1969).
127. P. L. Tardrew, J. C. H. Mao, and D. Kenney, *Appl. Microbiol.* **18,** 159 (1969).
128. P. H. Jones and co-workers, *J. Med. Chem.* **15,** 631 (1972).
129. Y. C. Martin and co-workers, *J. Med. Chem.* **15,** 635 (1972).
130. U.S. Pat. 3,884,902 (May 20, 1975), R. Hallas, J. R. Martin, and J. S. Tadamier (to Abbott Laboratories).
131. Ger. Pat. 2,330,361 (Jan. 3, 1974), J. S. Tadanier and J. R. Martin (to Abbott Laboratories).
132. U.S. Pat. 3,361,738 (Jan. 2, 1968), P. H. Jones and E. A. Rowley (to Abbott Laboratories).
133. U.S. Pat. 3,478,013 (Nov. 11, 1969), P. H. Jones and E. A. Rowley (to Abbott Laboratories).
134. A. A. Sinkula, *J. Pharm. Sci.* **63,** 842 (1974).
135. U.S. Pat. 3,558,594 (Jan. 26, 1971), P. H. Jones, R. G. Weigand, and H. C. Chun (to Abbott Laboratories).
136. U.S. Pat. 3,842,069 (Oct. 15, 1974), P. H. Jones and co-workers (to Abbott Laboratories).
137. U.S. Pat. 3,884,903 (May 20, 1975), P. H. Jones and co-workers (to Abbott Laboratories).
138. E. H. Flynn, H. W. Murphy, and R. E. McMahon, *J. Am. Chem. Soc.* **77,** 3104 (1955).
139. U.S. Pat. 3,681,325 (Aug. 1, 1972), L. A. Frieberg (to Abbott Laboratories).
140. P. H. Jones and E. K. Rowley, *J. Org. Chem.* **33,** 665 (1968).
141. U.S. Pat. 3,598,805 (Aug. 10, 1971), P. H. Jones (to Abbott Laboratories).
142. U.S. Pat. 3,629,232 (Dec. 21, 1971), P. H. Jones (to Abbott Laboratories).
143. U.S. Pat. 3,417,077 (Dec. 17, 1968), H. W. Murphy, V. C. Stephens, and J. W. Conine (to Eli Lilly and Co.).
144. H. Bojarska-Dahlig and W. Slawinski, *Rocz. Chem.* **46,** 2211 (1972).

145. W. Slawinski and co-workers, *Recueil* **94**, 236 (1975).
146. A. Hempel and co-workers, *Tetrahedron Lett.* 1599 (1975).
147. H. Bojarska-Dahlig and co-workers, *J. Antibiot.* **29**, 907 (1976).
148. U.S. Pat. 3,701,770 (Oct. 31, 1972), P. H. Jones and K. S. Iyer (to Abbott Laboratories).
149. U.S. Pat. 3,366,647 (Jan. 30, 1968), T. J. Perun (to Abbott Laboratories).
150. U.S. Pat. 3,357,999 (Dec. 12, 1967), T. J. Perun (to Abbott Laboratories).
151. T. J. Perun, *J. Org. Chem.* **32**, 2324 (1967).
152. J. Tadanier and co-workers, *J. Am. Chem. Soc.* **95**, 592 (1973).
153. J. Tadanier and co-workers, *J. Am. Chem. Soc.* **95**, 593 (1973).
154. P. Kurath and co-workers, *Experientia* **27**, 362 (1971).
155. P. Kurath and R. S. Egan, *Helv. Chim. Acta.* **54**, 523 (1971).
156. P. Kurath and co-workers, *Helv. Chim. Acta* **56**, 1557 (1973).
157. J. Tadanier and co-workers, *Helv. Chim. Acta* **56**, 2711 (1973).
158. H. Bojarska-Dahlig, I. Dziegielewska, and T. Glabski, *Recueil* **92**, 1305 (1973).
159. K. Krowicki and A. Zamojski, *J. Antibiot.* **26**, 569, 575, 582, 587 (1973).
160. K. Krowicki, *J. Antibiot.* **27**, 626 (1974).
161. H. Bojarska-Dahlig, T. Glabski, and I. Dziegielewska, *Rocz. Chem.* **48**, 155 (1974).
162. J. Tadanier and co-workers, *J. Org. Chem.* **39**, 2495 (1974).
163. R. A. Le Mahieu, J. F. Blount, and R. W. Kierstead, *J. Antibiot.* **28**, 705 (1975).
164. S. Djokic and Z. Tamburasev, *Tetrahedron Lett.* 1645 (1967).
165. E. H. Massey and co-workers, *Tetrahedron Lett.* 157 (1970).
166. U.S. Pat. 3,869,444 (Mar. 4, 1975), L. A. Freiberg (to Abbott Laboratories).
167. U.S. Pat. 3,681,326 (Aug. 1, 1972), A. M. Von Esch (to Abbott Laboratories).
168. U.S. Pat. 3,869,445 (Mar. 4, 1975), R. Hallas, J. S. Tadanier, and A. M. Von Esch (to Abbott Laboratories).
169. G. H. Timms and E. Wildsmith, *Tetrahedron Lett.* 195 (1971).
170. E. Wildsmith, *Tetrahedron Lett.* 29 (1972).
171. R. Ryden and co-workers, *J. Med. Chem.* **16**, 1059 (1973).
172. A. F. Cockerill and co-workers, *J. Chem. Soc., Perkin Trans. 2* 173 (1973).
173. R. S. Egan, L. A. Freiberg, and W. H. Washburn, *J. Org. Chem.* **39**, 2492 (1974).
174. R. A. Le Mahieu and co-workers, *J. Med. Chem.* **17**, 953 (1974).
175. R. A. Le Mahieu, M. Carson, and R. W. Kierstead, *J. Antibiot.* **28**, 704 (1975).
176. R. A. Le Mahieu and co-workers, *J. Med. Chem.* **18**, 849 (1975).
177. R. S. Jaret, A. K. Mallams, and H. F. Vernay, *J. Chem. Soc. Perkin Trans. 1* 1389 (1973).
178. L. A. Mitscher, R. L. Foltz, and M. I. Levenberg, *Org. Mass Spectrom.* **5**, 1229 (1971).
179. L. A. Mitscher, H. D. H. Showalter, and R. L. Foltz, *Chem. Comm.* 796 (1972).
180. K. L. Rinehart, Jr. and co-workers, *J. Antibiot.* **27**, 1 (1974).
181. P. V. Demarco, *Tetrahedron Lett.* 383 (1969).
182. P. V. Demarco, *J. Antibiot.* **22**, 327 (1969).
183. T. J. Perun and R. S. Egan, *Tetrahedron Lett.* 387 (1969).
184. T. J. Perun, R. S. Egan, and J. R. Martin, *Tetrahedron Lett.* 4501 (1969).
185. L. A. Mitscher and co-workers, *Tetrahedron Lett.* 4505 (1969).
186. T. J. Perun and co-workers, *Antimicrob. Agents Chemother.* 111 (1970).
187. J. R. Martin, T. J. Perun, and R. S. Egan, *Tetrahedron* **28**, 2937 (1972).
188. R. S. Egan and co-workers, *Tetrahedron* **29**, 2525 (1973).
189. R. S. Egan and co-workers, *J. Am. Chem. Soc.* **97**, 4578 (1975).
190. J. G. Nourse and J. D. Roberts, *J. Am. Chem. Soc.* **97**, 4584 (1975).
191. Y. Terui and co-workers, *Tetrahedron Lett.* 2583 (1975).
192. S. Omura and co-workers, *Tetrahedron Lett.* 2939 (1975).
193. T. Kaneda and co-workers, *J. Biol. Chem.* **237**, 322 (1962).
194. S. M. Friedman, T. Kaneda, and J. W. Corcoran, *J. Biol. Chem.* **239**, 2386 (1964).
195. J. Majer and co-workers, *Chem. Ind.* (*London*) 669 (1961).
196. J. W. Corcoran, *J. Biol. Chem.* **236**, PC 27 (1961).
197. U.S. Pat. 3,684,794 (Aug. 15, 1972), J. R. Martin (to Abbott Laboratories).
198. J. R. Martin and co-workers, *Tetrahedron* **29**, 935 (1973).
199. J. R. Martin and W. Rosenbrook, *Biochemistry* **6**, 435 (1967).
200. J. R. Martin, T. J. Perun, and R. L. Girolami, *Biochemistry* **5**, 2852 (1966).
201. R. A. Le Mahieu and co-workers, *J. Antibiot.* **29**, 728 (1976).
202. J. R. Martin and T. J. Perun, *Biochemistry* **7**, 1728 (1968).

203. J. R. Martin and R. S. Egan, *Biochemistry* **9**, 3439 (1970).
204. J. R. Martin and co-workers, *Tetrahedron* **31**, 1985 (1975).
205. A. K. Mallams, R. S. Jaret, and H. Reimann, *J. Am. Chem. Soc.* **91**, 7506 (1969).
206. R. S. Jaret, A. K. Mallams, and H. Reimann, *J. Chem. Soc., Perkin Trans. 1* 1374 (1973).
207. U.S. Pat. 3,883,507 (May 13, 1975), H. Reimann and R. S. Jaret (to Schering Corporation).
208. U.S. Pat. 3,669,953 (June 13, 1972), A. K. Mallams (to Schering Corporation).
209. U.S. Pat. 3,669,952 (June 13, 1972), A. K. Mallams (to Schering Corporation).
210. U.S. Pat. 3,634,393 (Jan. 11, 1972), S. Motola (to Schering Corporation).
211. I. Kawamoto and co-workers, *J. Antibiot.* **27**, 493 (1974).
212. R. S. Egan and co-workers, *J. Antibiot.* **27**, 544 (1974).
213. H. Brockmann and W. Henkel, *Chem. Ber.* **84**, 284 (1951).
214. H. Brockmann, H. Genth, and R. Strufe, *Chem. Ber.* **85**, 426 (1952).
215. H. Brockmann and R. Strufe, *Chem. Ber.* **86**, 876 (1953).
216. H. Brockmann, H. B. Konig, and R. Oster, *Chem. Ber.* **87**, 856 (1954).
217. H. Brockmann and R. Oster, *Chem. Ber.* **90**, 605 (1957).
218. R. Anliker and K. Gubler, *Helv. Chim. Acta* **40**, 119 (1957).
219. *Ibid.,* 1768 (1957).
220. H. Muxfeldt and co-workers, *J. Am. Chem. Soc.* **90**, 4748 (1968).
221. R. E. Hughes and co-workers, *J. Am. Chem. Soc.* **92**, 5267 (1970).
222. C. Tsai, J. J. Stezowski, and R. E. Hughes, *J. Am. Chem. Soc.* **93**, 7286 (1971).
223. H. Ogura, K. Furuhata, and H. Kuwano, *Tetrahedron Letters,* 4715 (1971).
224. H. Ogura and co-workers, *J. Am. Chem. Soc.* **97**, 1930 (1975).
225. S. Omura and co-workers, *J. Antibiot.* **29**, 316 (1976).
226. I. Maezawa, A. Kinumaki, and M. Suzuki, *J. Antibiot.* **27**, 84 (1974).
227. J. Majer and co-workers, *J. Antibiot.* **29**, 769 (1976).
228. H. Ogura and co-workers, *Chem. Pharm. Bull. (Tokyo)* **15**, 682 (1967).
229. R. Corbaz and co-workers, *Helv. Chim. Acta* **38**, 935 (1955).
230. R. Anliker and co-workers, *Helv. Chim. Acta* **39**, 1785 (1956).
231. V. Prelog and co-workers, *Helv. Chim. Acta* **45**, 4 (1962).
232. T. Hori and co-workers, *Chem. Comm.* 304 (1971).
233. I. Maezawa, T. Hori, and M. Suzuki, *Agr. Biol. Chem.* **38**, 91, 539 (1974).
234. I. Maezawa and co-workers, *J. Antibiot.* **26**, 771 (1973).
235. B. A. Sobin, A. R. English, and W. D. Celmer, *Antibiot. Ann.* **2**, 827 (1954–1955).
236. W. D. Celmer, H. Els, and K. Murai, *Antibiot. Ann.* 476 (1957–1958).
237. F. A. Hochstein and co-workers, *J. Am. Chem. Soc.* **82**, 3225 (1960).
238. W. D. Celmer, *J. Am. Chem. Soc.* **87**, 1797, 1799, 1801 (1965).
239. W. D. Celmer, *Antibiot. Ann.* 277 (1958–1959).
240. D. M. Trakhtenberg and co-workers, *Antibiotiki* **14**, 492 (1969).
241. J. R. Martin and co-workers, *J. Antibiot.* **27**, 570 (1974).
242. H. Grisebach and W. Hofheinz, *J. Roy. Inst. Chem.* **88**, 332 (1964).
243. E. Gaumann and co-workers, *Helv. Chim. Acta* **43**, 601 (1960).
244. W. Keller-Schierlein and G. Roncari, *Helv. Chim. Acta* **47**, 78 (1964).
245. S. Omura and co-workers, *J. Antibiot.* **22**, 629 (1969).
246. R. S. Egan and J. R. Martin, *J. Am. Chem. Soc.* **92**, 4129 (1970).
247. W. Richle and co-workers, *Helv. Chim. Acta* **55**, 467 (1972).
248. S. Omura and co-workers, *J. Antibiot.* **24**, 717 (1971).
249. J. Sawada and co-workers, *J. Antibiot.* **27**, 639 (1974).
250. J. R. Martin and co-workers, *Helv. Chim. Acta* **59**, 1886 (1976).
251. N. Nagahama and co-workers, *J. Antibiot.* **20A**, 261 (1967).
252. T. Furumai, N. Nagahama, and T. Okuda, *J. Antibiot.* **21A**, 85 (1968).
253. N. Nagahama and co-workers, *Chem. Pharm. Bull. (Tokyo)* **19**, 649 (1971).
254. N. Nagahama, I. Takamori, and M. Suzuki, *Chem. Pharm. Bull. (Tokyo)* **19**, 655, 660 (1971).
255. N. Miyairi and co-workers, *J. Antibiot.* **19A**, 56 (1966).
256. F. W. Tanner and co-workers, *Antibiot. Chemother.* **2**, 441 (1952).
257. J. F. Pagano, M. J. Weinstein, and C. M. McKee, *Antibiot. Chemother.* **3**, 899 (1953).
258. J. D. Dutcher and co-workers, *Antibiot. Chemother.* **3**, 910 (1953).
259. R. B. Woodward, L. S. Weiler, and P. C. Dutta, *J. Am. Chem. Soc.* **87**, 4662 (1965).
260. H. Achenbach and H. Grisebach, *Z. Naturforsch.* **19b**, 561 (1964).
261. H. Grisebach and H. Achenbach, *Z. Naturforsch.* **17b**, 6 (1962).

262. H. Grisebach and H. Achenbach, *Tetrahedron Lett.* 569 (1962).
263. W. D. Celmer, *J. Am. Chem. Soc.* **88**, 5028 (1966).
264. M. Muroi, M. Izawa, and T. Kishi, *Chem. Pharm. Bull. (Tokyo)* **24**, 463 (1976).
265. F. A. Hochstein and K. Murai, *J. Am. Chem. Soc.* **76**, 5080 (1954).
266. S. Omura and co-workers, *J. Am. Chem. Soc.* **97**, 4001 (1975).
267. Jpn. Kokai 76, 82,790 (July 20, 1976), (to Sanraku-Ocean KK).
268. G. Huber and co-workers, *Arzneim. Forsch.* **12**, 1191 (1962).
269. U.S. Pat. 3,817,836 (June 18, 1974), R. J. Theriault and E. Elmer (to Abbott Laboratories).
270. U.S. Pat. 3,932,383 (June 13, 1976), L. A. Freiberg (to Abbott Laboratories).
271. U.S. Pat. 3,948,884 (Apr. 6, 1976), R. J. Theriault (to Abbott Laboratories).
272. Brit. Pat. 785,098 (Jan. 2, 1956), (to Rhone-Poulenc).
273. R. Corbaz and co-workers, *Helv. Chim. Acta* **39**, 304 (1956).
274. R. Paul and S. Tchelitcheff, *Bull. Soc. Chim. France,* 443, 1059 (1957).
275. *Ibid.,* 150 (1960).
276. *Ibid.,* 189, 650 (1965).
277. S. Omura and co-workers, *J. Am. Chem. Soc.* **91**, 3401 (1969).
278. H. Takahira and co-workers, *J. Antibiot.* **18A**, 269 (1965).
279. Belg. Pat. 769,767 (Oct. 1, 1972), Y. Fujimoto and K. Nakano (to Kyowa Hakko Kogyo).
280. Belg. Pat. 769,766 (Oct. 1, 1972), Y. Fujimoto and K. Nakano (to Kyowa Hakko Kogyo).
281. T. Hata and co-workers, *J. Antibiot.* **6A**, 87 (1953).
282. T. Watanabe, T. Fujii, and K. Satake, *J. Biochem.* **50**, 197 (1961).
283. T. Watanabe, *Bull. Chem. Soc. Japan* **34**, 15 (1961).
284. T. Watanabe, H. Nishida, and K. Satake, *Bull. Chem. Soc. Japan* **34**, 1285 (1961).
285. S. Omura, H. Ogura, and T. Hata, *Tetrahedron Lett.* 609, 1267 (1967).
286. T. Hata and co-workers, *Chem. Pharm. Bull. (Tokyo)* **15**, 358 (1967).
287. S. Omura, M. Katagiri, and T. Hata, *J. Antibiot.* **20**, 234 (1967).
288. S. Omura and co-workers, *Chem. Pharm. Bull. (Tokyo)* **15**, 1529 (1967).
289. S. Omura and co-workers, *Chem. Pharm. Bull. (Tokyo)* **16**, 1167, 1181 (1968).
290. S. Omura, M. Katagiri, and T. Hata, *J. Antibiot.* **21**, 199, 272 (1968).
291. S. Omura, Y. Hironaka, and T. Hata, *J. Antibiot.* **23**, 511 (1970).
292. M. Hiramatsu and co-workers, *Bull. Chem. Soc. Japan* **43**, 1966 (1970).
293. S. Omura and co-workers, *Chem. Pharm. Bull. (Tokyo)* **16**, 1402 (1968).
294. S. Omura and co-workers, *Chem. Pharm. Bull. (Tokyo)* **18**, 1501 (1970).
295. L. A. Freiberg, R. S. Egan, and W. H. Washburn, *J. Org. Chem.* **39**, 2474 (1974).
296. S. Omura and co-workers, *Tetrahedron* **28**, 2839 (1972).
297. S. Omura and co-workers, *J. Am. Chem. Soc.* **97**, 6600 (1975).
298. T. Osono, K. Moriyama, and M. Murakami, *J. Antibiot.* **27**, 366 (1974).
299. S. Omura and co-workers, *J. Antibiot.* **27**, 370 (1974).
300. S. Omura, and co-workers, *J. Antibiot.* **27**, 147 (1974).
301. N. N. Girotra and N. L. Wendler, *Tetrahedron Lett.* 227 (1975).
302. S. Omura and co-workers, *Progr. Antimicr. Anticancer Chemother. Proc. 6th Int. Congr. Chemother.* **2**, 1043 (1969).
303. Ger. Pat. 2,230,729 (Jan. 18, 1973), S. Omoto, S. Inoue, and T. Niida (to Meiji Seika Kaisha).
304. S. Omura and co-workers, *J. Antibiot.* **21**, 532 (1968).
305. Neth. Pat. 7,305,775 (Oct. 30, 1973) (to Tanabe Seiyaku KK).
306. Ger. Pat. 2,319,100 (Oct. 30, 1973), R. J. Theriault (to Abbott Laboratories).
307. U.S. Pat. 3,769,273 (Oct. 30, 1973), E. H. Massey (to Eli Lilly and Co.).
308. A. Nakagawa and co-workers, *Chem. Pharm. Bull. (Tokyo)* **23**, 1426 (1974).
309. N. N. Girotra, A. A. Patchett, and N. L. Wendler, *Tetrahedron* **32**, 991 (1976).
310. T. Tsuruoka and co-workers, *J. Antibiot.* **24**, 452 (1971).
311. S. Inouye and co-workers, *J. Antibiot.* **24**, 460 (1971).
312. T. Tsuruoka and co-workers, *J. Antibiot.* **24**, 526 (1971).
313. S. Omoto and co-workers, *J. Antibiot.* **29**, 536 (1976).
314. Ger. Pat. 2,316,705 (Nov. 15, 1973), S. Inouye and co-workers (to Meiji Seika Kaisha).
315. Jpn. Kokai 73, 72,389 (Sept. 29, 1973), T. Niida and co-workers (to Meiji Seika Kaisha).
316. Belg. Pat. 832,813 (Dec. 16, 1975), S. Inouye and co-workers (to Meiji Seika Kaisha).
317. Jpn. Kokai 74, 93,384 (Sept. 5, 1974), S. Omoto and co-workers, (to Meiji Seika Kaisha).
318. Ger. Pat. 2,153,573 (Aug. 17, 1972), T. Tsuruoka and co-workers (to Meiji Seika Kaisha).
319. S. Inouye and co-workers, *Chem. Pharm. Bull. (Tokyo)* **20**, 2366 (1972).

320. Jpn. Kokai 72, 25,384 (Oct. 20, 1972), I. Machida and co-workers (to Nikken Chemicals Co. Ltd.).
321. M. Suzuki and co-workers, *Tetrahedron Lett.* 435 (1971).
322. M. Suzuki and co-workers, *J. Antibiot.* **24,** 904 (1971).
323. T. Furumai and co-workers, *J. Antibiot.* **27,** 95 (1974).
324. A. Kinumaki and co-workers, *J. Antibiot.* **27,** 107, 117 (1974).
325. Jpn. Kokai 73, 04,683 (Jan. 20, 1973) M. Suzuki, Y. Sugawara, and Y. Seki (to Tanabe Seiyaku).
326. Jpn. Kokai 73, 04,684 (Jan. 1, 1973), M. Suzuki, Y. Sugawara, and Y. Seki (to Tanabe Seiyaku).
327. Jpn. Kokai 73, 23,991 (Mar. 28, 1973), M. Suzuki and co-workers (to Tanabe Seiyaku).
328. T. Furumai and co-workers, *J. Antibiot.* **26,** 708 (1973).
329. T. Furumai and M. Suzuki, *J. Antibiot.* **28,** 770,775,783 (1975).
330. T. Furumai, K. Takeda, and M. Suzuki, *J. Antibiot.* **28,** 789 (1975).
331. M. Muroi, M. Izawa, and T. Kishi, *Experientia* **28,** 129 (1972).
332. M. Muroi and co-workers, *Experientia* **28,** 501, 878 (1972).
333. H. Ono and co-workers, *J. Antibiot.* **26,** 191 (1973).
334. M. Muroi and co-workers, *J. Antibiot.* **26,** 199 (1973).
335. M. Muroi, M. Izawa, and T. Kishi, *Chem. Pharm. Bull. (Tokyo)* **24,** 450 (1976).
336. K. Nakahama and co-workers, *J. Antibiot.* **27,** 425 (1974).
337. K. Nakahama, T. Kishi, and S. Igarasi, *J. Antibiot.* **27,** 487 (1974).
338. K. Nakahama and S. Igarasi, *J. Antibiot.* **27,** 605 (1974).
339. M. Muroi, M. Izawa, and T. Kishi, *J. Antibiot.* **27,** 449 (1974).
340. M. Shibata, M. Uyeda, and S. Mori, *J. Antibiot.* **28,** 434 (1975).
341. M. Shibata, M. Uyeda, and S. Mori, *J. Antibiot.* **29,** 824 (1976).
342. K. Nakahama, T. Kishi, and S. Igarasi, *J. Antibiot.* **27,** 433 (1974).
343. H. Ono, S. Harada, and T. Kishi, *J. Antibiot.* **27,** 442 (1974).
344. S. Harada and co-workers, *Antimicrob. Agents Chemother.* **4,** 140 (1973).
345. S. Omura and co-workers, *Tetrahedron Lett.* 4503 (1975).
346. H. A. Whaley and co-workers, *Antimicrob. Agents Chemother.* 45 (1963).
347. L. I. Feldman and co-workers, *Antimicrob. Agents Chemother.* 54 (1963).
348. R. Corbaz and co-workers, *Helv. Chim. Acta* **38,** 1202 (1955).
349. A. Kinumaki and M. Suzuki, *J. Antibiot.* **25,** 480 (1972).
350. H. Koshiyama and co-workers, *J. Antibiot.* **16A,** 59 (1966).
351. H. Koshiyama and co-workers, *J. Antibiot.* **22,** 61 (1969).
352. U.S. Pat. 3,950,516 (Apr. 13, 1976), T. Miyaki (to Bristol-Myers Co.).
353. H. Tsukiura and co-workers, *J. Antibiot.* **22,** 89 (1969).
354. H. Tsukiura and co-workers, *J. Antibiot.* **22,** 100 (1969).
355. T. Kusaka, H. Yamamoto, and T. Suzuki, *J. Takeda Res. Lab.* **29,** 239 (1970).
356. T. Suzuki, *Bull. Chem. Soc. Japan* **43,** 292 (1970).
357. T. Suzuki, E. Mizuta, and N. Sugita, *Chem. Lett.* 793 (1973).
358. T. Suzuki, *Chem. Lett.* 799 (1973).
359. H. Bickel and co-workers, *Helv. Chim. Acta* **45,** 1396 (1962).
360. G. H. Wagman and co-workers, *J. Antibiot.* **25,** 641 (1972).
361. H. Reimann and R. S. Jaret, *Chem. Comm.* 1270 (1972).
362. A. K. Ganguly and co-workers, *J. Antibiot.* **29,** 976 (1976).
363. Ger. Pat. 2,034,245 (Feb. 25, 1971), M. Shibata and co-workers (to Takeda Chemical Industries Ltd).
364. Jpn. Kokai 75, 34,637 (Oct. 11, 1975), M. Shibata and co-workers (to Takeda Chemical Industries Ltd.).
365. K. Hatano, E. Higashide, and M. Shibata, *J. Antibiot.* **29,** 1163 (1976).
366. T. Kishi and co-workers, *J. Antibiot.* **29,** 1171 (1976).
367. T. Furumai and co-workers, *J. Antibiot.* **30,** 443 (1977).
368. A. Kinumaki and co-workers, *J. Antibiot.* **30,** 450 (1977).
369. Jpn. Kokai 76, 36,471 (Mar. 27, 1976), M. Suzuki, K. Harada, and T. Yamaguchi (to Tanabe Seiyaku KK).
370. P. W. K. Woo, H. W. Dion, and Q. R. Bartz, *J. Am. Chem. Soc.* **83,** 3352 (1961).
371. P. W. K. Woo, H. W. Dion, and L. F. Johnson, *J. Am. Chem. Soc.* **84,** 1066 (1962).
372. P. W. K. Woo, H. W. Dion, and Q. R. Bartz, *J. Am. Chem. Soc.* **84,** 1512 (1962).
373. *Ibid.,* **86,** 2724, 2726 (1964).
374. J. Krc and R. B. Scott, *Microscope* **23,** 15 (1975).
375. D. V. Lefemine and co-workers, *Antimicrob. Agents Chemother.* 41 (1964).

376. M. P. Kunstmann and L. A. Mitscher, *Experientia* **21**, 372 (1965).
377. L. A. Mitscher and M. P. Kunstmann, *Experientia* **25**, 12 (1969).
378. M. P. Kunstmann, L. A. Mitscher, and E. L. Patterson, *Antimicrob. Agents Chemother.* 87 (1964).
379. H. Achenbach and W. Karl, *Chem. Ber.* **108**, 759 (1975).
380. H. Achenbach and W. Karl, *Chem. Ber.* **108**, 780 (1975).
381. H. Achenbach and W. Karl, *Chem. Ber.* **108**, 772 (1975).
382. K. Kono, T. Kasuga, and S. Mitsuhashi, *Jpn. J. Microbiol.* **10**, 109 (1966).
383. E. J. L. Lowbury and A. M. Hood, *J. Gen. Microbiol.* **9**, 524 (1953).
384. W. E. Grundy, *Exptl. Chemoth. Acad. Press* **3**, 171 (1964).
385. A. W. Linnane and J. M. Haslam, in B. L. Horecker and E. R. Stadtman, eds., *Current Topics in Cellular Regulation,* Vol. 2 Academic Press, New York, 1970, p. 101.
386. Y. Chabbert, *Ann. Inst. Pasteur (Paris)* **90**, 787 (1956).
387. L. P. Garrod, *Brit. Med. J.* **2**, 57 (1957).
388. P. A. Pattee and J. N. Baldwin, *J. Bacteriol.* **84**, 1049 (1962).
389. J. R. Weaver and P. A. Pattee, *J. Bacteriol.* **88**, 574 (1964).
390. S. Mitsuhashi, *Jpn. J. Microbiol.* **11**, 49 (1967).
391. T. D. Brock and M. L. Brock, *Biochim. Biophys. Acta* **33**, 274 (1959).
392. S. B. Taubman and co-workers, *Biochim. Biophys. Acta* **123**, 438 (1966).
393. K. Tanaka and H. Teraoka, *Biochim. Biophys. Acta* **114**, 204 (1966).
394. J. C. H. Mao, in S. Mitsuhashi, ed., *Drug Action and Drug Resistance in Bacteria,* Vol. 1, *Macrolide Antibiotics and Lincomycin,* University Park Press, Tokyo, 1971, p. 153.
395. S. Pestka, *Antimicrob. Agents Chemother.* **6**, 474 (1974).
396. S. Pestka and R. LeMahieu, *Antimicrob. Agents Chemother.* **6**, 479 (1974).
397. *AMA Drug Evaluations,* 1st ed., 1971, American Medical Association.
398. D. F. Johnson, Jr. and W. H. Hall, *New Eng. J. Med.* **265**, 1200 (1961).
399. W. D. Celmer, G. Els, and K. Murai, *Antibiot. Ann.* 476 (1957–1958).
400. M. Kondo and co-workers, *Antimicrob. Agents Chemother.* **4**, 149 (1973).
401. M. Kondo and co-workers, *Antimicrob. Agents Chemother.* **4**, 156 (1973).
402. Y. C. Martin and K. R. Lynn, *J. Med. Chem.* **14**, 1162 (1971).
403. S. Omura and co-workers, *J. Med. Chem.* **15**, 1011 (1972).
404. S. Rakhit and K. Singh, *J. Antibiot.* **27**, 221 (1974).

ALAN K. MALLAMS
Schering-Plough Corporation

NUCLEOSIDES

The group of nucleoside antibiotics comprises compounds which consist of a heterocyclic moiety (aglycone base) linked by a carbon–carbon or a carbon–nitrogen bond to a carbohydrate. They are obtained from predominantly microbial sources, and have the capacity to interfere with the growth or function of various biological systems. The antibiotics are, essentially, structural analogues of the naturally occurring nucleosides, but in a few instances (eg, aminoacyl and peptidyl nucleosides) they resemble end-portions of aminoacyl or peptidyl ribonucleic acid (RNA) (see Biopolymers).

The antibiotics can be grouped according to their structural resemblance to the natural nucleosides as either purine or pyrimidine analogues, and they can be further classified with respect to the location of the structural change in either the aglycone or the carbohydrate moiety. Within these categories, subdivisions can be established, depending upon whether the carbohydrate is of the tetrahydrofuran or tetrahydropyran form. The nucleoside antibiotics covered in this survey are summarized according to this scheme in Tables 1 and 2.

This survey does not list all the nucleosides so far encountered in nature. For instance, it does not detail information on the numerous RNA-derived nucleosides (eg, N-(purin-6-yl-carbamoyl) threonine riboside) that appear in the urine of mammals (1) or the cytokinin nucleosides that act as plant hormones (2). Some of these compounds might well possess antibiotic (growth inhibitory) activity. Furthermore, it does not refer to nucleosides whose structure has not been definitively established (eg, thraustomycin [51683-38-6] (3) or raphanatin [38165-56-9] (4)).

It may be added that various structural analogues of the natural purine or pyrimidine bases have been isolated on the basis of their growth inhibitory properties. Among these are emimycin [3735-45-4] (5), pathocidin [134-58-7] (6), isoguanine [3373-53-3] (7), agelasin [134-58-7] (8) and bacimethrin [3690-12-8] (9).

Nucleosides with Modifications in the Aglycone Portion

5-Azacytidine (**1**) (4-amino-1β-D-ribofuranosyl-1,3,5-triazine-2-one) was isolated from *S. ladakanus* (10–11) and its structure was determined by degradation, spectral analysis (10–11) and by synthesis (12–13). Activity against some bacterial strains (11,14), experimental tumors (11,15), and certain leukemias in man has been observed (16–17). The compound inhibits orotidylate decarboxylase (18) and protein synthesis (19–21), possibly as a result of incorporation into RNA, giving rise to defective messenger-RNA (21–23). The LD$_{50}$ ip (intraperitoneal) in mice is 115 mg/kg (15).

Oxazinomycin (**2**) (minimycin, 5β-D-ribofuranosyl-1,3-oxazine-2,4-dione) was isolated from *S. tanesashinensis* (24) and from *S. hygroscopicus* (25), and its structure determined by x-ray and spectral analysis (24–25). It is sol in H$_2$O, and methanol; sl sol in ethanol propanol, and acetone; insol in benzene, and ether (24–25); inhibitory activity against some gram-positive and gram-negative bacteria and against Ehrlich ascites carcinoma has been demonstrated. The LD$_{50}$ for mice is 10–30 mg/kg ip; 80–120 mg/kg iv (intravenous) (24–25).

Table 1. Nucleoside Antibiotics

Nucleoside antibiotics with modifications in the aglycone portion	
Pyrimidine analogues or antimetabolites	*Purine analogues or antimetabolites*
5-azacytidine (1)	bredinin (5)
oxazinomycin (2)	crotonoside (6)
pyrazofurin (3)	coformycin (7)
showdomycin (4)	2'-deoxycoformycin (8)
	formycin (9)
	formycin B (10)
	oxoformycin B (11)
	nebularine (12)
	spongosine (13)
	tubercidin (14)
	toyocamycin (15)
	sangivamycin (16)

Nucleoside antibiotics with modifications in the carbohydrate portion	
Pyrimidine derivatives	*Purine derivatives*
hikizimycin (17)	aristeromycin (23)
octosyl acids (18)	2'-amino-2'-deoxyguanosine (24)
pentopyranine A (19)	3'-amino-3'-deoxyadenosine (25)
pentopyranine C (20)	3'-acetamido-3'-deoxyadenosine (26)
spongothymidine (21)	arabinofuranosyl adenine (Ara-A) (27)
spongouridine (22)	cordycepin (28)
	decoyinine (29)
	nucleocidin (30)
	psicofuranine (31)

Nucleoside antibiotics carrying aminoacyl or peptidyl residues	
Pyrimidine derivatives	*Purine derivatives*
amicetin (32)	homocitrullylaminoadenosine (39)
bamicetin (33)	lysylaminoadenosine (40)
plicacetin (34)	puromycin (41)
blasticidin (35)	septacidin (42)
gougerotin (36)	
oxamicetin (37)	
polyoxins (38)	

Nucleoside antibiotics with modifications in the aglycone and carbohydrate portions
streptothricins (43)
exotoxin of *Bacillus thuringiensis* (44)

Pyrazofurin (3) (3β-D-ribofuranosyl-4-hydroxypyrazole-5-carboxamide; pyrazomycin) was isolated from *S. candidus* (26–27). It is active against vaccinia, herpes, measle, rhino, and influenza viruses *in vitro* (28) and Friend leukemia virus in mice (29) and effective against some experimental tumors (30–31). It inhibits orotidylic acid decarboxylase (28,31).

Pyrazofurin B is the α-anomer of pyrazofurin. In water, pyrazofurin is slowly converted to pyrazofurin B, which has only low antiviral and antitumor activity (32–33).

Showdomycin (**4**) (2-(β-D-ribofuranosyl)maleimide, 3β-D-ribofuranosyl-1H-pyrrole-2,5-dione) was isolated from *S. showdoensis* (34). It is active against gram-positive and gram-negative bacteria and against various experimental tumors *in vitro* (34–35). It is sol in H_2O, alcohol, and acetone; insol in ether and benzene; and it is unstable in base (34,36). Showdomycin was totally synthesized (37) after its structure was elucidated by degradation (36,38), spectral analysis (39), and x-ray crystallography (40). LD_{50} in mice is 25 mg/kg ip, 110 mg/kg iv (34). The antibiotic may act as an alkylating agent (36). It causes metaphase arrest in HeLa cells (35); inhibits deoxyribonucleic acid (DNA) synthesis but not RNA synthesis in *E. coli* K-12 (41); interferes with uridine monophosphate (UMP) kinase activity in Ehrlich ascites cells (42); alkylates uridine diphosphate (UDP) glucose dehydrogenase (42), and radiosensitizes *E. coli* (43). The LD_{50} in mice is 25 mg/kg ip and 110 mg/kg iv.

Bredinin (**5**) (4-carbamoyl-1β-D-ribofuranosylimidazolium-5-olate) was isolated from *Eupenicillium brefeldianum* (44–45), interferes with *in vitro* vaccinia virus replication, inhibits leukemia L5178 Y cells in culture (44,46) and is markedly immunosuppressive in mice (44). It is sol in H_2O, sl sol in lower alcohols, and insol in most organic solvents (44). The inhibition of cell growth is reversible by guanine, guanosine, and guanylic acid (46). The LD_{50} in mice is 5000 mg/kg ip and 1500 mg/kg iv.

Crotonoside (**6**) (2-hydroxy-9β-D-ribofuranosyl adenine; isoguanosine) was isolated from *Croton tiglium* seeds (47); its structure was determined by spectral analysis (48–49), degradation (49–50), and synthesis (51–52). The compound is toxic to mice at 50 mg/kg (53) and has vasodepressor action greater than that of adenosine (54–55).

Coformycin (**7**) [3-(β-D-ribofuranosyl)-6,7,8-trihydroimidazo [4,5-d][1,3] diazepin-8(R)-ol] was isolated together with formycin from *N. interforma* (56) and its structure was determined by x-ray analysis (57) and by total synthesis (58). Coformycin is a potent inhibitor of adenosine deaminase (59), and as a result enhances the potency of various analogues of adenosine formycin (60) that are subject to deamination.

2'-Deoxycoformycin (**8**) [(R)-3-(2-deoxy-β-D-*erythro*-pentofuranosyl)-3,6,-7,8-tetrahydroimidazo[4,5-d] [1,3] diazepin-8-ol] was isolated from *S. antibioticus*; its structure was determined by degradation, spectral and x-ray analysis (61). By inhibiting adenosine deaminase, it enhances the potency of inhibitors which are subject to deamination (62–64).

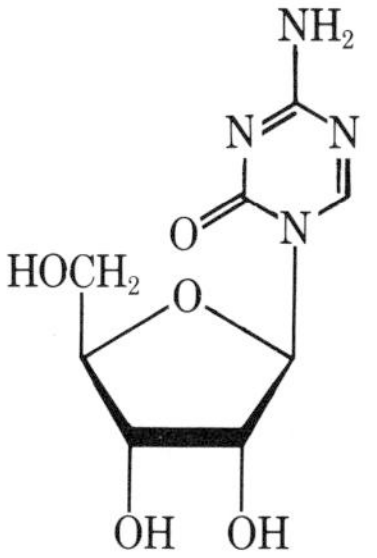

(1) 5-azacytidine   (2) oxazinomycin   (3) pyrazofurin   (4) showdomycin

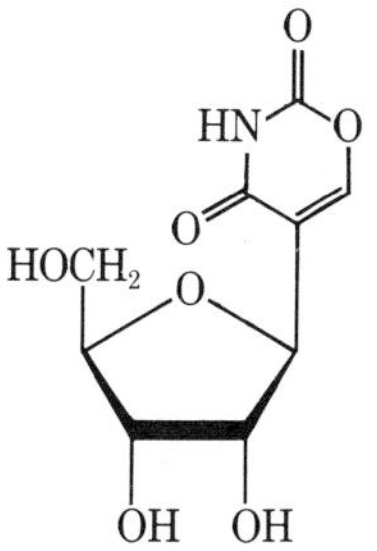

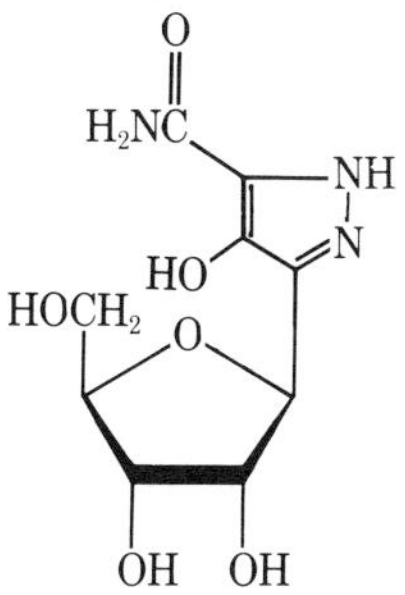

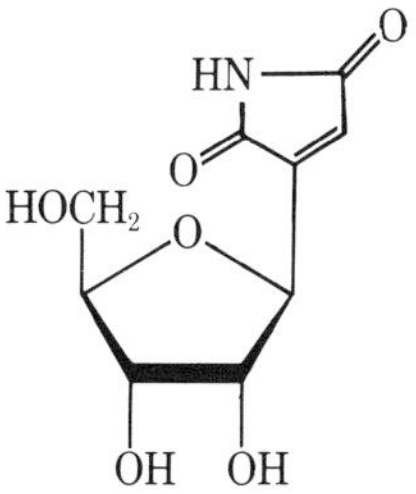

Table 2. Selected Properties of Nucleosides

Compound	CAS Registry No.	Structure no.	Mol formula	Mol wt	mp, °C	$[\alpha]_D^{(t)a}$, c^b	pK_a	UV max, nm, $(E_{1cm}^{1\%})$ solvent^c
3'-acetamido-3-deoxyadenosine	[21299-78-5]	(26)	$C_{12}H_{16}N_6O_4$	308.3	263–265	+8° (25), 1.0 in 0.1N HCl		260, (15,600), H_2O
amicetin	[17650-86-1]	(32)	$C_{29}H_{42}N_6O_9$	618.7	165–169, needles from cold H_2O; 243–244 dec, cryst from warm H_2O	+116.5° (25), 0.5 in 0.1 N HCl		305, (433), H_2O; 316, (433), 0.1 N HCl; 322, (470), 0.1 N NaOH
3'-amino-3'-deoxyadenosine	[2504-55-4]	(25)	$C_{10}H_{14}N_6O_3$	266.3	265–267 dec	−40° (25), 0.4 in DMF		259, (15,000), H_2O
2'-amino-2'-deoxyguanosine	[60966-26-9]	(24)	$C_{10}H_{14}N_6O_4$	282.3	252–254 dec	−56.6° (26), 0.5 in H_2O		same as guanosine
9-arabinofuranosyladenine (Ara-A)	[2006-02-2]	(27)	$C_{10}H_{13}N_5O_4$	267.3	257	−5° (27), 0.25 in H_2O		257.5, (12,700), pH 1; 259, (14,000), pH 13
aristeromycin	[19186-33-5]	(23)	$C_{11}H_{15}N_5O_3$	265.3	213–215 dec (nat prod); 238–242 (syn prod)	−52.5° (25), 1.0 in DMF		258, (14,500), 0.1 N HCl; 212, (20,600), 0.1 N HCl
5-azacytidine	[320-67-2]	(1)	$C_8H_{12}N_4O_5$	244.2	228–230	+39° (25), 1.0 in H_2O		241, (8,767), H_2O; 249, (3,077), 0.01 N HCl; 223, (24,200), 0.01 N KOH
bamicetin	[43043-14-7]	(33)	$C_{28}H_{40}N_6O_9$	604.7	240–241 dec	+121° (26), 0.5 in 0.1 N HCl		314, na, 0.1 N HCl; 322, na, 0.1 N NaOH; 302, na, H_2O
blasticidin S	[2079-00-7]	(35)	$C_{17}H_{26}N_8O_5$	422.5	235–236 dec	+108.4° (11), 1.0 in H_2O		274, (13,400), 0.1 N HCl; 266, (8,850), 0.1 N NaOH
bredinin	[50924-49-7]	(5)	$C_9H_{13}N_3O_6$	259.2	200 dec	−35° (27), 0.8 in H_2O	6.75	245, (260), 1 N HCl; 281, (495), 1 N HCl; 277, (660), 1 N NaOH
coformycin	[11033-22-0]	(7)	$C_{11}H_{16}N_4O_5$	284.3	182–184	+34° (24), 1.0 in H_2O	5.3	282, (290), H_2O; 264, (257), 0.1 N HCl; 284, (290), 0.1 N NaOH

Name	[CAS]	No.	Formula	MW	MP (°C)	$[\alpha]$	pK_a	UV λ_{max} nm (ε)
cordycepin	[73-03-0]	(28)	$C_{10}H_{13}N_5O_3$	251.3	230–231	−35° (25), 9.4 in H_2O		259, (13,100), pH 4; 260, (13,700), pH 11
crotonoside	[1818-71-9]	(6)	$C_{11}H_{13}N_5O_5$	295.2	237–241 dec	−60.38° (25), 1.0 in 0.1 N NaOH		259, (15,500), H_2O and pH 11
decoyinine	[2004-04-8]	(29)	$C_{11}H_{13}N_5O_4$	279.3	I 130–133^d II 156–159 dec	+43.5° (26), 1.0 in H_2O		282, (8,000), H_2O;
2'-deoxycoformycin	[53910-25-1]	(8)	$C_{11}H_{16}N_4O_4$	268.3	220–225	+76.4° (25), 1.0 in H_2O	5.2	283, (7,970), pH 11; 273, (7,570), pH 2
exotoxin	[23526-02-5]	(44)	$C_{22}H_{32}N_5O_{19}P$	701.5				
formycin	[6742-12-7]	(9)	$C_{10}H_{13}N_5O_4$	267.2	141–144	−35.5° (20), 1.0 in 0.1 N HCl	4.5 and 9.5	295, (390), H_2O; 234, (280), acid; 290, (340), acid; 235, (500), base; 305, (260), base
formycin B	[13877-76-4]	(10)	$C_{10}H_{12}N_4O_5$	268.2	254–255	−51.5° (20), 1.0 in H_2O	8.8	219, (348), H_2O; 280, (294), H_2O; 221, (543), 0.1 N HCl; 276, (300), 0.1 N HCl; 230, (643), 0.1 N NaOH; 292, (338), 0.1 N NaOH
gougerotin	[2096-42-6]	(36)	$C_{16}H_{25}N_7O_8$	443.4	200–215 dec	+45° (21), 1.0 in H_2O		267, (9,400), H_2O; 235, (9,300), H_2O; 275, (13,600), 0.1 N HCl; 267, (9,800), 0.1 N NaOH
hikizimycin	[12706-94-4]	(17)	$C_{21}H_{37}N_5O_{14}$	583.6	>300	−40.6° (23.5), 1.0 in H_2O		274, (8,000), 0.1 N HCl; 266, (5,600), H_2O; 237, (5,300), H_2O; 268, (5,500), 0.1 N NaOH; 238, (5,200), 0.1 N NaOH
homocitrulyl-aminoadenosine	[59204-62-5]	(39)	$C_{17}H_{27}N_9O_5$	437.5				
9-lysylamino-adenosine	[62949-62-5]	(40)	$C_{16}H_{26}N_8O_4$	394.5				
nebularine	[550-33-4]	(12)	$C_{10}H_{12}N_4O_4$	252.2	182–183	−48.6° (45), 1.0 in H_2O		262, (232), 0.1 N HCl; 263, (361), 0.1 N NaOH

Table 2 (*continued*)

Compound	CAS Registry No.	Structure no.	Mol formula	Mol wt	mp, °C	$[\alpha]_D^{a}$, c^{b}	pK_a	UV max, nm, $(E_{1cm}^{1\%})$ solvent^{c}
nucleocidin	[24751-69-7]	(30)	$C_{10}H_{13}FN_6O_6S$	364.3	143–144	−33.3° (24.5), 1.05 in 1:1 C_2H_5OH–0.1 N HCl		256, (15,500), H_2O
octosyl acid A	[55728-21-7]	(18)	$C_{13}H_{14}N_2O_{10}$	358.3	290–295 dec	+13.3° (20), 0.425 in 1 N NaOH	3.0, 4.3, and 9.4	220, (9,900), H_2O and 0.1 N HCl; 276, (10,700), H_2O and 0.1 N HCl; 272, (7,000), 0.1 N NaOH
octosyl acid B	[55728-22-8]	(18)	$C_{13}H_{16}N_2O_9$	344.3	200 dec			265, (7,700), H_2O and 0.1 N HCl; 265, (5,500), 0.1 N NaOH
octosyl acid C	[55728-23-9]	(18)	$C_{13}H_{12}N_2O_{10}$	356.3	192–198			220, (9,200), H_2O and 0.1 N HCl; 275, (9,200), H_2O and 0.1 N HCl; 272, (6,400), 0.1 N NaOH
oxamicetin	[52665-75-5]	(37)	$C_{29}H_{42}N_6O_{10}$	634.7	176–179	+66° (25), 0.4 in H_2O		305, (31,700), H_2O; 316, (26,600), 0.1 N HCl; 322, (21,900), 0.1 N NaOH
oxazinomycin	[32388-21-9]	(2)	$C_9H_{11}NO_7$	245.2	161 (prisms) 166 (needles)	+18° (25), 1.0 in H_2O		231.5, (168), H_2O; 230, (188), 0.01 N HCl
oxoformycin B	[19246-88-9]	(11)	$C_{10}H_{11}N_4O_6$	283.2				
pentopyranine A	[39057-02-8]	(19)	$C_9H_{13}N_3O_3$	211.2	258 dec	+31.5° (21), 2.0 in H_2O	4.2	278, (13,100), 0.1 N HCl; 270, (8,850), 0.1 N NaOH
pentopyranine B	[51257-56-8]		$C_9H_{13}N_3O_3$	211.2	242 dec	+12° (21), 4.2 in H_2O		278, (11,300), 0.01 N HCl; 270, (8,290), 0.01 N NaOH
pentopyranine C	[39007-97-1]	(20)	$C_9H_{13}N_3O_4$	227.2	143–145	+20° (21), 1.2 in H_2O	4.2	278, (12,200), 0.1 N HCl; 270, (8,450), 0.1 N NaOH
pentopyranine D	[51257-57-9]		$C_9H_{13}N_3O_4$	227.2	261 dec	+13.7° (21), 1.3 in H_2O		278, (12,000), 0.01 N HCl; 270, (8,370), 0.01 N NaOH
plicacetin	[43043-15-8]	(34)	$C_{25}H_{35}N_5O_7$	517.6	160–163	+181° (26), 2.7 in CH_3OH		257, na, 0.1 N HCl; 311.5, na, 0.1 N HCl; 249, na, H_2O; 321, na, H_2O; 329, na, 0.1 N NaOH
polyoxin A	[19396-03-3]	(38)	$C_{23}H_{32}N_6O_{14}$	616.5		−30° (20), 1.0 in H_2O	3.0, 7.3, and 9.6	262, (142), 0.05 N HCl; 264, (103), 0.05 N NaOH

Name	CAS	Ref.	Formula	MW	mp	$[\alpha]$	pKa	UV
polyoxin B	[19396-06-6]	(38)	$C_{17}H_{25}N_5O_{13}$	507.4		+34° (20), 1.0 in H_2O	3.0, 6.9, and 9.4	262, (172), 0.05 N HCl; 264, (130), 0.05 N NaOH
polyoxin C	[11043-74-6]	(38)	$C_{11}H_{15}N_3O_8$	317.3		−68° (20), 1.0 in H_2O	2.4, 8.1, and 9.5	262, (297), 0.05 N HCl; 264, (231), 0.05 N NaOH
polyoxin D	[22976-86-9]	(38)	$C_{17}H_{23}N_5O_{14}$	521.4		+30° (20), 1.0 in H_2O	2.6, 3.7, 7.3 and 9.4	218, (217), 0.05 N HCl; 276, (127), 0.05 N HCl; 271, 137, 0.05 N NaOH
polyoxin E	[22976-87-0]	(38)	$C_{17}H_{23}N_5O_{13}$	505.4		+19° (20), 1.0 in H_2O	2.8, 3.9, 7.4 and 9.3	218, (200), 0.05 N HCl; 276, (200), 0.05 N HCl; 271, (128), 0.05 N NaOH
polyoxin F	[23116-76-9]	(38)	$C_{23}H_{30}N_6O_{15}$	630.5		−18° (20), 1.0 in H_2O	2.7, 3.9, 7.2, and 9.3	215 sh, (257), 0.05 N HCl; 276, (181), 0.05 N HCl; 271, (118), 0.05 N NaOH
polyoxin G	[22976-88-1]	(38)	$C_{17}H_{25}N_5O_{12}$	491.4		+37° (20), 1.0 in H_2O	3.2, 7.3, and 9.3	262, (170), 0.05 N HCl; 264, (134), 0.05 N NaOH
polyoxin H	[24695-54-3]	(38)	$C_{23}H_{32}N_6O_{13}$	600.5		−38 (20), 1.0 in H_2O	3.3, 7.2, and 9.4	265, (127), 0.05 N HCl; 266, (103), 0.05 N NaOH
polyoxin I	[22886-33-5]	(38)	$C_{17}H_{22}N_4O_9$	500.4		−35° (20), 1.0 in H_2O	2.6, 6.2, and 9.3	262.5, (165), 0.05 N HCl; 264, (123), 0.05 N NaOH
polyoxin J	[22976-89-2]	(38)	$C_{17}H_{25}N_5O_{12}$	491.4		+31.7° (20), 1.0 in H_2O	3.0, 7.1, and 9.9	264, (7,940), 0.05 N HCl; 267, (6,310), 0.05 N NaOH
polyoxin K	[22886-46-0]	(38)	$C_{22}H_{30}N_6O_{13}$	586.5		−16.5° (20), 1.0 in H_2O	3.0, 7.2, and 9.3	259, (10,000), 0.05 N HCl; 262, (7,940), 0.05 N NaOH
polyoxin L	[22976-90-5]	(38)	$C_{16}H_{23}N_5O_{12}$	477.4		+34.4° (20), 1.0 in H_2O	3.0, 7.1 and 9.4	259, (10,000), 0.05 N HCl; 262, (7,940), 0.5 N NaOH
psicofuranine	[1874-54-0]	(31)	$C_{11}H_{15}N_5O_5$	297.3	212–214 dec	−53.7° (25), 1.0 in DMSO		259, (508), 0.01 N H_2SO_4; 261, (530), 0.01 N NaOH
puromycin	[53-79-2]	(41)	$C_{22}H_{29}N_7O_5$	471.5	175–177	−11° (25), 1.0 in C_2H_5OH		267.5, (19,500), 0.1 N HCl; 275, (20,300), 0.1 N NaOH
pyrazofurin	[31660-71-6]	(3)	$C_9H_{13}N_3O_6$	259.2	108–113	−47° (25), 1.25 in H_2O	6.7	263, (6,200), H_2O; 307, (8,100), pH 12
pyrazofurin B	[41855-21-4]		$C_9H_{13}N_3O_6$	259.2				
sangivamycin	[18417-89-5]	(16)	$C_{12}H_{15}N_5O_5$	309.3	260 dec	−45.7° (26), 1.0 in 1.0 N HCl		278, (15,100), C_2H_5OH; 229, (8,200), C_2H_5OH; 273, (12,800), pH 1; 228, (9,500), pH 1; 227, (14,100), pH 11; 277, (14,400), pH 11

Table 2 (*continued*)

Compound	CAS Registry No.	Structure no.	Mol formula	Mol wt	mp, °C	$[\alpha]_D^{(t)a}$, c^b	pK_a	UV max, nm, $(E_{1cm}^{1\%})$ solvent^c
septacidin	[62362-59-8]	(42)	$C_{30}H_{51}N_7O_7$	621.8	215–220 dec	+6.6° (23), 1.0 in DMF		264, (253), CH$_3$OH; 272, (275), 0.1 N NaOH
showdomycin	[16755-07-0]	(4)	$C_9H_{11}NO_6$	229.2	160–161	+49.9° (22.5), 1.0 in H$_2$O	9.29	220, (442), H$_2$O
spongosine	[24723-77-1]	(13)	$C_{11}H_{15}N_5O_5$	297.3	192–193 dec	−42.5° (25), 0.8 in 8% NaOH		274, (11,900), pH 1; 249, (8,350), pH 1; 268, (12,700), pH 13
spongothymidine	[605-23-2]	(21)	$C_{10}H_{14}N_2O_6$	258.3	246–247	+80° (25), 1.1 in 8% NaOH		268, (9,590), H$_2$O; 270, (7,870), pH 13
spongouridine	[3083-77-0]	(22)	$C_9H_{12}N_2O_6$	244.3	226–228	+126° (na), 1.0 in H$_2$O		263, (10,500), H$_2$O
streptothricin A	[3484-67-1]	(43)	$C_{49}H_{94}N_{18}O_{13}$	1143.4				
streptothricin B	[3484-68-2]	(43)	$C_{43}H_{82}N_{16}O_{12}$	1015.3				
streptothricin C	[3776-36-1]	(43)	$C_{37}H_{70}N_{14}O_{11}$	887.1				
streptothricin D	[3776-37-2]	(43)	$C_{31}H_{58}N_{12}O_{10}$	758.9			7.1, 8.2, and 10.1	
streptothricin E	[3776-38-3]	(43)	$C_{25}H_{46}N_{10}O_9$	630.7				
streptothricin F	[3808-42-2]	(43)	$C_{19}H_{34}N_8O_8$	502.5				
streptothricin X	[24543-64-4]	(43)	$C_{55}H_{106}N_{20}O_{14}$	1271.6				
toyocamycin	[606-58-6]	(15)	$C_{12}H_{13}N_5O_4$	291.3	247–250	−51.3° (25), 1.4 in H$_2$O; −45.7° (16), 1.05 in 0.1 N HCl		231, (9,300), C$_2$H$_5$OH; 278, (15,100), C$_2$H$_5$OH; 232, (16,000), 0.1 N HCl; 272, (12,200), 0.1 N HCl; 277, (10,200), pH 11; 277, (14,300), pH 11
tubercidin	[69-33-0]	(14)	$C_{11}H_{14}N_4O_4$	266.3	247–248 dec	−67° (17), 1.0 in 50% CH$_3$COOH	5.3	272, (12,200), 0.01 N HCl; 227, na, 0.01 N HCl; 270, (12,100), 0.01 N NaOH

^{a} Temperature °C is shown parenthetically.
^{b} c = concentration by volume, g/100 mL solvent.
^{c} na = not available.
^{d} Decoyinine resolidifies at 150°C.

188

Formycin (**9**) [7-amino-3-(β-D-ribofuranosyl)-1*H*-pyrazol [4,3-*d*]pyrimidine; formycin A] was isolated from *Nocardia interforma* (65) and from *S. lavendulae* (66). It is sol in H_2O and methanol; mod sol in ethanol; insol in acetone and ether. Structure proof was obtained by x-ray and spectral analysis (67–70), and by degradation (68). The antibiotic is effective against *X. oryzae* and *P. filamentosa* which infect the rice plant (65,71–72). It is also active against some experimental tumors *in vitro* and *in vivo* (65,72). Its LD_{50} iv and ip is 250–500 mg/kg. Formycin is biochemically activated by phosphorylation, and interferes with DNA synthesis as well as a host of other metabolic functions (73–74).

Formycin B (**10**) [1,6-dihydro-3-(β-D-ribofuranosyl)-7*H*-pyrazolo [4,3-*d*]pyrimidin-7-one; laurusin; oyamycin] was isolated from *N. interforma* (75) and *S. lavendulae* (66). It is sol in H_2O and insol in most organic solvents. Its structure was determined by degradation, spectral and x-ray analysis (68–70,76). It inhibits *X. oryzae*, a fungus which produces rice plant blight (66), and interferes with influenza A virus replication in chick chorioallantoic membrane (76–77). The LD_{50} in mice is about 100 mg/kg iv (12). Formycins A and B are interconvertible (78).

Oxoformycin B (**11**) [3-(β-D-ribofuranosyl)-1*H*-pyrazolo [4,3-*d*]-pyrimidine-5,7 (4*H*,6*H*)-dione] was isolated from *N. interforma* (78), and is not inhibitory to *X. oryzae* (77). It is derived from formycin B (78).

Nebularine (**12**) (9β-D-ribofuranosyl-9*H*-purine) was isolated from *Agaricus* (clitocybe) *nebularis* (Batsch) (79) and *S. yokosukanensis* (80). It is sol in H_2O and sl sol in organic solvents. Its structure was determined by degradation (81–82) and by synthesis (83–85). It inhibits the growth of *M. tuberculosis* and of *B. abortus* (79,86), is markedly cytotoxic to mammalian cells (81–82,87), is active against experimental tumors (88), and inhibits influenza B virus replication (89). Its LD_{50} sc (subcutaneous) to rats and guinea pigs is 220 and 15 mg/kg, respectively (90).

Spongosine (**13**) (9β-D-ribofuranosyl-2-methoxyadenine) was isolated from the sponge *Cryptotethia crypta* (91–92). Its structure was determined by degradation (92–94) and by synthesis (94–95).

Tubercidin (**14**) [4-amino-7β-D-ribofuranosyl-7*H*-pyrrolo [2,3-*d*]pyrimidine; 7-deazaadenosine; sparsamycin A] was isolated from *S. tubercidicus* (96), from *S. sparsogenes* (97) and *S. cuspidosporus* (98). It is sl sol in H_2O, readily sol in acid or alkali, and insol in most organic solvents (99–100). The structure of tubercidin was established by degradation (99–102), x-ray analysis (103–104), and by total synthesis (105). The antibiotic is a potent inhibitor of the growth of various microbial species, is highly cytotoxic to a variety of tumor cells, and interferes with the replication of some RNA and DNA viruses (for reviews see Refs. 106–107). Applied topically in a lipophilic base, tubercidin is effective against basal cell carcinoma in man (108). In the housefly it acts as a chemosterilant (109). The LD_{50} for mice ip is 35 mg/kg and for rats 1.5 mg/kg (110). In living cells, tubercidin is phosphorylated to the nucleoside triphosphate stage, and is incorporated into RNA and DNA. It interferes with a variety of cellular functions, resulting in the inhibition of RNA, DNA and protein synthesis (105–106).

Toyocamycin (**15**) (4-amino-7β-D-ribofuranosyl-7*H*-pyrrolo[2,3-*d*]pyrimidine-5-carbonitrile; 4-amino-5-cyano-7-(β-D-ribofuranosyl)-7*H*-pyrrolo [2,3-*d*] pyrimidine; unamycin B; vengicide) has been isolated from *S. toyocaensis* (111), various *Streptomyces* sp (112–115), *S. fungicidicus* (116), *S. vendargensis* (117), and *S. rimosus* (118). It is sol in acidic soln; sl sol in H_2O, methanol, ethanol, and acetone; insol in chloroform and ethyl acetate. Its structure was established by degradation (112, 119) and by total synthesis (120–121). Toyocamycin inhibits various *Candida, Trychophyton,* and *Mycobacterial* species (122), and is active against some experimental tumors *in vitro* (123). Severe local toxicity limits its value as an antitumor agent in man (124). Its LD_{50} in mice is 20 mg/kg ip (123) and 10 mg/kg iv (122).

Sangivamycin (**16**) (4-amino-7β-D-ribofuranosyl-7*H*-pyrrolo [2,3-*d*]pyrimidine-5-carboxamide; 4-amino-5-carboxamido-7-(β-D-ribofuranosyl)pyrrolo [2,3-*d*] pyrimidine) was isolated from *S. rimosus* (125) and its structure determined by degradation (126) and by total synthesis (121). It is sol in acidic H_2O, methanol, pyridine, and DMF; sl sol in H_2O and lower alcohols; and insol in most other organic solvents. The antibiotic is active against various experimental tumors *in vitro* and *in vivo* (125). An enzyme extract from a sangivamycin producing *streptomyces* sp converts the nitrile group of toyocamycin to the carboxamide group of sangivamycin (127–128).

Nucleosides with Modifications in the Carbohydrate Portion

Hikizimycin (**17**) (1-*N*-[2-*O*-(3-amino-3-deoxy-β-D-glucopyranosyl)-4-amino-4-deoxy-D-glycero-D-galacto-D-gluco-β-D-undecopyranosyl]cytosine) was isolated

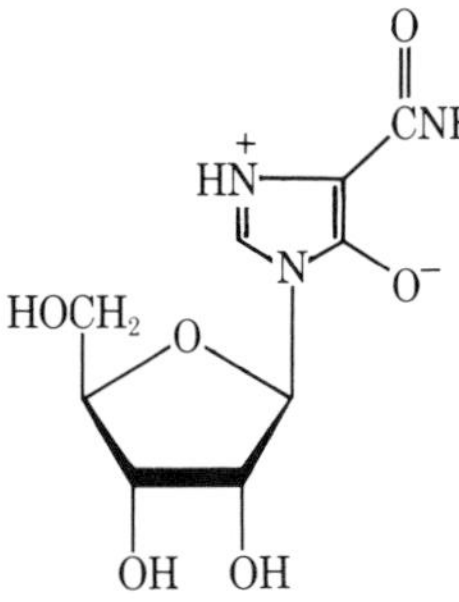

(**5**)
bredinin

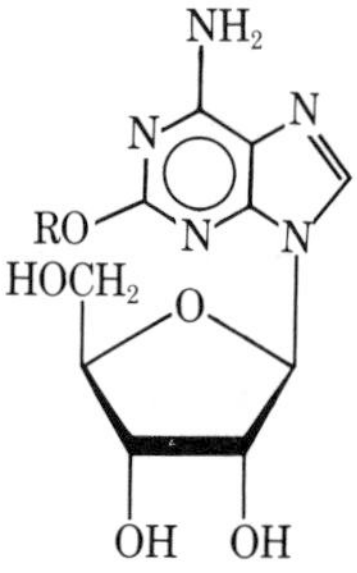

(**6**) R = H
crotonoside
(**13**) R = CH₃
spongosine

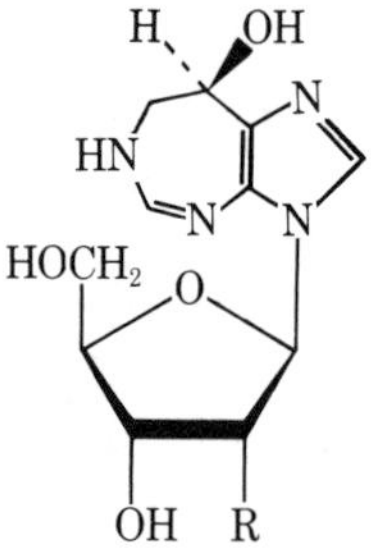

(**7**) R = OH
coformycin
(**8**) R = H
2′-deoxycoformycin

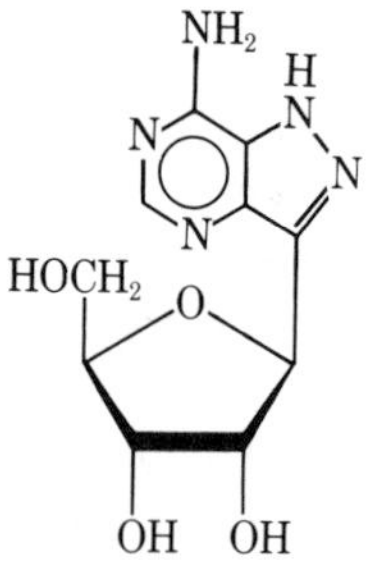

(**9**)
formycin

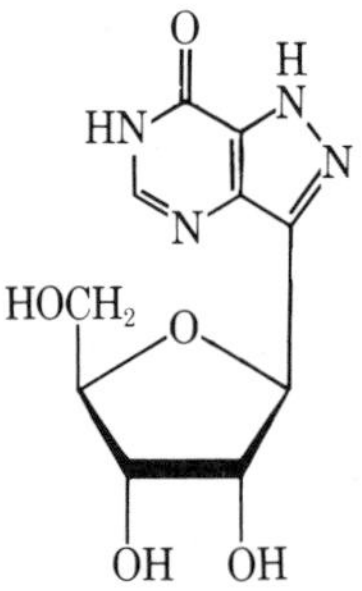

(**10**)
formycin B

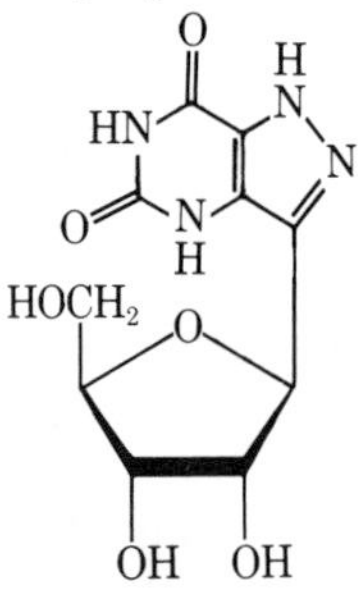

(**11**)
oxoformycin B

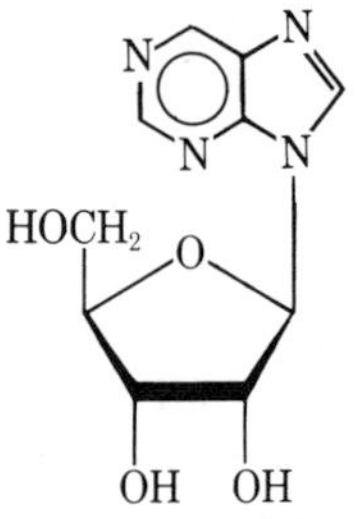

(**12**)
nebularine

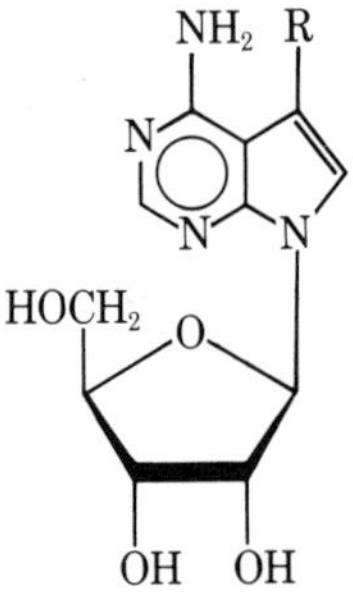

(**14**) R = H
tubercidin
(**15**) R = CN
toyocamycin

(**16**) R = CNH₂
sangivamycin

from *Streptomyces* sp (129) *Helminthosporium hikizimycin* (130) and its structure was determined by degradation and by spectral analysis (131–133). Heating of hikizimycin hydrobromide leads to color change at 214–215°C and darkening at 230°C without melting up to 300°C. The hydrobromide derivative is highly sol in H_2O, sl sol in methanol, and insol in other organic solvents. The compound inhibits the growth of some bacteria and fungi (129). It interferes with protein synthesis by inhibiting ribosomal peptidyl transferase activity (134).

Octosyl acids (**18**) have the following structures: (**a**) 1β-(3,7-anhydro-6-deoxy-D-*glycero*-D-*allo*-octafuranosyluronic acid)-5-carboxyuracil; (**b**) 1β-(3,7-anhydro-6-deoxy-D-*glycero*-D-*allo*-octafuranosyluronic acid)-5-hydroxymethyluracil; and (**c**) 1β-(3,7-anhydro-6-deoxy-D-*glycero*-L-*lyxo*-octofuranos-5-urosyluronic acid)-5-carboxyuracil. The antibiotics were isolated from *S. cacaoi* var. *asoensis*, and their structure determined by spectral analysis (135).

Pentopyranine A (**19**) [1-(2,3-dideoxy-α-L-*glycero*-pentopyranosyl)cytosine; 1α-(2,3-dideoxy-L-arabinopyranosyl cytosine] was isolated from *S. griseochromogenes* (136). Its structure was determined by degradation, spectral analysis (136–137), and by chemical synthesis (138).

Pentopyranine C (**20**) [1-(3-deoxy-α-L-*threo*-pentopyranosyl)cytosine; 1α-(3-deoxy-L-arabinopyranosyl)cytosine] was isolated from *S. griseochromogenes* (136). Its structure was determined by degradation and spectral analysis (137) and by chemical synthesis (139).

Pentopyranines B and D are two additional cytosine nucleosides which have been isolated from *S. griseochromogenes* together with pentopyranines A and C. By 1977, their structure has not been unequivocally established.

The pentopyranines have not shown inhibitory activity against the microbial and fungal systems in which they were examined. They have demonstrated some slight inhibition of ^3H-uridine incorporation into Ehrlich ascites cells.

Spongothymidine (**21**) (1β-D-arabinofuranosylthymine) was isolated from the sponge *Cryptotethia crypta* (140). Its structure was determined by degradation (141) and synthesis (142–143).

Spongouridine (**22**) (1β-D-arabinofuranosyluracil) was isolated from the sponge *Cryptotethia crypta* (144–145). Its structure was determined by degradation (144–145) and synthesis (146). Inhibitory activity against *E. coli* has been observed (147).

Aristeromycin (**23**) (1'R,2'S,3'R,4'R-9-[β-2'α,3'α-dihydroxy-4'β-(hydroxymethyl)cyclopentyl]adenine) was isolated from *S. citricolor* (148). Its structure determined by nmr, x-ray analysis (149), and total synthesis (150–151). Aristeromycin is sol in H_2O, acetic acid DMSO, and DMF; and insol in many other organic solvents. It is active against *X. oryzae* and *P. oryzae* which cause blast disease of rice (1), and against H. Ep. no. 2 cells *in vitro* (152).

2'-Amino-2'-deoxyguanosine (**24**) (9β-D-2'-amino-2-deoxy*erythro*pentofuranosyl guanine) was isolated from *Aerobacter* KY 3071 (153); and its structure was determined by degradation and spectral analysis (153). It shows activity against *E. coli* KY 8323 and HeLa cells *in vitro*, and against solid sarcoma 180 *in vivo* (153).

3'-Amino-3'-deoxyadenosine (**25**) [9-(3'-amino-3'-deoxyribofuranosyl)adenine] was isolated from *Helminthosporium* sp (154) and from *Cordyceps militaris* (155). Its structure was determined by degradation, spectral analysis (154–155), and by synthesis (156). The antibiotic showed activity against *Cryptococcus neoformans* and

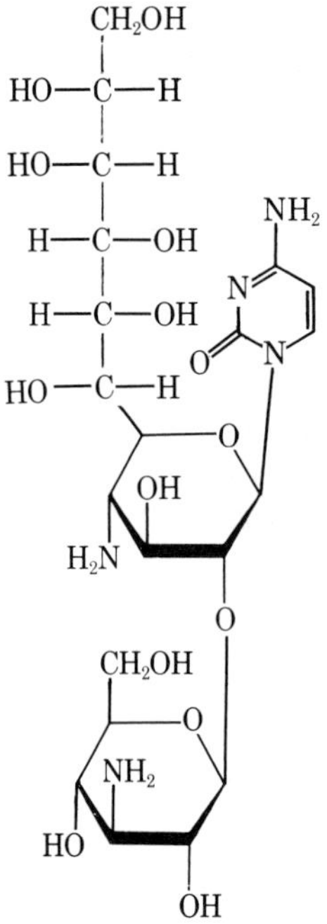

(18)
octosyl acid

(17)
hikizimycin

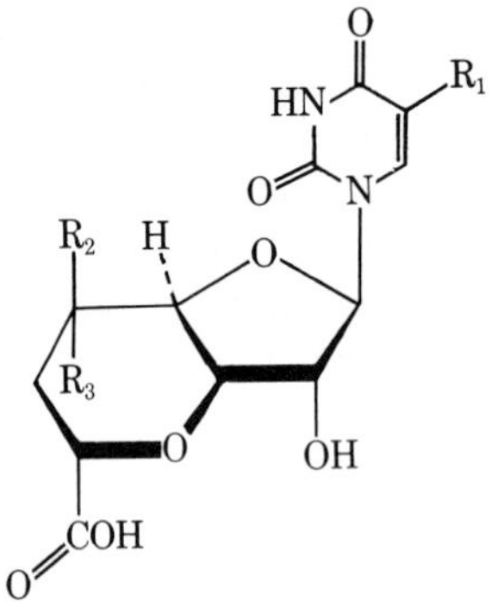

	R₁	R₂	R₃
(a)	$\overset{O}{\overset{\|}{C}}OH$	OH	H
(b)	CH_2OH	OH	H
(c)	$\overset{O}{\overset{\|}{C}}OH$	R₂, R₃ = O	

(as-fused ring system)

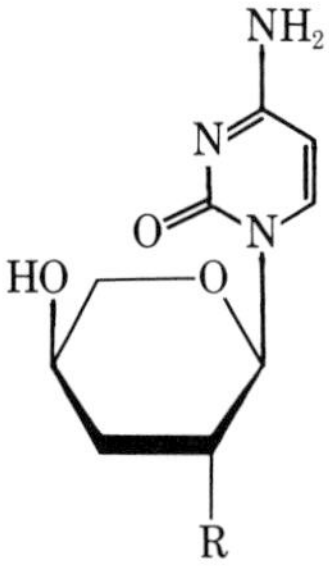

(19) R = H
pentopyranine A
(20) R = OH
pentopyranine C

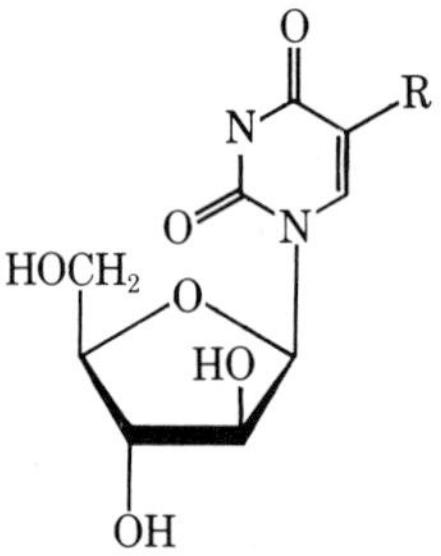

(21) R = CH₃
spongothymidine
(22) R = H
spongouridine

Candida albicans (3), and against some experimental tumors *in vitro* (156) and *in vivo* (157). It inhibits RNA and DNA synthesis in Ehrlich ascites cells, and RNA polymerase activity *in vitro* (74). Its LD$_{50}$ in mice is 28 mg/kg ip (154).

3'-Acetamido-3'-deoxyadenosine (**26**) (9β-D-3'-acetamido-3'-deoxy*erythro*-pentofuranosyladenine) was isolated from *Helminthosporium* sp 215; and its structure was determined by degradation and spectral analysis (158). It has been synthesized (159).

Spongoadenosine (**27**) (9β-D-arabinofuranoxyladenine; Ara-A; vidarabine) was isolated from *S. antibioticus* (160), subsequent to its chemical synthesis (161–164). It has shown activity against certain DNA viruses (165–166), bacteria (167) and experimental tumors (168), particularly when administered in conjunction with co-formycin or 2'-deoxycoformycin which prevent its rapid deamination (169–171). Enzymes inhibited by arabinosyl adenine include DNA polymerase (172–173) ribonucleotide reductase (174–175), and polynucleotide phosphorylase (176). Incorporation of the compound into polynucleotides leads to chain termination (177–178). The LD_{50} in mice is ip 4.68 mg/kg and po (*per os* oral) 7.8 mg/kg.

Cordycepin (**28**) (3'-deoxyadenosine; 9β-D-3'-deoxyerythropentofuranosyl adenine) was isolated from *Cordyceps militaris* (179–180) and from *Aspergillus nidulans* (181). Its structure was determined by degradation and spectral analysis (182–185) and by total synthesis (186–188). Cordycepin is sol in H_2O, hot ethanol, and methanol; and insol in many other organic solvents. Inhibitory activity of the compound against *B. subtilis* and *M. tuberculosis* (179) and against various tumor cell lines *in vitro* (181) and *in vivo* (189) has been observed. Among its biochemical effects are interference with RNA synthesis (190–193) and with purine *de novo* synthesis at the level of phosphoribosyl pyrophosphate amidotransferase (194) and ribose phosphate pyrophosphokinase (195).

Decoyinine (**29**) (9-(6-deoxy-β-D-erythro-hex-5-en-2-ulofuranosyl)-6-aminopurine; angustmycin A) was isolated from *S. hydroscopicus* var. *decoyicus* and var. *angustmyceticus* (196–198) and its structure determined by degradation and spectral analysis (196–197,199), and by synthesis (200–201). It has been demonstrated to inhibit mycobacteria (196), gram-positive bacteria (202), and some experimental tumors (203). The oral and parenteral LD_{50} for mice is 2.5 mg/kg (204). Decoyinine interferes with the enzymatic conversion of xanthosine-5'-phosphate to guanosine-5'-phosphate (205–206) and with ribose phosphate pyrophosphokinase activity (207).

Nucleocidin (**30**) [9-(4-fluoro-5-O-sulfamoyl-β-D-*erythro*-pentofuranosyl)adenine] was isolated from *S. calvus* (205–210). It was found to be active against trypanosomes (equiperdum, congolense, equinum, gambiense) in rats and mice (211), *M. pneumoniae* (212), and various gram-positive and gram-negative bacteria (209). Nucleocidin is sol in acid, methanol, and acetone; and insol in most other organic solvents. Its structure was determined by degradation, physical–chemical data (213–216), and synthesis (217).

Psicofuranine (**31**) (9β-D-psicofuranosyladenine; 6-amino-9β-D-psicofuranosyl purine; angustmycin C) was isolated from *S. hygroscopicus* var. *decoyicus* (218–220). Its structure was determined by degradation (221), spectral analysis (202), and synthesis (218,223–224). Psicofuranine has restricted solubility in H_2O and lower alcohols. It has demonstrated activity against *M. tuberculosis* (219) and protects mice against *S. hemolyticus*, *S. aureus*, and *E. coli* infections (225). It is also effective against various experimental tumors, and its LD_{50} in mice is 1700 mg/kg ip (226). In man the compound produces pericarditis (227–228). Psicofuranine interferes with the enzymatic amination of xanthosine-5'-phosphate to guanosine-5'-phosphate (229–231).

Nucleosides with Aminoacyl or Peptidyl Residues

Amicetin (**32**) (allomycin; sacromycin) was isolated from *S. vinaceus-drappus* (232–233), *S. fasciculatis* (234), and *S. plicatus* (235). Its structure was determined by degradation (236–239) and partial synthesis (230–242). Amicetin is sol in H_2O and dilute acid; and insol in most organic solvents. The antibiotic has been shown active against gram-positive and gram-negative bacteria, as well as against mycoplasma

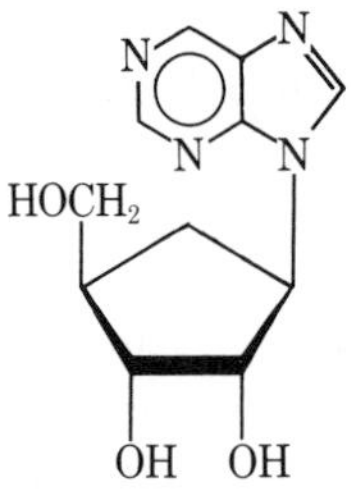

(23)
aristeromycin

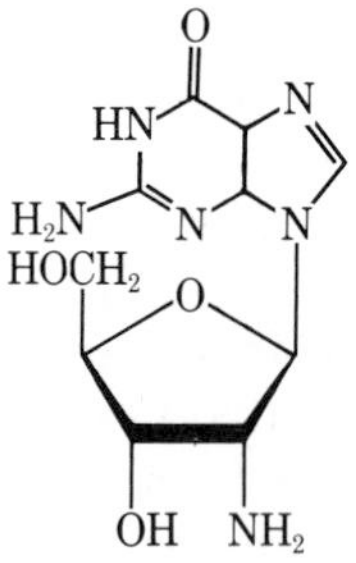

(24)
2′-amino-2′-deoxyguanosine

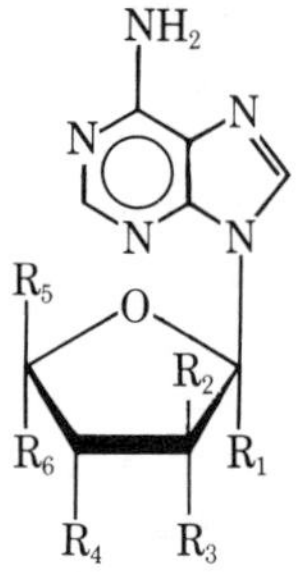

	R_1	R_2	R_3	R_4	R_5	R_6
(25) 3′-amino-3′-deoxyadenosine	H	H	OH	NH_2	CH_2OH	H
(26) 3′-acetamido-3′-deoxyadenosine	H	H	OH	$NHCCH_3$ ($\overset{O}{\parallel}$)	CH_2OH	H
(27) arabinofuranosyladenine (Ara-A)	H	OH	H	OH	CH_2OH	H
(28) cordycepin	H	H	OH	H	CH_2OH	H
(29) decoyinine	CH_2OH	H	OH	OH	$R_5,R_6 = CH_2$	
(30) nucleocidin	H	H	OH	OH	CH_2OSNH_2 ($\overset{O}{\underset{O}{\parallel\parallel}}$)	F
(31) psicofuranine	CH_2OH	H	OH	OH	CH_2OH	H

(232,243–246) and it inhibits the growth of some experimental tumors *in vitro* (247) and *in vivo* (248). Its inhibitory activity is due to interference with peptide bond formation (249–251).

Bamicetin (**33**) was isolated from *S. plicatus* (252) and its structure determined by degradation (252–253). It is active against some microorganisms, including *E. coli* (252) and *M. fortuitum* (254).

Plicacetin (**34**) (amicetin B) was isolated from *S. plicatus* (252) and another *Streptomyces* sp (255). Its structure was determined by degradation (252,256) and total synthesis. Activity against some mycobacteria has been observed (252).

Blasticidin S (**35**) ((S)-4-[[3-amino-5-[(aminoiminomethyl)methylamino]-1-oxopentyl]amino]-1-(4-amino-2-oxo-1-(2H)-pyrimidinyl)-1,2,3,4-tetradeoxy-β-D-*erythro*-hex-2-enopyranuronic acid; 1-(1′-cytosinyl)-4-[L-3′-amino-5′-(1″-Nmethylguanidino)-valerylamino]-1,2,3,4-tetradeoxy-β-D-*erythro*-hex-2-enuronic acid) was isolated from *S. griseochromogenes* (257) and from *S. morookaensis* (258) together with other members of the group including Blasticidin A, B, C (259). It is sol in water and acetic acid; and insol in most organic solvents. Its structure was determined by degradation (259), spectral and x-ray analysis (260–261), and partial synthesis (262–264). The antibiotic inhibits various gram-positive and gram-negative bacteria, and is particularly effective against *P. oryzae* (265) and against stripe virus (266), which infect the rice plant. Blasticidin S inhibits protein synthesis by interfering with peptide chain elongation (73–74).

Gougerotin (**36**) 1-(4-amino-2-oxo-1(2H)-pyrimidinyl)-1,4-dideoxy-4-[D-2-[2-(methylamino)acetamido]hydracrylamido]glucopyranuronamide; asteromycin (267); aspiculamycin (268) was isolated from *S. gougerotii* (269), and its structure was elucidated by degradation (270–272) and total synthesis (273). It is active *in vitro* against a variety of gram-positive and gram-negative microorganisms (269) and against some RNA and DNA viruses (274). Its LD_{50} in mice is 57 mg/kg iv and 250 mg/kg ip (3). The compound inhibits protein synthesis by interfering with peptide chain elongation (73–74).

Oxamicetin (**37**) is an antibiotic closely related to amicetin. It is freely sol in acidic H_2O, methanol, ethanol, and butanol; and insol in other common organic solvents (275). The mp of its hydrochloride is 205–210°C. The antibiotic was isolated from *Arthrobacter oxamicetus* (276), and its structure determined by degradation, spectral analysis (277), and partial synthesis (278–279). It is active against gram-positive and gram-negative bacteria and, when given sc (subcutaneous), it protected mice against *S. aureus* and *E. coli* infections. The LD_{50} iv in mice is 200 mg/kg (275).

Polyoxins (**38**) are 12 peptide nucleosides (A–L) of the same general structure (280). The family was isolated from *S. cacaoi* var. *asoensis* (281–283). The heterocycle is uracil, thymine, 5-hydroxymethyluracil, or uracil-5-carboxylic acid. The antibiotics, except C or I, are active against phytopathogenic fungi, particularly *Pellicularia filimentosa sasakii*, causing sheath blight of the rice plant (280). The inhibition appears to result from interference with cell wall chitin synthesis (284).

Homocitrullyaminoadenosine (**39**) was isolated from *Cordyceps militaris* (285). Degradation and spectral data (285) are suggestive of the proposed structure, but do not prove it (73). The compound interferes with the transfer of amino acids from aminoacyl transfer-RNA (t-RNA) to the growing peptide chain (286).

Lysylaminoadenosine (**40**) was isolated from *Cordyceps militaris* (287). Its structure was derived by degradation and spectral data (287), but these are not conclusive (73).

Puromycin (**41**) (6-dimethylamino-9-[3-deoxy-3-(1-methoxy-L-phenylalanylamino)-β-D-ribofuranosyl]-β-purine; (*S*)-3′-[[2-amino-3-(4-methoxyphenyl)-1-oxopropyl]amino]-3′-deoxy-N,N-dimethyladenosine; stylomycin; originally called Achromycin) was isolated from *S. alboniger* (288). Its structure was established by degradation (289) and total synthesis (290). Puromycin has demonstrated *in vitro* activity against gram-positive and gram-negative bacteria (288), *in vivo* activity against various species of trypanosomes (288,291–293), entamoeba (294–296), oxyurids and tapeworms (297), and against various experimental tumors *in vitro* and *in vivo* (298–299). It appears to act as a functional analogue of aminoacyl-t-RNA (structural resemblance to aminoacyl terminal region), and reacts with peptidyl-t-RNA to form

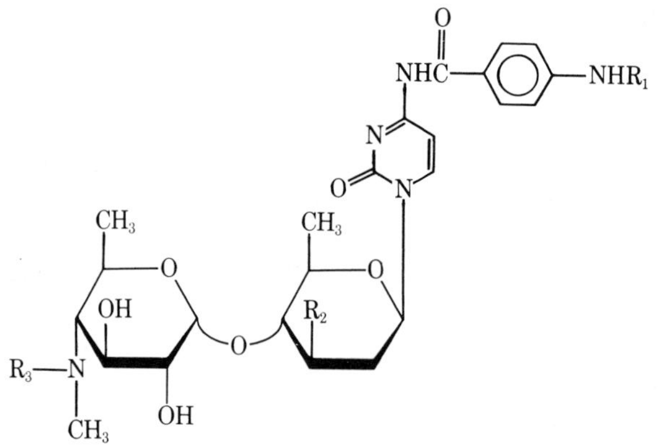

	R₁	R₂	R₃
(**32**) amicetin	$\underset{NH_2}{\overset{\overset{\displaystyle O}{\parallel}}{CC(CH_3)CH_2OH}}$	H	CH₃
(**33**) bamicetin	$\underset{NH_2}{\overset{\overset{\displaystyle O}{\parallel}}{CC(CH_3)CH_2OH}}$	H	H
(**34**) plicacetin	H	H	CH₃
(**37**) oxamicetin	$\underset{NH_2}{\overset{\overset{\displaystyle O}{\parallel}}{CC(CH_3)CH_2OH}}$	OH	CH₃

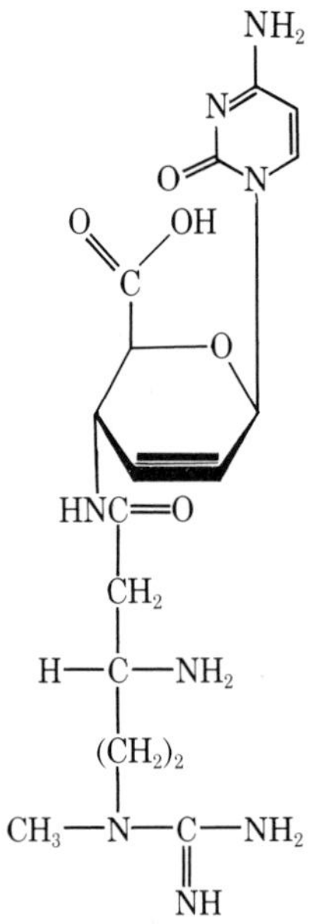

(**35**)
blasticidin S

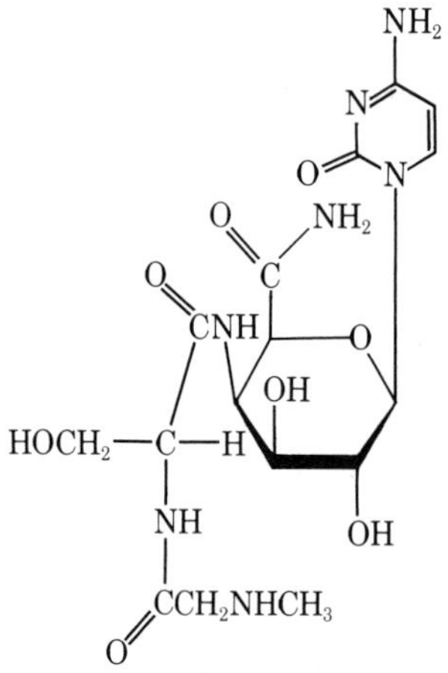

(**36**)
gougerotin

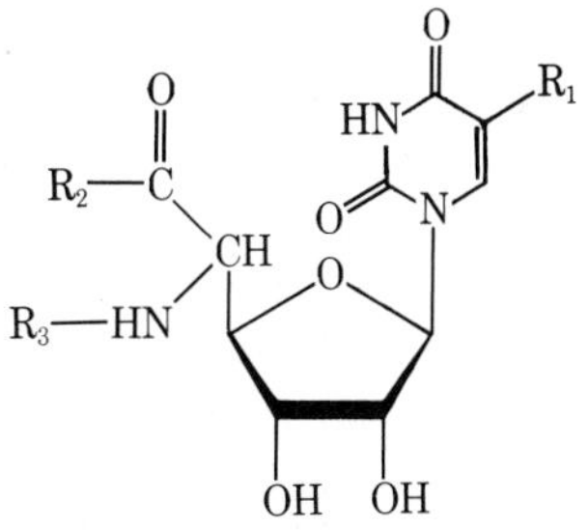

(38)
polyoxin A–L

	R₁	R₂	R₃	R₄
A	CH₂OH	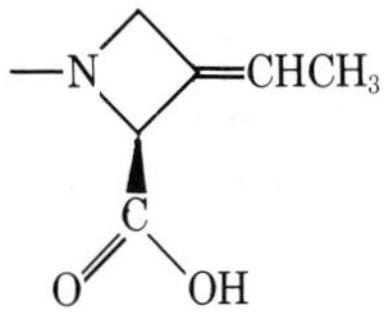 (azetidine ring with =CHCH₃ and C(=O)OH)	a	OH
B	CH₂OH	OH	a	OH
C	CH₂OH	OH	H	
D	COOH	OH	a	OH
E	COOH	OH	a	H
F	COOH	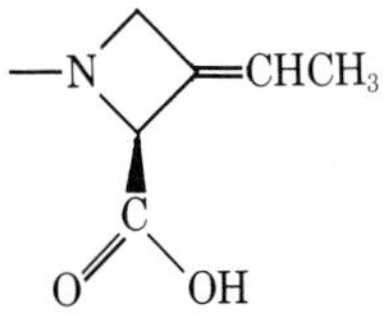 (azetidine ring with =CHCH₃ and C(=O)OH)	a	OH
G	CH₂OH	OH	a	H
H	CH₃	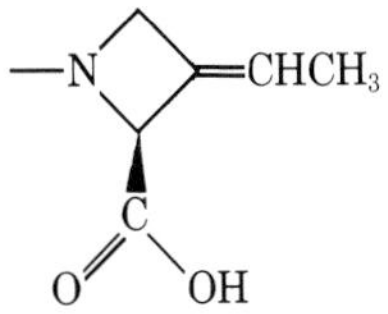 (azetidine ring with =CHCH₃ and C(=O)OH)	a	OH
I	CH₂OH	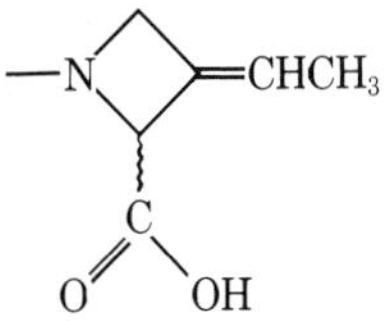 (azetidine ring with =CHCH₃ and C(=O)OH)	H	
J	CH₃	OH	a	OH
K	H	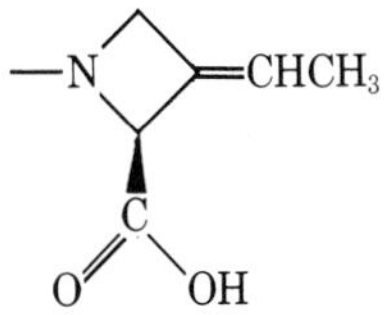 (azetidine ring with =CHCH₃ and C(=O)OH)	a	OH
L	H	OH	a	OH

a for polyoxins A, B, D–H, and J–L:

$$R_3 = $$

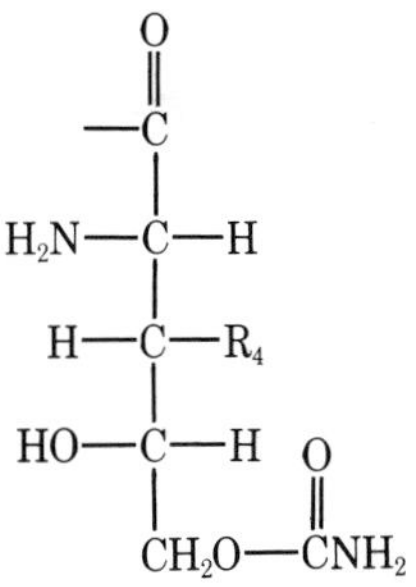

(structure showing amino acid / sugar chain:
—C(=O)—
H₂N—C—H
H—C—R₄
HO—C—H   O
CH₂O—CNH₂)

peptidyl puromycin, which terminates chain elongation and causes the release of the incomplete peptide chains from the messenger RNA–ribosome complex (73–74). Its LD_{50} in mice is approximately 350 mg/kg iv and 550 mg/kg ip (291,300).

The aminonucleoside of puromycin [58-60-6] (3'-amino-3'-deoxy-N,N-dimethyladenosine) was obtained by chemical synthesis (301). It is also effective against trypanosomal infections in mice (302–303), but it produces a chracteristic nephrotic syndrome (304). The compound appears to act primarily by inhibition of t-RNA synthesis (305–306).

Septacidin (**42**) was isolated from *S. fimbriatus* and its structure established by degradation and spectral analysis (307–308). It inhibits the growth of several filamentous fungi, Earle's L cells in culture, and carcinoma 755 in mice (307). The LD_{10} in mice of 0.88 mg/(kg·d) for a week (307).

Nucleosides with Modifications in Both the Aglycone and Carbohydrate Moieties

Streptothricins (**43**) (racemomycins (309), yazumycins (310)) differ from each other in the number of L-β-lysine residues in the peptide side chain ranging from 1 to 7 (311), eg, streptothricin F, n = 1; hydrochloride $[\alpha]_D^{25}$ −51.3 (C = 1.4, H$_2$O) (see Table 2); sol in H$_2$O and dilute mineral acids; insol in ether and chloroform. The antibiotic was isolated from *S. lavendulae* (312), and its structure proven by degradation (311,313–314).

Exotoxin of Bacillus Thuringiensis (**44**) has been isolated. Its structure was determined by degradation and spectral analysis (315–318), and by total chemical synthesis (319). Selective insecticidal properties have been ascribed to the compound (317,320).

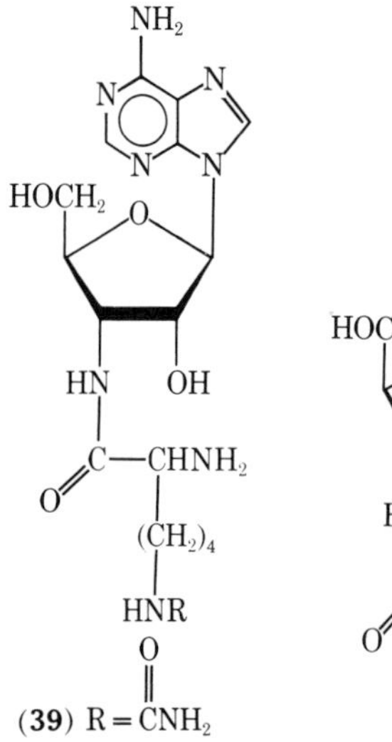

(**39**) R = CNH$_2$
homocitrullylaminoadenosine
(**40**) R = H
lysylaminoadenosine

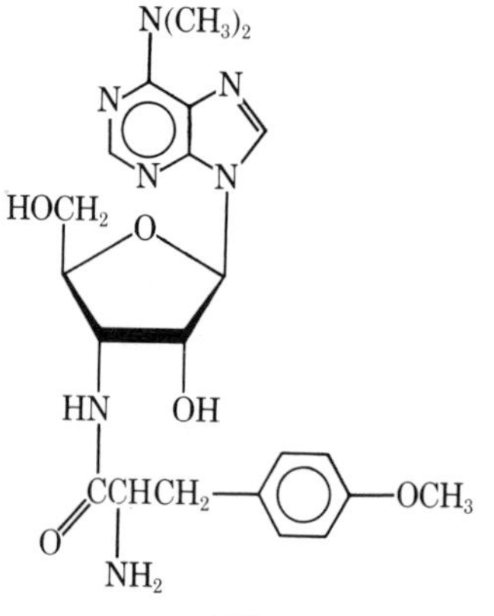

(**41**)
puromycin

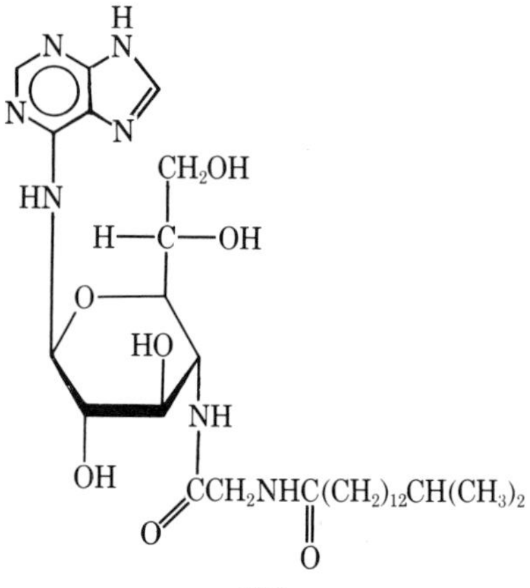

(**42**)
septacidin

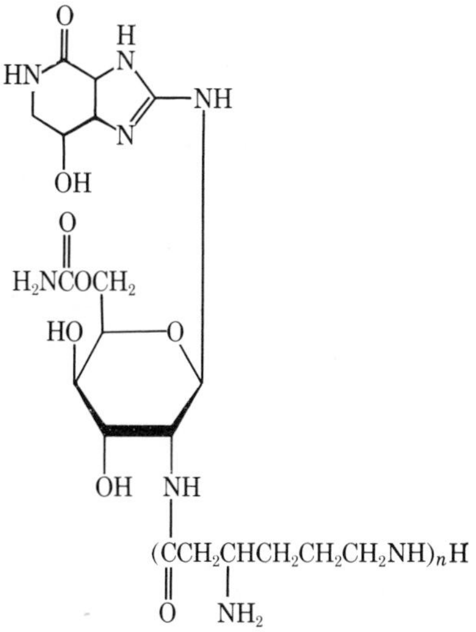

(43)
streptothricin

	n
A	6
B	5
C	4
D	3
E	2
F	1
X	7

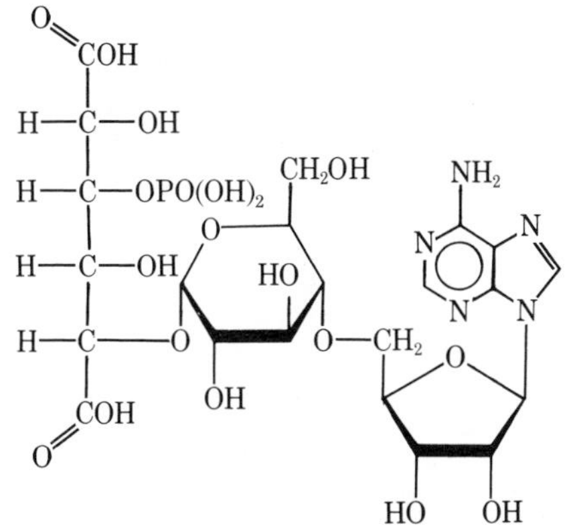

(44)
exotoxin of *Bacillus thuringiensis*

Economic Potential

Some of the nucleoside antibiotics are selective inhibitors of bacterial growth and others effectively interfere with viral replication. Many of them are capable of inhibiting parasitic infections in experimental animals (see Chemotherapeutics), and some are used in the treatment of fungus infections of the economically important rice plant (see Fungicides). Various nucleoside analogues are used in cancer chemotherapy (see Chemotherapeutics), and the cardiovascular (see Cardiovascular agents), immunosuppressive and cytokinin activity of some of the compounds points towards additional areas of use. There can be no doubt that the further evaluation of nucleoside antibiotics will reveal as yet unrecognized forms of activity. This group of agents, in addition to having been of great value in elucidating basic information on cellular biochemistry, has demonstrated its utility or potential for the treatment of pathogenic microorganisms.

BIBLIOGRAPHY

1. G. Chheda in, *Handbook of Biochemistry and Molecular Biology*, 3rd ed. Vol. 1, 1975, p. 251.
2. R. H. Hall, *Progr. Nucleic Acid Res. Mol. Biol.* **10,** 57 (1970).
3. H. Kneifel, W. A. König, G. Wolf, and H. Zähner, *J. Antibiot.* **27,** 20 (1974).
4. C. W. Parker and D. S. Letham, *Biochem. Biophys. Res. Commun.* **49,** 460 (1972).
5. M. Terao and co-workers, *J. Antibiot.* **13A,** 401 (1960).
6. K. Anzai and S. Suzuki, *J. Antibiot.* **14,** 253 (1961).
7. I. R. Spies, *J. Am. Chem. Soc.* **61,** 350 (1939).

8. E. Cullen and J. P. Devlin, *Can. J. Chem.* **53,** 1690 (1975).
9. F. Tanaka and co-workers, *J. Antibiot.* **14A,** 161 (1961).
10. M. E. Bergy and R. R. Herr, *Antimicrob. Agents Chemother.* 625 (1966).
11. L. J. Haňka and co-workers, *Antimicrob. Agents Chemother.* 619 (1966).
12. A Pískala and F. Šorm, *Collect. Czech. Chem. Commun.* **29,** 2060 (1964).
13. M. W. Winkley and R. Robins, *J. Org. Chem.* **35,** 491 (1970).
14. A. Čihák and F. Šorm, *Collect. Czech. Chem. Commun.* **30,** 2091 (1965).
15. F. Šorm and J. Veselý, *Neoplasma* **11,** 123 (1964).
16. M. Karon and co-workers, *Blood* **42,** 359 (1973).
17. K. B. McCredie and co-workers, *Blood* **40,** 975 (1972).
18. J. Veselý, A. Čihák, and F. Šorm, *Biochem. Pharmacol.* **17,** 519 (1968).
19. J. Doskočil, V. Pačes, and F. Šorm, *Biochim. Biophys. Acta* **145,** 771 (1967).
20. A. Čihák, J. Vesely, and F. Šorm, *Biochim. Biophys. Acta* **134,** 486 (1967).
21. I. B. Levitan and T. E. Webb, *Biochim. Biophys. Acta* **182,** 491 (1969).
22. A. Čihak, J. Vesely, and F. Šorm, *Biochim. Biophys. Acta* **166,** 277 (1968).
23. V. Pačes, J. Doskočil, and F. Šorm, *FEBS Lett.* **1,** 55 (1968).
24. T. Haneishi and co-workers, *J. Antibiot.* **24,** 797 (1971).
25. Y. Kusakabe and co-workers, *J. Antibiot.* **25,** 44 (1972).
26. K. Gerzon and co-workers, *2nd International Congress on Heterocycles, Chem. Abstr. C30 Montpelier, France, 1969.*
27. R. H. Williams and co-workers, *158th Meeting of the American Chemical Society, Abstr. Micr. 38, New York, 1969.*
28. F. J. Streightoff and co-workers, *9th Conference Antimicrobial Agents Chemotherapy Abstr. 18, Washington, D.C., 1969.*
29. D. C. DeLong and co-workers, *7th International Congress on Chemotherapy, Prague, Czechoslovakia, 1971.*
30. M. J. Sweeney and co-workers, *Cancer Res.* **33,** 2619 (1973).
31. G. E. Gutowski and co-workers, *Ann. N.Y. Acad. Sci.* **255,** 544 (1975).
32. G. E. Gutowski and co-workers, *Biochem. Biophys. Res. Commun.* **51,** 312 (1973).
33. E. Wenkert, E. W. Hagaman, and G. E. Gutowski, *Biochem. Biophys. Res. Commun.* **51,** 318 (1973).
34. H. Nishimura and co-workers, *J. Antibiot.* **17A,** 148 (1964).
35. S. Matsuura, O. Shiratori, and K. Katagiri, *J. Antibiot.* **17A,** 234 (1964).
36. K. R. Darnall, L. B. Townsend, and R. K. Robins, *Proc. Nat. Acad. Sci. U.S.A.* **57,** 548 (1967).
37. L. Kalvoda, J. Faraks, and F. Sorm, *Tetrahedron Lett.* 2297 (1970).
38. V. Nakagawa and co-workers, *Tetrahedron Lett.* 4105 (1967).
39. R. K. Robins and co-workers, *J. Heterocycl. Chem.* **3,** 110 (1966).
40. Y. Tsukuda and co-workers, *Chem. Commun.* 975 (1967).
41. Y. Komatusu and K. Tanaka, *Agric. Biol. Chem.* **32,** 1021 (1968).
42. S. Roy-Burman, P. Roy-Burman, and D. W. Visser, *Cancer Res.* **28,** 1605 (1968).
43. Y. Titani and Y. Katsube, *Biochim. Biophys. Acta* **192,** 367 (1969).
44. K. Mizuno and co-workers, *J. Antibiot.* **27,** 775 (1974).
45. K. Mizuno and co-workers, *J. Ferment. Technol.* **53,** 609 (1975).
46. K. Sakaguchi and co-workers, *J. Antibiot.* **28,** 798 (1975).
47. E. Cherbuliez and K. Bernhard, *Helv. Chim. Acta* **15,** 464 (1932).
48. Ref. 47, p. 878.
49. R. Falconer, J. M. Gulland, and L. F. Story, *J. Chem. Soc.* 1784 (1939).
50. J. R. Spies and N. L. Drake, *J. Am. Chem. Soc.* **57,** 774 (1935).
51. J. Davoll, *J. Am. Chem. Soc.* **73,** 3174 (1951).
52. J. A. Montgomery and K. Hewson, *J. Org. Chem.* **33,** 432 (1968).
53. H. E. Skipper and co-workers, *Cancer Res.* **19,** 425 (1959).
54. D. A. Clarke and co-workers, *J. Pharmacol. Exp. Ther.* **106,** 291 (1952).
55. E. Mihich, D. A. Clarke, and F. S. Philips, *J. Pharmacol. Exp. Ther.,* **111,** 335 (1954).
56. T. Tsuruoka and co-workers, *Meiji Shika Kenkyu Nempo* **9,** 17 (1967).
57. H. Nakamaru and co-workers, *J. Am. Chem. Soc.* **96,** 4327 (1974).
58. M. Ohno and co-workers, *J. Am. Chem. Soc.* **96,** 4326 (1974).
59. T. Sawa and co-workers, *J. Antibiot.* **20A,** 227 (1967a).
60. T. Shomura and co-workers, *Meiji Shika Kenkyu Nempo* **9,** 21 (1967).
61. P. W. K. Woo and co-workers, *J. Heterocycl. Chem.* **11,** 641 (1974).
62. G. A. LaPage, L. W. Worth, and A. P. Kimball, *Cancer Res.* **36,** 1481 (1976).

63. C. E. Cass and T. H. Au-Yeung, *Cancer Res.* **36,** 1486 (1976).
64. D. G. Johns and R. H. Adamson, *Biochem. Pharmacol.* **25,** 1441 (1976).
65. M. Hori and co-workers, *J. Antibiot.* **17A,** 96 (1964).
66. S. Aizawa and co-workers, *Agric. Biol. Chem.* **29,** 375 (1965).
67. G. Koyama and co-workers, *Tetrahedron Lett.* 597 (1966).
68. K. Kawamura and co-workers, *J. Antibiot.* **19A,** 91 (1966).
69. S. Watanabe and co-workers, *J. Anbitiot.* **19A,** 93 (1966).
70. R. K. Robins and co-workers, *J. Heterocycl. Chem.* **3,** 110 (1966).
71. H. Umezawa and co-workers, *J. Antibiot.* **18A,** 178 (1965).
72. M. Ishizuka and co-workers, *J. Antibiot.* **21A,** 5 (1968).
73. J. J. Fox, K. A. Watanabe, and A. Bloch, *Progr. Nucleic Acid Res. Mol. Biol.* **5,** 251 (1966).
74. R. J. Suhadolnik, *Nucleoside Antibiotics,* Interscience Publishers, a division of John Wiley & Sons, Inc., New York, 1970.
75. G. Koyama and H. Umezawa, *J. Anbitiot.* **18A,** 175 (1965).
76. T. Takeuchi and co-workers, *J. Antibiot.* **29A,** 297 (1967).
77. T. Kunimoto and co-workers, *J. Antibiot.* **21A,** 468 (1968).
78. T. Sawa and co-workers, *J. Antibiot.* **21A,** 334 (1968).
79. L. Ehrenberg and co-workers, *Sven. Kem. Tidsskr.* **58,** 269 (1946).
80. K. Isono and S. Suzuki, *J. Anbitiot.* **13A,** 270 (1960).
81. N. Löfgren and B. Lüning, *Acta Chem. Scand.* **7,** 225 (1953).
82. N. Löfgren, B. Lüning, and H. Hedström, *Acta Chem. Scand.* **8,** 670 (1954).
83. G. B. Brown and V. S. Weliky, *J. Biol. Chem.* **204,** 1019 (1953).
84. J. J. Fox and co-workers, *J. Am. Chem. Soc.* **80,** 1669 (1958).
85. T. Hashizume and H. Iwamura, *Tetrahedron Lett.* 643 (1966).
86. L. Ehrenberg and co-workers, *Sven. Farm. Tidsskr.* **50,** 645 (1946).
87. J. J. Biesele, M. C. Slautterback, and M. Margolis, *Cancer* **8,** 87 (1955).
88. K. Sugiura and M. M. Sugiura, *Cancer Res.* **18**(2), 246 (1958).
89. I. Tamm, K. Folkers, and C. H. Shunk, *J. Bacteriol.* **72,** 59 (1956).
90. A. P. Traunted and H. E. D'Amato, *Fed. Proc.* **14,** 391 (1955).
91. W. Bergmann and R. J. Feeney, *J. Am. Chem. Soc.* **72,** 2809 (1950).
92. W. Bergmann and R. J. Feeney, *J. Org. Chem.* **16,** 981 (1951).
93. W. Bergmann and D. C. Burke, *J. Org. Chem.* **21,** 226 (1956).
94. W. Bergmann and M. F. Stempien, Jr., *J. Org. Chem.* **22,** 1575 (1957).
95. H. J. Schaeffer and H. J. Thomas, *J. Am. Chem. Soc.* **80,** 3738 (1958).
96. K. Anzai and S. Marumo, *J. Antibiot.* **10A,** 20 (1957).
97. U.S. Pat. 3,336,289 (1967), W. J. Wechter and A. R. Hanze.
98. E. Higashide and co-workers, *Takeda Kenkyusho Nempo* **25,** 1 (1966).
99. S. Suzuki and S. Marumo, *J. Antibiot.* **13A,** 360 (1960).
100. S. Suzuki and S. Marumo, *J. Antibiot.* **14A,** 34 (1961).
101. Y. Mizuno and co-workers, *J. Org. Chem.* **28,** 3329 (1963).
102. Y. Mizuno and co-workers, *J. Org. Chem.* **28,** 331 (1963).
103. J. Abola and M. Sundaralingam, *Acta Crystallogr. Sect. B* **29,** 697 (1973).
104. R. M. Stroud, *Acta Crystallogr. Sect. B* **29,** 690 (1973).
105. R. L. Tolman, R. K. Robins, and L. B. Townsend, *J. Heterocycl. Chem.* **4,** 230 (1967).
106. Ref. 74, p. 315.
107. A. Bloch in E. J. Ariens, ed., *Drug Design,* Academic Press, Inc., New York, 1973.
108. G. H. Burgess and co-workers, *Cancer* **34,** 250 (1974).
109. R. E. Kohls, A. J. Lemin, and P. W. O'Connell, *J. Econ. Entomol.* **59,** 745 (1966).
110. S. P. Owen and C. G. Smith, *Cancer Chemother. Rep.* **36,** 19 (1964).
111. H. Nishimura and co-workers, *J. Antibiot.* **9A,** 60 (1956).
112. K. Ohkuma, *J. Antibiot.* **13A,** 361 (1960).
113. H. Yamamoto and co-workers, *Takeda Kenkyusho Nempo* **16,** 26 (1957).
114. K. Kikuchi, *J. Antibiot.* **8A,** 145 (1955).
115. K. Katagiri, K. Sato, and S. Nishiyama, *Shionogi Kenkyusho Nempo* **7,** 715 (1957).
116. M. Matsuoka and H. Umezawa, *J. Antibiot.* **13A,** 114 (1960).
117. Swiss Pat. 331988 (1953), A. A. Stheeman and A. P. Struyk.
118. U.S. Pat. 3,116,222 (1963), K. V. Rao, W. S. Harsh, and D. W. Renn.
119. K. Ohkuma, *J. Antibiot.* **14A,** 343 (1961).
120. R. L. Tolman, R. K. Robins, and L. B. Townsend, *J. Am. Chem. Soc.* **91,** 2102 (1969).
121. R. L. Tolman, R. K. Robins, and L. B. Townsend, *J. Am. Chem. Soc.* **90,** 524 (1968).

122. M. Matsuoka, *J. Antibiot.* **13A,** 121 (1960).
123. M. Saneyoshi, R. Tokuzen, and F. Fukuoka, *Gann* **56,** 219 (1965).
124. W. L. Wilson, *Cancer Chemother. Rep.* **52,** 301 (1968).
125. K. V. Rao and D. W. Renn, *Antimicrob. Agents Chemother.* **1963,** 77.
126. K. V. Rao, *J. Med. Chem.* **11,** 939 (1968).
127. M. E. Smulson and R. J. Suhadolnik, *J. Biol. Chem.* **242,** 2872 (1967).
128. R. J. Suhadolnik and T. Uematsu, *J. Biol. Chem.* **245,** 4365 (1970).
129. K. Uchida and co-workers, *J. Antibiot.* **24,** 259 (1971).
130. Jpn. Kokai 70 39,038 (1970), K. Uchida.
131. K. Uchida and B. C. Das, *Biochimie* **55,** 635 (1973).
132. K. Uchida, E. Breitmaier, and W. A. Koenig, *Tetrahedron* **31,** 2315 (1975).
133. K. Uchida, *Agric. Biol. Chem.* **40,** 395 (1976).
134. K. Uchida and H. Wolf, *J. Antibiot.* **27,** 783 (1974).
135. K. Isono, P. F. Crain, and J. A. McCloskey, *J. Am. Chem. Soc.* **97**(4), 943 (1975).
136. H. Seto, N. Ōtake, and H. Yonehara, *Agric. Biol. Chem.* **37,** 2421 (1973).
137. H. Seto, N. Ōtake, and H. Yonehara, *Tetrahedron Lett.* **38,** 3991 (1972).
138. K. A. Watanabe and co-workers, *J. Org. Chem.* **39,** 2482 (1974).
139. T. M. K. Chiu and co-workers, *J. Org. Chem.* **38,** 3622 (1973).
140. W. Bergmann and R. J. Feeney, *J. Am. Chem. Soc.* **72,** 2809 (1950).
141. D. C. Burke, *J. Org. Chem.* **20,** 643 (1955).
142. J. J. Fox, N. Yung, and A. Bendich, *J. Am. Chem. Soc.* **79,** 2775 (1957).
143. I. L. Doerr, J. F. Codington, and J. J. Fox, *J. Med. Chem.* **10,** 247 (1967).
144. W. Bergmann and D. C. Burke, *J. Org. Chem.* **20,** 1501 (1955).
145. D. A. Buthala, *Proc. Soc. Exp. Biol. Med.* **115,** 69 (1964).
146. D. M. Brown, A. Todd, and S. Varadarajan, *J. Chem. Soc.* 2388 (1956).
147. I. L. Doerr, J. F. Codington, and J. J. Fox, *J. Org. Chem.* **30,** 467 (1965).
148. T. Kusaka and co-workers, *J. Anbitiot.* **21A,** 255 (1968).
149. T. Kishi and co-workers, *Chem. Commun.* 852 (1967).
150. Y. F. Shealy and J. D. Clayton, *J. Am. Chem. Soc.* **88,** 3885 (1966).
151. Y. F. Shealy and J. D. Clayton, *J. Am. Chem. Soc.* **91,** 3075 (1969).
152. L. L. Bennet, Jr., P. W. Allan, and D. L. Hill, *Mol. Pharmacol.* **4,** 208 (1968).
153. T. Nakanishi, F. Tomita, and T. Suzuki, *Agric. Biol. Chem.* **38,** 2465 (1974).
154. N. N. Gerber and H. A. Lechevalier, *J. Org. Chem.* **27,** 1731 (1962).
155. A. J. Guarino and N. M. Kredich, *Biochim. Biophys. Acta* **68,** 317 (1963).
156. B. R. Baker, R. E. Schaub, and H. M. Kissman, *J. Am. Chem. Soc.* **77,** 5911 (1955).
157. L. H. Pugh and N. N. Gerber, *Cancer Res.* **23,** 640 (1963).
158. R. J. Suhadolnik, B. M. Chassy, and G. R. Waller, *Biochim. Biophys. Acta* **179,** 258 (1969).
159. B. R. Baker, R. E. Schaub, and H. M. Kissman, *J. Am. Chem. Soc.* **77,** 5911 (1955).
160. Belg. Pat. 671,557 (1967), (to Parke, Davis and Company).
161. W. W. Lee, A. Benitez, L. Goodman, and B. R. Baker, *J. Am. Chem. Soc.* **82,** 2648 (1960).
162. E. J. Reist and co-workers, *J. Org. Chem.* **27,** 3274 (1962).
163. R. Baker, and H. G. Fletcher, *J. Org. Chem.* **26,** 4605 (1961).
164. C. P. J. Glaudemans and H. G. Fletcher, Jr., *J. Org. Chem.* **28,** 3004 (1963).
165. F. M. Schabel, Jr., *Chemotherapy* **13,** 321 (1968).
166. F. A. Miller and co-workers, *Antimicrob. Agents Chemother.* 136 (1968).
167. M. Hubert-Habart and S. S. Cohen, *Biochim. Biophys. Acta* **59,** 468 (1962).
168. J. J. Brink and G. A. LePage, *Cancer Res.* **24,** 312 (1964).
169. T. Sawa, and co-workers *J. Antibiot.* **20,** 227 (1967).
170. C. E. Cass and T. H. Au-Yeung, *Cancer Res.* **36,** 1486 (1976).
171. G. A. LePage, L. S. Worth, and A. P. Kimball, *Cancer Res.* **36,** 1481 (1976).
172. J. L. York and G. A. LePage, *Can. J. Biochem.* **44,** 331 (1966).
173. J. J. Furth and S. S. Cohen, *Cancer Res.* **28,** 2061 (1968).
174. J. L. York and G. A. LePage, *Can. J. Biochem.* **44,** 19 (1966).
175. E. C. Moore and S. S. Cohen, *J. Biol. Chem.* **242,** 2116 (1967).
176. J. M. Lucas-Lenard and S. S. Cohen, *Biochim. Biophys. Acta* **123,** 471 (1966).
177. M. R. Atkinson and co-workers, *Biochemistry* **8,** 4897 (1969).
178. R. L. Momparler, *Biochem. Biophys. Res. Commun.* **34,** 465 (1969).
179. K. G. Cunningham and co-workers, *J. Chem. Soc.* **1951,** 2299.
180. S. Frederiksen, H. Milling, and H. Klenow, *Biochim. Biophys. Acta* **95,** 189 (1965).
181. E. A. Kaczka and co-workers, *Biochem. Biophys. Res. Commun.* **14,** 452 (1964).

182. H. R. Bentley K. G. Cunningham, and F. S. Spring, *J. Chem. Soc.* 2301 (1951).
183. E. A. Kaczka and co-workers, *Biochem. Biophys. Res. Commun.* 14, 456 (1964).
184. R. J. Suhadolnik and J. G. Cory, *Biochim. Biophys. Acta* 91, 661 (1964).
185. S. Hanessian, D. C. DeJongh, and J. A. McCloskey, *Biochim. Biophys. Acta* 117, 480 (1966).
186. A. R. Todd and T. L. V. Ulbricht, *J. Chem. Soc.* 3275 (1960).
187. W. W. Lee and co-workers, *J. Am. Chem. Soc.* 83, 1906 (1961).
188. E. Walton and co-workers, *J. Am. Chem. Soc.* 86, 2952 (1964).
189. D. V. Jagger, N. M. Kredich, and A. J. Guarino, *Cancer Res.* 21, 216 (1961).
190. H. T. Shigeura and G. E. Boxer, *Biochem. Biophys. Res. Commun.* 17, 758 (1964).
191. H. T. Shigeura and C. N. Gordon, *J. Biol. Chem.* 240, 806 (1965).
192. H. Klenow, *Biochim. Biophys. Acta* 76, 354 (1963b).
193. R. J. Suhadolnik, S. I. Finkel, and B. M. Chassy, *J. Biol. Chem.* 243, 3532 (1968).
194. F. Rottman and A. J. Guarino, *Biochim. Biophys. Acta* 89, 465 (1964).
195. K. Overgaard-Hanse, *Biochim. Biophys Acta* 80, 504 (1964).
196. H. Yüntsen and co-workers, *J. Antibiot.* 9A, 195 (1956).
197. H. Hoeksema, G. Slomp, and E. E. van Tamelen, *Tetrahedron Lett.* 1964, 1787.
198. U.S. Pat. 3,207,750 (Sept. 21, 1965), C. DeBoer and co-workers.
199. H. Yüntsen, *J. Antibiot.* 11A, 233 (1958).
200. E. J. Prisbe and co-workers, *J. Org. Chem.* 41, 1836 (1976).
201. J. R. McCarthy, Jr., R. K. Robins, and M. J. Robins, *J. Am. Chem. Soc.* 90, 4993 (1968).
202. N. Tanaka, N. Miyairi, and H. Umezawa, *J. Antibiot.* 13A, 265 (1959).
203. N. Tanaka and co-workers, *J. Antibiot.* 14A, 98 (1961).
204. Fr. Pat. 1,465,395 (1967), C. DeBoer and co-workers.
205. N. Tanaka, *J. Antibiot.* 16A, 163 (1963).
206. A. Bloch and C. A. Nichol, *Fed. Proc. Fed. Am. Soc. Exp. Biol.* 23, 324 (1964).
207. A. Bloch, and C. A. Nichol, *Biochem. Biophys. Res. Commun.* 16, 400 (1964).
208. E. J. Backus, H. D. Tresner, and T. H. Campbell, *Antibiot. Chemother.* 7, 532 (1957).
209. S. O. Thomas and co-workers, *Antibiot. Annu.* 716 (1956–1957).
210. R. I. Hewitt and co-workers, *Antibiot. Annu.* 722 (1956–1957).
211. E. J. Tobie, *J. Parasitol.* 43, 291 (1957).
212. S. Arai and co-workers, *J. Antibiot.* 19A, 118 (1966).
213. G. O. Morton and co-workers, *J. Am. Chem. Soc.* 91, 1535 (1969).
214. C. W. Waller and co-workers, *J. Am. Chem. Soc.* 79, 1011 (1957).
215. J. B. Patrick and W. E. Meyer, *156th Meeting, American Chemical Society, Atlantic City, N.J., September, 1968, Abstracts Medi, 24.*
216. D. A. Shuman, R. K. Robins, and M. J. Robins, *J. Am. Chem. Soc.* 91, 3391 (1969).
217. I. D. Jenkins, J. P. Verheyden, and J. G. Moffatt, *J. Am. Chem. Soc.* 98, 3346 (1976).
218. W. Schroeder, and H. Hoeksema, *J. Am. Chem. Soc.* 81, 1767 (1959).
219. H. Yuntsen, H. Yonehara, and H. Ui, *J. Antibiot.* 7A, 113 (1954).
220. H. Sakai, H. Yuntsen, and F. Ishikawa, *J. Antibiot.* 7A, 116 (1954).
221. H. Yuntsen, *J. Antibiot.* 11A, 244 (1958b).
222. J. R. McCarthy, Jr., R. K. Robins, and M. J. Robins, *J. Am. Chem. Soc.* 90, 4993 (1968).
223. J. Farkas and F. Sorm, *Tetrahedron Lett.* 813 (1962).
224. J. Farkas and F. Sorm, *Collect. Czech. Chem. Commun.* 28, 882 (1963).
225. C. Lewis, H. R. Reames, and L. E. Rhuland, *Antibiot. Chemother.* 9, 421 (1959).
226. J. S. Evans and J. E. Gray, *Antibiot. Chemother.* 9, 675 (1959).
227. R. C. Yates and K. B. Olson, *N. Engl. J. Med.* 265, 274 (1961).
228. G. Costa and J. F. Holland, *Cancer Chemother. Rep.* 8, 33, 1960.
229. L. J. Hanka, *J. Bacteriol.* 80, 30 (1960).
230. T. T. Sukuyama, *J. Biol. Chem.* 241, 4745 (1966).
231. N. Zyk, N. Citri, and H. S. Moyed, *Biochemistry* 8, 2787 (1969).
232. C. DeBoer, E. L. Caron, and J. W. Hinman, *J. Am. Chem. Soc.* 75, 499 (1953).
233. J. W. Hinman, E. L. Caron, and C. DeBoer, *J. Am. Chem. Soc.* 75, 5864 (1953).
234. M. H. McCormick and M. M. Hoehn, *Antibiot. Chemother.* 3, 718 (1953).
235. T. H. Haskett and co-workers, *J. Am. Chem. Soc.* 80, 743 (1958).
236. E. H. Flynn and co-workers, *J. Am. Chem. Soc.* 75, 5867 (1953).
237. T. H. Haskell, *J. Am. Chem. Soc.* 80, 747 (1958).
238. C. L. Stevens, P. Blumbergs, and F. A. Daniher, *J. Am. Chem. Soc.* 85, 1552 (1963).
239. S. Hanessian, and T. H. Haskell, *Tetrahedron Lett.* 2451 (1964).
240. C. L. Stevens and co-workers, *J. Am. Chem. Soc.* 86, 5695 (1964).

241. C. L. Stevens, P. Blumbergs, and D. L. Wood, *J. Am. Chem. Soc.* **86**, 3592 (1964).
242. C. L. Stevens and co-workers, *J. Org. Chem.* **31**, 2822 (1966).
243. K. Tatsuoka and co-workers, *Yakugaku Zasshi* **75**, 1206 (1955).
244. T. Araki and co-workers, *Annu. Rep. Takeda Res. Lab.* **14**, 112 (1955).
245. S. Arai and co-workers, *J. Antibiot.* **19A**, 118 (1966).
246. E. A. Brosbe and co-workers, *Antimicrob. Agents Chemother.* 733 (1964).
247. C. G. Smith, W. L. Lummis, and J. E. Grady, *Cancer Res.* **19,** 847 (1959).
248. J. H. Burchenal and co-workers, *Proc. Soc. Exp. Biol. Med.* **86,** 891 (1954).
249. A. Bloch and C. Coutsogeorgopoulos, *Biochemistry* **5,** 3345 (1966).
250. R. E. Monro and D. Vazquez, *J. Mol. Biol.* **28,** 161 (1967).
251. S. Pestka, *Arch. Biochem. Biophys.* **89,** 136 (1970).
252. T. H. Haskell and co-workers, *J. Am. Chem. Soc.* **80,** 743 (1958).
253. T. H. Haskell, *J. Am. Chem. Soc.* **80,** 747 (1958).
254. E. A. Brosbe and co-workers, *Am. Rev. Res. Dis.* **88,** 112 (1963).
255. P. Sensi and co-workers, *Antibiot. Chemother.* **7,** 645 (1957).
256. T. H. Haskell, *J. Am. Chem. Soc.* **80,** 747 (1958).
257. S. K. Takeuchi and co-workers, *J. Antibiot.* **11A,** 1 (1958).
258. T. Tsuruoka and T. Niida, *Meiji Shika Kenkyu Nempo* **23,** (1963).
259. K. Funkunaga and co-workers, *Bull. Agric. Chem. Soc. Jpn.* **19,** 181 (1955).
260. H. Yonehara and N. Otake, *Tetrahedron Lett.* 3785 (1966); J. J. Fox and K. A. Watanabe, *Tetrahedron Lett.* 897 (1966).
261. S. Onuma, Y. Nawata, and Y. Saito, *Bull. Chem. Soc. Jpn.* **39,** 1091 (1966).
262. R. S. Goody, K. A. Watanabe and J. J. Fox, *Tetrahedron Lett.* 293 (1970).
263. J. J. Fox and K. A. Watanabe, *Pure Appl. Chem.* **28,** 475 (1971).
264. T. Kondo, H. Nakai, and T. Goto, *Tetrahedron* **29,** 1801 (1973).
265. T. Misato and coworkers, *Nippon Shokubutsu Byori Gakkaiho* **24,** 302 (1959).
266. T. Hirai and co-workers, *Phytopathology* **58,** 602 (1968).
267. T. Ikeuchi and co-workers, *J. Antibiot.* **25,** 548 (1972).
268. F. W. Lichtenthaler, T. Morino, H. M. Menzei, *Tetrahedron Lett.* 665 (1975).
269. T. Kanzaki and co-workers, *J. Antibiot.* **15A,** 93 (1962).
270. J. J. Fox and co-workers, *Antimicrob. Agents Chemother.* 518 (1964).
271. H. Iwasaki, *Zasshi Yakugaku* **82,** 1358 (1962).
272. J. J. Fox, Y. Kuwada, and K. A. Watanabe, *Tetrahedron Lett.* 6029 (1967).
273. K. A. Watanabe, E. V. Falco, and J. J. Fox, *J. Am. Chem. Soc.* **94,** 3272 (1972).
274. L. Thiry, *J. Gen. Virol.* **2,** 143 (1968).
275. M. Konishi and co-workers, *J. Antibiot.* **26,** 752 (1973).
276. K. Tomita and co-workers, *J. Antibiot.* **26,** 765 (1973).
277. M. Konishi and co-workers, *J. Antibiot.* **26,** 757 (1973).
278. T. Ogawa and M. Matsui, *J. Chem. Soc. Chem. Commun.* **1975,** 992.
279. F. W. Lichtenthaler and T. Kulikowshi, *J. Org. Chem.* **41,** 600 (1976).
280. K. Isono, K. Asahi, and S. Suzuki, *J. Am. Chem. Soc.* **91,** 7490 (1969).
281. K. Isono and co-workers, *Agric. Biol. Chem.* **29,** 848 (1965).
282. K. Isono and co-workers, *Agric. Biol. Chem.* **31,** 190 (1967).
283. K. Isono and S. Suzuki, *Agric. Biol. Chem.* **32,** 1193 (1968).
284. A. Endo and T. Misato, *Biochem. Biophys. Res. Commun.* **37,** 718 (1969).
285. N. M. Kredich and A. J. Guarino, *J. Biol. Chem.* **236,** 3300 (1961).
286. A. J. Guarino, M. L. Ibershof, and R. Swain, *Biochim. Biophys. Acta* **72,** 62 (1963).
287. A. J. Guarino and N. M. Dredich, *Fed. Proc. Fed. Am. Soc. Exp. Biol.* **23,** 371 (1964).
288. J. N. Porter and co-workers, *Antibiot. Chemother.* **2,** 409 (1952).
289. C. W. Waller and co-workers, *J. Am. Chem. Soc.* **75,** 2025 (1953).
290. B. R. Baker and co-workers, *J. Am. Chem. Soc.* **77,** 12 (1955c).
291. R. I. Hewitt and co-workers, *Am. J. Trop. Med. Hyg.* **2,** 254 (1953).
292. E. J. Tobie, *Am. J. Trop. Med. Hyg.* **3,** 852 (1954).
293. C. Trincao and co-workers, *Am. J. Trop. Med. Hyg.* **5,** 784 (1956).
294. D. J. Taylor, H. W. Bond, and J. F. Sherman, *Antibiot. Annu.* 745 (1954–1955).
295. D. E. Eyles and N. Coleman, *Antibiot. Chemother.* **4,** 649 (1954).
296. J. Faiguenbamm and M. Alba, *Bol. Chil. Parasitol.* **9,** 94 (1954).
297. A. R. Gumble and co-workers, *Antibiot. Annu.* 260 (1955–1956).
298. W. Troy and co-workers, *Antibiot. Annu.* 186 (1953–1954).
299. K. Sugiura, *Antibiot. Annu.* 924 (1959–1960).

300. Ref. 294, p. 757.
301. B. R. Baker, R. E. Schaub, and J. H. Williams, *J. Am. Chem. Soc.* **77,** 7 (1955).
302. R. I. Hewitt and co-workers, *Antibiot. Chemother.* **4,** 1222 (1954).
303. E. J. Tobie and B. Highman, *Am. J. Trop. Med. Hyg.* **5,** 504 (1956).
304. S. Frenk and co-workers, *Proc. Soc. Exp. Biol. Med.* **89,** 424 (1955).
305. G. P. Studzinski and K. O. L. Ellem, *Cancer Res.* **28,** 1773 (1968).
306. J. M. Taylor and C. P. Stanners, *Biochim. Biophys. Acta* **155,** 424 (1968).
307. J. D. Dutcher, M. H. Von Saltza, and F. E. Pansy, *Antimicrob. Agents Chemother.* **83,** (1963).
308. H. Agahigian and co-workers, *J. Org. Chem.* **30,** 1085 (1965).
309. H. Taniyama, J. Sawada, and T. Kitagawa, *Chem. Pharm. Bull.* **19,** 1627 (1971).
310. H. Taniyama, J. Sawada, and T. Kitagawa, *J. Antibiot.* **24,** 390 (1971).
311. A. S. Khokhlor and K. I. Shutova, *J. Antibiot.* **25,** 501 (1972).
312. S. A. Waksman and H. B. Woodruff, *Proc. Soc. Exp. Biol. Med.* **49,** 207 (1942).
313. E. E. van Tamelen and co-workers, *J. Am. Chem. Soc.* **83,** 4295 (1961).
314. A. W. Johnson and J. W. Westley, *J. Chem. Soc.* 1642 (1962).
315. E. McConnell, and A. G. Richards, *Can. J. Microbiol.* **5,** 161 (1959).
316. H. de Barjac and R. Dedonder, *C. R. Acad. Sci.* **260,** 7050 (1965).
317. G. Benz, *Experientia* **22,** 81 (1966).
318. K. Sebesta, K. Horska, and J. Van Kova, *Collect. Czech. Chem. Commun.* **34,** 891 (1969).
319. L. Kalvoda, M. Prystas, and F. Sorm, *Tetrahedron Lett.* **47,** 4671 (1973).
320. A. M. Heimpel, *Annu. Rev. Entomol.* **12,** 287 (1967).

ALEXANDER BLOCH
Roswell-Park Memorial Institute

OLIGOSACCHARIDES

During the last two decades, four members of the oligosaccharide group of antibiotics have been isolated. These are everninomicins (1), curamycins (2), avilamycins (3), and flambamycins (4). They represent very complex structures and possess many asymmetric centers. Extensive chemical degradations and spectroscopic evidence led to the structural elucidation of everninomicin B (5), C (6), and D (7), the first among this class of antibiotics whose structures have been determined. At present some of these compounds are under detailed biological and toxicological evaluation for possible clinical testing. Following the above mentioned degradation experiments, the structure of flambamycin has recently been elucidated. Curamycin (8) and avilamycin (9) have been degraded and the structures of some of the constituent monosaccharides have been established. The molecular formulas and melting points of several oligosaccharides are listed in Table 1.

Everninomicins have proved to be active against a wide variety of gram-positive aerobic and anaerobic bacteria as well as neiseria and mycobacteria (1). Everninomicin B and D are the two main constituents of the antibiotic complex produced by *Micromonospora carbonacea* var. *carbonaceae* NRRL 2972, and most of the initial microbiological studies were carried out on them. Both of these compounds were active against a variety of strains of *Staphylococcus, Streptococcus* bacillus and *Mycobacteria* also including penicillin-resistant strains. The activities of these antibiotics were inhibited by serum and it was estimated that everninomicin B and D were strongly protein bound to the extent of 75 and 95%, respectively. In spite of this high serum

Table 1. Molecular Formulas and Melting Points of Oligosaccharides

Compound	CAS Registry Number	Molecular formula	mp, °C
avilamycin	[11051-71-1]	$C_{63}H_{94}Cl_2O_{35}$	188–189
curamycin	[63939-09-3]	$C_{53-55}H_{82-82}Cl_2O_{32-33}$	198
everninomicin B	[53296-30-3]	$C_{66}H_{99}Cl_2NO_{36}$	184–185
everninomicin C	[53296-29-0]	$C_{63}H_{93}Cl_2NO_{34}$	181–184
everninomicin D (1)	[39340-46-0]	$C_{66}H_{99}Cl_2NO_{35}$	169–171
everninomicin D$_1$ (2)	[55539-06-5]	$C_{66}H_{101}Cl_2NO_{36}$	
everninonitrose pyranosyl (1 → 4) digitolactone methyl ether (3)	[40983-35-5]	$C_{30}H_{41}Cl_2NO_{14}$	186–188
flambamycin (5)	[42617-24-3]	$C_{61}H_{90}Cl_2O_{34}$	202–203
olgose (4)	[55539-05-4]	$C_{37}H_{62}O_{22}$	212–215

protein binding both of these compounds showed (10) excellent *in vivo* activities in experimental infections in mice, eg, ED_{50s} was less than 5 mg/kg for protection against infection caused by gram-positive strains.(ED_{50S} is the minimum effective for 50% survival.) It has been shown that these antibiotics are, (a) bactericidal for group A streptococci and bacteriostatic for other organisms; and b) lack cross-resistance with other antimicrobials (11). Activities against mycoplasma (12) and a small group of anerobes (13) have been reported. Everninomicins and their derivatives have no activity against *Enterobacteriacae* or *Pseudomonas*. Serum and urine levels in dogs following intravenous administration were high indicating a serum half-life of about 90 min for everninomicin D. Absorption following intramuscular administration of everninomicin D, to both man and dogs, was slow and erratic. Recent studies with everninomicin B in dogs, rats and mice showed that it behaved similarly to everninomicin D. Studies indicated that one of the ways these antibiotics were eliminated was via urinary excretion.

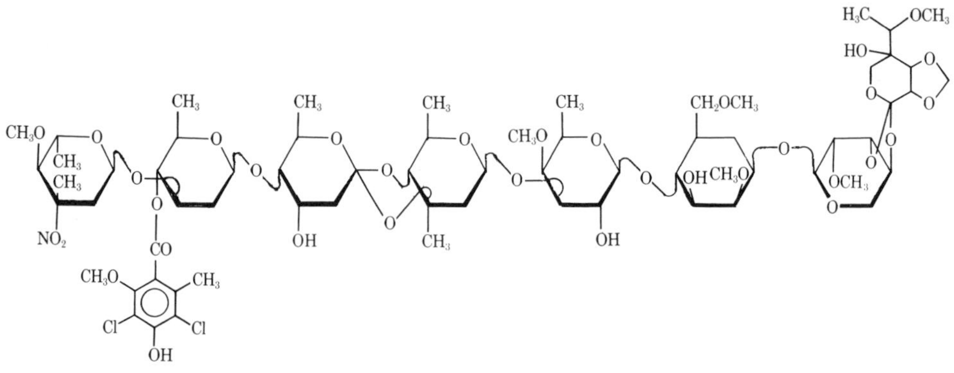

(1) everninomicin D

EVERNINOMICINS

Physical Properties

Everninomicin D is a colorless crystalline solid, $\lambda_{max}^{methanol}$ 289 nm ($\epsilon = 22$), $\lambda_{max}^{NaOH/methanol}$ 295 nm ($\epsilon = 80.8$), $[\alpha]_D^{26}$ −34.2° (chloroform) neutralization equivalent

1558, pK_a 7.3. In the ir it shows absorption for hydroxyl, ester, and nitro (1538 cm^{-1}) groups (7).

Chemical Properties

The strategy in the structural elucidation of everninomicin D was to hydrolyze the antibiotic into its various components, determine their structures and absolute stereochemistries and find the sequence in which they were linked. The details of the structural elucidation of the individual components have been reported (see General bibliography).

Everninomicin D (1) is hydrolyzed with aqueous acid to everninomicin D$_1$ (2) (7). On treatment with diazomethane, (2) undergoes smooth cleavage to the methyl ether of everninonitrose pyranosyl (1 → 4) digitolactone (3) and olgose (4) (see General bibliography).

Compound (3) is a colorless crystalline solid, $[\alpha]_D$ −57.9°, γ max 1754 (carbonyl), 1555 (nitro) and 3472 cm^{-1} (hydroxyl).

OLGOSE

Olgose (4) is a colorless crystalline solid, $[\alpha]_D$ −21.8° (7). In the ir there is no carbonyl absorption and there is no selective absorption in the uv.

FLAMBAMYCIN

Flambamycin (5) is produced by *Streptomyces hygroscopicus* DS 2320. It shows high activity *in vitro* against gram-positive bacteria and neiserria. As in everninomicins, flambamycin also showed the presence of two ortho ester carbon atoms at δ119.8 and 120.9 in the ^{13}C nmr spectrum.

CURAMYCIN AND AVILAMYCIN

The structures and the structure-activity relationships of curamycin and avilamycin, have not yet been established.

The structure-activity relationship in this group of antibiotics is not completely understood. It is clear, however, from the work done on everninomicins that the presence of the free phenolic hydroxyl group and ortho ester linkages are essential for biological activity. Everninomicin D could be reduced chemically (14) or electrochemically (15) to hydroxylamino derivatives which gave high blood levels when administered intramuscularly to dogs.

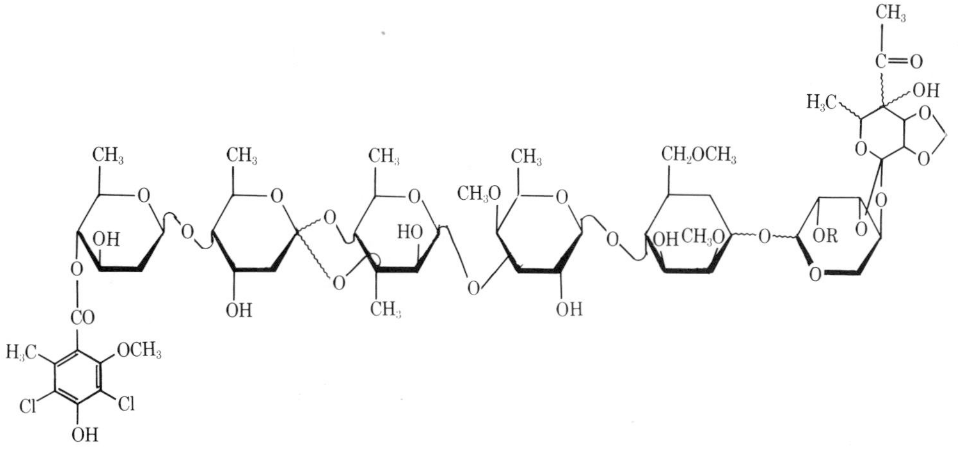

flambamycin

(5) R = —COCH(CH₃)₂

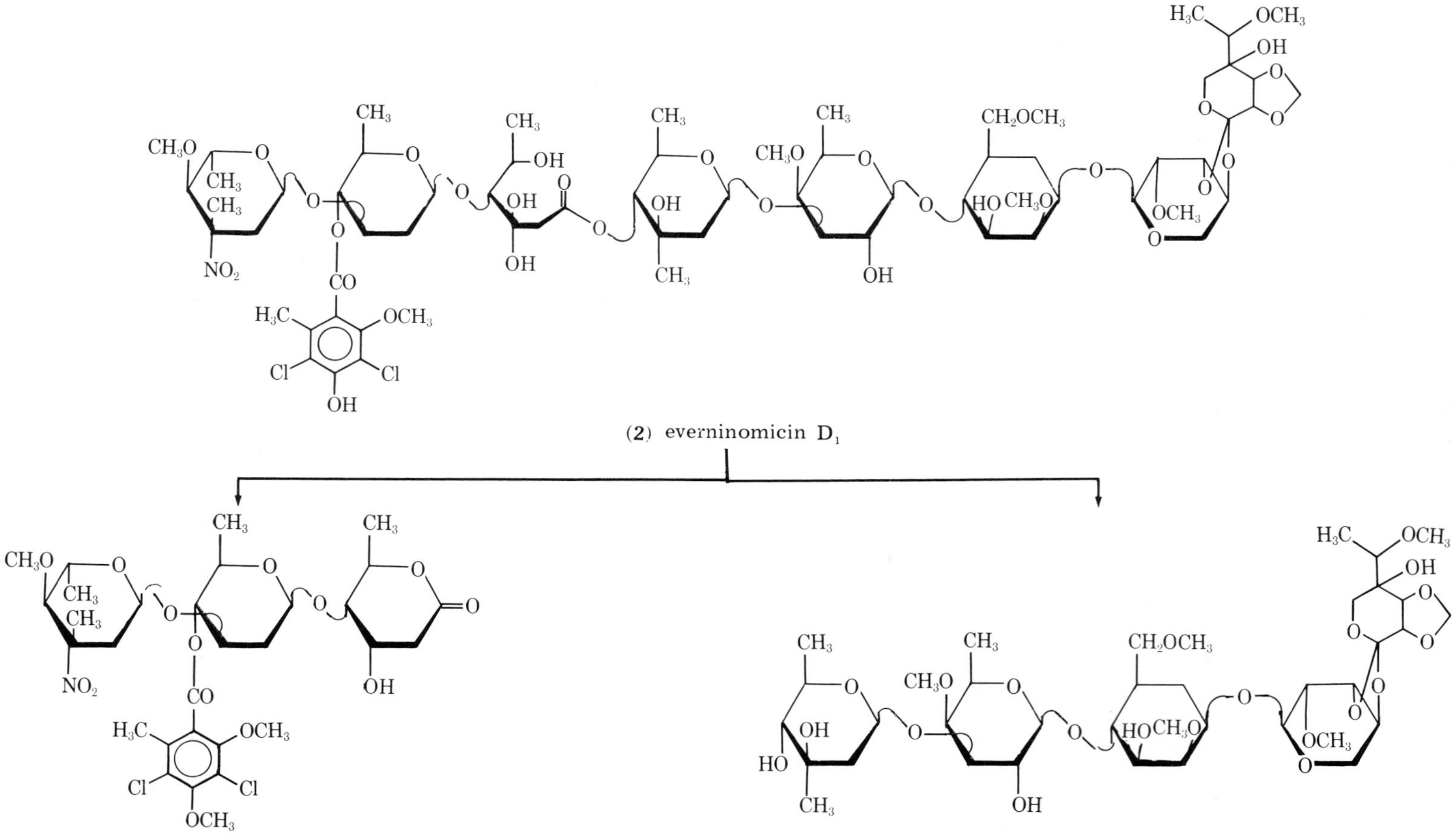

(2) everninomicin D_1

(3) everninonitrosepyranosyl

$(1 \rightarrow 4)$digitolactone, methylether

(4) olgose

BIBLIOGRAPHY

1. M. J. Weinstein, G. M. Luedemann, E. M. Oden, and G. H. Wagman, *Antimicrob. Agents Chemother.* 24 (1964).
2. O. L. Galmarini and V. Deulofeu, *Tetrahedron* **15,** 76 1961.
3. Ger. Pat. 1,116,864 (Nov. 9, 1961), E. Gaeumann, V. Prelog, and E. Vischer (to Ciba, Ltd.).
4. L. Ninet, F. Benazet, Y. Charpentie, M. Dubost, J. Flovent, J. Lunel, D. Mancy, and J. Preud'homme, *Experientia* **30,** 1720 1974.
5. A. K. Ganguly and A. K. Saksena, *J. Antibiot.* **28,** 707 1975.
6. A. K. Ganguly and S. Szmulewicz, *J. Antibiot.* **28,** 710 1975.
7. A. K. Ganguly, O. Z. Sarre, D. Greeves, and J. Morton, *J. Am. Chem. Soc.* **97,** 1982 1975.
8. E. G. Gros, V. Deulofeu, O. L. Galmarini and B. Flydman, *Experientia,* **24,** 323 1968; V. Deulofen and E. G. Gros, *An. Quim.* **68,** 789 1972.
9. F. Buzzetti, F. Eisenberg, H. N. Grant, W. Keller-Schierlein, W. Voser, and H. Zahner, *Experientia* **24,** 320 (1968).
10. J. Black, B. Calesnick, F. G. Falco, and M. J. Weinstein, *Antimicrob. Agents Chemother.* 38 (1964).
11. W. E. Sanders and C. C. Crowe, *Abs. Proc. 13th Intersciences Conf. Antimicrob. Agents Chemotherapy, Washington, D.C.,* 1973, Abs. 139.
12. J. A. Waitz, E. L. Moss, F. Sabatelli, F. Menzel, and C. G. Drube, *Abs. Proc., 13th Intersciences Conf. Antimicrob. Agents Chemotherapy, Washington, D.C.,* 1973, Abs. 140.
13. V. L. Sutter and S. M. Finegold, *Antimicrob. Agents Chemother.* 736 (1976).
14. U.S. Pat. 3,915,956 (Oct. 28, 1975), A. K. Ganguly and O. Z. Sarre (to Schering Corp.).
15. U.S. Pat. 3,998,708 (Dec. 21, 1976), P. Kabasakalian, S. Y. Kalliney, A. K. Ganguly, and A. Westcott (to Schering Corp.).

General References

Structural elucidations are described in the following references.

H. P. Faro, A. K. Ganguly, and D. H. R. Barton, *Chem. Commun.* 823 (1971).
A. K. Ganguly, O. Z. Sarre, and H. Reimann, *J. Am. Chem. Soc.* **90,** 7129 (1968).
A. K. Ganguly, O. Z. Sarre, and J. Morton, *Chem. Commun.* 1488 (1969).
A. K. Ganguly and O. Z. Sarre, *Chem. Commun.* 911, 1149 (1969).
A. K. Ganguly, O. Z. Sarre, and S. Szmulewicz, Chem. Commun., 746 (1971).
A. K. Ganguly and A. K. Saksena, *Chem. Commun.* 531 (1973).
A. K. Ganguly, O. Z. Sarre, D. Greeves, and J. Morton, *J. Am. Chem. Soc.,* **95,** 942 (1973).
D. M. Lemal, P. D. Pacht, and R. B. Woodward, *Tetrahedron,* **18,** 1275 (1962).
W. D. Ollis, C. Smith, and D. E. Wright, *Chem. Commun.* 882 (1974).
A. K. Ganguly, S. Szmulewicz, O. Z. Sarre, and V. M. Girijavallabhan, *Chem. Commun.* 609 (1976).
A. K. Ganguly, O. Z. Sarre, A. T. McPhail, and K. D. Onan, *Chem. Commun.,* 313 (1977).

ASHIT K. GANGULY
Schering Corp.

PEPTIDES

The large group of natural products with antimicrobial properties contain a variety of chemical structures. One logical classification based on biogenetic derivation was proposed by Abraham and Newton (1). These authors defined 3 major groups derived from (1) amino acids, (2) acetates or propionates, and (3) sugars. They subdivided the members of group (1) further according to the number of amino acids involved in their structure as shown in Table 1. The peptide subgroup, the subject of this section, can be subdivided (2) as shown in Figure 1.

Linear Peptides. Relatively few natural antibiotics are linear peptides and the exceptions such as gramicidins A, B, and C, and amphomycin (and its related antibiotics) form a small independent group. However, certain synthetic polypeptides, such as the poly-α-amino acids including poly-L-lysine (3), poly-L-α,γ-diaminobutyric acid (4), and poly-L-aspartic acid (5), all have significant antimicrobial activity. Their specific antimicrobial activity is usually so low in comparison with antibiotics from

Table 1.   Some Antibiotics Derived from Amino Acids

From a single amino acid	CAS Registry No.	From two amino acids	CAS Registry No.	From several amino acids[a]	CAS Registry No.
alanosine	[5854-93-3]	actithiazic acid	[539-35-5]	amphomycin	[1402-82-0]
alazopeptin	[1397-84-8]	albonoursin	[1222-90-8]	bacitracin	[1405-87-4]
anticapsin	[28978-07-6]	apoaranotin	[19885-52-0]	bleomycins	[11056-06-7]
armentomycin	[11043-31-5]	aranotin	[19885-51-9]	cactinomycin	[8052-16-2]
azaleucine	[4746-36-5]	aspergillic acid	[490-02-8]	capreomycins	[11003-38-6]
azaserine	[115-02-6]	aureothricin	[574-95-8]	colistin	[1066-17-7]
azetidine-2-carbonic acid	[2517-04-6]	cephalosporins (see page 871)		dactinomycin	[50-76-0]
				enduracidin	[11115-82-5]
azirinomycin	[31772-89-1]	chaetomin	[1403-36-7]	gramicidin A	[11029-61-1]
azotomycin	[7644-67-9]	gliotoxin	[67-99-2]	gramicidin J(S)	[113-73-5]
O-carbamylserine	[2105-23-9]	holomycin	[488-04-0]	mikamycins	[11006-76-1]
cyclohexenyl-l-glycine	[38147-79-4]	holothin	[488-03-9]	polymyxins	[1406-11-7]
		mycelianamide	[22775-52-6]	stendomycin	[11006-78-3]
cycloserine	[68-41-7]	oryzachlorin	[12678-20-5]	thiopeptin	[12609-84-6]
dehydroleucine		penicillins (see page		thiostrepton	[1393-48-2]
diazooxonorleucine	[764-17-0]	871)		tyrocidines	[8011-61-8]
		pulcherriminic acid	[957-86-8]	viomycin	[32988-50-4]
2,5-dihydrophenylalanine	[29821-30-5]	rhodotorulic acid	[18928-00-2]	virginiamycins	[11006-76-1]
		thienemycin (see page			
duazomycin A	[2508-89-6]	871)			
duazomycin B	[7644-67-9]	thioaurin	[1401-63-4]		
hadacidin	[689-13-4]	thiolutin	[87-11-6]		
N^5-hydroxyarginine	[42599-90-6]	thiomycin	[1393-47-1]		
threomycin	[12794-09-1]				

[a] Includes only those compounds produced on commercial scale (consult Table 4 for additional compounds).

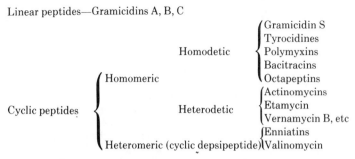

Figure 1. Structural types of peptide antibiotics.

microorganisms, and their therapeutic index is so poor, that their therapeutic potential has been less than peptide antibiotics from microorganisms.

Cyclic Peptides. Most antibiotic peptides contain cyclic structures distinct from those involving the disulfide bridges such as those found in insulin and oxytocin. In the cyclic antibiotic peptides the terminal carboxyl group of an otherwise linear peptide participates in the cyclization by condensation with an amino or a hydroxyl function at some position along the peptide chain.

In a *homomeric* cyclic peptide the ring is composed entirely of atoms from amino acids and in a *heteromeric* cyclic peptide one (or more) component of the ring is not an amino acid. The *homomeric* group can be of the *homodetic* type in which the amino acids in the ring are joined only through amide bonds, or of the *heterodetic* type, in which two or more amino acids present in the ring are joined through bonds other than amide bonds, eg, lactones involving the hydroxyl of threonine or serine. Examples of the heteromeric cyclic peptides are the depsipeptides, enniantins, and valinomycin, where the hetero units contributing to the formation of the ring are α- or β-hydroxy-aliphatic acids.

Unique Characteristics of Peptide Antibiotics

Peptide antibiotics differ in many respects from the proteins and peptides having hormonal or other functions in higher animals and plants. Among the major differences are:

Low molecular weight. Most peptide antibiotics have molecular weights in the range 500–1500, whereas hormonal peptides and proteins frequently are much larger (see Hormones).

Absence of usual amino acids. Most peptide antibiotics have between 6 and 12 amino acid residues, and some of the amino acid residues including methionine and histidine, which are frequently found in peptides and proteins of plant and animal origin, are infrequently noted.

Presence of unusual amino acids. Many peptide antibiotics contain amino acid residues or derivatives of amino acids not found in proteins and peptide hormones of animal or plant origin. Some of these are listed in Table 2.

Presence of lipids and other moieties. Many peptide antibiotics contain lipids and other residues of nonamino acid character (see Table 2) which differentiate these peptides from peptides of plant or animal origin.

Table 2.   Fatty Acids and Unusual Amino Acids Found in Peptide Antibiotics

Antibiotic	CAS Registry No.	Acid
Fatty acids		
amphomycin		3-anteisotridecenoic acid; 3-isododecenoic acid
destruxin B	[2503-26-6]	D-α-hydroxymethylvaleric acid
enniatins	[11113-62-5]	D-α-hydroxyisovaleric acid
enduracidins		10-methylundeca-2(*cis*)-4(*trans*)-dienoic acid; (+)-10-methyldodeca-2(*cis*)-4(*trans*)-dienoic acid
polymyxins		6-methyloctanoic acid; 6-methylheptanoic acid
sporidesmolides	[11113-90-9]	L-α-hydroxyisovaleric acid
Amino acids		
actinomycins	[1402-38-6]	N-methyl-L-valine; sarcosine; N-methyl-L-alanine; N-methyl-L-isoleucine
amphomycin		D-pipecolic acid; α,β-diaminobutyric acid; β-methylaspartic acid
bottromycins	[1393-68-6]	L-β,β-dimethyl-α-aminobutyric acid; α-amino-β-phenylbutyric acid; β-methylphenylalanine; L-*cis*-3-methylproline
capreomycins		β-lysine
cerexins		L-threo-γ-hydroxylysine
enniatins	[11113-62-5]	N-methyl-L-valine; N-methyl-L-isoleucine
etamycin	[299-20-7]	L-α,N-dimethylleucine; 3-hydroxypicolinic acid; L-phenylsarcosine
ilamycins	[11006-41-0]	N-methyl-γ-formyl-L-norvaline; δ-dehydronorleucine; N-methyl-L-luecine; L-3-nitrotyrosine
nisins	[1414-45-5]	β-methylalanine; β-methyllanthionine; lanthionine; dehydroalanine; dehydrobutyrine
quinomycins	[11113-76-1]	quinoxalinecarboxylic acid; N-methyl-L-valine; N-methyl-L-isoleucine; N,N'-dimethylcystine; L-N-methyl-β-methylisoleucine
telomycin	[19246-24-3]	L-β-hydroxyleucine; L-*trans*-3-hydroxyproline; β-methyltryptophan
vernamycins	[11113-94-3]	L-phenylglycine; 3-hydroxypicolinic acid; 4-keto-L-pipecolic acid; N-methyl-L-phenylalanine; N-methyl-L-*p*-methylaminophenylalanine; N-methyl-L-*p*-dimethylaminophenylalanine

Presence of D-amino acid residues.   Most peptide antibiotics contain D-amino acid residues, a characteristic which differentiates these compounds from peptides of plant and animal origin (which contain only L-amino acid residues). Sometimes the antibiotic contains both D- and L-isomers of the same amino acid.

Resistance to hydrolysis by proteolytic enzymes.   Practically all of the peptide antibiotics are resistant to attack by proteolytic enzymes of plant and animal origin which are effective in hydrolyzing plant and animal peptides. In a few instances the microorganisms producing the peptide antibiotics have been found to produce enzymes degrading these antibiotics, and these constitutive enzymes are frequently inactive on peptides of plant and animal origin.

Biosynthesis by enzymes rather than ribosomes.   Nearly all of the peptide antibiotics (nisin and subtilin are exceptions) examined so far have been shown to be of enzymatic origin, rather than ribosomal origin which further differentiates the peptide antibiotics from the proteins and peptides found in plants and animals.

Biosynthesis of families of peptide antibiotics.   Most of the peptide antibiotics are produced as families of closely related substances by the microorganisms involved. Substitution by related amino acids has frequently occurred without major change in antibiotic activity. Examples of these substitutions are: N-methyl-L-alanine and N-methyl-L-isoleucine for N-methyl-L-valine in the actinomycins; N-methyl-p-dimethylaminophenylalanine and N-methyl-L-phenylalanine for N-methyl-p-methylaminophenylalanine in the vernamycins; D-phenylalanine for D-leucine and L-phenylalanine for L-leucine in the octapeptins.

Established Antibiotics

The basic principles that are used in the large-scale production of peptide antibiotics by fermentation processes are described in more general articles (see Fermentation).

Only those antibiotics that have established applications as antibacterial, antifungal, or antitumor agents in clinical medicine or agriculture will be discussed in any detail. These include the antibiotics listed in Table 3 which are currently produced by fermentation processes on a tonnage scale (with the exception of dactinomycin and cactinomycin which are produced on a kilogram scale). Although there are 21 peptides listed, the duplications (eg, mikamycins, pristinamycins, and virginiamycins are closely related, as are capreomycins and viomycins, and siomycin and thiostrepton) reduce the number to 13 really separate entities, and one of these, stendomycin, is no longer manufactured on a commercial scale.

A more general survey of antibiotic peptides is presented in Table 4 where 230 of the compounds which appear to merit the designation of antibiotic peptides are listed. Although most of them have been examined in relatively crude form, several have been rather exhaustively studied and in some instances both structures and chemical synthesis have been worked out. Some are still being evaluated in clinical medicine or agriculture and they may in time find useful application.

In the discussion of the individual antibiotic groups which follows, methods of bioassay have been referred to only briefly. These can be found, collectively, and in detail, in several handbooks of which Kavanagh's *Analytical Microbiology* (242) is perhaps the most useful. Note should also be made of the marked effect on the nature of the antibiotic produced exerted by changing the strain of the microorganism. For example, more than 20 different types of peptide antibiotics are produced by different strains of *Bacillus subtilis*.

Peptide Antibiotics Produced by *Bacillus* Species.   Those peptide antibiotics produced by *Bacillus* species listed in Table 5 include several that are chemically closely related although produced by taxonomically different species: bacitracin from *Bacillus licheniformis* and *Bacillus subtilis*; and polymyxins from *Bacillus polymyxa*, *Bacillus aerosporus*, *Bacillus colistinus*, and *Bacillus circulans*. Examination of the descriptions of the fermentation conditions for production of the same antibiotic type by the different culture shows that different media, incubation temperatures, and aeration rates are frequently used to obtain maximum antibiotic productivity. It is thus likely that there are several enzyme systems available for the production of any one of these compounds.

Table 3.   Source and Biological Activity of Peptide Antibiotics Currently Manufactured on Industrial Scale for Therapeutic and Agricultural Use [a]

Compound	Microbial source	Antibiotic activity[b]	Manufacturer, 1977[c]	Some uses, 1977
amphomycin	*Streptomyces canus*	G+	1	topical antibacterial
bacitracin	*Bacillus subtilis*	G+	1, 2, 3, 4, 5, 6, 7, 8, 9, 10	topical antibacterial; animal feed supplement
bleomycins	*Streptomyces verticillus*	G+, G−, and TB; antitumor	11	antitumor
cactinomy-cin	*Streptomyces chrysomallus*	G+; antitumor	12	antitumor
capreomycin	*Streptomyces capreolus*	TB	13	anti-TB
colistin	*Bacillus colistinus*	G−	3, 4, 14, 15, 16	systemic antibacterial
dactinomy-cin	*Streptomyces antibioticus*	G+; antitumor	17, 18, 19	antitumor
enduracidin	*Streptomyces fungicidus*	G+ and TB	20	animal feed supplement
gramicidin A	*Bacillus brevis*	G+	1, 7, 21	topical antibacterial
gramicidin J(S)	*Bacillus brevis*	G+ and G−	22, 23	topical antibacterial
mikamycins	*Streptomyces mitakaensis*	G+	14, 24	animal feed supplement
polymyxins	*Bacillus polymyxa*	G−	4, 6, 8	systemic and topical antibacterial
pristinamy-cins [11006-76-1]	*Streptomyces pristinae spiralis*	G+	17	systemic antibacterial
siomycin A [12656-09-6]	*Streptomyces sioyaensis*	G+	25	veterinary
stendomycin	*Streptomyces endus*	G+ and TB; antifungal	26 (at one time)	agricultural (withdrawn)
thiopeptin	*Streptomyces tateyamensis*	G+ and TB	27, 28	animal feed supplement
thiostrepton	*Streptomyces azureus*	G+	29	veterinary
tyrocidine	*Bacillus brevis*	G+	1	topical antibacterial
tyrothricin [1404-88-2]	*Bacillus brevis*	G+ and G−	1, 7, 21, 30	topical antibacterial
viomycin	*Streptomyces floridae*	TB	31	anti-TB
virginiamycin	*Streptomyces virginiae*	G+	32	systemic antibacterial; animal feed supplement

[a] Cactinomycin is also known as actinomycin C; dactinomycin is also known as actinomycin D; colistin is a member of the polymyxin group; capreomycin and viomycin are members of the same group; mikamycin, pristinamycin, and virginiamycin are all members of the same group; tyrothricin is a mixture of gramicidin A and tyrocidine; siomycin and thiostrepton are members of the same group.
[b] G+ = gram-positive bacteria; G− = gram-negative bacteria; TB = tubercle bacillus bacteria.
[c] Manufacturers, by number on page 1028.

The Polymyxins.   The announcement by Ainsworth and co-workers (243), Shepherd and co-workers (244), and Benedict and Langlykke (245) in 1947 of aerosporin and polymyxin from *Bacillus polymyxa* strains led to an understanding that a group of closely related antibiotics was involved. The generic name polymyxin was adopted

Table 4. Some Antibiotic Peptides Produced by Microorganisms

Name	CAS Registry No.	Synonym or related substance	Producing microorganisms	Antimicrobial and other activities[a] G+	G–	My	AF	AT	Other	Chemical structure proposed	Synthesis completed	Ref.
actinine	[407-64-7]	mycetin	Streptomyces felis	+	+			+				6
actinogan	[1338-58-5]		Streptomyces sp					+				7
actinomycellin	[1394-87-2]		Streptomyces sp	+								8
actinomycins	[1402-38-6]		Streptomyces antibioticus; S. chysomallus; S. galbus; S. kitasawaensis; S. latanus; S. michiganensis; S. murinus; S. parvullus; S. parvus	+				+		+	+	
actinoidin	[39319-82-9]		Nocardia actinoides	+								10
actinomycetin	[1402-37-5]		Streptomyces albus	+		+						11
actinonin	[13434-13-4]		Streptomyces felis	+	+				APh			12
actinoxanthin	[59680-34-1]		Actinomyces globisporus	+				+				13
aerosporin	[1406-11-7]	polymyxin A	Bacillus polymyxa	+	+					+	+	14
alamethicin	[27061-78-5]		Trichoderma viride	+	+			+		+		15
albomycin	[1414-39-7]	grisein; sideromycin	Streptomyces subtropicalis	+		+				+		16
alboverticillin	[65454-60-6]		Streptomyces alboverticillatus	+	+	+						17
almarcetin	[65454-06-0]		Streptomyces albus	+	+							18
althiomycin	[12656-40-5]	matamycin; actinothiocin	Streptomyces althioticus	+	+					+		19
alvein	[9008-49-5]		Bacillus albei	+								20
alveomycin	[65454-07-1]	sideromycin	Streptomyces sp	+	+							21
amidinomycin	[3572-60-9]		Streptomyces sp	+	+							22
amidomycin	[552-33-0]		Streptomyces sp				+		AV			23
aminomycin	[11016-07-2]	valinomycin	Streptomyces sp	+		+	+			+	+	24
amphomycin	[1402-82-0]	glumamycin; asparatocin	Streptomyces canus; S. lavendulae	+		+				+		25
anthelvencin	[11011-24-8]	netropsin	Streptomyces venezuelae	+	+				AV			26
antiamoebin	[12692-85-2]	stilbellin	Stilbella sp	+	+				AP			27
arsimycin	[65454-08-2]		Streptomyces arsitiensis; S. roseus	+								28

Table 4 (*continued*)

Name	CAS Registry No.	Synonym or related substance	Producing microorganisms	Antimicrobial and other activities[a]						Chemical structure proposed	Synthesis completed	Ref.
				G+	G−	My	AF	AT	Other			
aspartocin	[4117-65-1]	amphomycin	*Streptomyces griseus* var. *spiralis*	+								29
aspochracin	[22029-09-0]	4.2.3	*Aspergillus ochraceus*	+					INS	+		30
avenacein	[1398-16-9]	enniatin	*Fusarium avenaceum*	+		+						31
ayfivin	[1405-87-4]	bacitracin	*Bacillus licheniformis*	+								32
azomultin	[65454-10-6]	kikumycin	*Streptomyces noboritoensis*	+	+							33
bacillin	[29393-20-2]	tetaine	*Bacillus pumilus*	+	+							34
bacillomycins	[1395-21-7]	fungistatin XG	*Bacillus subtilis*				+					35
bacillocin	[65454-05-9]		*Bacillus subtilis*				+					36
bacilysin	[29393-20-2]	tetaine	*Bacillus pumilus*	+	+							37
bacitracin	[1405-87-4]	ayfivin	*Bacillus subtilis*	+	+					+		38
beauvericin	[46048-05-5]		*Beauvaria bassiana*	+						+		39
berninamycin	[37326-21-9]	valinomycin	*Streptomyces berniensis*	+	+					+		40
bleomycins		U-27810	*Streptomyces verticillus*	+				+		+		41
bottromycin			*Streptomyces bottropensis*	+	+				PPLO	+		42
bresein	[37233-57-1]	tyrocidine	*Bacillus brevis*	+								43
brevin	[9008-51-9]		*Bacillus brevis*	+					AV			44
brevolin	[1403-13-0]	4.5.1.2	*Bacillus brevis*	+	+							45
bryamycin	[1403-14-1]	thiostrepton	*Streptomyces hawaiiensis*	+						+		46
capreomycin	[11003-38-6]	viomycin	*Streptomyces capreolus*			+				+		47
carcinomycin	[65454-12-8]	gammycin	*Streptomyces carcinomyceticus; S. gannmycicus*					+				48
carzinocidin	[1403-27-6]		*Streptomyces kitasawaensis*					+				49
cephalomycin	[11005-92-8]		*Streptomyces tashiensis* var. *cephalomyceticus*			+			AV			50
cerein B$_2$	[65454-14-0]		*Bacillus brevis*		+							51
cerexin	[65454-17-3]		*Bacillus cereus*	+								52
chrystallomycin	[37226-23-6]	amphomycin	*Streptomyces violaceae*	+						+		53
chymostatin A	[51759-76-3]		*Streptomyces hygroscopicus*		+							54
cinnamycin	[1405-39-6]		*Streptomyces cinnamomeus*	+		+						55
circulins	[9008-54-2]	polymyxins	*Bacillus circulans*	+	+	+				+		56
colisan	[11051-89-1]		*Bacillus* sp	+		+				+	+	57
colistin		polymyxins	*Bacillus colistinus*		+				AP		+	58
comirin	[1391-05-5]		*Pseudomonas antimycetica*				+					59
congocidine	[554-32-5]	netropsin	*Streptomyces ambofaciens*	+	+					+		60
cryomycin	[37306-12-0]		*Streptomyces psychrophylus*	+	+							61

217

Table 4 (continued)

Name	CAS Registry No.	Synonym or related substance	Producing microorganisms	G+	G-	My	AF	AT	Other	Chemical structure proposed	Synthesis completed	Ref.
glumamycin	[1402-82-0]	amphomycin	Streptomyces zaomyceticus	+						+		95
gramicidin A			Bacillus brevis	+						+	+	96
gramicidin J		gramicidin S	Bacillus brevis Nagano	+						+	+	97
gramicidin S	[1391-82-8]	tyrocidine	Bacillus brevis Gause Brazhnikova	+						+	+	98
grisein		albomycin	Streptomyces griseus	+	+					+		99
griseococcin	[65454-37-7]	netropsin	Streptomyces griseus	+						+		100
griseoviridin	[53216-90-3]	F-1370-8	Streptomyces griseus	+	+				AV	+		101
grisonomycin	[65454-39-9]	A-10073; sideromycin	Streptomyces griseus	+	+							102
griselimycin	[26034-16-2]		Streptomyces griseus; Streptomyces coelicus	+		+						103
grizin	[11097-04-4]	grisine; grisemin	Streptomyces griseus	+	+							104
hoydamycin	[65454-42-4]		Streptomyces sp	+	+		+					105
iaquirina	[65454-44-6]		Streptomyces iakyrus	+	+	+						106
ikarugamycin	[36531-78-9]		Streptomyces phaeochromogenes	+	+				TRI	+		107
ilamycin	[10409-85-5]	rufomycin	Streptomyces islandicus	+		+				+		108
isariin	[64667-10-3]		Isaria cretacia	+		+				+		109
iturin	[11006-64-7]		Bacillus subtilis	+	+		+			+		110
iyomycin	[50646-98-5]		Streptomyces phaeoverticillatus	+				+				111
janiemycin	[12688-25-4]	enduracidin	Streptomyces macrosporus	+		+						112
jolipeptin	[37913-77-2]	polymyxin	Bacillus polymyxa var. colistinus	+	+							113
kikumycin A	[65454-09-3]	R-719	Streptomyces phaechromogenes	+	+			+	AV	+		114
kobenomycin	[65454-11-7]		Streptomyces kobensis	+								115
komamycin			Streptomyces pyridomyceticus				+					116
laspartomycin	[12676-61-8]	amphomycin	Streptomyces viridochromogenes var. komabensis	+								117
lateritin	[65454-13-9]	enniatin	Fusarium lateritium	+		+				+		118
laterosporin	[1392-15-0]		Bacillus laterasporin	+	+							119
lathumycin	[53025-07-3]		Streptomyces lathumensis	+								120
leucinamycin	[11033-65-1]		Streptomyces cinnamomeus	+	+		+		TRI	+		121
leucinostatin	[39405-64-6]		Penicillium lilacinum			+	+					122
leucopeptin	[65454-15-1]		Streptomyces hachijoensis var. takahaziensis	+	+	+	+			+		123
levomycin	[1403-88-9]	echinomycin	Streptomyces sp	+	+	+	+					124
licheniformin	[1392-23-0]		Bacillus licheniformis	+		+						125

No.	Antibiotic	CAS No.	Synonym	Source	1	2	3	4	5	6	7	8
126	lymphomycin	[54578-02-8]		Streptomyces sp	+	+			+	+		
127	lysotoxin	[65454-18-4]	xanthomycin	Streptomyces lysotoxis	+	+	+		AP	+	+	+
128	malformin A	[3022-92-2]		Aspergillus niger	+	+	+			+		+
129	marcesin	[1403-94-7]		Marasimus ramealis	+				+			
130	marinamycin	[11006-43-2]		Streptomyces mariensis	+		+					
131	matamycin	[65454-24-2]	althiomycin	Streptomyces bellus	+	+			+			
132	matchamycin	[65454-21-9]		Streptomyces amagasakaensis	+	+						
133	melanomycin	[65454-27-5]		Streptomyces melanogenes	+				AP	+		
134	mesenterin	[1392-42-3]	ostreogrycin	Nocardia mesenterica	+	+						
135	micrococcin P	[1392-45-6]		Bacillus pumilis	+	+						
136	micropolysporin	[65454-30-0]	55-AB	Micropolyspora caesia	+		+			+		
137	mikamycin			Streptomyces mitakaensis	+				+			
138	mitomalcin	[11043-99-5]	vernamycin	Streptomyces malayensis	+	+				+		
139	monamycin	[11115-98-3]		Streptomyces jamaicensis	+	+			+	+		
140	mycobacillin	[18524-67-9]		Bacillus subtilis	+			+				
141	mycosubtilin	[1392-60-5]		Bacillus subtilis	+	+		+				
142	negamycin	[33404-78-3]	leucylnegamycin	Streptomyces sp	+	+			+	+		
143	neocarzinostatin	[9014-02-2]		Streptomyces carzinostaticus	+	+				+		
144	nisin		subtilin	Streptococcus cremoris; Streptococcus lactis	+	+			+	+		
145	nocardamin	[26605-16-3]		Nocardia sp	+		+		+		+	
146	noformacin	[155-38-4]	MK-61	Nocardia formica	+				AV		+	
149	nosiheptide	[56377-79-8]	thiostrepton	Streptomyces actuosus	+	+						
147	octapeptin	[39342-08-0]	EM-49	Bacillus circulans	+	+	+		AP	+	+	
148	ostreogrycin	[11006-76-1]	mikamycin; vernamycin	Streptomyces ostreogriseus	+	+	+		+	+	+	
150	parvulin	[62339-77-9]	amphomycin	Streptomyces parvullus	+				+			
151	peptidolipin NA	[65454-53-7]		Nocardia asteroides	+	+	+			+		
152	peptimycin	[11006-46-5]		Streptomyces mauvecolor	+		+		+			
153	phalamycin	[1392-86-5]		Streptomyces noursei	+	+	+			+		
154	phenomycin	[12624-22-5]		Streptomyces fervens var. phenomyceticus	+		+		+			
155	phleomycin	[11006-33-0]	bleomycin	Streptomyces verticillus	+	+	+	+	+	+	+	
156	phthiomycin	[1392-88-7]		Streptomyces luteochromogenes	+	+	+			+	+	
157	phytoactin	[11005-09-7]		Streptomyces sp	+			+		+		
158	phytostreptin	[11016-19-6]	polyaminohygrostr-eptin	Streptomyces lavendulae	+	+				+		
159	polycillin			Bacillus subtilis					+			
160	polymyxins	[7177-48-2]	colistin; circulins	Bacillus polymyxa					+		+	
161												+

Table 4 (*continued*)

Name	CAS Registry No.	Synonym or related substance	Producing microorganisms	Antimicrobial and other activities[a]						Chemical structure proposed	Synthesis completed	Ref.
				G+	G−	My	AF	AT	Other			
polypeptin	[59866-84-1]	polymyxin	*Bacillus krzemieniewski*	+	+							162
pristinamycins		vernamycins; ostreogrycins; virginiamycins; mikamycins	*Streptomyces pristinaespiralis*	+						+	+	163
pumilin	[1405-19-2]		*Bacillus pumilus*	+								164
quinomycin		echinomycin	*Streptomyces aureus*	+	+	+				+		165
rhizobacidin	[65454-54-8]		*Bacillus subtilis*	+								166
rhizomycin	[12626-13-0]		*Streptomyces novoverticillis*	+					APh			167
rufomycin	[65454-56-0]		*Streptomyces atratus*	+			+			+		168
sambucin	[18719-76-1]	enniatin	*Fusarium sambucinum*	+		+				+		169
saramycetin	[11130-70-4]	X-5079C	*Streptomyces saraceticus*				+					170
serratamolide	[5285-25-6]		*Serratia marcescens*	+						+		171
sideromycin	[56509-18-3]											172
siomycin		thiostrepton	*Streptomyces sioyaensis*	+		+						173
sporangiomycin	[37244-77-2]		*Planomonospora parontospora* var. *antibiotica*	+								174
sporidesmolide			*Pithomyces chartarum*	+						+		175
staphylomycins	[11006-76-1]	virginiamycins; mikamycins; ostreogrycins	*Streptomyces virginiae*	+						+		176
stendomycin			*Streptomyces endus; Streptomyces antimycoticus*	+	+	+						177
stilbellin	[65454-55-9]	antamoebin	*Stilbella* sp	+					AP			178
streptogramin	[11006-76-1]	vernamycin	*Streptomyces graminofaciens*	+		+				+		179
subsporin	[65454-57-1]		*Bacillus subtilis*	+			+					180
subtilins	[1393-38-0]	nisins	*Bacillus subtilis*	+						+		181
subtilysin	[9014-01-1]	surfactin	*Bacillus subtilis*	+	+					+		182
succinimycin	[65454-58-2]	sideromycin	*Streptomyces olivochromogenes*	+								183
sulfactin	[59-52-9]	thiostrepton	*Streptomyces roseus*	+								184
sulfomycin	[65454-59-3]		*Streptomyces viridochromogenes* var. *sulfomycin*	+					PPLO	+		185, 186
surfactin	[24730-31-2]	subtilysin	*Bacillus subtilis*	+	+					+		187
suzukacillin	[11017-50-8]		*Trichoderma viride*	+								188

220

Antibiotic	CAS/Code No.	Synonym	Source organism								No.
syringomycin	[11140-67-3]		*Pseudomonas syringae*	+						+	189
taitomycin	[65454-16-2]		*Streptomyces afghaniensis; Streptomyces griseosporus*	+	+						190
telomycin	C-159		*Streptomyces canus*	+	+						192
tetaine	[29393-20-2]	bacilysine	*Bacillus pumilus*	+	+	+					191
theiomycetin	[1407-06-3]		*Streptomyces lavendulae*	+	+						193
thermothiocin	[11032-08-9]		*Thermoactinopolyspora coremialis*	+							194
thiopeptin		thiostrepton	*Streptomyces tateyamensis*	+		+					195
thiostrepton		siomycin	*Streptomyces azureus; Streptomyces hawaiiensis*	+				+			196
threomycin			*Streptomyces sp*	+		AV			+		197
toximycin	[1404-85-9]		*Bacillus subtilis*		+		+				198
trichotoxin	[65454-19-5]		*Trichoderma viridae*	+	+	+	+				199
tric(u)lamin	[65454-22-0]		*Streptomyces triculaminicus*		+		+				200
triostin	[512-64-1]	echinomycin; quinomycin	*Streptomyces aureus*	+	+	+		+			201
tsushimycin	[11054-63-0]	amphomycin	*Streptomyces pseudogriseolus*	+							202
tuberactinomycin	[11075-36-8]	viomycin	*Streptomyces griseoverticillatus var. tuberacticus*			+					203
tyrocidine			*Bacillus brevis*	+							204
tyrothricin		gramicidin S	*Bacillus brevis*	+	+						205
ussamycin			*Streptomyces lavendulae*	+		+		+			206
valinomycin	[65454-25-3]	aminomycin	*Streptomyces fulvissimus; Streptomyces tsusimaensis*	+	+	+					207
vancomycin	[2001-95-8]		*Streptomyces orientalis*	+		+					208
vernamycins	[1404-90-6]	ostreogrycins; mikamycins; PA-114	*Streptomyces loidensis*	+		+					209
violacetin	[554-32-5]	netropsin	*Streptomyces pureochromogenes*	+	+	+					210
viomycin		tuberactinomycin	*Streptomyces abikoensis; Streptomyces floridae; Streptomyces puniceus; Streptomyces vinaceus; Streptomyces californicus*	+		+		+			211
viridomycin	[52970-22-6]		*Streptomyces viridaris; Streptomyces roseoviridis*	+		+					212
viscosin	[27127-62-4]		*Pseudomonas viscosa*			AV					213
yakusimycin	[65454-28-4]		*Streptomyces antibioticus*	+			+				214
yemenimycin	[12764-56-6]		*Streptomyces albus*	+		+					215, 216

221

Table 4 (continued)

Name	CAS Registry No.	Synonym or related substance	Producing microorganisms	Antimicrobial and other activities[a]						Chemical structure proposed	Synthesis completed	Ref.
				G+	G−	My	AF	AT	Other			
zaomycin	[1405-08-9]	amphomycin	Streptomyces zaomyceticus	+								217
zorbamycin	[11056-20-5]	bleomycin	Streptomyces bikiniensis	+	+		+	+				218
zorbonamycin	[65454-31-1]	bleomycin	Streptomyces bikiniensis	+	+		+	+				219
A 59	[65454-34-4]	siomycin	Streptomyces sp	+		+						220
A 116	[39386-83-9]		Streptomyces endus	+								221
AO 341	[65454-36-6]		Streptomyces candidus	+								222
ASK 753	[54650-03-2]	sideromycin	Streptomyces sp	+	+		+					223
B 43	[61230-33-9]		Bacillus circulans	+	+							224
B 344	[65454-38-8]		Bacillus subtilis	+	+		+					225
EM 49	[11098-13-8]	octapeptins	Bacillus circulans	+	+		+					226
F 1370A	[65454-40-2]	etamycin	Streptomyces congonensis	+		+						227
ICI 13595	[65454-43-5]		Paecylomyces sp						TRP			228
K 16	[1010-38-4]		Streptomyces rimosus						TRP			229
KM 208	[29393-20-2]	bacilysin	Bacillus sp	+	+							230
LA 5352	[65454-41-3]	sideromycin	Streptomyces sp	+								231
LA 5937	[65454-45-7]	sideromycin	Streptomyces sp	+								231
M 81	[640-15-3]		Streptomyces griseus var. psychrophiluy	+	+							232
N 44-A 21	[65454-46-8]		Streptomyces sp	+								233
PA 114	[11006-76-1]	staphylomycin; mikamycin	Streptomyces olivaceus	+								234
RP 9671	[65454-47-9]		Streptomyces actuosus	+		+						235
RP 11072	[11005-33-1]		Streptomyces caelicus	+		+						236
S 520	[55598-63-5]		Streptomyces diastaticus			+						237
TL 119	[55599-68-3]		Bacillus subtilis	+						+		238
X 5079C	[65454-48-0]	saramycetin	Streptomyces saraceticus				+					170
61-26	[55762-77-1]		Bacillus sp	+			+					239
333-25	[59217-95-7]	octapeptins	Bacillus circulans	+	+							240
333-29	[65454-49-1]		Bacillus pumilus	+								241

[a] G+ = gram-positive bacteria; G− = gram-negative bacteria; My = mycobacteria; AF = antifungal; AT = antitumor; APh = antiphage (or antibacteriophage); AV = antiviral; TRI = antitrichomonas; AP = antiprotozoal; INS = insecticide; PPLO = antiPPLO (or antimycoplasma); TRP = antirypanosomal.

Table 5.   Peptide Antibiotics from *Bacillus* Species

From *Bacillus subtilis*

bacillomycin	fungocin	subtenolin
bacillocin	iturin	subtilin
bacitracin	mycosubtilin	subtilysin
colisan	mycobacillin	surfactin
fluvomycin	policillin	toximycin
fungistatin	rhizobacidin	B 344
	subsporin	

From *Bacillus polymyxa*

aerosporin	gatavaline	polypeptin
colistin	polymyxin	

From *Bacillus brevis*

bresein	cerein	gramicidin J(S)
brevin	edeine	tyrocidine
brevolin	esein	tyrothricin
	gramicidin A	

From *Bacillus circulans*

circulin	EM 49	octapeptin

From *Bacillus licheniformis*

ayfivin	bacitracin	licheniformin

From *Bacillus pumilus*

bacillin	micrococcin P	tetaine
bacilysin	pumulin	

From *Bacillus cereus*

cerexin

From *Bacillus colistinus*

colistin

From *Bacillus mesentericus*

esperin

(246) and aerosporin was renamed polymyxin A and polymyxin became polymyxin D. Both of these antibiotics were nephrotoxic and this clinical defect led to the search for other antibiotic-producing strains of *B. polymyxa* and the development of four new polymyxins B, C, E, and F. Polymyxins B and E produced negligible toxic effects within the limits of the therapeutic dosage range (247).

Other polymyxins were discovered during evaluation of other strains of *Bacillus polymyxa*. In 1950, Koyama (248) isolated an antibiotic which he named colistin from a microorganism initially identified as a strain of *Bacillus colistinus* and now classified *Bacillus polymyxa* var. *garyphalus*. In 1958, a strain of *B. polymyxa* from a soil sample taken in Moscow yielded an antibiotic which was designated as polymyxin M (249).

Polymyxin B and E are produced in aerated submerged culture in a medium containing glucose, autolyzed yeast, and $(NH_4)_2HPO_4$. Strain selection is of fundamental importance in obtaining satisfactory antibiotic yields and titers of polymyxins of the order of 500 mg/L have been obtained after a 48 h fermentation time.

A high proportion of gummy polysaccharide is simultaneously produced by the bacteria and is broken down by a short hydrolysis period with dilute acid. The polymyxin is isolated from the culture filtrate by procedures such as precipitation, solvent extraction, and adsorption using either charcoal or cationic-exchange resins (250).

In a typical extraction, polymyxin B is precipitated from the neutralized filtrate as the azobenzene-4-sulfonate and recovered by centrifugation. Treatment of the dried salt with triethylamine sulfate in an azeotropic mixture of methanol and acetone gives the crude polymyxin sulfate. This is purified first by precipitation of the base (251) and then by recrystallization of the naphthalene-2-sulfonate (252). The base is regenerated, converted to the neutral sulfate, and lyophilized.

All of the polymyxins are basic polypeptides whose basicities are associated with the uncommon basic amino acid, α,γ-diaminobutyric acid. They form water-soluble salts with mineral acids with only the phosphates being isolated in crystalline form. The normal form of pharmaceutical presentation of the sulfates and the hydrochlorides is amorphous solids. The water insolubility of the naphthalene-2-sulfonates and azobenzene-4-sulfonates is of advantage in purification of the polymyxins and crystalline forms can be obtained from aqueous alcohols. The picrates, reineckates, helianthates, Polar Yellow and other acid dyestuff salts, long-chain alkyl sulfates, etc, are very insoluble in water and are useful in the various purification procedures.

The polymyxins are irreversibly inactivated in alkaline solution or by treatment with acetic anhydride or other acylating agents. Accompanying the alkaline inactivations are characteristic changes in the specific optical rotations and the optical rotatory dispersion curves, which can be observed, even in the case of the water-insoluble polymyxin bases, by the use of nickel complexes of the antibiotics and measurements at pH 9.3 (253).

Intramuscular injection of polymyxins is painful and tends to result in an inflammatory reaction at the site of injection. When polymyxins are treated with formaldehyde and sodium bisulfite they are converted into their sodium N-sulfomethyl derivatives, which are relatively free from causing pain upon injection and still retain most of their antibacterial activities. The potency of these derivatives depends on regeneration *in vivo* to the parent compound so the nephrotoxicity is not significantly reduced. The degree of N-sulfomethylation varies: most preparations of Coli-Mycin (Warner-Chilcott) have about 50% of the maximum 7 sulfomethyl groups.

Commercial samples of polymyxin B are separable by countercurrent distribution into two components to which the names polymyxin B_1 and B_2 were given (254). Further studies showed that other polymyxin preparations are also mixtures and there are 10 compounds involved. Acid hydrolysis of each shows the presence of a fatty acid as well as several amino acids. In many instances the structures of the individual pairs of the two major components are found to differ only in the nature of the accompanying aliphatic acid. All of the polymyxins have a chain of three amino acids attached to a cyclic heptapeptide via the α-amino group of an α,γ-diaminobutyric acid residue. The terminal α-amino group of the chain is acylated with one or other of the two major fatty acid components mentioned above. The structures of the individual antibiotics are presented in Table 6.

Included in the list of structures is that of circulin A, an antibiotic from *Bacillus circulans* (56). The structures of the Japanese antibiotic colistin and of polymyxin E were found to be identical (58). Similarly, identical structures were established for the components of polymyxin A and the Russian polymyxin M (161). Consequently, the original 5 polymyxins, A, B, C, D, and E, still remain the only known polypeptide antibiotics derived from strains of variants of *Bacillus polymyxa*. However, related compounds named the octapeptins have been found in Streptomycetes (Table 7) which suggests that the biosynthetic capability for this type of microbial metabolite does cross genus lines.

Table 6. The Structures of the Members of the Polymyxin Group [a]

$$
\begin{array}{c}
NH_2\ (\gamma) \\
| \\
Dab \rightarrow Y \\
\end{array}
$$

R $\xrightarrow{\alpha}$ Dab $\longrightarrow$ Thr $\xrightarrow{\alpha}$ X $\xrightarrow{\alpha}$ Dab
| $\nearrow^\alpha$
NH$_2$ (γ)   Dab $\rightarrow$ Y $\searrow$ Z
                                                     $\downarrow$
                                                     Dab —— NH$_2$ (γ)
                                                     $\swarrow$
                                        $\gamma\nwarrow$ Thr $\leftarrow$ Dab
                                                     |
                                                     NH$_2$ (γ)

Polymyxin	CAS Registry No.	R	X	Y	Z
A$_1$ (= M1)	[65454-50-4]	MOA	D-Dab	D-Leu	Thr
A$_2$ (= M2)	[65454-51-5]	IOA	D-Dab	D-Leu	Thr
B$_1$	[4135-11-9]	MOA	Dab	D-Phe	Leu
B$_2$	[34503-87-2]	IOA	Dab	D-Phe	Leu
D$_1$	[10072-50-1]	MOA	D-Ser	D-Leu	Thr
D$_2$	[34167-45-8]	IOA	D-Ser	D-Leu	Thr
E$_1$ (colistin A)	[7722-44-3]	MOA	Dab	D-Leu	Leu
E$_2$ (colistin B)	[7239-48-7]	IOA	Dab	D-Leu	Leu
circulin A	[5854-98-8]	MOA	Dab	D-Leu	Ile

[a] Dab = α,γ-diaminobutyric acid; MOA = (+)-6-methyloctanoic acid; IOA = isooctanoic acid.

Polymyxins A and D each contain two D-amino acid residues, where polymyxins B and E have one. This difference may be responsible for the higher nephrotoxicity with the A and D compounds. The higher proportions of hydroxyamino acids found in A and D are reflected in the water solubility of the bases of these polymyxins, in contrast with that of polymyxins B and E and circulin A, which precipitate when aqueous solutions are neutralized.

Although Vogler and co-workers (250) were able to chemically synthesize polymyxins B$_1$ and E$_1$ (colistin A) and circulin A, and Wilkinson polymyxin A$_1$ (251), the procedures are more costly than the microbiological process. However, their elegant work, summarized in Figure 2, is a very good example of the strategy that can be used. The three protected peptides (1), (2), and (3) were synthesized by classical methods, using the azide procedure to avoid racemization. The BOC group was removed from (1) by treatment with trifluoroacetic acid, and then (1) was treated with the azide derived from peptide (2). The resulting octapeptide ester was in turn converted to the azide (via the hydrazide) and coupled with peptide (3) to give the protected open-chain decapeptide ester (4). The Bu^t and BOC groups were removed with trifluoroacetic acid and the product (5) cyclized in highly dilute solution in a mixture of dioxane and dimethylformamide, using a large excess of dicyclohexyl carbodiimide. The N-protecting benzyloxycarbonyl residues were removed by reduction with sodium in liquid ammonia and the product was purified by countercurrent distribution to give a 10–15% yield of polymyxin B$_1$ at the cyclization–reduction stage. Even lower yields were encountered at the cyclization stage during the syntheses of circulin A and polymyxin A$_1$. In their early work on the synthesis Vogler and co-workers (253) prepared a number of analogues with a larger cyclic portion in the molecule and found these had little antimicrobial activity.

Table 7.   The Octapeptin Group of Streptomyces Antibiotics

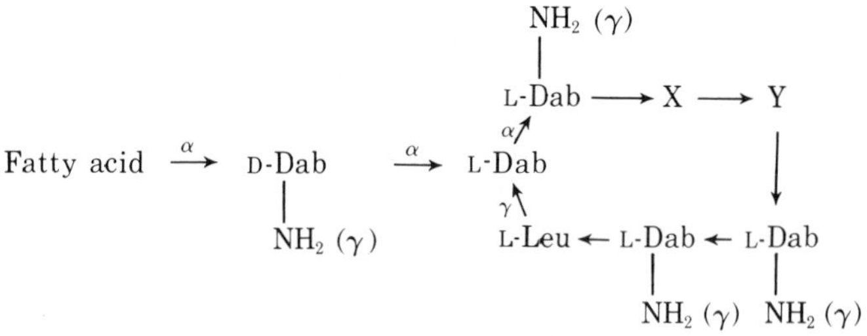

$$
\begin{array}{c}
\text{NH}_2\,(\gamma) \\
| \\
\text{L-Dab} \longrightarrow X \longrightarrow Y \\
\alpha\nearrow \\
\text{Fatty acid} \xrightarrow{\alpha} \text{D-Dab} \xrightarrow{\alpha} \text{L-Dab} \\
| \qquad\qquad \gamma\nwarrow \\
\text{NH}_2\,(\gamma) \qquad \text{L-Leu} \leftarrow \text{L-Dab} \leftarrow \text{L-Dab} \\
| \qquad\quad | \\
\text{NH}_2\,(\gamma)\quad \text{NH}_2\,(\gamma)
\end{array}
$$

Octapeptin	Synonym	Dab[a] D	Dab[a] L	X	Y	Fatty acids
A_1	EM 49β	1	4	D-Leu	L-Leu	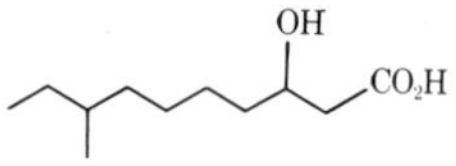 (structure with OH, CO$_2$H)
A_2	EM 49α	1	4	D-Leu	L-Leu	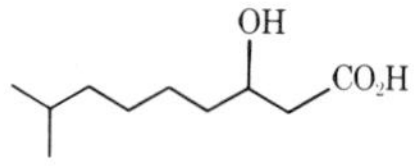 (structure with OH, CO$_2$H)
A_3	EM 49α	1	4	D-Leu	L-Leu	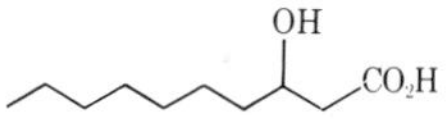 (structure with OH, CO$_2$H)
B_1	EM 49δ	1	4	D-Leu	L-Phe	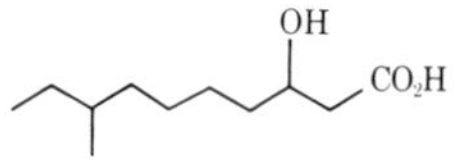 (structure with OH, CO$_2$H)
B_2	EM 49γ	1	4	D-Leu	L-Phe	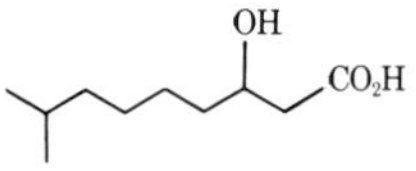 (structure with OH, CO$_2$H)
B_3	EM 49γ	1	4	D-Leu	L-Phe	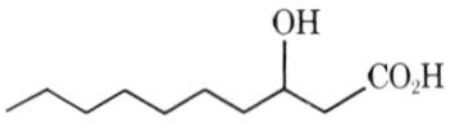 (structure with OH, CO$_2$H)
C_1	Bu-1880		5	Leu	Phe	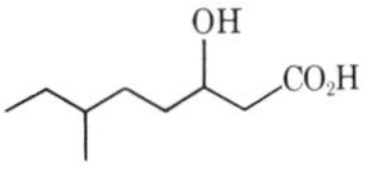 (structure with OH, CO$_2$H)
	333-25	1	4	D-Phe	L-Leu	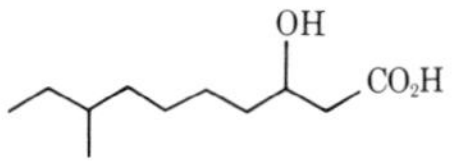 (structure with OH, CO$_2$H)
	Y-8495	+		+	+	+

[a] Dab = α,γ-diaminobutyric acid.

The polymyxins inhibit the growth of a number of gram-negative organisms including *Pseudomonas, Escherichia, Klebsiella, Enterobacter, Salmonella, Shigella,* and *Haemophilus* species, and are not inhibitors of growth of *Proteus* and gram-positive bacteria. Preparations of sulfates of polymyxin B and of colistin (polymyxin E) are used for local, topical, oral, and intravenous medication, and the sodium *N*-sulfomethyl derivatives are used for intramuscular and intrathecal administration. A wide range of mixed antibiotic formulations is marketed some of which are listed in Table 8.

The sulfates of polymyxin B and colistin have been used orally for gastrointestinal infections and bowel sterilization prior to surgery, but because of poor absorption, they are not used for systemic infections. Dosage levels are of the order of 75–100 mg/d

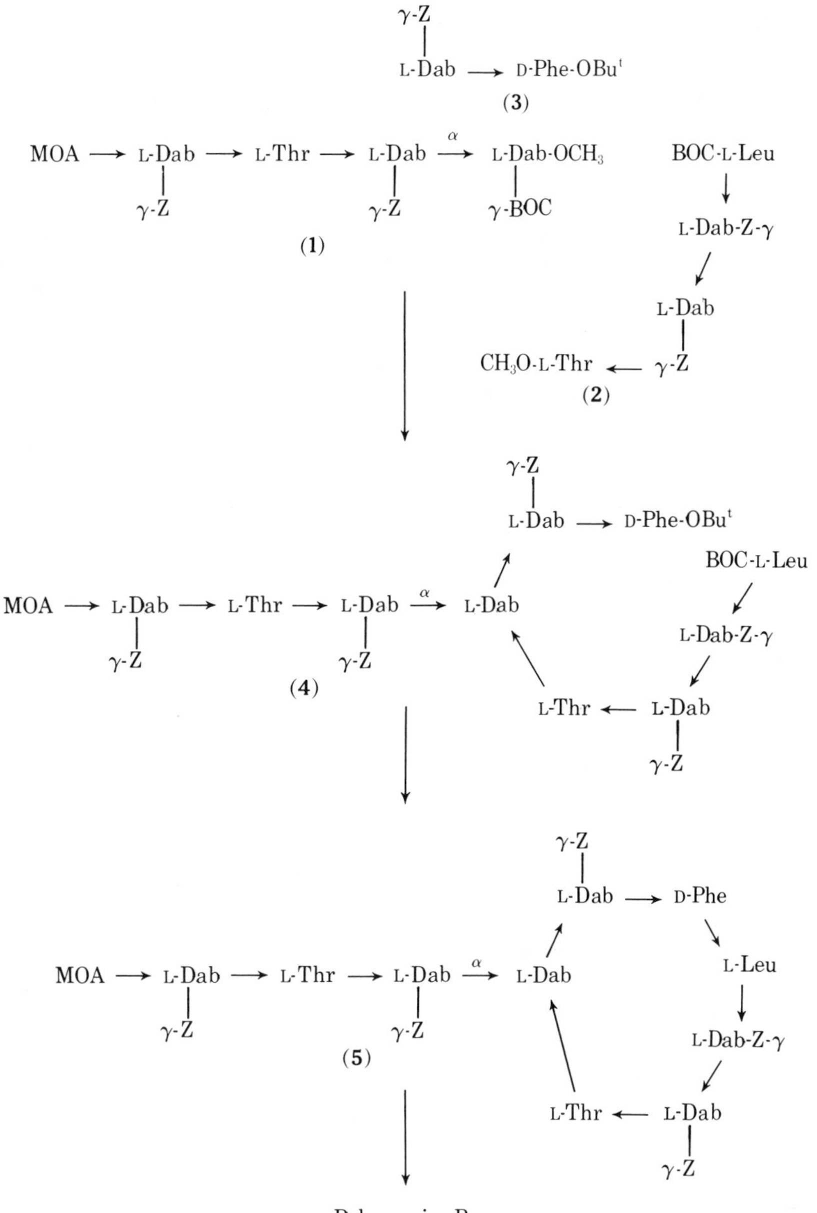

$$\begin{array}{c}\gamma\text{-Z}\\ |\\ \text{L-Dab}\longrightarrow \text{D-Phe-OBu}^t\\ (\textbf{3})\end{array}$$

MOA $\longrightarrow$ L-Dab $\longrightarrow$ L-Thr $\longrightarrow$ L-Dab $\xrightarrow{\alpha}$ L-Dab·OCH$_3$ BOC·L-Leu

with γ-Z under first L-Dab, γ-Z under second L-Dab, γ-BOC under L-Dab·OCH$_3$

(**1**)

BOC·L-Leu $\downarrow$ L-Dab-Z-γ $\searrow$ L-Dab

CH$_3$O·L-Thr $\longleftarrow$ γ-Z

(**2**)

$$\begin{array}{c}\gamma\text{-Z}\\ |\\ \text{L-Dab}\longrightarrow \text{D-Phe-OBu}^t\end{array}$$

BOC·L-Leu

MOA $\longrightarrow$ L-Dab $\longrightarrow$ L-Thr $\longrightarrow$ L-Dab $\xrightarrow{\alpha}$ L-Dab

L-Dab-Z-γ

(**4**)

L-Thr $\longleftarrow$ L-Dab

with γ-Z

$$\begin{array}{c}\gamma\text{-Z}\\ |\\ \text{L-Dab}\longrightarrow \text{D-Phe}\end{array}$$

L-Leu

MOA $\longrightarrow$ L-Dab $\longrightarrow$ L-Thr $\longrightarrow$ L-Dab $\xrightarrow{\alpha}$ L-Dab

L-Dab-Z-γ

(**5**)

L-Thr $\longleftarrow$ L-Dab

with γ-Z

Polymyxin B$_1$

Figure 2. The synthesis of polymyxin B$_1$ (250). MOA = (+)-6-methyloctanoic acid; Z = benzyloxycarbonyl; OBu^t = 3-*tert*-butoxy; BOC = 3^t-butyloxycarbonyl.

for adults when given *per os* (orally) with corresponding reduction in level and use of divided doses for children.

For local or topical use (see Table 8) in otic solutions or ointments the concentrations are usually 0.1–0.25% (wt/vol or wt/wt) of the polymyxin sulfates. Ophthalmic

Table 8. Therapeutic Dosage Forms for Some Peptide Antibiotics

Type of preparation	Antibiotics present	Trade names	Manufacturer
ophthalmic ointment	bacitracin; oxytetracycline [79-57-2]	Terramycin ophthalmic	Pfizer
	chloramphenicol; polymyxin B [1404-26-8]	Chloromycetin–Polymyxin	Parke, Davis
	bacitracin	Baciguent	Upjohn
	polymyxin B; neomycin [1404-04-2]	Statrol	Alcon
	polymyxin B; zinc bacitracin [1405-89-6]	Polysporin ophthalmic	Burroughs-Wellcome
	polymyxin B; zinc bacitracin; neomycin	Neopolycin	Dow
	polymyxin B; bacitracin; neomycin	Mycitracin	Upjohn
	polymyxin B; zinc bacitracin; neomycin	Neosporin	Burroughs-Wellcome
		Pyocidin	SMP
		Polyspectrum	Allergan
	neomycin; polymyxin B; hydrocortisone	Cortisporin	Burroughs-Wellcome
	neomycin; polymyxin B; dexamethsasone	Maxitrol	Alcon
	chloramphenicol; polymyxin B; hydrocortisone	Ophthocort	Parke, Davis
otic solutions	polymyxin B	Aerosporin otic	Burroughs-Wellcome
	neomycin; polymyxin	Cortisporin otic	Burroughs-Wellcome
	neomycin; polymyxin; hydrocortisone	Otocort	Lemmon
	neomycin; tyrothricin	Otalgine	Purdue-Frederick
	neomycin; colistin	Coly-Mycin S	Warner-Chilcott
	neomycin; polymyxin; nystatin [1400-61-9]; fludrocortisone	Florotic	Squibb
vaginal tablet	oxytetracycline; polymyxin	Terramycin vaginal tablets	Pfizer
general purpose ointment	bacitracin	Baciguent	Upjohn
general purpose topical solution	bacitracin	Bacitracin powder for solution	Pfizer
antimicrobial ointment	polymyxin; gramicidin; neomycin	Neosporin ointment	Burroughs-Wellcome
	polymyxin; neomycin; bacitracin	Mycitracin ointment	Upjohn
	polymyxin; neomycin; zinc bacitracin; benzalkonium chloride	Biotres ointment	Central

ointments may contain 0.2% (wt/vol). Polymyxin B in isotonic saline (0.5%) is used intrathecally and sterile, pyrogen-free polymyxin B sulfate is available for intravenous infusion in cases of severe systemic infection (usually requiring hospitalization). Although the acute intravenous toxicity is reduced by sulfomethylation with formaldehyde and sodium metabisulfite, this toxicity is of little therapeutic importance because the polymyxin B sulfates have a satisfactory therapeutic index. The main advantage of the sulfomethyl derivatives is the reduction of pain at the site of intramuscular injection and thus making parenteral therapy tolerable to the patient.

Barnett and co-workers (255) have discussed the relationship between the degree of sulfomethylation and therapeutic response and have noted a correlation of the intravenous LD_{50} values of various preparations and their therapeutic efficiency. The data showed that detoxification by sulfomethylation is minimal and that derivatives with LD_{50} (iv in mice) of the order of 100 mg/kg are a reasonable compromise. Burroughs-Wellcome & Company's Thiosporin (sodium sulfomethyl polymyxin B), Warner Chilcott Laboratories' Coli-Mycin, and the Colimycine Intramusculaire from Laboratorie Roger Bellon all have some differences in degree of sulfomethylation and different LD_{50} values and thus should be considered as somewhat different products. They are useful when administered intramuscularly or intrathecally to combat acute enteritis, urinary and respiratory tract infections, bacteremia, peritonitis, and meningitis caused by *Pseudomonas* sp *Escherichia coli*, *Enterobacter aerogenes*, and *Klebsiella* sp.

The potency of polymyxin B sulfate is expressed in terms of units based on a master standard assigned the arbitrary value of 10,000 units per milligram of polymyxin B sulfate. The potency of colistin is expressed in terms of a master standard with a value of 30,000 units/mg of colistin base (equivalent to 20,000 units/mg of colistin sulfate). These potencies are usually determined using *Brucella bronchiseptica* as test organism in the agar diffusion bioassay. Samples containing the sulfomethyl derivatives are treated in pH 2.0 glycine buffer to convert them to the polymyxin base before the bioassay.

In addition to the dosage forms mentioned in Table 8, polymyxin is available as a powder for reconstitution for use in injections (Aerosporin brand Polymyxin sulfate from Burroughs-Wellcome & Co. and Polymyxin B sulfate from Pfizer) and the above mentioned sodium sulfomethyl derivatives (Thiosporin from Burroughs-Wellcome & Co.; Coly-mycin Injectable from Warner-Chilcott Laboratories; and Dynamyxin from Pfizer, Inc.).

The Bacitracins. Bacitracin is a complex mixture of water-soluble peptides produced by certain strains of *Bacillus subtilis* (38,256) and *Bacillus licheniformis* (32). The latter produces an antibiotic originally named ayfivin and later shown to be the same as bacitracin (257).

This group of related peptides is produced by growing *B. subtilis* var. *Tracy* in media containing soybean products, eg, soybean meal, soybean flour, soybean grits, and a source of fermentable carbohydrate. Yields of the order of 500 units/mL (about 9 mg/mL) are obtained in the 40 h incubation period (38). The antibiotic activity is recovered from the fermented medium by extraction with *n*-butanol (258), by precipitation with basic dyes (259), by precipitation with methylenedisalicylic acid (260), or by adsorption on cationic-exchange resins followed by elution with dilute ammonium hydroxide (261).

Commercial bacitracin is a white amorphous powder which is soluble in water, ethanol, methanol, and *n*-butanol, and insoluble in acetone, ethyl ether, and chloroform. The USP unit of bacitracin is defined as the bacitracin activity given by 26 μg of the dried FDA master standard; commercial-grade material has a potency of about 50 units/mg, and some material has been isolated which as a potency of about 100 units/mg. Biological standardization is based on an agar diffusion bioassay with *Micrococcus flavus* or *Sarcina subflava* as test organisms (242).

Bacitracins are usually stable at temperatures between 25 and 27°C when the moisture content is less than 1%. Aqueous solutions at pH 5.7 deteriorate rapidly at room temperature and slowly when refrigerated. Even more instability has been noted at pH 9. The insoluble salts, such as zinc bacitracin and bacitracin methylenedisalicylate, are more stable than the parent compound, especially when dry. They are also less bitter than the parent and can be compounded in oral preparations. Bacitracin methylene-disalicylate contains 2 mol of methylenedisalicylic acid per mol of bacitracin and the commercial material has a potency of about 18 bacitracin units/mg. Its solubility in water is about 5% while that of bacitracin (potency about 60 units/mg) has a solubility of about 0.5%.

Commercial bacitracin was separated by countercurrent distribution into a number of components designated as bacitracins A, B, C, D, E, F, and G (262). Bacitracin F was later found to be an artifact of low antibacterial activity and high nephrotoxicity formed from bacitracin A at alkaline or neutral pH (263).

The structures presented in Figure 3 have been proposed for bacitracin (264–266). The initial proposal accounted for the detection of only 3 basic centers, the liberation of 1 mol of NH_3 on hydrolysis, and the location of isoleucine as the N-terminal amino acid. However, it was not consistent with the absence of a free-thio group and the identification of the peptides containing the sequence Phe–Ile in the partial hydrolyzates.

The D-aspartic acid was found to be present as the α-amide and the β-carboxyl group of the L-aspartic acid was found to be linked to the ϵ-amino group of lysine. These and other observations led to the revised structure shown in Figure 3.

Bacitracin B is considered to be a fermentation product and bacitracins C, D, and E may be formed during the purification of the bacitracin mixture from the fermented medium (267). Bacitracin B contains a L-valine residue and its final structure is still to be determined (267).

Bacitracins inhibit the growth of gram-positive bacteria and have found use in topical preparations, eg, lotions, creams, ointments, for the control of these organisms in skin infections. Although changes in purification methods have reduced the nephrotoxicity, intramuscular injections of bacitracin may frequently be followed by renal damage and this use is restricted to hospitalized patients without a record of renal damage. In the latter group of patients a high fluid intake is usually recommended when bacitracin is injected, and progressive renal damage (with diminished renal output) requires prompt withdrawal of the antibiotic. The oral route is safe for treatment of intestinal amebiases as bacitracin is not absorbed from the gastrointestinal tract. The major use of bacitracin in clinical therapy is in combination with other antibiotics in creams, lotions, and ointments (see Table 8) where the concentration may range from 250 to 1000 USP units per gram or milliliter.

Bacitracin as either the zinc bacitracin or the bacitracin methylenedisalicylate has been widely used as a growth promotant for poultry, swine, and other farm animals. The usual level added to the feed is 1–3 g/t, and the major portion of the bacitracin produced (see Table 3) is used for this purpose (see Pet and livestock feeds).

Tyrothricin, Gramicidin, and Tyrocidine. Tyrothricin was the first antibiotic to be discovered as the result of planned investigation of the metabolic products of soil microorganisms. Dubos isolated the active material from a *Bacillus brevis* fermentation (268) and showed it to be a mixture of two materials (205).

Tyrothricin is produced when the *B. brevis* culture is grown in several types of

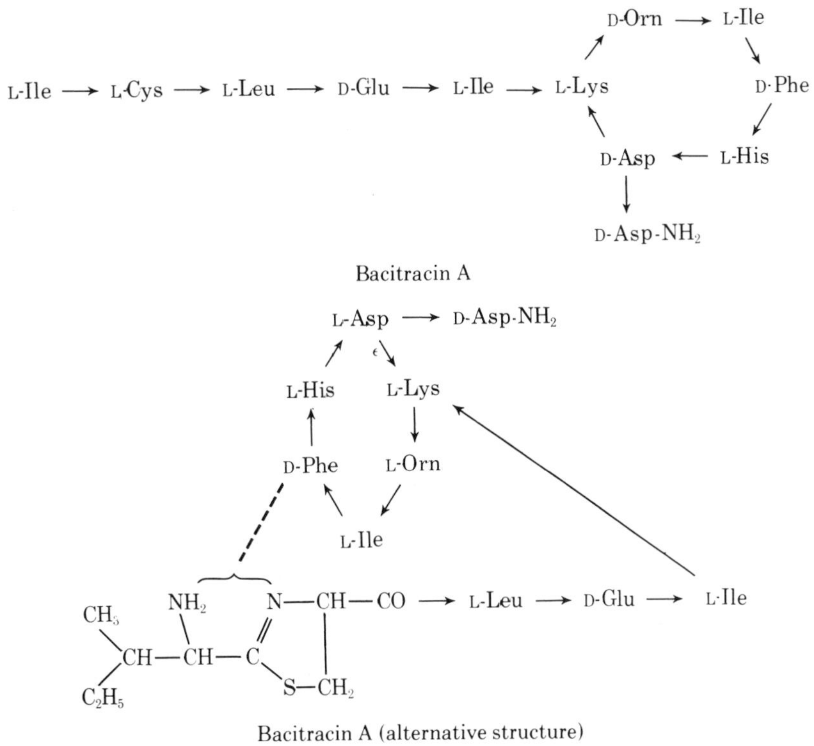

D-Orn ⟶ L-Ile

L-Ile ⟶ L-Cys ⟶ L-Leu ⟶ D-Glu ⟶ L-Ile ⟶ L-Lys   D-Phe

D-Asp ⟵ L-His

D-Asp-NH₂

Bacitracin A

L-Asp ⟶ D-Asp-NH₂

L-His   L-Lys

D-Phe   L-Orn

L-Ile

CH₃
      NH₂   N—CH—CO ⟶ L-Leu ⟶ D-Glu ⟶ L-Ile
    CH—CH—C
C₂H₅   S—CH₂

Bacitracin A (alternative structure)

Figure 3. Structures proposed for bacitracin A (264–266).

media (269) under aerated culture. Maximum titers of the order of 3 g/L can be obtained after a few days of fermentation, and the yields vary with incubation conditions. Isolation of the antibiotic activity from the fermented media usually involves a procedure similar to that outlined in Figure 4. The antibacterial activity is precipitated when the pH of the fermented medium is adjusted to pH 4.5–4.8 with HCl. The precipitate is dried and then extracted with ethanol. Sodium chloride is added to the ethanolic solution and the purified tyrothricin precipitates. The precipitate is then extracted with an acetone–ethyl ether mixture which dissolves the neutral gramicidin and the insoluble fraction is the basic tyrocidine (270).

Commercial tyrothricin (see Table 3 for producers) is a purified unresolved mixture of these two components with a gramicidin content of about 20%. The white amorphous powder is practically insoluble in water and soluble in pyridine, methanol, ethanol, acetic acid, and ethylene glycol. The solubility of tyrothricin in ethanol and ethylene glycol makes it feasible to prepare stable emulsions for clinical use by adding the requisite amount of a stock solution to isotonic saline or distilled water. Clear aqueous solutions may be obtained by using formaldehyde or cationic surface-active agents as solubilizers.

Gramicidin, the isoluble neutral fraction isolated by treating tyrothricin with an acetone–ethyl ether mixture, can be crystallized from acetone or dioxan. This material is also known as *gramicidin Dubos* and was separated by countercurrent

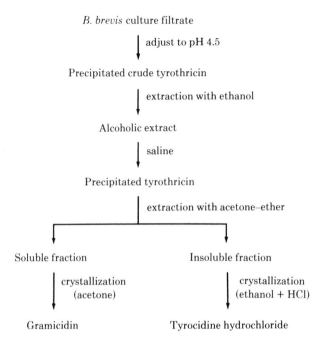

B. brevis culture filtrate

adjust to pH 4.5

Precipitated crude tyrothricin

extraction with ethanol

Alcoholic extract

saline

Precipitated tyrothricin

extraction with acetone–ether

Soluble fraction   Insoluble fraction

crystallization   crystallization
(acetone)   (ethanol + HCl)

Gramicidin   Tyrocidine hydrochloride

Figure 4.   Flow sheet for the extraction of tyrocidine and gramicidin A from *Bacillus brevis*.

distribution into 4 components (271). Gramicidin A was found in one preparation to be the major component with gramicidins B and C amounting to about 10% of the weight of the starting material and gramicidin D to much less than this. Although each fraction was isolated in apparently crystalline form, each was further resolved into two closely related peptides (272–273). Chemical studies showed these 6 gramicidins to be linear pentadecapeptides differing only in the nature of the amino acids at positions 1 and 11 (see Table 9). Although these peptides do not have free-amino or free-carboxyl groups, they are not cyclic peptides; the terminal amino group is formylated and the carboxyl is blocked as the ethanolamide. The valine and isoleucine gramicidins A have been prepared by chemical synthesis (96).

Tyrocidine, prepared by fractionation of tyrothricin, crystallizes as a monohydrochloride from ethanol (containing HCl). As in the case of gramicidin, this material, although crystalline, is not homogeneous and can be separated by countercurrent distribution into three major components, tyrocidines A, B, and C (270). The structures of these closely related compounds are presented in Figure 5.

Gramicidin S was isolated from a strain of *B. brevis* Gauze-Brazhnikova (98). The term gramicidin S is deceptive in that the antibiotic is structurally different from gramicidin and more closely related to tyrocidine. It is produced by the particular strain of *B. brevis* when grown in a variety of media and can be recovered from the fermented medium by acidification of the cell-free liquid to pH 4.7. The gramicidin S precipitates and can be collected by filtration and dried. The dried solids are dissolved in ethanol, the solution treated with activated charcoal, filtered, and concentrated. The crystalline gramicidin S forms colorless needles. These are insoluble in water and soluble in ethanol and methanol.

Table 9.   The Structures of the Gramicidins A, B, and C

$$\text{CHO} \qquad\qquad \overset{15}{\text{HOCH}_2\text{CH}_2\text{NH}}—\overset{}{\text{Tyr}}—\overset{14}{\text{D·Leu}}—\overset{13}{\text{Trp}}—\overset{12}{\text{D·Leu}}$$

$$\underset{1}{\text{X}}—\underset{2}{\text{Gly}}—\underset{3}{\text{Ala}}—\underset{4}{\text{D·Leu}}—\underset{5}{\text{Ala}}—\underset{6}{\text{D·Val}}—\underset{7}{\text{Val}}—\underset{8}{\text{D·Val}}—\underset{9}{\text{Trp}}—\underset{10}{\text{D·Leu}}—\underset{11}{\text{Y}}$$

	X	Y
valine–gramicidin A	Val	Trp
isoleucine–gramicidin A	Ile	Trp
valine–gramicidin B	Val	Phe
isoleucine–gramicidin B	Ile	Phe
valine–gramicidin C	Val	Tyr
isoleucine–gramicidin C	Ile	Tyr

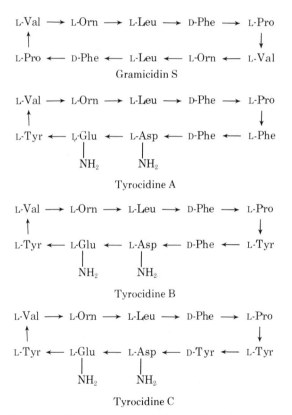

Figure 5.   Structures of gramicidin S and tyrocidines (274).

The structure was deduced by analyzing the products of total and partial acid hydrolysis (98), and a total chemical synthesis was achieved by Schwyzer and Sieber (275). The two gramicidins J_1 and J_2, isolated by Otani and co-workers (97) from other strains of *B. brevis* are now recognized as being identical with gramicidin S (276).

Studies of gramicidin S and tyrocidine syntheses by cell-free enzymes established that only soluble enzyme systems are involved in the total synthesis of these cyclic peptides in contrast to the ribosomal systems previously reported (277). Extracts of gramicidin S-producing strains of *B. brevis* on filtration through Sephadex G-200 gave two complimentary factors that synthesized gramicidin S when supplied with ATP, Mg^{2+}, and the constituent amino acids (278). Factor I has a molecular weight of 280,000 and factor II 100,000. The lighter factor activates and racemizes D- and L-phenylalanine, and the heavy factor activates the other four amino acids (279).

Tyrothricin is very effective in experimental infections against many gram-positive pathogens (280). Unfortunately, it has a hemolytic action, due mainly to the tyrocidine, and is not suited for systemic chemotherapy. The antibacterial activities of both gramicidin and tyrocidine are inhibited by the presence of plasma, and parenteral administration has not been seriously considered. The clinical application of tyrothricin, gramicidin, and tyrocidine has been restricted to local and topical uses. A variety of pharmaceutical formulations including ointments, creams, and lotions are mentioned in Table 8. At one time tyrothricin was used in lozenges, troches, and dentifrices, but these applications have been discontinued.

Subtilin is a mixture of basic polypeptides produced by a particular strain of *Bacillus subtilis*. They have been isolated in pure form following chromatography (182,281) and the structure of subtilin A determined (Fig. 6) (282). It is a peptide containing lanthionine and β-methyllanthionine, and the dehydroamino acids dehydroalanine and dehydrobutyrine. It is chemically related to nisin an antibiotic produced by streptococci (see Fig. 6) (144). Both inhibit the growth of gram-positive organisms with subtilin having broader activity while nisin's activity is restricted to streptococci. Nisin is produced on a commercial basis for use as a food preservative in a few European countries.

Peptide Antibiotics from *Streptomyces* Species. In Table 4 are 150 peptide antibiotics (a minimum) which have been isolated from different species of *Streptomyces*. The number is increasing rapidly as different species are screened and more sensitive and specific analytical methods are developed. Only a limited number have proved valuable as therapeutic agents and these are discussed individually below.

Viomycin and the related capreomycin are tuberculostatic antibiotics isolated from cultures of *Streptomyces puniceus* (211) and *Streptomyces capreolus* (47), respectively. These antibiotics may be recovered from the fermented medium by adsorption (from the filtrate) on charcoal, by precipitation with various acidic dyestuffs, or by use of cationic-exchange resins (283). The viomycin and capreomycin are strongly basic water-soluble peptides, readily forming highly colored crystalline salts such as the hydrochloride, the sulfate, or the naphthalene-2-sulfonate. They are stable in acid solution, and somewhat unstable under alkaline conditions.

The unit (USP) of viomycin is defined as 1 μg of the pure base and the activity of viomycin preparations is expressed in terms of such units. Capreomycin potency is expressed in terms of μg of the free base. Standardizations of both antibiotics are conducted using bioassays with *Klebsiella pneumoniae*, *Mycobacterium butyricum*, or *Bacillus subtilis* as test organisms (both turbidimetric and agar diffusion assay systems have been used).

Structures proposed for viomycins and capreomycins are shown in Figure 7.

Particular interest in viomycin and capreomycin lies in their tuberculostatic activity. Among the toxic manifestations noted are nephrotoxicity, ototoxicity (auditory),

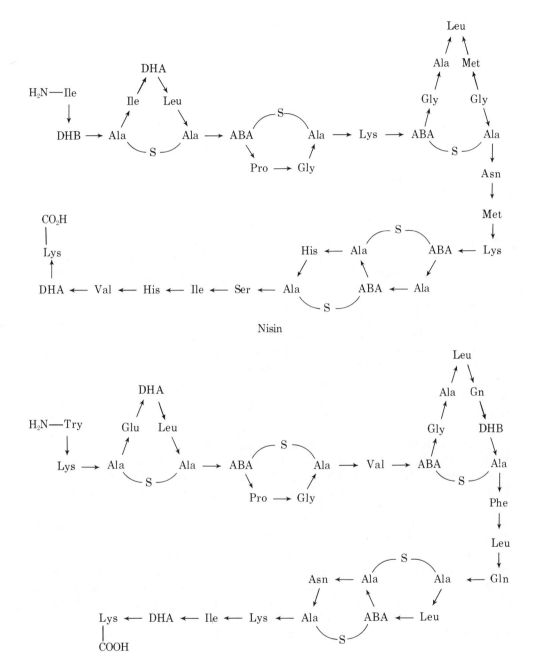

Figure 6. Structures proposed for nisin and subtilin (144,282). ABA = aminobutyric acid; Asn = asparagine; ABA-S-Ala = β-methyllanthionine; DHA = dehydroalanine; Ala-S-Ala = lanthionine; DHB = dehydrobutyrine; Gln = glutamine.

235

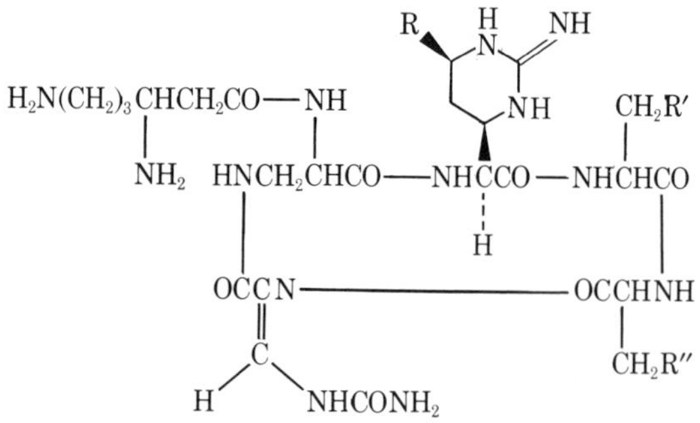

Figure 7.   Structures proposed for viomycin and capreomycins (47). Viomycin: R = R′ = R″ = H; capreomycin IB: R = R′ = H, R″ = NH_2; capreomycin IA: R = H, R′ = OH, R″ = NH_2.

abnormal liver function, leukocytosis, leukopenia, and hypersensitivity, and as a result, these drugs are not very frequently used for treatment of tuberculosis unless other therapy has not been satisfactory. The usual dosage regimen has included 1 g/d (not to exceed 20 mg/kg) given intramuscularly for 60 to 120 d followed by 1 g two or three times per week with a total treatment of 18–24 mo.

Amphomycin is a mixture of closely related peptides (see Table 10) produced by *Streptomyces canus*. It inhibits the growth of gram-positive bacteria and is included in topical preparations (ointments and creams) for this purpose: Amcort contains calcium amphomycin, neomycin sulfate, and hydrocortisone acetate in a cream base. Amphomycin has a low potential for producing sensitivity reactions, and organisms develop resistance to it very slowly. Unlike bacitracin, amphomycin is water-stable, and therefore, ideally suited for use in a hydrophilic base. Amphomycin cannot be used in injectable formulations as it causes hemolysis of the red blood cells.

Thiostrepton, a crystalline sulfur-containing antibiotic, was isolated from cultures of *Streptomyces azureus* (284–285). A tentative structure has been determined by chemical degradation studies and x-ray crystallographic observations (196,286–287). The antibiotic crystallizes readily from a mixture of methanol and chloroform, and is insoluble in water and lower alcohols. It has high potency against gram-positive bacteria and is used in treatment of bovine mastitis. A related antibiotic, siomycin (produced by *Streptomyces sioyaensis* (173,288), is a mixture of compounds with apparent peptide sequences in common with thiostrepton. This mixture which is active against gram-positive bacteria has found veterinary application in Japan. The third member of this sulfur-containing peptide antibiotic group is the thiopeptins, produced by *Streptomyces tateyamensis*.They can be differentiated (195) from thiostrepton, siomycin, pepthiomycins (289), thermothiocin (194), sporangiomycin (174), and sulfomycins (196) on the basis of sulfur content and mobility in several chromatographic systems.

Thiopeptins are active against gram-positive bacteria and *Mycoplasma laidlawii*. They are nontoxic when administered to poultry and swine *per os,* highly stable when added to animal feed, and well tolerated by poultry and swine. Thiopeptin-supplemented feed contributes to the improvement of weight gain, feed efficiency in chickens and swine, and the egg performance in layers. It is widely used in Japan as a livestock feed supplement.

Table 10. Constituents of the Amphomycin Group of Antibiotics from Streptomycetes[a]

$CH_3CH_2CH(CH_2)_5CH{=}CHCH_2CO$—Asp —MeAsp—Asp— Gly —Asp —Gly—Dab[e]—Val—Pro
        |
        CH_3
                                        ┌—Pip—Dab[t]—┐

Antibiotic	Fatty acids	Aspartic acid	β-Methyl-aspartic acid	Pro-line	Gly-cine	Va-line	D-Pipe-colic acid	α,β-Diamino-butyric acid
ampho-mycin	3-anteisotridecenoic; 3-isododecenoic	3	1	1	2	1	1	2[b]
asparto-cin	3-anteisopenta-decenoic; 3-isopenta-decenoic	4	+	1	2	1	+	+
chrystallo-mycin	unidentified	8 (3)[c]	?	+	6 (2)	3 (1)	3 (1)	+[d]
gluma-mycin	3-anteisotri-decenoic	3	1	1	2	1	1	2
lasparto-mycin[e]	2-isopentadecenoic	4	−	1	4	−	+	1
tsushi-mycin	3-anteisotridecenoic	4[f]		1	2	1	+	+[d]
zaomycin	isoundecenoic			similar to tsushimycin				

[a] Dab[e] = D-erythro-α,β-diaminobutyric acid; Dab[t] = L-threo-α,β-diaminobutyric acid; Pip = D-pipecolic acid.
[b] L-Threo- and D-erythro-α,β-diaminobutyric acid.
[c] Values in parentheses are corrected, probable values.
[d] Basic amino acids.
[e] Contains also threonine and isoleucine.
[f] Including β-methylaspartic acid.

The enduracidins are a group of chlorine containing peptide antibiotics produced by *Streptomyces fungicidicus*. Chemical studies showed that hydrolyzates contained aspartic acid, threonine and/or *allo*-threonine, serine, glycine, alanine, citrulline, ornithine, 4-hydroxyphenylglycine, 3,5-dichloro-4-hydroxyphenylglycine, αS-amino-β-4R-(2-iminoimidazolidinyl)-propionic acid, and αR-amino-β-4R-(2-iminoimida-zolidinyl)-propionic acid as well as a lipophilic component (290). Enduracidin A contains 10-methylundeca-2(*cis*)-4(*trans*)-dienoic acid and enduracidin B contains (+)-10-methyldodeca-2(*cis*)-4(*trans*)-dienoic acid . The structure proposed for enduracidin B is presented in Figure 8. Enduracidin and the related janeimycins (112) inhibit cell wall formation in gram-positive bacteria and also inhibit growth of Mycobacteria. Enduracidin is well tolerated by poultry and swine and not absorbed when given *per os*. It has found commercial application in Japan as a feed supplement for poultry and swine.

Stendomycin, an antifungal peptide antibiotic produced by *Streptomyces endus* (177) is a mixture of closely related compounds (291). Their amino acid sequence was elucidated mainly through the study of peptides from partial acid hydrolysis. In all members of the stendomycin family the *N*-terminal amino acid, proline, is acylated

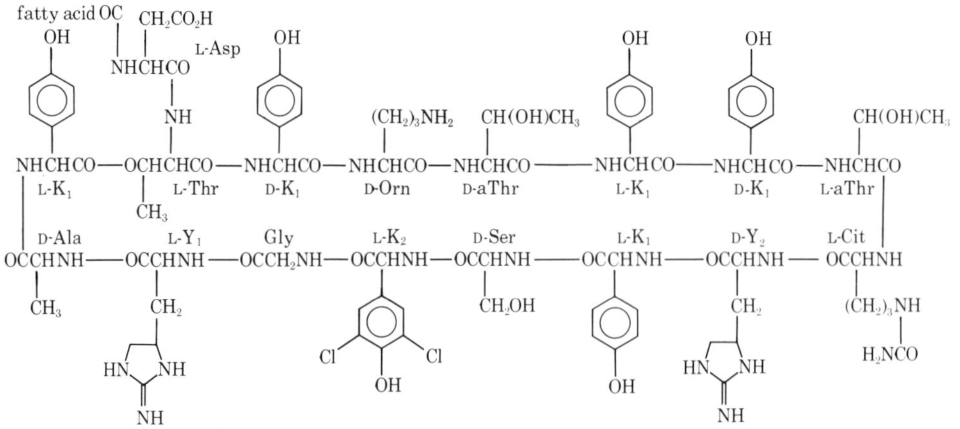

Figure 8. Structure proposed for enduracidin (71). Cit = citrulline; K_1 = (4-hydroxyphenyl)glycine; K_2 = (3,5-dichloro-4-hydroxyphenyl)glycine; Y_1 = $2S$-α-amino-$4R$-β-(2-iminoimidazolidinyl)-propionic acid; Y_2 = $2R$-α-amino-$4R$-β-(2-iminoimidazolidinyl)-propionic acid.

by a branched-chain fatty acid and the C-terminal amino acid, a cyclic derivative of arginine, forms a lactone bond with the hydroxyl group of one of the *allo*-threonine residues. The structures proposed by Bodanszky and co-workers (291) are presented in Figure 9. Stendomycin was manufactured for some years by the Eli Lilly Company for commercial use as an antifungal agent in agriculture. It is not now available for this purpose.

The antitumor compound neocarzinostatin is an acidic single-chain molecule, cross-linked by two disulfide bridges, and consists of 109 amino acid residues. It is produced by *Streptomyces carzinostaticus* (143) and inhibits the growth of gram-positive bacteria as well as many tumors in experimental animals. The principal effect of neocarzinostatin is arrest of mitosis and the mechanism of action is inhibition of DNA synthesis and possibly degradation of existing DNA. The structure proposed by Meienhofer and co-workers (143) is presented in Figure 10. Clinical tests are promising for treatment of tumors in the rectum and stomach and carcinoma of the bladder and penis (see Chemotherapeutics, antimitotic).

The bleomycins are a group of peptide antibiotics produced by *Streptomyces verticillus* and extracted from the fermented media by the successive application of cation-exchange resin chromatography, carbon chromatography, and alumina chromatography (292). The bleomycin complex thus obtained contains copper (ie, the copper-chelated form) and is a mixture of bleomycins A_1, demethyl–A_2, A_2'–a, A_2'–b, A_2'–c, A_5, A_6, B_1', B_2, and B_4 which have been purified by chromatography on a CM-Sephadex column using a gradient of ammonium formate or sodium chloride (293–294). The cupric ion in the copper-chelated bleomycins can be removed by treatment with H_2S and both copper-chelated and copper-free bleomycins show almost the same activity in inhibiting the growth of bacterial and animal cells. A mixture of copper-free bleomycins consisting mainly of A_2 (55–70%) and B_2 (25–32%) was shown to be superior to A_2 alone in its effect on human squamous cell carcinoma and has been used clinically.

All bleomycins are water soluble and soluble in methanol. They are essentially

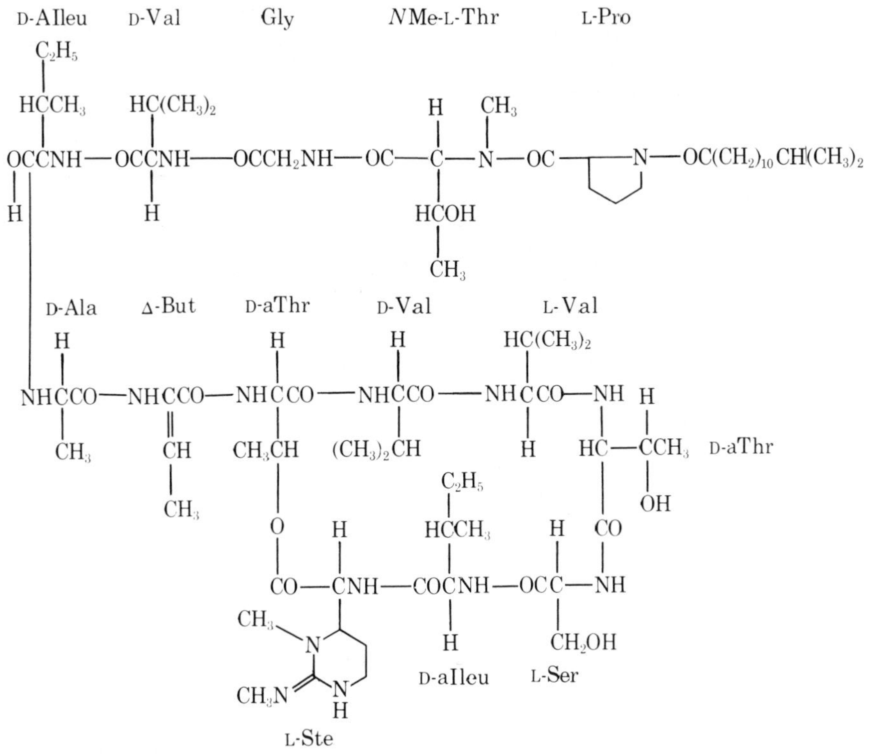

D-Alleu   D-Val   Gly   NMe-L-Thr   L-Pro

C_2H_5

HĊCH$_3$ HC(CH$_3$)$_2$ H   CH$_3$

OCĊNH—OCĊNH—OCCH$_2$NH—OC—Ċ—N—OC———N—OC(CH$_2$)$_{10}$CH(CH$_3$)$_2$

H   H   HĊOH

CH$_3$

D-Ala   Δ-But   D-aThr   D-Val   L-Val

H   H   H   H   HC(CH$_3$)$_2$

NHĊCO—NHĊCO—NHĊCO—NHĊCO—NHĊCO—NH H

CH$_3$ CH   CH$_3$ĊH   (CH$_3$)$_2$ĊH   H   HĊ—ĊCH$_3$ D-aThr

CH   O   H C_2H_5 H   CO   OH

CH$_3$ HĊCH$_3$ H CO

CO—ĊNH—COCNH—OCĊ—NH

CH$_3$ H   CH$_2$OH

N   D-alleu   L-Ser

CH$_3$N   N
         H

L-Ste

Figure 9.   Structure proposed for stendomycin (273). Ste = stendomycidine; alleu = alloisoleucine.

Ala—Ala—Pro—Thr—Ala—Thr—Val—Thr—Pro—Ser—Ser—Gly—Leu—Ser—Asp—Gly—Thr—
Val—Val—Lys—Val—Ala—Gly—Ala—Gly—Leu—Gln—Ala—Gly—Thr—Ala—Tyr—Asp—Val—
Gly—Gln—Cys—Ala—Ser—Val—Asn—Thr—Gly—Val—Leu—Trp—Asn—Ser—Val—Thr—Ala—
Ala—Gly—Ser—Cys—Asx—Pro—Ala—Asn—Phe—Ser—Leu—Thr—Val—Arg—Arg—Ser—Phe—
Glu—Gly—Phe—Leu—Phe—Asp—Gly—Thr—Arg—Trp—Gly—Thr—Val—Asx—Cys—Thr—Thr-
—Ala—Ala—Cys—Gln—Val—Gly—Leu—Ser—Asp—Ala—Ala—Gly—Asp—Gly—Glu—Pro—Gly—
Val—Ala—Ile—Ser—Phe—Asn

Figure 10.   Proposed sequence for neocarzinostatin (143).

insoluble in other organic solvents. The structures proposed for bleomycins A$_2$, A$_2'$–b, and B$_2$ are presented in Figure 11. The members of this group differ from each other in the terminal amine moiety: B$_2$ contains agmatine; A$_2$ contains (3-aminopropyl)-dimethylsulfonium.

All bleomycins inhibit the growth of gram-positive and gram-negative bacteria and mycobacteria. They also cause induction of bacteriophage in a lysogenic strain and inhibit vaccinia virus replication in infected HeLa cells and in mice.

Bleomycin sulfate is considered as a palliative treatment and/or adjuvant to surgery and radiation therapy for squamous cell carcinoma (head and neck, skin, larynx and paralarnyx, penis, cervix, and vulva), lymphomas, testicular carcinoma, and some renal carcinomas. The dosages range from 0.25 to 0.5 units/kg given im (intramuscular)

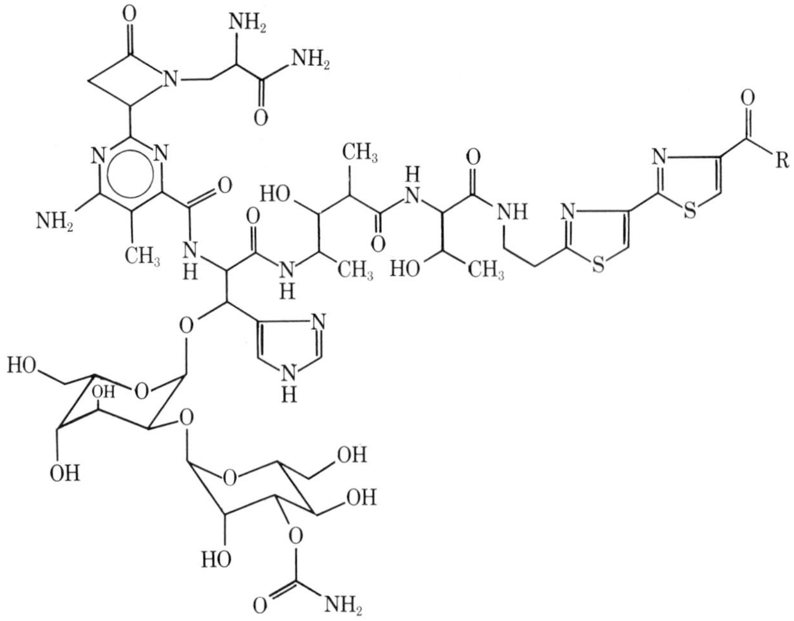

A_2, R = $NHCH_2CH_2CH_2\overset{+}{S}\begin{smallmatrix}CH_3\\CH_3\end{smallmatrix}$

B_2, R = $NHCH_2CH_2CH_2CH_2NHC\begin{smallmatrix}NH\\NH_2\end{smallmatrix}$

A'_2-b, R = $NHCH_2CH_2CH_2NH_2$

Bleomycinic acid, R = OH

Figure 11. Structure proposed for bleomycin.

or iv (intravenous) weekly or twice weekly, and because of the possibility of anaphylaxis, all lymphoma patients should be started with 5 units or less for the first 2 doses. Among the side effects are pulmonary (found in about 50% of the patients) which is usually a pneumonitis occasionally progressing to a pulmonary fibrosis, skin changes (also found in about 50% of the patients) including mouth ulcers, alopecia, hyperpigmentation, ulceration, hyperkeratosis, rash and nail changes, fever, nausea, and vomiting. As renal, hepatic, and central nervous system toxicity may occur at any time after initiation of therapy, these systems must be monitored. There has been no evidence of bone marrow or immunological depression.

Some 300 analogues of bleomycins have been prepared by various methods including directed fermentations and chemical modifications of bleomycins and none of these appear to be less toxic and more useful than bleomycins A_2 and B_2 (41).

The Antibiotic Cyclodepsipeptides. The cyclodepsipeptides or peptolides are often produced by the microorganisms as families of chemically related compounds. Separation of the congeners may be difficult or impossible, and even when it is possible, some are obtained only in small amounts, sufficient for identification of their structure, but not for determination of their physical properties. The triostin, quinoxaline, and sporidesmolide groups are examples of this situation. When the components cannot be separated, their structure can sometimes be inferred, but the physical properties reported are those for the mixture.

The cyclodepsipeptides can be divided into a group of peptide lactones and a group of true cyclodepsipeptides. In the former, the lactone linkage is through a hydroxy amino acid. They are either totally composed of amino acids or have a hetero moiety attached outside the lactone ring. Two members of this group, the triostins and the quinomycins, have been modified by crossbridging (see Fig. 12 for the structure of echinomycin related to triostin). The best methods for identifying these compounds include mass spectroscopy, nmr studies, and amino acid analyses (69).

The actinomycins are of therapeutic interest since they are the drug of choice for treatment of Wilm's tumor and have found use in therapy of other tumors. The actinomycins are peptide derivatives of a chromophore, actinocin (see Fig. 13), a phenoxazonecarboxylic acid liberated from all actinomycins under mild hydrolytic conditions. The acid is linked to two 16-membered peptide lactones via the amino group of threonine residues. In actinomycin D (also known as dactinomycin) the peptide lactone contains D-valine, L-proline, sarcosine, N-methyl-L-valine, and L-threonine. In actinomycin C_3 (also known as cactinomycin), D-*allo*-isoleucine residues replace the D-valine. The lactone bridge between the hydroxyl group of the L-threonine and the carboxyl group of the terminal N-methyl-L-valine is a common feature of these antibiotics.

The mode of action of the actinomycins in biological systems has been ascribed to the inhibition of DNA-dependent RNA synthesis, and special interest in these substances lies in their cytostatic activity. Their value as antitumor agents and their activity against lymphogranulomatosis is being studied. With Wilm's tumor (in children) the usual dosage is 0.015 mg/kg iv daily for 5 d and a second course of therapy may be attempted after an interval of at least 2 weeks. Treatment schedules for rhabdomyosarcoma and carcinoma of the testis and uteris in adults usually include 0.5 mg given iv daily for a maximum of 5 d. The adverse and potentially severe reactions encountered during treatment with the actinomycins require careful supervision (see Chemotherapeutic, antimitotic). Chemical synthesis of actinomycin analogues and chemical modification of the naturally occurring actinomycins has not resulted in significant improvement of the therapeutic index (9,295).

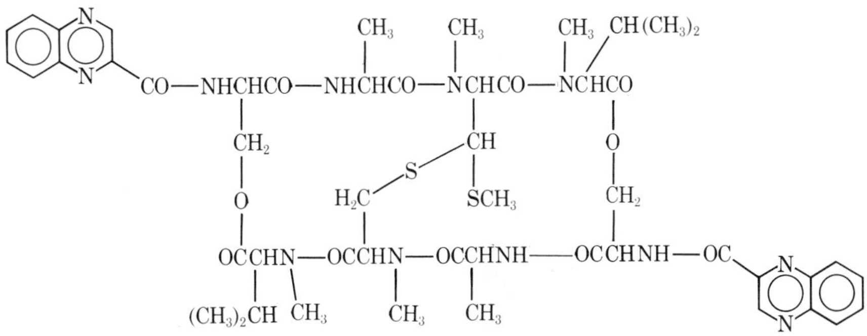

Figure 12.   Structure proposed for echinomycin.

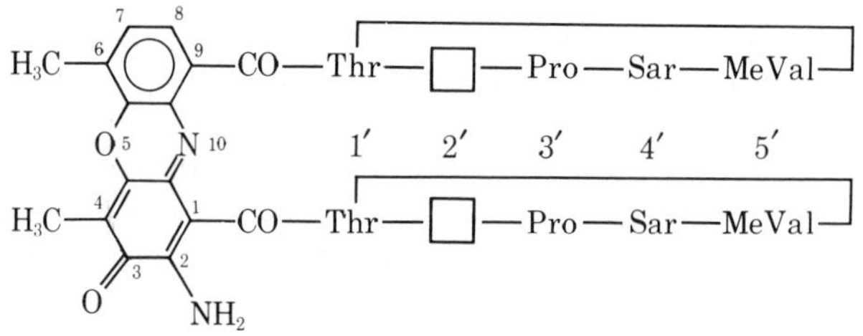

Figure 13.   Basic structure of actinomycins. Actinomycin D, $2'$—□— = D-Val; Sar = N-methylglycine.

A second group of peptide lactones are the synergistic family of antibiotics. The components can be separated into two groups, usually identified as A and B (Table 11). These antibiotics are unique in so far as, in their activity against gram-positive organisms, the members of the group A are synergistic with group B. The total complexes are therefore more active microbiologically than the individual components (296–298). Although the antibiotics of both groups inhibit protein synthesis, they differ considerably in their structures: those of group A are macrolides and those of group B are cyclic polypeptides having a lactone structure (see Table 12). These have either a 19- or 22-membered lactone ring associated with the hydroxyl function of a threonine residue and a chromophore, a heterocyclic acid such as 3-hydroxypicolinic acid, which acylates the amino group of threonine. The remaining portion of the lactone ring is invariably formed by a peptide chain consisting, in part, of uncommon amino acids.

These antibiotics have limited use in clinical medicine: pristinamycin (Pyostacine) is used in France and in several other countries to treat cases of infections due to *Staphylococcus aureus* (particularly those resistant to penicillin G), *Streptococcus faecalis,* and *Hemophilus influenzae* (299). The related staphylomycin mixture was used at one time in Belgium for similar purposes.

Mikamycin (Table 12) and virginiamycin (staphylomycin) are currently being used in Japan, Europe, and the United States as animal growth promotants. Addition of 1–3 g of the mikamycin mixture (A and B) or virginiamycin per metric ton of poultry feed produces a definite increase in growth rate and feed efficiency in chickens and turkeys.

Table 11.   A Summary of the Names of the Components of the Synergistic Family of Antibiotics

Antibiotic complex	Group A (macrolide) component	Group B (peptide) component
streptogramin	streptogramin A [21411-53-0]	streptogramin B [3131-03-1]
staphylomycin (virginiamycin)	staphylomycin M [21411-53-0]	staphylomycin S [23152-29-6]
ostreogrycin (antibiotic E 129)	ostreogrycin A [21411-53-0]	ostreogrycin B [3131-03-1]
mikamycin	mikamycin A [21411-53-0]	mikamycin B [3131-03-1]
pristinamycin (antibiotic 7293 R.P.)	pristinamycin II_A [21411-53-0]	pristinamycin I_A [3131-03-1]
vernamycin	vernamycin A [21411-53-0]	vernamycin B_α [3131-03-1]
synergistin [11006-76-1] (antibiotic PA 114)	synergistin A [11126-45-7]	synergistin B [65454-52-6]

Table 12.   The Streptogramin Family of Streptomycete Antibiotics

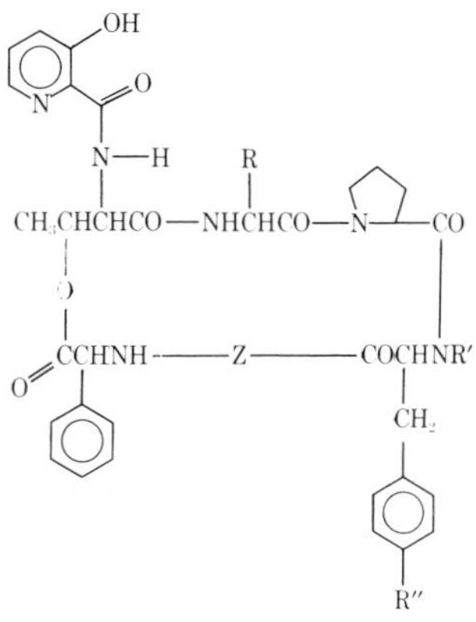

Name	R	R'	R''	Z
virginiamycin S [9040-14-6]	C_2H_5	CH_3	H	4-oxopipecolic acid
virginiamycin S$_4$ [33477-37-1]	CH_3	CH_3	H	4-oxopipecolic acid
virginiamycin S$_2$ [33477-38-2]	C_2H_5	H	H	4-hydroxypipecolic acid
virginiamycin S$_3$ [33477-39-2]	C_2H_5	CH_3	H	3-hydroxy-4-oxopipecolic acid
patricin B [38188-91-9]	C_2H_5	CH_3	H	pipecolic acid
streptogramin B mikamycin B PA 114 B$_1$ pristinamycin I$_A$ vernamycin B$_\alpha$ ostreogrycin B [3131-03-1]	C_2H_5	CH_3	$N(CH_3)_2$	4-oxopipecolic acid
pristinamycin I$_C$ vernamycin B$_\gamma$ ostreogrycin B$_1$ [28979-74-0]	CH_3	CH_3	$N(CH_3)_2$	4-oxopipecolic acid
pristinamycin I$_B$ vernamycin B$_\beta$ ostreogrycin B$_2$ [57206-54-9]	C_2H_5	CH_3	$NHCH_3$	4-oxopipecolic acid
vernamycin B$_\delta$ [29139-17-1]	CH_3	CH_3	$NHCH_3$	4-oxopipecolic acid
ostreogrycin B$_3$ [31508-69-7]	C_2H_5	CH_3	$N(CH_3)_2$	3-hydroxy-4-oxopipecolic acid
vernamycin C doricin [14014-70-1]	C_2H_5	CH_3	$N(CH_3)_2$	aspartic acid
patricin A [2105-09-1]	C_2H_5	CH_3	H	proline

The true cyclodepsipeptides contain both amino and hydroxy acids. Two classes can be distinguished: those containing alternating hydroxy and amino acid residues, and those consisting largely of amino acids, with the lactone linkage through hydroxy acids or hydroxy amino acids. The structures proposed for some of these compounds are presented in Table 13. Several of this group have chelation properties that are quite unique and these serve as the special agents in ion-selective sensors. Valinomycin is one of these used in potassium electrodes.

Microbial Peptides as Antimetabolites

Woolley (315) defined an antimetabolite as a structural analogue of an essential metabolite, vitamin, hormone, or amino acid, etc, which is able to cause signs of deficiency of the essential metabolite in some living thing or in some biological reaction. This definition was based on the theory that antimetabolites act as isosteric enzyme inhibitors (316). Accordingly, reversible inhibition would be relieved by the addition to the test system of either the product or an excess of substrate. In the case of irreversible inhibition, only addition of product would be effective, and thus experimental reversibility has become commonly accepted as evidence for antimetabolite activity even though this was not explicitly required for the original definition.

Table 13.   The True Antibiotic Cyclodepsipeptides

Name	CAS Registry No.	Structures	Ref.
angolide	[2441-03-4]	cyclo-(D-*allo*-isoleucyl-L-α-hydroxyisovaleryl-L-isoleucyl-L-α-hydroxyisovaleryl)	300
beauvericin		cyclo-(*N*-methyl-L-phenylalanyl-D-α-hydroxyisovaleryl)$_3$	301
destruxin A	[6686-70-0]	D-2-hydroxy-4-pentenoyl-L-prolyl-L-isoleucyl-*N*-methyl-L-valyl-*N*-methyl-L-alanyl-β-alanyl lactone	302
destruxin B		D-α-hydroxy-γ-methylvaleryl-L-propyl-L-isoleucyl-*N*-methyl-L-valyl-*N*-methyl-L-alanyl-β-alanyl lactone	303
enniatin A	[2503-13-1]	cyclo-(*N*-methyl-L-isoleucyl-D-α-hydroxyisovaleryl)$_3$	304
enniatin B	[917-13-5]	cyclo-(*N*-methyl-L-valyl-D-α-hydroxyisovaleryl)$_3$	305
isariin		D-β-hydroxydodecanoyl-L-valyl-L-alanyl-D-leucyl-L-valylglycyl lactone	306
peptidolipine NA		D-β-hydroxyeicosanoyl-L-threonyl-L-valyl-D-alanyl-L-prolyl-D-*allo*-isoleucyl-L-alanyl lactone	307
pithomycolide	[2601-84-5]	cyclo-(D-β-hydroxy-β-phenylpropionyl-D-β-hydroxy-β-phenyl-propionyl-L-α-hydroxyisovaleryl-*N*-methyl-L-alanyl-L-alanyl)	308
serratamolide		cyclo-(D-β-hydroxydecanoyl-L-seryl)$_2$	309
sporidesmolide I	[2900-38-1]	cyclo-(L-α-hydroxyisovaleryl-D-valyl-D-leucyl-L-α-hydroxyiso-valeryl-L-valyl-*N*-methyl-L-leucyl)	310
sporidesmolide II	[3200-75-7]	cyclo-(L-α-hydroxyisovaleryl-D-*allo*-isoleucyl-D-leucyl-L-α-hy-droxyisovaleryl-L-valyl-*N*-methyl-L-leucyl)	311
sporidesmolide III	[1803-67-4]	cyclo(L-α-hydroxyisovaleryl-D-valyl-D-leucyl-L-α-hydroxyiso-valeryl-L-valyl-L-leucyl)	311
surfactin		3-hydroxy-13-methyltetradecanoyl-L-glutamyl-L-leucyl-D-leucyl-L-valyl-L-aspartyl-D-leucyl-L-leucyl lactone	312
valinomycin		cyclo-(L-lactyl-L-valyl-D-α-hydroxyisovaleryl-D-valyl)$_3$	313
viscosin		*N*-(D-β-hydroxydecanoyl-L-leucyl-D-glutamyl)-D-*allo*-threonyl-D-valyl-L-leucyl-D-seryl-L-leucyl-D-seryl-L-isoleucyl lactone	314

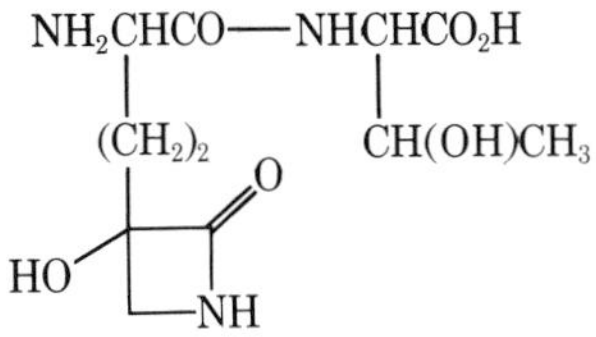

Tabtoxin

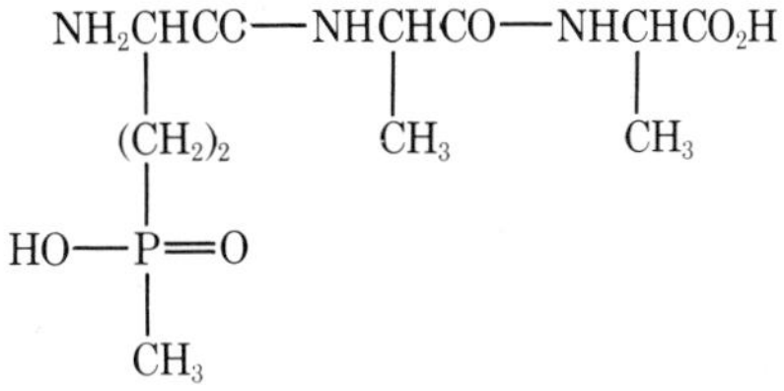

Phosphinothricyl-alanyl–alanine

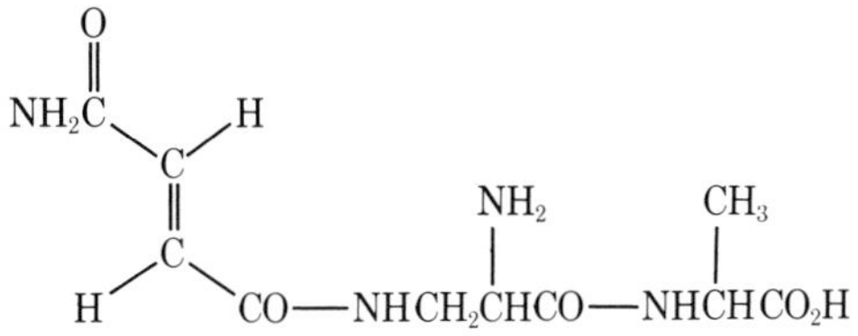

Fumarylcarboxamido-L-2,3-diamino-propionyl-L-alanine

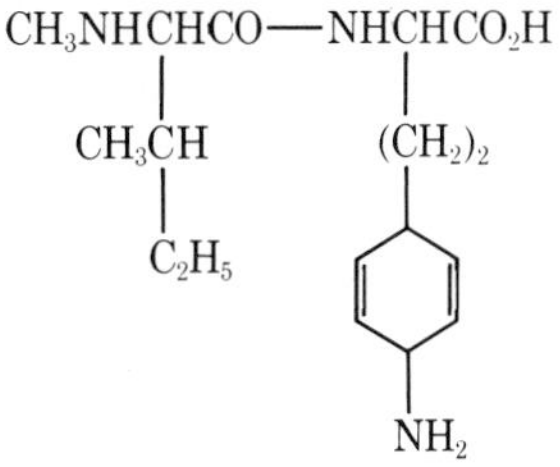

Stravidin

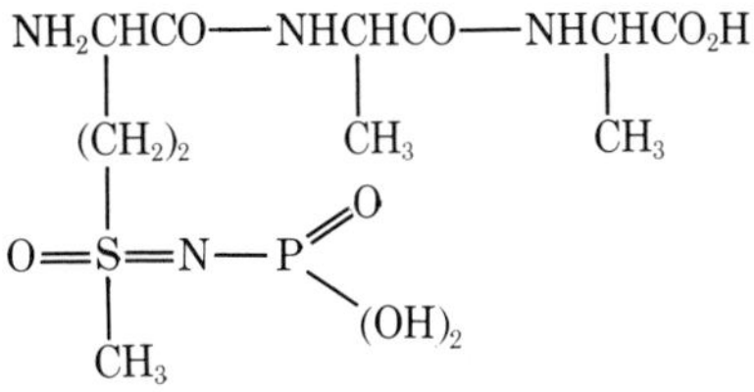

L-(N^5-Phosphono)methionine-(*S*)-sulfoximinyl-L-alanyl-L-alanine

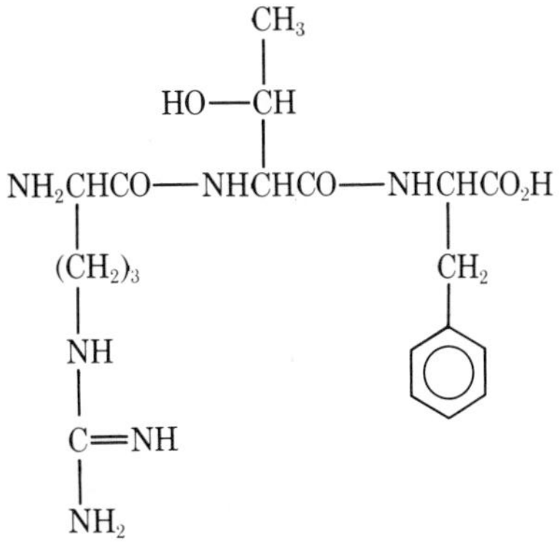

L-Arginyl-D-*allo*-threonyl-L-phenylalanine

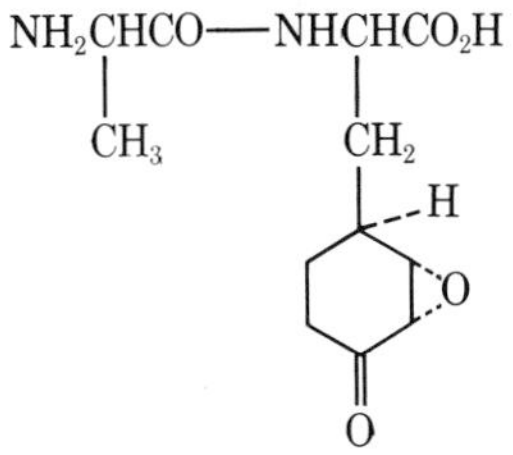

Bacilysin

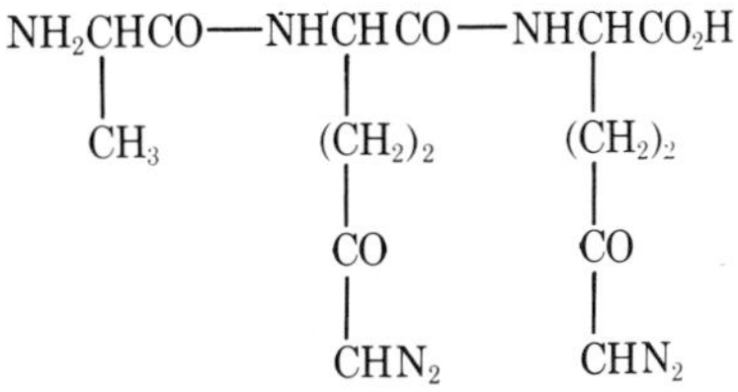

Alazopeptin

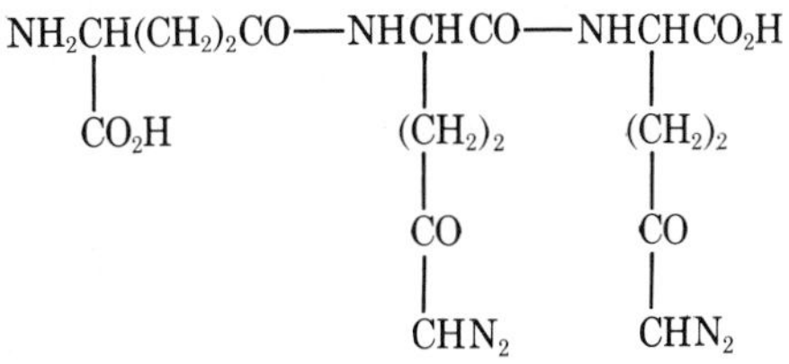

Duazomycin B

Figure 14. Structures of some peptide antimetabolites (317).

Table 14. Some Microbial Peptides Which Act as Antimetabolites in Biological Systems

Compound	Trivial name	Source	Reversant	Ref.
2-amino-4-(3-hydroxy-2-oxo-3-azetidinyl)butanoyl-L-threonine [40957-90-2]	wild fire toxin; tabtoxin	*Pseudomonas* sp; *Pseudomonas tabaci*	L-glutamine	318
2-amino-4-methylphosphinobutanoyl-L-alanyl-L-alanine	phosphinothricyl-alanylalanine	*Streptomyces viridochromogenes*	L-glutamine	319
fumarylcarboxamido-L-2,3-diaminopropionyl-L-alanine		*Streptomyces collinus*	D-glucosamine; N-acetylglucosamine	320
(S,S)-N-methylisoleucyl-L-2-amino-4-(4-amino-2,5-cyclohexadien-1-yl)butanoic acid [21754-03-0]	stravidin; MSD-235 S_3	*Streptomyces avidinii; Streptomyces lavendulae*	D-biotin	321
L-(N^5-phosphono)methionine-(S)-sulfoximinyl-L-alanyl-L-alanine		*Streptomyces* sp	L-glutamine	322
L-arginyl-D-*allo*-threonyl-L-phenylalanine		*Keratinophyton terrum*	L-histidine; L-threonine	322
L-alanyl-L-2,3-epoxy-4-oxohexahydrophenylalanine [29393-20-2]	bacilysin; tetaine	*Bacillus subtilis; Bacillus pumilus*	L-glutamine; D-glucosamine	324
L-alanyl-(6-diazo-5-oxo)-L-norleucyl-(6-diazo-5-oxo)-L-norleucine [1397-84-8]	alazopeptin	*Streptomyces griseoplanus*	L-glutamine; purine bases; purine nucleosides	325
5-L-glutamyl-(6-diazo-5-oxo)-L-norleucyl-(6-diazo-5-oxo)-L-norleucine [7644-67-9]	duazomycin B	*Streptomyces ambofaciens*	L-glutamine	326
(S)-alanyl-3-[α-(S)-chloro-3-(S)-hydroxy-2-oxo-3-azetidinylmethyl]-(S)-alanine		*Streptomyces* sp	L-glutamine	327

246

Pruess and Scannell (317) have catalogued some 75 microbially produced antimetabolites and noted that 10 are di- or tri-peptides. These are listed in Table 14 together with the reversants that have been reported. (Their structures are presented in Fig. 14.) In most instances these compounds have antibiotic activity only when the test organisms are grown in chemically defined media which are either lacking in the reversant or have only very low levels of the reversant present. The potential utility of these compounds for therapeutic or other purposes has rarely been demonstrated since in most *in vivo* situations the reversants are present in sufficiently high concentrations to preclude observation of antimicrobial activity.

Manufacturers of Peptide Antibiotics

The following is a list of worldwide producers of peptide antibiotics: (*1*) H. Lundbeck and Company, Valby, Denmark; (*2*) Apothekernes Laboratorium für Specialpraeparater A/S, Oslo, Norway; (*3*) Asahi Chemical Industry, Tokyo, Japan; (*4*) Dumex A/S, Copenhagen, Denmark; (*5*) IMC Chemicals Group, Inc., Terre Haute, Ind.; (*6*) Novo Industri A/S, Bagsvaerd, Denmark; (*7*) S. B. Penick and Company, Lyndhurst, N. J.; (*8*) Pfizer, Inc., New York; (*9*) G. Richter, Budapest, Hungary; (*10*) Societe Chimique Pointet Girard, Velleneuve La Garenne, France; (*11*) Nihon Nohyaku Company, Tokyo, Japan; (*12*) Farbenfabriken Bayer A.G., Wuppertal, West Germany; (*13*) Dista Products Ltd., Liverpool, England; (*14*) Banyu Pharmaceutical Company, Tokyo, Japan; (*15*) Koyaku Antibiotics Research Co. Ltd., Tokyo, Japan; (*16*) Kyowa Hakko Kogyo Company, Tokyo, Japan; (*17*) Rhone-Poulenc S.A., Paris, France; (*18*) Merck & Co., Inc., Rahway, N. J.; (*19*) Reanal, Budapest, Hungary; (*20*) Takeda Chemical Industries, Osaka, Japan; (*21*) Wallerstein Laboratories, Inc., Morton Grove, Ill.; (*22*) Meiji Seika Kaisha Ltd., Tokyo, Japan; (*23*) Nikken Chemicals Company Ltd., Tokyo, Japan; (*24*) Kanegafuchi Chemical Industries, Osaka, Japan; (*25*) Shionogi and Company Ltd., Osaka, Japan; (*26*) Eli Lilly and Company, Indianapolis, Ind.; (*27*) Fujisawa Pharmaceutical Company, Osaka, Japan; (*28*) Kaken Chemical Company, Tokyo, Japan; (*29*) E. R. Squibb and Sons, Inc., Princeton, N. J.; (*30*) Biochemie G.m.b.H., Kundl/Tirol, Austria; (*31*) Toyo Jozo Company Ltd., Tokyo, Japan; and (*32*) Recherche et Industrie Therapeutique, Genval, Belgium.

BIBLIOGRAPHY

"Polypeptide Antibiotics" in *ECT* 2nd ed., Vol. 16, pp. 306–345, by S. Wilkinson, The Wellcome Research Laboratories, Beckenham, Kent, England.

1. E. P. Abraham and G. G. F. Newton, *Br. Med. Bull.* **16**, 3 (1960).
2. R. Schwyzer and co-workers, *Helv. Chim. Acta* **46**, 1975 (1963).
3. M. Sela and E. Katchalski, *Adv. Protein Chem.* **14**, 391 (1959); E. Katchalski and co-workers, "Polyamino Acids as Protein Models," in H. Neurath, ed., *The Proteins,* 2nd ed., Vol. II, Academic Press, Inc., New York, 1976.
4. M. J. Fridecky and W. H. McGregor, *J. Med. Chem.* **9**, 255 (1966).
5. M. A. Pisano and co-workers, *Antimicrob. Agents Chemother. 1966,* 457 (1967).
6. G. DeAngeles, *Alteno Parmense* **28**, 248 (1957).
7. K. E. Price and co-workers, *Antimicrob. Agents Chemother. 1962,* 543 (1963).
8. P. Cercos, *Publ. Ternica No. 16,* Inst. Fifotecnic, 1948, p. 147.
9. S. A. Waksman, ed., *The Actinomycins,* Interscience Publishers, a division of John Wiley & Sons, Inc., New York, 1968.

10. N. N. Lomakina and co-workers, *Antibiotiki (Moscow)* **6**, 609 (1961).

11. J. M. Ghuysen, *C. R. Seances Soc. Biol. Paris* **148**, 169 (1954).

12. J. J. Gordon, B. K. Kelly, and G. A. Miller, *Nature (London)* **195**, 701 (1962); J. J. Gordon and co-workers, *J. Chem. Soc.* 819 (1975).

13. A. S. Khoklov and co-workers, *J. Antibiot. Ser. A* **22**, 541 (1969).

14. G. Brownlee, *Ann. N.Y. Acad. Sci.* **51**, 875 (1949).

15. A. W. Burgess and S. J. Leach, *Biopolymers* **12**, 2691 (1973).

16. J. Turkova, O. Mikes, and F. Sorm, *Collect. Czech. Chem. Commun.* **29**, 280 (1964).

17. K. Maeda and co-workers, *J. Antibiot. Ser. A* **11**, 30 (1958).

18. M. J. Bachler and co-workers, *Antimicrob. Agents Chemother. 1964*, 53 (1965).

19. H. N. Kirst and co-workers, *J. Antibiot. Ser. A* **18**, 286 (1965).

20. K. Gilliver, A. M. Holmes, and E. P. Abraham, *Br. J. Exp. Pathol.* **30**, 209 (1949).

21. G. Schmidt-Kastner and J. Schmid, *Med. Chem. Abhandl. Med. Chem. Forschungestaetter Far-benfabriken Bayer AG* **7**, 528 (1963).

22. T. Takaisawa and co-workers, *J. Antibiot. Ser. A* **21**, 567 (1968); S. Nakamura and co-workers, *J. Antibiot. Ser. A* **13**, 362 (1960).

23. L. C. Vining and W. A. Taber, *Can. J. Chem.* **35**, 1109 (1951); M. M. Shemyakin and co-workers, *Tetrahedron Lett.* 351 (1963).

24. Ger. Pat. 926,806 (Apr. 25, 1955), H. Brockmann and co-workers.

25. B. Heinemann and co-workers, *Antibiot. Chemother. (Washington D.C.)* **3**, 1239 (1953); M. Bodanszky, G. F. Sigler, and A. Bodanszky, *J. Am. Chem. Soc.* **95**, 2352 (1973).

26. G. W. Probst, M. M. Hoehn, and B. L. Woods, *Antimicrob. Agents Chemother. 1965*, 798 (1966).

27. P. V. Deshmukh, *Hind. Antibiot. Bull.* **10**, 299 (1968).

28. Ger. Pat. 1,090,380 (Oct. 6, 1960), J. Reitstotter.

29. W. K. Hausmann and co-workers, *Antimicrob. Agents Chemother. 1963*, 352 (1964).

30. Jpn. Kokai 71 21,789 (June 21, 1971), S. Tamura and co-workers.

31. T. H. Farmer, *J. Chem. Soc.* 1072 (1949).

32. A. Arriagada and co-workers, *Br. J. Exp. Pathol.* **30**, 425 (1949).

33. Jpn. Kokai 70 6,073 (Feb. 1970), (to Kaken Chemical Company).

34. J. W. Foster and H. B. Woodruff, *J. Bacteriol.* **51**, 363 (1946); R. B. Walton and E. L. Rickes, *J. Bacteriol.* **84**, 1148 (1962).

35. R. A. Turner, *Arch. Biochem. Biophys.* **60**, 364 (1956).

36. Jpn. Kokai 61 1,149 (May 7, 1961), (to Nippon Agricultural Drug Co.).

37. J. E. Walker and E. P. Abraham, *Biochem. J.* **118**, 563 (1970).

38. I. M. Lockhart and E. P. Abraham, *Biochem. J.* **58**, 633 (1954); R. J. Hickey, *Prog. Ind. Microbiol.* **5**, 93 (1964).

39. M. Bernardini and co-workers, *Phytochemistry* **14**, 1865 (1975).

40. U.S. Pat. 3,689,639 (Jan. 23, 1969), M. E. Bergey, J. H. Coats, and F. Reusser (to Upjohn Company); J. M. Liesch and co-workers, *J. Am. Chem. Soc.* **98**, 299 (1976).

41. H. Umezawa, *Gann Monogr.*, 19 (1976).

42. J. M. Waisvisz and co-workers, *J. Am. Chem. Soc.* **79**, 4520, 4522, 4524 (1957).

43. G. G. Zharikova and co-workers, *Dokl. Akad. Nauk. SSSR* **204**, 465 (1972).

44. K. Gillver, *Br. J. Exp. Pathol.* **30**, 214 (1949).

45. J. Kawamata and Y. Motomura, *J. Antibiot. Ser. A* **7**, 25 (1954).

46. M. J. Cron and co-workers, *Antibiot. Chemother. (Washington D.C.)* **6**, 63 (1956).

47. E. B. Herr, *Antimicrob. Agents Chemother. 1962*, 201 (1963); B. G. Bycroft and co-workers, *Nature (London)* **231**, 301 (1971).

48. Y. Harada and S. Tanaka, *J. Antibiot. Ser. A* **9**, 113 (1956).

49. Y. Harada, T. Nara, and F. Okamoto, *J. Antibiot. Ser. A* **9**, 6 (1956).

50. A. Matsumae, *J. Antibiot. Ser. A* **13**, 143 (1960).

51. E. Borowski and co-workers, *Bull. State Inst. Mar. Trop. Med. Gdansk* **7**, 119 (1956).

52. J. Shoji, T. Kato, and R. Sakazaki, *J. Antibiot.* **29**, 1268, 1275, 1281 (1976).

53. G. F. Gauze and co-workers, *Antibiotiki (Moscow)* **2**, 9 (1957); N. N. Lomakina and M. G. Brazhnikova, *Biokhimiya* **24**, 425 (1959).

54. H. Umezawa and co-workers, *J. Antibiot.* **23**, 425 (1970).

55. R. G. Benedict and co-workers, *Antibiot. Chemother. (Washington D.C.)* **2**, 591 (1952).

56. D. H. Peterson and L. M. Reineke, *J. Biol. Chem.* **181**, 95 (1949).

57. S. A. Leon and F. Bergmann, *Biotechnol. Bioeng.* **10**, 429 (1968).

58. T. Suzuki and co-workers, *J. Biochem.* (*Tokyo*) **54**, 173 (1963); S. Wilkinson and L. A. Lowe, *J. Chem. Soc.* **1964**, 4107.

59. J. J. Gordon, B. K. Kelly, and G. A. Miller, *Biochem. J.* **64**, 6P (1956); W. G. G. Forsyth, *Biochem. J.* **59**, 500 (1955).

60. C. Cosar and co-workers, *C. R. Acad. Sci.* **234**, 1498 (1952); J. Joseph, *C. R. Acad. Sci.* **243**, 961 (1956).

61. N. Yoshida, Y. Tani, and K. Ogata, *J. Antibiot.* **25**, 653 (1972); N. Yoshida and K. Ogata, *J. Antibiot.* **27**, 138 (1974).

62. W. O. Godtfredsen, S. Vangedahl, and D. W. Thomas, *Tetrahedron* **26**, 4931 (1970).

63. H. Tsukiura and co-workers, *J. Antibiot. Ser. A* **17**, 39 (1964).

64. S. Kuyama and S. Tamura, *Agric. Biol. Chem.* **29**, 168 (1965).

65. Jpn. Kokai 70 26,715 (Sept. 2, 1970), Y. Tshida.

66. A. M. Casazza and co-workers, *Antimicrob. Agents Chemother. 1966*, 593 (1967).

67. M. Bodanszky and J. T. Sheehan, *Antimicrob. Agents Chemother. 1963*, 38 (1964).

68. T. G. Pridham and co-workers, *Phytopathology* **46**, 568 (1956); O. L. Shotwell and co-workers, *J. Am. Chem. Soc.* **80**, 3912 (1958).

69. J. Berger and co-workers, *Experientia* **13**, 434 (1957); R. Corbaz and co-workers, *Helv. Chim. Acta* **40**, 199 (1957); A. Dell and co-workers, *J. Am. Chem. Soc.* **97**, 2497 (1975).

70. G. Roncari, Z. Kurylo-Borowska, and L. C. Craig, *Biochemistry* **5**, 2153 (1966); Z. Kurylo-Borowska and W. Szer, *Biochim. Biophys. Acta* **418**, 63 (1976).

71. H. Iwasaki and co-workers, *Chem. Pharm. Bull.* **21**, 1184 (1973).

72. E. Gaumann and co-workers, *Experientia* **3**, 202 (1947); Pl. A. Plattner and co-workers, *Helv. Chim. Acta* **46**, 927 (1963).

73. Y. Suhara and co-workers, *J. Antibiot. Ser. A* **16**, 107 (1963).

74. C.-Y. Hsu and G. M. Wiseman, *Can. J. Microbiol.* **17**, 1223 (1971).

75. G. G. Zharikova and co-workers, *Dokl. Akad. Nauk SSSR* **204**, 465 (1972); R. A. Radzhapov and co-workers, *Nauchn. Dokl. Vyssh. Shk. Biol. Nauki,* 99 (1968).

76. H. Ogawa and T. Ito, *Nippon Nogei Kagaku Kaishi* **26**, 432 (1952).

77. B. Heinemann and co-workers, *Antibiot. Annu.* **1954–1955**, 728; J. C. Sheehan, H. E. Zachau, and W. B. Lawson, *J. Am. Chem. Soc.* **80**, 3349 (1958).

78. J. Charney and co-workers, *Antibiotics Annu.* **1955–1956**, 228; R. E. Harman and co-workers, *J. Am. Chem. Soc.* **80**, 5173 (1958).

79. M. Bodanszky, *Acta Chem. Acad. Sci. Hung.* **3**, 237 (1952).

80. I. R. Shimi and S. Shoukry, *J. Antibiot. Ser. A* **19**, 110, 250 (1966).

81. T. Emery and J. B. Neilands, *J. Am. Chem. Soc.* **83**, 1626 (1961).

82. Belg. Pat. 625,238 (1963), (to CIBA Ltd.).

83. H. Bickel and co-workers, *Helv. Chim. Acta* **43**, 2105 (1960).

84. A. Ballio and co-workers, *Nature* (*London*) **194**, 769 (1962); A. Ballio and co-workers, *Proc. Roy. Soc. London Ser. B* **158**, 48 (1963); **161**, 384 (1964).

85. F. Carvajal, *Antibiot. Chemother.* (*Washington D.C.*) **3**, 765 (1953).

86. A. H. Cook, S. F. Cox, and T. H. Farmer, *Nature* (*London*) **162**, 61 (1948).

87. G. L. Hobby and co-workers, *J. Clin. Invest.* **28**, 927 (1949).

88. A. P. Cercos and A. Castronovo, *An. Soc. Cient. Argent.* **152**, 68 (1951).

89. Fr. Pat. 1,164,181 (Oct. 7, 1958), M. A. Couchoud.

90. J. Shoji and co-workers, *J. Antibiot.* **28**, 122 (1975).

91. U.S. Pat. 3,642,984 (Feb. 15, 1972), M. E. Bergey and C. DeBoer (to Upjohn).

92. N. Nakajima, S. Chihara, and Y. Koyama, *J. Antibiot.* **25**, 243 (1972).

93. K. V. Rao, D. W. Renn, and I. Truumees, *Antimicrob. Agents Annu.* 72 (1960).

94. Jpn. Kokai 60 21,395 (Sept. 1960), (to Ono Pharmaceutical Company).

95. M. Shibata and co-workers, *J. Antibiot. Ser. A* **15**, 1 (1960); M. Fujino and co-workers, *Bull. Chem. Soc. Jpn.* **38**, 515 (1965).

96. B. Witkop and co-workers, *Agnew. Chem.* **76**, 793 (1967); R. Sarges and B. Witkop, *J. Am. Chem. Soc.* **87**, 2011, 2020, 2027 (1965).

97. S. Otani and Y. Saito, *Proc. Jpn. Acad.* **30**, 191 (1954).

98. G. F. Gauze and M. G. Brazhnikova, *Lancet* **247**, 715 (1944); R. Consden and co-workers, *Biochem. J.* **41**, 598 (1947); R. Consden and co-workers, *Biochem. J.* **39**, 362 (1945).

99. D. M. Reynolds, A. Schatz, and S. A. Waksman, *Proc. Soc. Exp. Biol. Med.* **64**, 50 (1947); F. A. Kuehl and co-workers, *J. Am. Chem. Soc.* **73**, 1770 (1951).

100. T. Takeuchi and co-workers, *J. Antibiot. Ser. A* **15**, 141 (1962).

101. J. Ehrlich and co-workers, *Antibiot. Ann.* 709 (1954–1955); M. C. Falloma *Can. J. Chem.* **42,** 511 (1964).
102. Ger. Pat. 1,070,782 (Dec. 10, 1959), E. Gaumann and H. Bickel (to Ciba, Ltd.).
103. T. Terlain and co-workers, *Bull. Soc. Chim.* **6,** 2357 (1971).
104. N. A. Krasil'nikov and co-workers, *Microbiologia* **26,** 418 (1957).
105. I. R. Shimi, A. Deweda, and S. Shoukry, *J. Antibiot.* **23,** 388 (1970).
106. F. D. A. Lyra and co-workers, *Rev. Inst. Antibiot. Univ. Fed. Pernambuco Recife* **4,** 33, 67 (1962).
107. K. Jomon and co-workers, *J. Antibiot.* **25,** 271 (1972).
108. T. Takita, *J. Antibiot. Ser. A* **16,** 211 (1963); **17,** 129 (1964).
109. W. A. Taber and L. C. Vining, *Can. J. Microbiol.* **9,** 136 (1963).
110. F. Peypouk and co-workers, *Tetrahedron* **29,** 3455 (1973).
111. T. Hoshino and co-workers, *J. Antibiot. Ser. A* **20,** 36 (1967); S. Nomura and co-workers, *J. Antibiot. Ser. A* **17,** 104 (1964).
112. E. Meyers and co-workers, *J. Antibiot.* **23,** 502 (1970).
113. M. Ito and Y. Koyama, *J. Antibiot.* **25,** 147, 304 (1972).
114. M. Kikuchi and co-workers, *J. Antibiot. Ser. A* **18,** 243 (1965).
115. S. Okamoto and co-workers, *J. Antibiot. Ser. A* **21,** 320 (1968).
116. Jpn. Kokai 70 8,636 (Mar. 27, 1970), T. Oda, T. Mori, and Y. Kamemoto (to Kowa Company Ltd.).
117. H. Naganawa and co-workers, *J. Antibiot. Ser. A* **21,** 55 (1968).
118. A. H. Cook, S. F. Cox, and T. H. Farmer, *Nature (London)* **162,** 61 (1948).
119. E. M. Barnes, *Br. J. Exp. Pathol.* **30,** 100 (1949).
120. Neth. Pat. 106,644 (June 17, 1963), (to N. V. Koningklijke Nederlandse Gist-en Spiritus Fabriek).
121. K. Mizuno and co-workers, *J. Antibiot. Ser. A* **20,** 194 (1967).
122. Jpn. Kokai 74 41,594 (Apr. 18, 1974), T. Ari.
123. S. Kondo and co-workers, *J. Antibiot. Ser. A* **17,** 262 (1964).
124. H. E. Carter, C. P. Schaffner, and D. Gottlieb, *Arch. Biochem. Biophys.* **53,** 282 (1954).
125. R. K. Callow and T. S. Work, *Biochem. J.* **51,** 558 (1952).
126. N. Ishida and co-workers, *J. Antibiot. Ser. A* **22,** 218 (1969).
127. Jpn. Kokai 63 20,298 (Oct. 2, 1963), K. Arima and K. Takiguchi.
128. N. Takahashi and R. W. Curtis, *Plant Phys.* **36,** 30 (1961); M. Bodanszky and G. L. Stahl, *Proc. Nat. Acad. Sci. U.S.A.* **71,** 2791 (1974).
129. R. Cambee and co-workers, *J. Chem. Soc.* **1963,** 4120.
130. M. Soeda and M. Mitomi, *J. Antibiot. Ser. A* **15,** 182 (1962).
131. P. Margalith, G. Beretta, and M. T. Timbal, *Antibiot. Chemother. (Washington D.C.)* **9,** 71 (1959).
132. A. Kimura and H. Nishimura, *J. Antibiot.* **23,** 461 (1970).
133. R. Sugawara, A. Matsumae, and T. Hata, *J. Antibiot. Ser. A* **10,** 133 (1957).
134. M. Ueda and H. Umezawa, *J. Antibiot. Ser. A* **8,** 164 (1955).
135. P. Brooks, A. T. Fuller, and J. Walker, *J. Chem. Soc.* **1957,** 689.
136. A. Blinov and co-workers, *Antibiotiki (Moscow)* **11,** 587 (1966).
137. M. Arai and co-workers, *J. Antibiot. Ser. A* **9,** 193 (1956); **11,** 14 (1958).
138. T. J. McBride and co-workers, *Proc. Soc. Exp. Biol. Med.* **130,** 1188 (1969).
139. C. H. Hassall and K. E. Magnus, *Nature (London)* **184,** 1223 (1959).
140. S. K. Majumdar and S. K. Bose, *Biochem. J.* **74,** 596 (1960).
141. R. B. Walton and H. B. Woodruff, *J. Clin. Invest.* **28,** 294 (1949).
142. M. Hamada and co-workers, *J. Antibiotics* **23,** 170 (1970).
143. N. Ishida and co-workers, *J. Antibiot. Ser. A* **18,** 68 (1965); J. Meienhofer and co-workers, *Science* **178,** 875 (1972).
144. E. Gross and J. L. Morell, *J. Am. Chem. Soc.* **93,** 4634 (1971).
145. A. Stoll and co-workers, *Z. Path. Bakt.* **14,** 225 (1951).
146. D. A. Harris and H. B. Woodruff, *Antibiot. Annu.* 609 (1953–1954).
147. W. L. Parker and M. L. Rathnum, *J. Antibiot.* **28,** 379 (1975).
148. A. H. Ball and co-workers, *Biochem. J.* **68,** 24P (1958).
149. H. Depaire and co-workers, *Tetrahedron Lett.* **1977,** 1403.
150. *Gyogys zerkutato Intezet Hung. Teljes,* 422 (June 1970).
151. M. Giunand and G. Miche, *Biochim. Biophys. Acta* **125,** 75 (1966).
152. M. Murase and co-workers, *J. Antibiot. Ser. A* **14,** 113 (1961).
153. R. Brown and E. Hazen, *Antibiot. Chemother. (Washington D.C.)* **3,** 818 (1953).
154. S. Nakamura and co-workers, *J. Antibiot. Ser. A* **20,** 210 (1967).

155. K. Maeda and co-workers, *J. Antibiot. Ser. A* **9,** 82 (1956).
156. K. Maeda and co-workers, *J. Antibiot. Ser. A* **6,** 183 (1953).
157. J. S. Ziffer and co-workers, *Phytopathology* **47,** 539 (1957).
158. R. Sprague, *Plant Dis. Rep.* **42,** 1208 (1958).
159. S. Omura and co-workers, *Agric. Biol. Chem.* **29,** 548 (1965).
160. K. Vogler and R. Studer, *Experientia* **22,** 345 (1966).
161. S. Wilkinson, *Antimicrob. Agents Chemother. 1966,* 651 (1967).
162. W. K. Hausmann and L. C. Craig, *J. Biol. Chem.* **198,** 405 (1952).
163. J. Preud'homme and co-workers, *C. R. Acad. Sci.* **260,** 1309 (1965).
164. D. S. Bhate, *Nature (London)* **175,** 816 (1955).
165. K. Katagiri and K. Sugiura, *Antimicrob. Agents Chemother. 1961,* 162 (1962).
166. C. Casas-Campillo, *Ciencia (Mexico City)* **11,** 21 (1951).
167. T. Tsurvoka and co-workers, *Meiji Seika Kenkyu Nempo* (11), 26 (1970).
168. M. Shibata and co-workers, *Agric. Biol. Chem.* **26,** 228 (1962); M. Fujino and co-workers, *Chem. Pharm. Bull.* **12,** 1390 (1964).
169. M. S. Lacey, *J. Gen. Microbiol.* **4,** 122 (1950).
170. J. Berger and co-workers, *Antimicrob. Agents Chemother. 1961,* 436 (1962).
171. H. H. Wasserman, J. J. Kegge, and J. E. McKeon, *J. Am. Chem. Soc.* **84,** 2978 (1962).
172. H. Bickel and co-workers, *Helv. Chim. Acta* **43,** 2118 (1960).
173. H. Nishimura and co-workers, *J. Antibiot. Ser. A* **14,** 255 (1961).
174. J. E. Thiemann and co-workers, *J. Antibiot. Ser. A* **21,** 525 (1968).
175. D. W. Russell, *J. Chem. Soc.* 753 (1962).
176. P. DeSomer and P. J. Van Dijck, *Antibiot. Chemother. (Washington D.C.)* **5,** 632 (1955).
177. R. Q. Thompson and M. S. Hughes, *J. Antibiot. Ser. A* **16,** 187 (1963).
178. K. Sasaki and co-workers, *J. Antibiot.* **24,** 67 (1971).
179. J. Charney and co-workers, *Antibiot. Annu.* 171 (1953–1954).
180. M. Ebata and co-workers, *J. Antibiot. Ser. A* **22,** 467 (1969).
181. H. N. Hirschhorn, M. A. Bussa, and J. D. Thayer, *Proc. Soc. Exp. Biol. Med.* **67,** 429 (1948); S. F. Howell and J. D. Thayer, *Proc. Soc. Exp. Biol. Med.* **67,** 432 (1948). ·
182. A. Stracher and L. C. Craig, *J. Am. Chem. Soc.* **81,** 696 (1959).
183. A. W. Bernheimer and L. S. Avigad, *J. Gen. Microbiol.* **61,** 361 (1970).
184. T. H. Haskell and co-workers, *J. Antibiot. Ser. A* **16,** 67 (1963).
185. R. Junowicz-Kocholaty, W. Kocholaty, and A. Kelner, *J. Biol. Chem.* **168,** 765 (1947).
186. Y. Egawa and co-workers, *J. Antibiot. Ser. A* **22,** 12 (1969).
187. K. Arima, A. Kakinuma, and G. Tamura, *Biochem. Biophys. Res. Commun.* **31,** 488 (1968).
188. Y. Ooka and co-workers, *Agric. Biol. Chem.* **30,** 700 (1966).
189. S. L. Sinden, *Diss. Abstr.* **27,** 4048 (1967).
190. M. Shimo and co-workers, *J. Antibiot. Ser. A* **12,** 1 (1959).
191. S. Krynski and co-workers, *Acta Pol. Pharm.* **12,** 85 (1955); E. Borowski and co-workers, *Acta Biochem. Pol.* **4,** 241 (1957).
192. M. Misiek and co-workers, *Antibiot. Annu.* 852 (1957–1958); J. C. Sheehan and co-workers, *J. Am. Chem. Soc.* **85,** 2867 (1963).
193. M. Shibata, *Takeda Kenkyusho Nempo* **18,** 44 (1959).
194. C. Coronelli and co-workers, *Ann. Microbiol. Enzimol.* **13,** 125 (1963).
195. N. Miyari and co-workers, *J. Antibiot. Ser. A* **23,** 113 (1970).
196. M. Bodanszky and co-workers, *J. Am. Chem. Soc.* **86,** 2478 (1964); B. Andrew, D. Hodgkin, and M. A. Viswamitra, *Nature (London)* **225,** 233 (1970).
197. Y. Kimura and co-workers, *144th Meeting of the Japan Antibiotics Research Association, Mar. 26, 1965.*
198. G. J. Stessel, C. Leben, and G. W. Keitt, *Phytopathology* **43,** 23 (1953).
199. C. T. Hou, A. Ciegler, and C. W. Hesseltine, *Appl. Microbiol.* **23,** 183 (1972).
200. S. Suzuki and co-workers, *J. Antibiot. Ser. A* **20,** 126 (1972).
201. H. Otsuka and J. Shoji, *J. Antibiot. Ser. A* **19,** 128 (1966).
202. J. Shoji and co-workers, *J. Antibiot. Ser. A* **21,** 439 (1968).
203. H. Yoshioka and co-workers, *Tetrahedron Lett.* **1971,** 2043; A. Nagata, *J. Antibiot. Ser. A* **21,** 681 (1968).
204. T. P. King and L. C. Craig, *J. Am. Chem. Soc.* **77,** 6627 (1955).
205. R. J. Dubos and R. D. Hotchkiss, *J. Exp. Med.* **73,** 629 (1944).
206. O. G. de Lima and co-workers, *Rev. Inst. Antibiot. Univ. Fed. Pernambuco Recife* **5,** 19 (1963).

207. H. Brockmann and G. Schmidt-Kastner, *Chem. Ber.* **88,** 57 (1955).
208. M. H. McCormick and co-workers, *Antibiot. Annu.* **1955–1956,** 606.
209. U.S. Pat. 2,990,325 (June 27, 1961), R. Donovick and co-workers.
210. K. Aiso and co-workers, *J. Antibiot. Ser. A* **8,** 33 (1955).
211. A. Finlay and co-workers, *Am. Rev. Tuberc.* **62,** 1 (1951); Q. R. Bartz and co-workers, *Am. Rev. Tuberc.* **62,** 7 (1951).
212. Q. R. Bartz and co-workers, *Antibiot. Annu.* 777 (1954–1955).
213. I. N. Blinov and co-workers, *Khim. Prir. Soedin.* **11,** 490 (1975).
214. T. Ohno, S. Tajima, and K. Toki, *J. Agric. Chem. Soc. Jpn.* **27,** 665 (1953).
215. Jpn. Kokai 73 30,398 (Sept. 19, 1973), A. Shohjiroh and co-workers.
216. I. R. Shimi, A. Dewedar, and N. Abdallah, *J. Antibiot.* **24,** 283 (1971).
217. Y. Hinuma, *J. Antibiot. Ser. A* **7,** 124 (1954).
218. A. G. Argoudelis, M. E. Bergey, and T. R. Pyke, *J. Antibiot. Ser. A* **24,** 543 (1971).
219. J. H. Coats and J. Roesser, *J. Bacteriol.* **105,** 880 (1971).
220. S. Kondo and co-workers, *J. Antibiot. Ser. A* **14,** 194 (1961).
221. U.S. Pat. 3,061,514 (Oct. 30, 1962), A. Saeger and co-workers (to Eli Lilly & Co.).
222. U.S. Pat. 3,377,244 (Apr. 6, 1968), H. A. Whaley and co-workers (to American Cyanamid).
223. I. R. Shimi, G. M. Imam, and B. M. Haroun, *J. Antibiot. Ser. A* **22,** 106 (1969).
224. J. Shoji and co-workers, *J. Antibiot.* **29,** 813 (1976).
225. M. Sen and P. Nandi, *Ind. J. Chem.* **1,** 135 (1963).
226. E. Meyers and co-workers, *J. Antibiot.* **26,** 444 (1973).
227. Ger. Pat. 1,072,773 (Jan. 7, 1960), F. Lindner and co-workers.
228. G. W. Kenner and R. C. Sheppard, *Nature (London)* **181,** 48 (1958).
229. Neth. Pat. 105,150 (Jan. 15, 1963), (to Nederlandse Centrale Organizatie Voor Toegepast Natuurewetenshoppelijk Onderzock); J. G. Batelaan, *Tetrahedron Lett.* **1972,** 3103, 3107.
230. K. Atsumi and co-workers, *J. Antibiot.* **28,** 77 (1975).
231. P. Sensi and M. T. Timbal, *Antibiot. Chemother. (Washington D.C.)* **9,** 160 (1959).
232. M. Yoshida and co-workers, *J. Antibiot.* **27,** 128 (1974).
233. Jpn. Kokai 69 9,444 (June 3, 1969), S. Otani, S. Horie, and T. Yokouchi.
234. W. D. Celmer and B. A. Sobin, *Antibiot. Annu.* **1955–1956,** 437.
235. Belg. Pat. 614,211 (Aug. 21, 1962), (to Rhone Poulenc SA).
236. Fr. Pat. 1,393,208 (June 8, 1961), (to Rhone Poulenc SA).
237. J. Shoji and co-workers, *J. Antibiot. Ser. A* **23,** 429, 432 (1970).
238. J. Shoji and co-workers, *J. Antibiot.* **28,** 126 (1975).
239. Ref. 238, p. 129.
240. Ref. 238, p. 516.
241. Ref. 238, p. 809.
242. F. Kavanagh, ed., *Analytical Microbiology,* Vol. I, Academic Press, Inc., New York, 1963; Vol. II, 1973.
243. G. C. Ainsworth and co-workers, *Nature (London)* **160,** 263 (1947).
244. R. G. Sheperd and co-workers, *Bull. Johns Hopkins Hosp.* **87,** 43 (1947).
245. R. G. Benedict and A. F. Langlykke, *J. Bacteriol.* **54,** 24 (1947).
246. P. G. Stansly and G. Brownlee, *Nature (London)* **162,** 611 (1949).
247. T. S. G. Jones, *Ann. N.Y. Acad. Sci.* **51,** 909 (1949).
248. G. F. Gauze and co-workers, *Chem. Abstr.* **54,** 2025 (1960).
249. S. A. Il'inskaya and V. S. Rossovskaya *Antibiotiki (Moscow)* **3,** 10 (1958); A. S. Khokhlov and co-workers, *Antibiotiki* **5,** 3 (1960).
250. K. Vogler and co-workers, *Helv. Chim. Acta* **48,** 1161, 1371 (1965); R. O. Studer and co-workers, *Helv. Chim. Acta* **49,** 974 (1957).
251. S. Wilkinson, unpublished work.
252. Brit. Pat. 658,766 (Oct. 10, 1951), S. Wilkinson (to Wellcome Foundation, Ltd.).
253. K. Vogler and co-workers, *Helv. Chim. Acta* **43,** 1751 (1960); **44,** 131 (1961); R. Studer and K. Vogler, *Helv. Chim. Acta* **45,** 819 (1962); R. Studer and co-workers, *Helv. Chim. Acta* **46,** 612 (1963); K. Vogler and co-workers, *Helv. Chim. Acta* **46,** 2824 (1963).
254. W. K. Hausmann and L. C. Craig, *J. Am. Chem. Soc.* **76,** 4892 (1954).
255. M. Barnett and co-workers, *Br. J. Pharmacol.* **23,** 552 (1964).
256. F. L. Meleney and co-workers, *Science* **102,** 376 (1945).
257. G. G. F. Newton and E. P. Abraham, *Biochem. J.* **47,** 257 (1950).

258. U.S. Pat. 2,609,324 (Sept. 2, 1952), M. Senkus and P. C. Markunas (to Commercial Solvents Corp.); U.S. Pat. 2,828,246 (Mar. 25, 1958), T. E. Freaney and L. P. Allen (to Commercial Solvents Corp.).
259. U.S. Pat. 2,556,375 (June 12, 1951), P. P. Regna and I. A. Solomons (to Chas. Pfizer & Co.).
260. U.S. Pat. 2,834,711 (May 13, 1958), E. Zinn and F. Chornock (to Commercial Solvents Corp.).
261. U.S. Pat. 2,776,240 (Jan. 1, 1957), R. W. Shortridge (to Commercial Solvents Corp.).
262. L. C. Craig and co-workers, *J. Biol. Chem.* **199,** 259 (1952); G. G. F. Newton and E. P. Abraham, *Biochem. J.* **53,** 597 (1953); J. R. Weisiger and co-workers, *J. Am. Chem. Soc.* **77,** 721, 3123 (1955).
263. L. C. Craig and co-workers, *J. Biol. Chem.* **200,** 765 (1953); G. G. F. Newton and E. P. Abraham, *Biochem. J.* **53,** 604 (1953).
264. I. M. Lockhart and co-workers, *Biochem. J.* **61,** 534 (1955); **58,** 633 (1954); W. K. Hausmann and co-workers, *J. Am. Chem. Soc.* **77,** 721, 723 (1955); W. K. Hausmann and co-workers, *J. Biol. Chem.* **199,** 865 (1952); W. Konigsberg and L. C. Craig, *J. Org. Chem.* **27,** 934 (1962).
265. D. L. Swallow and E. P. Abraham, *Biochem. J.* **72,** 326 (1959).
266. R. E. Galardy and co-workers, *J. Biol. Chem.* **249,** 1823 (1971).
267. G. G. F. Newton and E. P. Abraham, *Biochem. J.* **53,** 597 (1953).
268. R. J. Dubos, *J. Exp. Med.* **70,** 1, 11, 249 (1939).
269. U.S. Pat. 2,602,043 (July 1, 1952), W. R. Mitchell (to Commercial Solvents Corp.).
270. A. R. Battersby and L. C. Craig, *J. Am. Chem. Soc.* **74,** 4019, 4023 (1952).
271. J. D. Gregory and L. C. Craig, *J. Biol. Chem.* **172,** 839 (1948); L. C. Craig and co-workers, *Cold Springs Harbor Symp. Quant. Biol.* **14,** 24 (1949).
272. L. K. Ramachandran, *Biochemistry* **2,** 1138 (1963).
273. E. Gross and B. Witkop, *Biochemistry* **4,** 2495 (1965).
274. A. Paladini and L. C. Craig, *J. Am. Chem. Soc.* **76,** 688 (1954); T. P. King and L. C. Craig, *J. Am. Chem. Soc.* **77,** 6624, 6627 (1955); T. P. King and L. C. Craig, *Biochemistry* **4,** 11 (1965).
275. R. Schwyzer and P. Sieber, *Helv. Chim. Acta* **40,** 624 (1957).
276. K. Kurahashi, *J. Biochem. (Tokyo)* **56,** 101 (1964); S. Otani and Y. Saito, *J. Biochem. (Tokyo)* **56,** 103 (1964).
277. W. Gevers and co-workers, *Proc. Nat. Acad. Sci. U.S.A.* **60,** 269 (1968); H. Kleinkauf and co-workers, *Proc. Nat. Acad. Sci. U.S.A.* **62,** 226 (1969); S. Otani and co-workers, *Biochem. Biophys. Res. Commun.* **33,** 620 (1968); T. Ljones and co-workers, *FEBS Lett.* **1,** 339 (1968).
278. W. Gevers and co-workers, *Proc. Nat. Acad. Sci. U.S.A.* **63,** 1335 (1969).
279. H. Kleinkauf and co-workers, *8th Int. Congr. Biochem.,* (1970).
280. R. D. Hotchkiss and R. J. Dubos, *J. Biol. Chem.* **140,** 791, 793, 803 (1940); **141,** 155 (1941); U.S. Pat. 2,453,534 (Nov. 9, 1948), H. S. Olcott and H. L. Frankel-Conrat (to U.S. Department of Agriculture).
281. A. Stracher and L. C. Craig, *J. Am. Chem. Soc.* **81,** 696 (1959); G. Alderton and N. Snell, *J. Am. Chem. Soc.* **81,** 701 (1959).
282. E. Gross and co-workers, *Z. Physiol. Chem.* **354,** 810 (1973).
283. W. M. Stark and co-workers, *Antimicrob. Agents Chemother.* **1962,** 596 (1963).
284. J. F. Pagano and co-workers, *Antibiot. Annu.* **1955–1956,** 554.
285. T. B. Platt and W. R. Frazier, *Antimicrob. Agents Chemother.* **1960,** 205 (1961).
286. M. Bodanszky and co-workers, *J. Am. Chem. Soc.* **86,** 2478 (1964).
287. M. Bodanszky and co-workers, *J. Antibiot. Ser. A* **16,** 76 (1963).
288. H. Nishimura and co-workers, *J. Antibiot. Ser. A* **14,** 255 (1961).
289. K. Mizuno and co-workers, *J. Antibiot.* **21,** 429 (1968).
290. M. Hori and co-workers, *Chem. Pharm. Bull.* **21,** 1171 (1973); E. Higashide and co-workers, *J. Antibiot.* **21,** 126 (1968).
291. M. Bodanszky and co-workers, *J. Am. Chem. Soc.* **91,** 2351 (1969).
292. H. Umezawa and co-workers, *J. Antibiot. Ser. A* **19,** 200 (1966).
293. H. Umezawa, *Pure Appl. Chem.* **28,** 665 (1971).
294. Ref. 292, p. 210.
295. J. Meienhofer and E. Atherton, *Adv. Appl. Microbiol.* **16,** 203 (1973).
296. A. R. Todd, *Int. Symp. Organic Chem. Nat. Prod. (Brussels)* (1962); K. Okabe, *J. Antibiot. Ser. A* **12,** 86 (1959).
297. K. Watanabe, *J. Antibiot. Ser. A* **13,** 62 (1960).
298. Y. A. Chabbert and J. F. Acar, *Ann. Inst. Pasteur Paris* **107,** 777 (1964).
299. M. Barber and P. Waterworth, *Br. Med. J.,* 603 (1964); J. Monnier and R. Bourse, *Ther. Sem. Hop.* **38,** 19 (1962).

300. D. W. Russell, *J. Chem. Soc. C* **1965**, 4664; C. G. MacDonald and J. S. Shannon, *Tetrahedron Lett.* 3113 (1964).

301. A. A. Kiryushin and co-workers, *Khim. Prir. Soedin.* **I**, 58 (1965); R. L. Hammill and co-workers, *Tetrahedron Lett.* 4255 (1969); Yu. A. Ovichinnikov and co-workers, *Tetrahedron Lett.* 159 (1971).

302. A. Suzuki and co-workers, *Org. Mass Spectrom.* **4**, 175 (1970); A. Suzuki and co-workers, *Agric. Biol. Chem.* **30**, 517 (1966); Y. Kodaira, *Agric. Biol. Chem.* **26**, 137 (1962).

303. S. Kuyama and S. Tamura, *Agric. Biol. Chem.* **29**, 168 (1965); S. Tamura and co-workers, *Agric. Biol. Chem.* **28**, 137 (1964).

304. Pl. A. Plattner and co-workers, *Helv. Chim. Acta* **31**, 594 (1948); M. M. Shemyakin and co-workers, *Tetrahedron* **19**, 581 (1963).

305. Pl. A. Plattner and co-workers, *Helv. Chim. Acta* **31**, 594, 665 (1948); **46**, 927 (1963); M. M. Shemyakin and co-workers, *Tetrahedron Lett.* 885 (1963).

306. W. A. Wolstenholme and L. C. Vining, *Tetrahedron Lett.* 7285 (1966); L. C. Vining and W. A. Taber, *Can. J. Chem.* **40**, 1579 (1962); A. A. Kiryushkin and co-workers, *Khim. Prir. Soedin.* **2**, 203 (1966).

307. M. Guirard and co-workers, *C. R. Acad. Sci.* **259**, 1267 (1964); M. Guirard and co-workers, *Biochim. Biophys. Acta* **125**, 75 (1966); M. Barber and co-workers, *Tetrahedron Lett.* 1331 (1963).

308. L. H. Briggs and co-workers, *J. Chem. Soc.* 5626 (1964).

309. H. H. Wasserman and co-workers, *J. Am. Chem. Soc.* **84**, 2978 (1964); **83**, 4107 (1961).

310. D. W. Russell, *J. Chem. Soc.* 753 (1962).

311. W. S. Bertaud and co-workers, *Tetrahedron* **21**, 677 (1965); W. S. Bertaud and co-workers, *J. Gen. Microbiol.* **32**, 385 (1963); M. M. Shemyakin and co-workers, *Zh. Obshch. Khim.* **35**, 1399 (1965).

312. A. Kikinuma and co-workers, *Agric. Biol. Chem.* **33**, 971, 1523, 1669 (1969); K. Arima and co-workers, *Biochem. Biophys. Res. Commun.* **31**, 488 (1968).

313. H. Brockmann and G. Schmidt-Kastner, *Chem. Ber.* **88**, 57 (1955); H. Brockmann and H. Geeren, *Ann.* **603**, 216 (1957); R. Brown and co-workers, *Antibiot. Chemother. (Washington D.C.)* **12**, 482 (1962); M. M. Shemyakin and co-workers, *Tetrahedron Lett.* 1921 (1963).

314. M. Hiramoto and co-workers, *Tetrahedron Lett.* 1087 (1970); M. Hiramoto and co-workers, *Biochem. Biophys. Res. Commun.* **36**, 194 (1969); T. Ohno and co-workers, *Bull. Agric. Chem. Soc.* **27**, 665 (1953).

315. D. W. Woolley in R. M. Hochster and J. H. Quastel, eds., *Metabolic Inhibitors,* Vol. I, Academic Press, Inc., New York, 1963, p. 445.

316. D. W. Woolley, *A Study of Antimetabolites,* John Wiley & Sons, Inc., New York, 1952.

317. D. L. Pruess and J. F. Scannell, *Adv. Appl. Microbiol.* **17**, 19 (1973).

318. P. A. Taylor and co-workers, *Biochim. Biophys. Acta* **286**, 107 (1972); W. W. Stewart, *Nature (London)* **229**, 174 (1971); S. L. Sinden and R. D. Durbin, *Nature (London)* **219**, 379 (1968).

319. E. Bayer and co-workers, *Helv. Chim. Acta* **55**, 224 (1972).

320. B. B. Molloy and co-workers, *J. Antibiot.* **25**, 137 (1972).

321. K. H. Baggaley and co-workers, *Chem. Commun.* 101 (1969); E. O. Stapley and co-workers, *Antimicrob. Agents Chemother. 1963,* 20 (1964).

322. D. L. Pruess and co-workers, *J. Antibiot.* **26**, 261 (1973); J. F. Scannell and co-workers, in J. Meienhofer, ed., *Chemistry and Biology of Peptides,* Ann Arbor Science Publications, Inc., Ann Arbor, Mich., 1975, p. 415.

323. W. A. König and co-workers, *Chem. Ber.* **106**, 816 (1973).

324. H. J. Rogers and co-workers, *Biochem. J.* **97**, 573 (1965); J. E. Walker and E. P. Abraham, *Biochem. J.* **118**, 557 (1970).

325. S. E. DeVoe and co-workers, *Antibiot. Annu.* 730 (1956–1957); E. L. Patterson and co-workers, *Antimicrob. Agents Chemother. 1966,* 115 (1967).

326. K. V. Rao and co-workers, *Antibiot. Annu.* 943 (1960); K. V. Rao, *Antimicrob. Agents Chemother.* 179 (1963).

327. J. P. Scannell and co-workers, *J. Antibiot.* **28**, 1 (1975).

General References

M. W. Miller, *The Pfizer Handbook of Microbial Metabolites,* 2nd ed., Academic Press, Inc., New York, 1978.

R. M. Evans, *The Chemistry of Antibiotics Used in Medicine,* Pergamon Press, London, 1965.

E. Schröder and K. Lübke, "Occurrence and Action of Biologically Active Polypeptides," in *The Peptides,* Vol. II, Academic Press, Inc., New York, 1966.

E. Gross and J. Meienhofer, *The Peptides; Analysis, Synthesis, and Biology,* Academic Press, Inc., New York, 1978.

D. Gottlieb and P. D. Shaw, eds., *Antibiotics,* Springer-Verlag, Berlin, Ger., 1967.

M. Bodanszky and D. Perlman, "Are Peptide Antibiotics Small Proteins?" *Nature* (*London*) **204,** 840 (1964).

D. Perlman and M. Bodanszky, "Biosynthesis of Peptide Antibiotics," *Ann. Rev. Biochem.* **40,** 449 (1971).

R. Reiner, *Antibiotica und Ausgewählte Chemotherapeutica,* Georg Thieme Verlag, Stuttgart, Ger., 1974.

A. I. Laskin and H. A. Lechevalier, eds., *CRC Handbook of Microbiology,* Vol. III, *Microbial Products,* CRC Press, Cleveland, Ohio, 1973.

E. Katz and A. L. Demain, "The Peptide Antibiotics of *Bacillus:* chemistry, Biogenesis, and Possible Functions," *Bacteriol. Rev.* **41,** 449 (1977).

D. PERLMAN
University of Wisconsin

PHENAZINES

Although a great many phenazine compounds are produced by microorganisms, by no means all of these substances can qualify as antibiotics because of their low or even untested antimicrobial activities. On the other hand, numerous phenazine derivatives have been obtained only by chemical synthesis, and although some of these substances have good antibacterial activities, they are not antibiotics in that they are not produced by microorganisms. Some derivatives first obtained synthetically have subsequently been encountered in natural sources (eg, 2-phenazinol). This article deals primarily with those phenazines, produced by microorganisms, that in low concentrations can inhibit the growth of some microorganisms. Among those phenazines given trivial names are myxin, lomofungin, iodinin, griseoluteins A and B, griseoluteic acid, hemipyocyanin and pyocyanin, tubermycins A and B, chlororaphin and oxychlororaphin, and aeruginosins A and B.

Microbial Phenazines

As early as 1860, Fordos reported (1) the production of the dark blue pigment pyocyanin, and Guignard and Sauvageau in 1894 (2) described the production of the pigment chlororaphin. Since then, over 30 variously substituted phenazines, many with antibiotic properties, have been isolated from natural sources. Microorganisms constitute the exclusive source of these compounds. The phenazine derivatives have been reported to be produced by bacteria belonging to the genera *Pseudomonas* (3–9) and *Brevibacterium* (10–12), by myxobacteria of the genus *Sorangium* (13), by actinomycetes of the genera *Streptomyces* (14–18), *Streptosporangium* (19), *Microbispora* (Waksmania) (15,20), as well as by members of a group of *Nocardiaceae* (reclassified as *Actinomadura dassonvillei*) (21–22).

There is considerable overlap in the production pattern with several microorganisms producing the same compound, and in other cases the same microorganism may produce 3–10 phenazine derivatives (16,21,23–24). Many of the isolated phenazines possess varying degrees of antibiotic properties, a feature that has been related to their interaction with deoxyribonucleic acid, presumably by intercalation of the planar aromatic ring system.

Chemical Relationships. The phenazine antibiotics bear the following common skeleton:

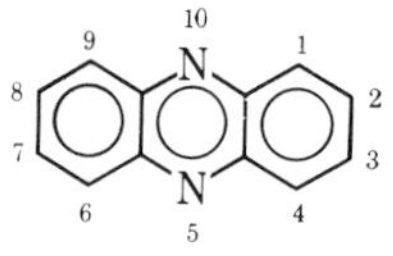

Chemical Abstracts Service Numbering System 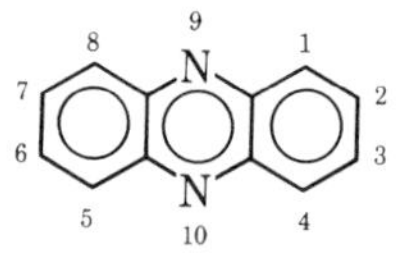   older numbering system (Beilstein)

Inspection of the known phenazine structures, as pointed out by Holstein and Marshall (25), reveals a symmetrical pattern: *C* or *O* substituents are often found at the 1, 4, 6, and 9 positions with identical substituents often attached at the diagonally opposed positions, 1,6 or 4,9. This sort of substituted ring system has encouraged the study of the biosynthetic origin of the phenazine nucleus. A dimerization of oppositely oriented aromatic precursors was strongly suggested. Review articles (20,22,26–28) on phenazine antibiotics are available.

With the exception of internal salts, such as aeruginosins A and B, phenazines can generally be extracted from fermentation broths with water-immiscible solvents such as chloroform. Concentrated extracts often yield crystalline material easily, although mixtures might have to be separated if the organism produces multi-components. Colors range from pale yellow through red to blue and purple. Sodium hydrosulfite treatment produces fading in the absence, or intensification of color in the presence of a 1-carboxyl group in the phenazine. Ultraviolet absorption spectra, with peaks between 250 and 300 nm, are often very characteristic; nmr, mass spectra, and x-ray crystal structure analysis have been used in recent years for characterization.

Biological Aspects.   *Biological Activity.* Inhibitory activities of phenazine antibiotics have been described against gram-positive and gram-negative bacteria, yeasts, fungi, animal tumors, helminths (29), selected protozoa such as *Trichomonas* (30), amoeba (31), noxious plants (32), acarids (33), and HeLa cells (34). One of the antibiotics, lomofungin, has been claimed to promote the growth of animals when used as a feed supplement (35). Although several phenazine antibiotics appeared at one time or another to have promising chemotherapeutic potential as antibacterials, anticancer agents, or antiprotozoal agents, only one, cuprimyxin (Unitop, Roche) is presently being sold as a topical formulation as verterinary medicine for dermal and otic use in dogs and cats, and additional uses are being developed. Table 1 describes some chemical and biological properties of phenazine antibiotics.

Biosynthesis. Biosynthetic pathways for various phenazine antibiotics have been studied: for pyocyanin (25,27.107–114), for iodinin (12,20,65,97,115–119), for chlororaphin (44), for phenazine-1-carboxylic acid (24–25,99,113,116), for phenazine-1-carboxamide (oxychlororaphin) (24,92,120), and for miscellaneous phenazine antibiotics and their intermediates (4,16,21,23,96,117).

Although shikimate is known to act as a precursor of several phenazines, and studies with mutants suggest that the branch point is in the shikimate-to-chorismate region, the mode of assembly of the phenazine ring system is still unknown (96,97).

Results from feeding labeled D-(^{14}C) shikimic acid to three types of bacteria (25,116) showed that phenazine synthesis proceeds by the symmetrical condensation of two identical C-6 or C-1 N-substituted chorismic acid molecules. These results have been confirmed and the same assembly mode has been proposed for iodinin (115). The proposed biosynthetic pathway for phenazine pigments based on data obtained with mutants of *Pseudomonas phenazinium* is shown in Figure 1 (117,121–122).

Mode of Action. Phenazine-producing *Pseudomonads* show a branched biosynthetic pathway leading to production of aromatic amino acids *or* the phenazine compounds. The latter may be produced in larger quantities than the former (123). Using semipurified enzymes from 4 bacterial species, Levitch (123) found that the enzyme 3-deoxy-D-arabino-heptulosonate-7-phosphate (DAHP) synthetase, which catalyzes the first reaction of aromatic amino acid biosynthesis, was inhibited by phenazine-1-carboxylic acid (tubermycin B), iodinin, and pyocyanin from 1 to 83% varying with the antibiotic and the bacterium which produced it.

Hollstein and Van Gemert in 1971 (124) studied by visible spectrophotometry the interaction with DNA of phenazine-1-carboxylic acid, phenazine-1-carboxamide (oxychlororaphin), pyocyanin, 1,6-dimethoxyphenazine and its mono- and di-*N*-oxides, 1,6-phenazinediol, iodinin, and myxin. They found that the phenazine derivatives inhibited DNA template-controlled RNA synthesis whereby iodinin approaches the inhibitory intensity of actinomycin. It was suggested that the inhibition, at least in part, was due to intercalation as has been proposed for other tricyclic planar aromatic antibiotics.

Myxin

This potent broad-spectrum antibiotic, also referred to as antibiotic 3C, was isolated in 1966 (125–127) from broth of a *Sorangium* sp (strain 3C) of a myxobacter.

Chemical and Physical Properties. At 120–130°C myxin decomposes into the inactive orange pigment 6-methoxy-1-phenazinol 10-oxide. On drying above 149°C it may explode (128). The uv absorption maximum (126–127) in 0.1*N* HCl is at 283 nm (ε 5400) and the visible is at 505 nm (ε 6500); in 0.1*N* NaOH, the maxima are at 272, 348, 390, and 590 nm. Myxin is slightly soluble in water, carbon tetrachloride, and petroleum ether, but is more readily soluble in methanol, acetone, ether, chloroform,

Table 1. Chemical and Biological Properties of Phenazine Antibiotics

Compound; CAS Registry No.	Structure; Molecular formula	Microbial sources	mp, °C; Color; λ max	Antimicrobial activity MIC[a], μg/mL	Toxicity,[b] LD$_{50}$, mg/kg	Refs.
aeruginosin A [21668-67-7]	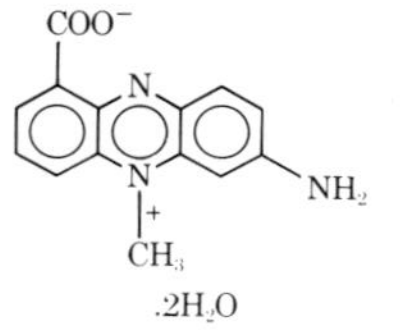 $C_{14}H_{11}N_3O_2$	*Pseudomonas aeruginosa*; *Ps. aeruginosa* var. *erythrogenes*	red; 235, 282, 396, and 515 nm	in mixture with aeruginosin B, exerted a moderate activity against tobacco mosaic virus; bacteriostatic vs *S. aureus* and *Mycobacterium* at 100, *C. albicans*, 400		6,36–41
aeruginosin B [6508-65-2]	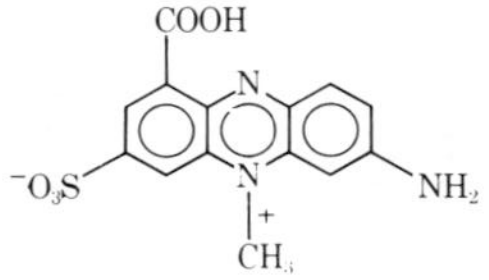 $C_{14}H_{11}N_3O_5S$	*Pseudomonas aeruginosa*; *Ps. aeruginosa* var. *erythrogenes*	red; similar abs spec to aeruginosin A	moderate activity against tobacco mosaic virus		5–6,36–38,40–41
chlororaphin [46801-26-7]	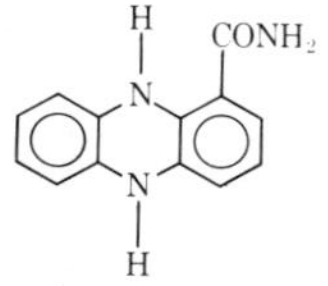 $C_{13}H_{11}N_3O$		228–230; green			42–46
griseoluteic acid [489-76-9]	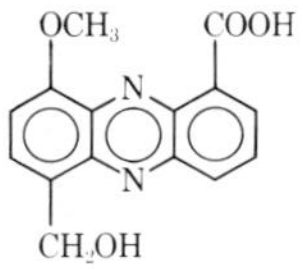 $C_{15}H_{12}N_2O_4$	*Streptomyces griseoluteus*; unidentified streptomycete	269 and 369 nm	only very weak antibacterial activity or inactive, vs *B. subtilis*		18,47–51

griseolutein A
[573-84-2]

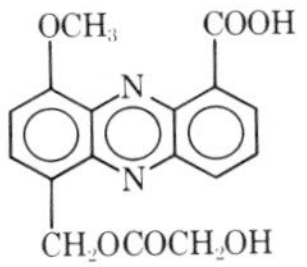

OCH$_3$ H, COOH
CH$_2$OCOCH$_2$OH

C$_{17}$H$_{14}$N$_2$O$_6$

Streptomyces griseo-luteus; unidentified streptomycete

193; red-dish yellow; 267 and 368 nm

bacteriostatic vs *S. aureus* and *S. paradysenteriae*, 0.8; *B. subtilis* 0.1; *B. anthracis* 0.4; *E. coli*, 6.3; *S. typhosa* 3.1; *S. typhimurium*, 25; *P. vulgaris*, 0.2; *Ps. aeruginosa* 12.5; in agar diffusion assay, griseolutein A is five times as active vs *B. subtilis* as B; MIC conc by tube dil assay were 6, 0.2 and 0.2 for *E. coli*, *S. aureus*, and *Salm. gallinarum*

>500 sc; slightly less toxic than griseolutein B, A is more toxic than B (<12.5 vs >125 ip; <100 vs 100 sc, respectively) ED$_{50}$ 0.1 mg/kg ip and >25 mg/kg sc vs *S. aureus* infection in mice

18,47–54

50

51

griseolutein B
[62842-51-7]

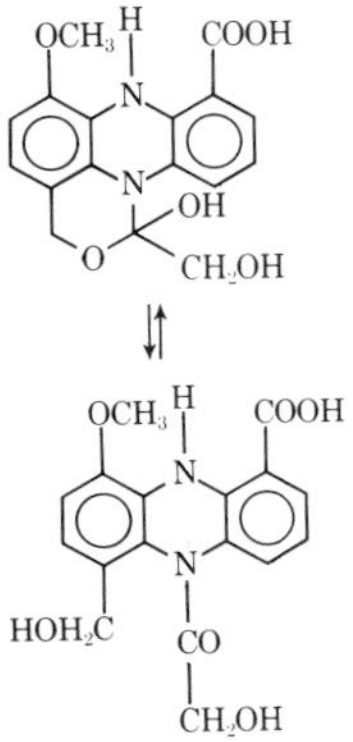

OCH$_3$ H N COOH
OH
CH$_2$OH
HOH$_2$C

⇌

OCH$_3$ H N COOH
CO
CH$_2$OH
HOH$_2$C

C$_{17}$H$_{16}$N$_2$O$_6$

Streptomyces griseo-luteus; unidenti-fied strepto-mycete

>220 dec; yellow; 281 and 342 nm

bacteriostatic vs *S. aureus* and *B. anthracis*, 0.2–0.4; *B. subtilis*, 0.2–0.4; *S. dysenteriae*, *S. paratyphi*, *S. schott-muelleri*, *M. avium* at 1–4; *E. coli*, 5; *S. typhosa*, 5–10; *S. typhimurium*, 25–50; *P. vulgaris* and *Ps. aeruginosa*, 25–50; *Pneumo-coccus*, 10–25; *S. hemolyticus*, 100; MIC conc by tube dil assay were 11, 0.2 and 0.7 for *E. coli*, *S. aureus*, and *Salm. gallinarum narum*

200 iv, 450 sc, >800 po; MLD in mice sc >1600; ED$_{50}$ vs *S. aureus* infected mice is about 37 mg/kg; ED$_{50}$ 0.95 mg/kg ip, 23.5 sc, and 850 po vs *S. aureus* infection in mouse; diacetyl derivative of gris-eolutein B vs *S. aureus* infection is 1/5 as active as B by ip route, equal by sc, and five times as active po

47–52, 55–57

259

Table 1 (*continued*)

Compound; CAS Registry No.	Structure; Molecular formula	mp, °C; Color; λ max	Microbial sources	Antimicrobial activity MIC[a], μg/mL	Toxicity,[b] LD_{50}, mg/kg	Refs.
hemipyocyanin [528-71-2]	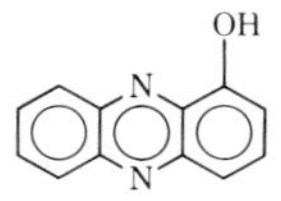 $C_{12}H_8N_2O$	158; yellow; 264, 352, 360, 384, and 425 nm	Ps. aeruginosa; Streptomyces thioluteus	weakly active against bacteria and fungi; has insecticidal properties; bacteriostatic vs B. subtilis at 50; S. aureus, 20–100; Mycobacterium, 10; C. albicans, 50; F. avenaceum, 100	less toxic in animals than pyocyanin	9,16,22, 26,37, 58–60
9-hydroxy-6-(hydroxymethyl)-1-phenazine carboxylic acid (antibiotic T-4138) [60160-03-4]	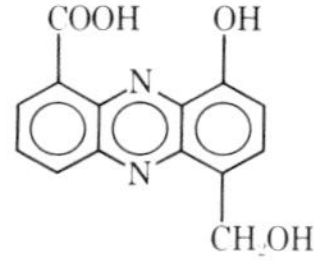 $C_{14}H_{10}N_2O_4$	269 and 369 nm	Streptomyces recifensis	effective against both gram-positive and gram-negative bacteria		17
1-hydroxy-methyl-6-carboxy-phenazine [62842-52-8]	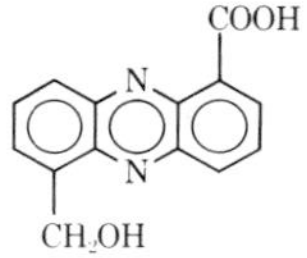 $C_{14}H_{10}N_2O_3$	251 and 364 nm	Streptomyces griseoluteus	almost no antibacterial activity		18,47
iodinin [68-81-5]	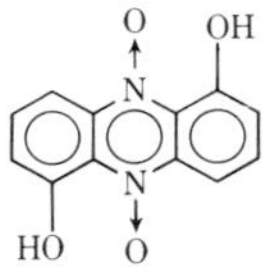 $C_{12}H_8N_2O_4$	230 dec; purple; 291 and 355 nm	Brevibacterium sp; Nocardia sp; Streptomyces thioluteus; Streptosporangium amethystogenes; Ps. aureofaciens; Arthrobacter	inhibits Streptococcus hemolyticus at 0.5, Sarcina lutea and Corynebacterium fimi, 0.08; Mycobacterium smegmatis, 1.5; Actinoplanes sp., 0.1; Nocardia coeliaca, Saccharo-	>1000 po	3–4,11– 12,15, 19,45, 61–67

Name [CAS]	Formula	Producing organism	Properties	Biological activity	Toxicity	References
(continued)		*paraffineus;* *Ps. phenazinium*		myces cerevisiae, and *Trichophyton mentagrophytes,* 0.4; *E. coli, P. vulgaris* > 2.0; 100 ppm gives 60% inhibition of bacterial leaf blight of rice plants; in agar diffusion test, limiting conc in µg/mL were: *B. subtilis,* 10; *B. globifer,* 0.4; *S. lutea,* 0.4; *E. coli* 0; *P. morganii,* 0.4	0.25 sc in mice, 10 ip in mice	35,68–72
lomofungin [26786-84-5]	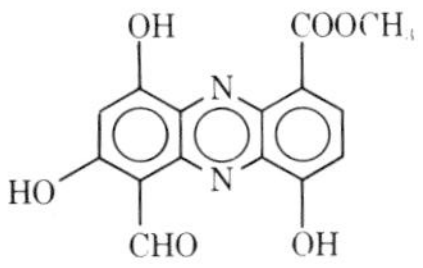 $C_{15}H_{10}N_2O_6$	*Streptomyces lomondensis*	> 320 dec; olive yellow	see text		
1-methoxy-4-methyl-9-carboxy-phenazine [29067-78-5]	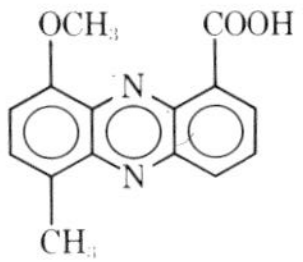 $C_{15}H_{12}N_2O_3$	*Streptomyces griseoluteus*	124–126; yellow; 267, 346, and 363 nm	almost no antibacterial activity		18,47
6-methoxy-1-phenazinol [13129-58-3]	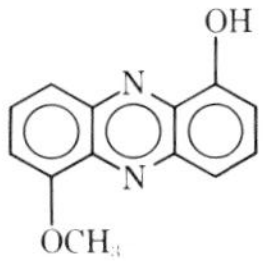 $C_{13}H_{10}N_2O_2$	*Streptomyces thioluteus*	192; orange; 237, 371, and 438 nm	weak antibacterial activity		16
myxin [13449-75-7]	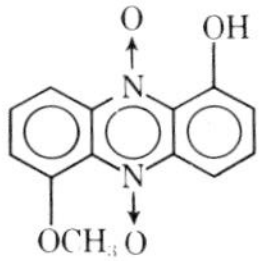 $C_{13}H_{10}N_2O_4$	*Sorangium* sp	130–135 dec; red	see text		13,29–30, 73–91

261

Table 1 (continued)

Compound; CAS Registry No.	Structure; Molecular formula	Microbial sources	mp, °C; Color; λ max	Antimicrobial activity MIC[a], μg/mL	Toxicity,[b] LD$_{50}$, mg/kg	Refs.
oxychlororaphin [550-89-0]	$C_{13}H_9N_3O$	*Ps. chlororaphis* NRRL B-977; *Ps. aeruginosa*, *Bacillus pyocyaneus*	243; yellow	inhibits at about 100 μg/mL the growth of *S. aureus, Streptococcus hemolyticus, S. typhi, P. vulgaris,* and *E. coli*; inhibits 5 pathogenic fungi in agar dilution tests at 12.5–50; 4 *Streptomyces* sp inhibited by 12.5–25	mice tolerate 500 mg/kg ip in olive oil	26,37,42–45,92–93
1,6-phenazinediol [69-48-7]	$C_{12}H_8N_2O_2$	*Brevibacterium crystalloiodinum*; *M. bispora; Ps. iodina; Streptomyces thioluteus; Ps. phenazinium*	274; golden yellow; 272, 372, and 440–445 nm	*S. lutea,* 5; *C. fimi,* 5; *C. ulmi,* 15; *M. smegmatis,* 25; *Actinoplanes* sp, 10; *E. coli, B. proteus,* >75; plant pathogenic fungi, 5–7.5; *Zygosacch. salsus,* 3		4,11,14–15,94–97
1,6-phenazinediol-5-oxide [69-86-3]	$C_{12}H_8N_2O_3$	*Microbispora aerata; Ps. iodina; Streptomyces thioluteus*	248–250 dec; orange; 283, 394, and 487 nm	intermediate between that of iodinin and phenazinediol, eg, *S. lutea,* 5–6; *C. fimi,* 5–6; *C. ulmi,* 3; *M. smegmatis,* 5; *Actinoplanes* sp, 5; *E. coli, B. proteus,* > 9 ·		4,21,23,96
pyocyanin [85-66-5]	$C_{13}H_{10}N_2O$	*Ps. aeruginosa* ATCC 9027; *Cyanococcus chromospirans*	133; dark blue; 244, 310 and 328 nm	*S. aureus* 12.5; *S. pyogenes* (hemolyticus) 25; *B. subtilis* 6.0; *C. diphtheriae* 25; *S. dysenteriae* 12.5; *N. gonorrhoea* 17; *P. pestis* 17; *V.*	MLD = 100 ip (mouse); tested clinically vs gonorrhoea, in ophthalmology, stoma-	9,26–27,36–37,59,92

Name [CAS]	Structure	Producing organism	Physical data	Antimicrobial spectrum	Toxicity	References
				... tology, and diphtheria in 1947		
tubermycin A [33103-22-9]	alkyl-substituted with a carboxyl function, $C_{17}H_{16}N_2O_2$	Streptomyces misakiensis	174; yellow; 256 and 365 nm	comma 4; 100 vs E. coli, S. typhimurium, Shigella, Mycobact. tuberculosis; 200 vs B. proteus; inhibits 3 Mycobacteria at 1–20; 3 gram-positive bacteria at 50; >50 against B. subtilis, E. coli, and fungi	160 iv mice	98
tubermycin B [2538-68-3]	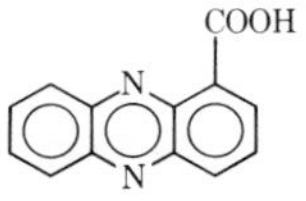 $C_{13}H_8N_2O_2$	Ps. aureofaciens, Ps. aeruginosa, Streptomyces misakiensis, Nocardiaceae	238; yellow; 251 and 364 nm	inhibits growth of some plant pathogens and mycobacterium, and algae and noxious plants; completely inhibits S. aureus, B. subtilis, Mycobacterium B at 50; at 100, completely inhibited Sarcina flava, Actinomyces griseus, and C. albicans; and at 200 Fusarium avenaceum; however, MIC >50 for S. aureus, M. flavus, B. subtilis, E. coli, A. oryzae, P. chrysogenum, C. albicans, and S. cerevisiae, but 10–50 for 3 Mycobacteria	400 iv mice	7, 21, 25, 32, 37, 92, 98–106

[a] MIC, minimum inhibitory concentration; ip, intraperitoneal; iv, intravenous; po, oral; sc, subcutaneous.
[b] MLD, minimum lethal dose; ED, effective dose.

263

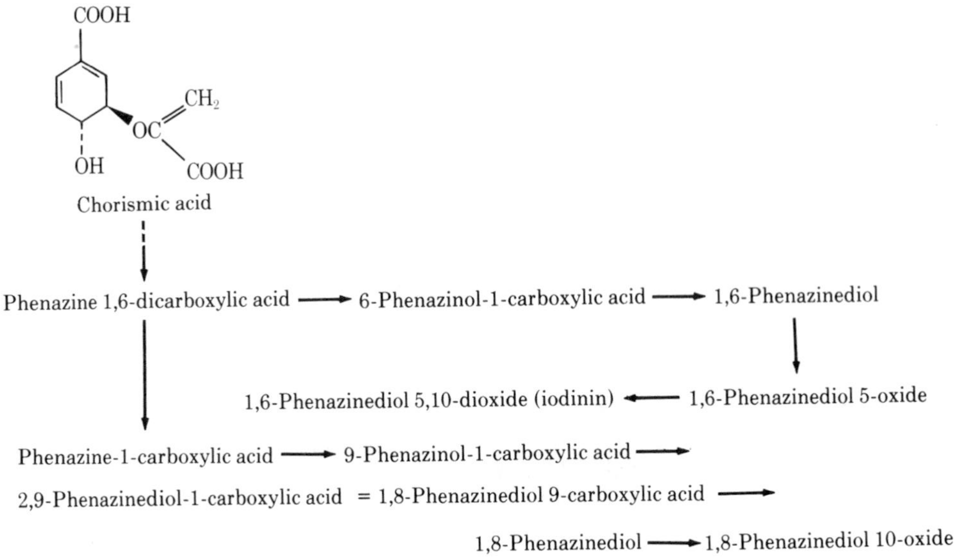

COOH

CH₂

OC

OH   COOH

Chorismic acid

Phenazine 1,6-dicarboxylic acid ⟶ 6-Phenazinol-1-carboxylic acid ⟶ 1,6-Phenazinediol

1,6-Phenazinediol 5,10-dioxide (iodinin) ⟵ 1,6-Phenazinediol 5-oxide

Phenazine-1-carboxylic acid ⟶ 9-Phenazinol-1-carboxylic acid ⟶

2,9-Phenazinediol-1-carboxylic acid = 1,8-Phenazinediol 9-carboxylic acid ⟶

1,8-Phenazinediol ⟶ 1,8-Phenazinediol 10-oxide

Figure 1. Biosynthesis of iodinin.

and toluene. The crystal structure of myxin is monoclinic (129). The packing is unusual in that there is apparently a nonbonded intermolecular oxygen–oxygen distance of 0.2577 nm. Many myxin-related phenazine derivatives (87–91) have been synthesized, some of which have the added advantage over the parent antibiotic of better solubility properties (130–131). Among the substances prepared were 1-hydroxy-6-amino-alkoxyphenazine 5,10-dioxides. The highly active antimicrobial agent 6-methoxy-1-phenazinol 5,10-dioxide cupric complex (132–134) provided a commercially useful phenazine antibiotic for the first time. The structure for this complex is given below:

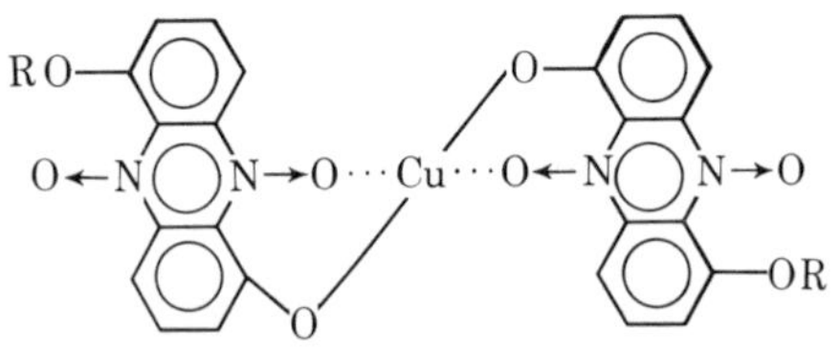

R = methyl [28069-65-0]
R = ethyl [28069-66-1] (ca 1/10 as active)

Stabilization of the myxin copper complex in a variety of dosage forms was achieved (135) by the addition of 2–20% molar excess of copper ions to the specific dosage form: ie, 0.5% of the cupric complex and 0.019% of cupric acetate trihydrate with 0.2% sodium acetate trihydrate to provide pH 5.7–6.2. A safe purification procedure for myxin involving an iron(III) complex has been reported (136).

Biological Aspects. Among the organisms sensitive *in vitro* to as little as 3.6 μg per assay disk were 11 plant-pathogenic bacteria, 21 out of 23 other species of gram-positive, gram-negative, and acid-fast bacteria, 34 out of 51 fungi, 12 streptomyces and 8 out of 12 yeasts (125–127). The activity against *Staphylococcus aureus* was shown to be bactericidal. Although data on toxicity to animals and plants were not yet available, the authors felt they had an unusually interesting potential therapeutic agent.

Synthetic myxin has high *in vitro* antibacterial activity, but it also has a high toxicity in mice (LD$_{50}$ about 40 mg/kg ip) (137). Doses of myxin at 3.75 mg/kg ip give little protection against heavy bacterial infections.

An extensive description of the use of the cupric complex of myxin is given in References 133–134 for mastitis in cattle, and topical bacterial, yeast, fungal, and protozoan infections in mammals. Pharmaceutical ointments and other formulations are described in detail, including the need for the antibiotic complex particles to have an initial size distribution of 5–20 μm to provide an increased surface area and to afford sufficient solubility. Since the material is sensitive to heat, shock, and static electricity, conventional means of deaggregation are unacceptable because of the explosion hazard. However, by the use of ultrasonic deaggregation (138), any copper complex aggregates can be safely reduced to their micronized form in the required particle size range (see Ultrasonics).

Experimentally-induced topical microbial infections of dogs—cutaneous *Microsporum canis*, otic *C. albicans,* and ophthalmic *S. aureus*—were effectively treated with cupric complex of myxin (139). Snyder and Imhoff (140) in trials with cuprimyxin (Unitop Topical 0.5% Cream, Roche) for bacterial and fungal skin lesions in dogs and cats, found a 97% incidence of improvement of clearing of the pyoderma.

Snyder and Maestrone (141) compared the *in vitro* antimicrobial activity of cuprimyxin with four other commercial veterinary products against four bacteria, two fungi and one yeast. Cuprimyxin showed significant *in vitro* sensitivity zones for all organisms tested, and the best overall inhibition pattern of all the products tested.

Mode of Action. Studies with growing cells of two bacteria, using radioactive labeled myxin, showed that the primary effect of myxin was on the cellular DNA (142–143). Additional results suggest the lethal effect of myxin is not due to inhibition of DNA synthesis directly, but is probably the result of irreparable damage to the DNA template (144).

In a detailed study comparing the interaction of myxin and other phenazine antibiotics with polydeoxyribonucleotides, Hollstein and Van Gemert (124) found two types of binding with widely varying association constants, but no binding to single-stranded polydeoxyribonucleotides. Myxin inhibited DNA template-controlled RNA synthesis, in a manner at least in part, due to intercalation. Hartman and co-workers (145) reported that in *Salmonella* myxin causes frameshift mutations.

Manufacture. Because of the low overall yields and difficulties of the total chemical synthesis, the antibiotic is prepared (146) by chemical methylation of iodinin, which in turn is made by fermentation (61). Selected strains of *Brevibacterium iodinum* are grown in suitable nutrients and antifoam agents in large cylindrical tanks provided with aeration and agitation devices, similar to the instrumented equipment used in general for large-scale antibiotic fermentations (see Fermentation). The highly insoluble antibiotic is excreted into the broth, and after centrifugation it is obtained by extraction of the sludge with organic solvents (such as chloroform), concentration and crystallization, or by centrifugation and successive washing of the sludge with water and water-miscible solvents. Iodinin of 95% purity or greater is thus obtained in yields exceeding 4 g/L of fermented medium.

For conversion to myxin, the iodinin is suspended in a mixture of hexamethyl-phosphoric triamide and dimethylsulfoxide. Potassium *tert*-butoxide is added and the reaction mixture is stirred at 25°C for 24 h. The mixture is cooled to 5°C, then dimethylsulfate is added with stirring. After stirring overnight at 25°C, the mixture is poured into ice water, and the precipitated myxin is filtered, washed with water, and refiltered. The crude myxin is dissolved in 50% aqueous sulfuric acid and complexed with ferric chloride (136,146). The resulting black solid is filtered and washed with glacial acetic acid and chloroform. The black solid complex is broken with acetone and crystallized myxin is filtered and washed with water to give a 65% yield, based on iodinin (146). The copper complex of myxin is prepared as previously described (132–133). Its stabilization in pharmaceutical dosage forms is reported (135).

Less than 100 kg/yr of cuprimyxin is currently being manufactured, with up to 20,000 L-sized fermenters used intermittently for iodinin production, and 200 L chemical reaction vessels for the methylation and metal salt complexation steps.

In view of their extreme sensitivity to violent decomposition when exposed to heat, high friction, or static charges, myxin and copper myxin are handled with great care in the manufacturing plant. Located in an out-of-the-way area, and of such a size as to minimize damage to personnel and facilities in the event of an accident, the equipment is fully grounded, and the large volumes of solvents required are transferred through closed systems by drum pumps to overhead volumetric tanks with overflow lines to the original container. Protective clothing and air masks are provided to the operators when they handle solids or transfer hazardous liquids. All solvents are pretreated to remove potentially hazardous materials from the process prior to recovery. Very little is discharged into the plant sewer system except for dilute acids or water containing minimal amounts of miscible solvents.

Lomofungin (Lomondomycin)

Lomofungin, formerly referred to as antibiotic U-24,792, was isolated at the Upjohn laboratories from submerged aerobic-fermentation culture broth of a new species, *Streptomyces lomondensis* var. *lomondensis* (NRRL 3252) (35,68–69). Although early findings indicated its activity against fungi and gram-positive and gram-negative bacteria, as well as a growth promoter of animals when added to feed supplements, it has not found any commercial use to date. It has, however, proven to be a useful biochemical tool in the study of yeast nucleic acids.

Chemical and Physical Properties. Crystalline lomofungin is soluble to less than 1 mg/mL in water, methanol, cyclohexane, acetone, ether, and ethyl acetate, but very soluble in acetone and methyl ethyl ketone at a pH of about 2.0. At pH 10–12, it is soluble in water (10 mg/mL), and in dimethylformamide (727 mg/mL). UV, ir, and nmr spectra are given in References 35 and 68.

Biological Aspects. *In vitro,* lomofungin was reported to inhibit 11 gram-positive and gram-negative bacteria at 16–125 μg/mL. Among a wide spectrum of human pathogenic fungi, 16 out of 18 were inhibited by 100 μg/mL agar, and 2 by 1 mg/mL (35,69). *In vivo,* lomofungin is quite toxic, with an LD_{50} of 10 mg/kg ip in mice (72).

Mode of Action.   Lomofungin is used in studies of yeast and bacterial RNA metabolism and enzyme synthesis, since other antibiotics, such as actinomycin D, do not inhibit yeast RNA synthesis or do so only at high concentrations (147). Lomofungin strongly inhibits the synthesis of ribosomal RNA and polydisperse RNA, but has comparatively less effect on synthesis of 5 sRNA (soluble RNA) and tRNA (transfer RNA) (148–150). Earlier studies showed that RNA synthesis was inhibited by a direct interaction of the antibiotic with the polymerase (149,151–153). With isolated *E. coli* RNA polymerase, lomofungin (as well as 8-hydroxyquinoline) could inhibit polymerase activity solely by chelating Mn^{2+} and Mg^{2+} (147,154). This inhibition was believed to occur in the absence of any direct contact between the RNA polymerase or DNA template and the inhibitor.

Iodinin

This deep purple, copper-glinting pigment was first isolated in 1938, from a culture called *Chromobacterium iodinum* (3), subsequently renamed *Brevibacterium iodinum* (12), and later from broths of numerous other bacteria. Although it has long been known to possess antibacterial activity (45,62) and also been claimed to have antihypertensive activity (155), it has not found any direct practical application as an antibiotic except as an intermediate in the manufacture of myxin (146).

Chemical and Physical Properties.   Iodinin dissolves in aq NaOH solution to a blue solution and shows greenish color in ethanol with $FeCl_3$. It is slightly soluble in chloroform, carbon disulfide, petroleum ether, glacial acetic acid, acetone, dioxane, and benzene; soluble in concentrated sulfuric acid and in aqueous sodium hydroxide; and insoluble in water, ethanol, and ether.

On methylation with dimethylsulfate in alkali (76) or with diazomethane (77) it yields the antibiotic myxin. In the latter case, smaller amounts of the dimethoxy-derivative as well as of the mono *N*-oxide are also produced. Yeast cells reduce iodinin to the orange pigment 1,6-phenazinediol 5-oxide, and crude enzymatic preparations from *Pseudomonas iodina* convert this orange pigment back to iodinin on overnight incubation at 28°C (20). Two yeasts (*H. anomala* and *S. cerevisiae*) as well as *Nocardia coeliaca* reduce 1,6-phenazinediol 5-oxide to the less active phenazinediol (4).

Biological Aspects.   Iodinin has been reported to be produced by *Chromobacterium iodinum* (3,12), *Brevibacterium crystalloiodinum* (11), *Streptomyces thioluteus* (4,16), *Microbispora* (Waksmania) *aerata* (15), *Actinomadura dassonvillei* (21–22), *Arthrobacter paraffineus* ATCC 15591 (64–65), *Nocardia hydrocarbonoxydans* ATCC 15104 (65), *Corynebacterium hydrocarboclastus* ATCC 15592 (65), *Micrococcus paraffinolyticus* ATCC 15582 (65), *Brevibacterium maris* (66), *Brevibacterium stationis* (66), *Streptosporangium amethystogenes* var. *nonreducans* (19), *Pseudomonas aureofaciens* (67), and *Pseudomonas phenazinium* (97). Frequently other phenazine derivatives are isolated along with the iodinin (16).

Uses and Indications.   Iodinin is claimed to be effective as an antihypertensive agent when administered daily to hypertensive patients at dosages of about 0.1–300 mg/kg of body weight, preferably by the oral route in divided dosages three to four times daily (155). Since the oral LD_{50} of iodinin is greater than 1 g/kg body weight, a therapeutic index of safety was claimed.

At 100 ppm, iodinin gave 60% inhibition against bacterial leaf blight of rice plants by pot test; in the same test, phenazine 5-oxide gave 97% inhibition (63).

Table 2. Chemical Features and Microbial Sources of Phenazine Derivatives

Compound; CAS Registry No.	Structure; Molecular formula	Microbial sources	mp, °C; Color; λ max	References
8-amino-1-phenazinol [62842-50-6]	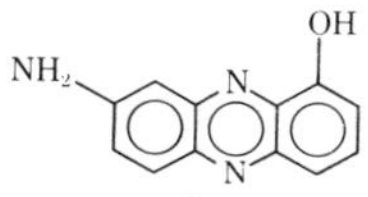 $C_{12}H_9N_3O$	an unidentified bacterium, gram-negative rod, strain V 15295	180 (methyl ether), 243; bright orange (methyl ether); 275, 376, and 480 nm	23
2,9-dihydroxy-1-phenazine carboxylic acid [23448-75-1]	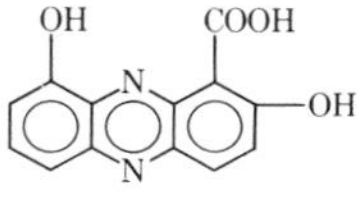 $C_{13}H_8N_2O_4$	Ps. phenazinium; unidentified gram-negative bacterium	>270; 271, 379, and 420 nm	23,96
1,6-dimethoxy-phenazine [13398-79-3]	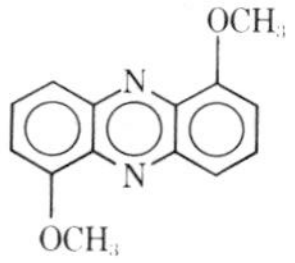 $C_{14}H_{12}N_2O_2$	S. luteoreticuli; S. thioluteus	248–249; 271, 367, and 430 nm	16,156
2-hydroxy-1-phenazine carboxylic acid [4015-25-6]	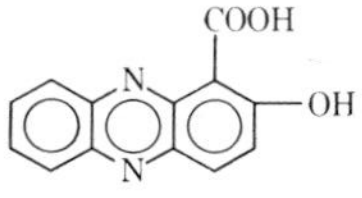 $C_{13}H_8N_2O_3$	Ps. aureofaciens; unidentified gram-negative bacterium, strain V 15295	252 and 363 nm	8,23,37,112
6-hydroxy-1-phenazine carboxylic acid [29453-77-8]	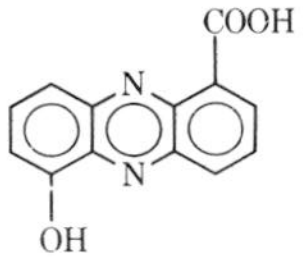 $C_{13}H_8N_2O_3$	Ps. phenazinium	272, 368, and 378 nm	10,96
9-hydroxy-1-phenazine-carboxylic acid [23462-26-2]	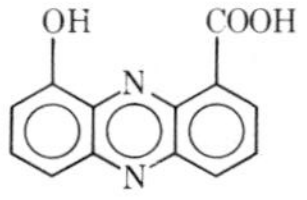 $C_{13}H_8N_2O_3$	an unidentified bacterium, gram-negative rod, strain V 15295	>270; 268 and 370 nm	23,96

Compound [CAS]	Structure	Source	Physical data	Ref.
1-methoxy-phenazine [2876-17-7]	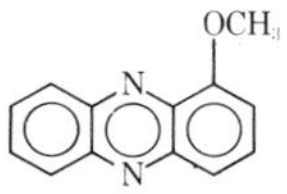 $C_{13}H_{10}N_2O$	Streptomyces luteoreticuli	170–171	156
6-methoxy-1-phenazine carboxylic acid, methyl ester [39011-76-2]	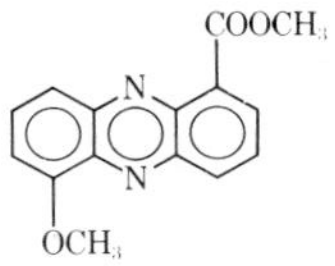 $C_{15}H_{12}N_2O_3$	S. luteoreticuli	150–151; yellow	157
1-phenazine-carboxylic acid, methyl ester [3225-19-2]	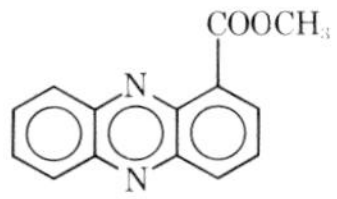 $C_{14}H_{10}N_2O_2$	S. luteoreticuli	126–127; 248 and 364 nm	156
phenazine-1,6-dicarboxylic acid [23462-25-1]	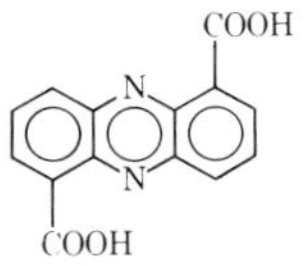 $C_{14}H_8N_2O_4$	an unidentified bacterium, gram-negative rod, strain V 15295	>300; 250 and 370 nm	23
1,8-phenazinediol [18258-40-7]	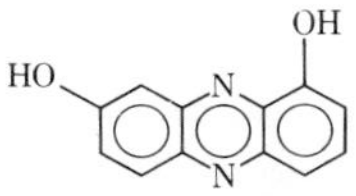 $C_{12}H_8N_2O_2$	Ps. phenazinium; unidentified gram-negative bacterium	230; yellow brown; 269, 385, 432 (K$^+$) nm	23,96
1,8-phenazinediol 10-oxide [23448-76-2]	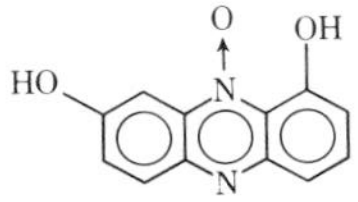 $C_{12}H_8N_2O_3$	Ps. phenazinium; unidentified gram-negative bacterium	235–240 dec; dark red; 283, 403, and 470 (H$^+$) nm	23,96
2-phenazinol [4190-95-8]	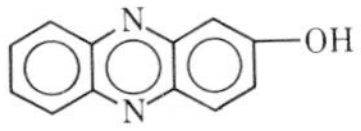 $C_{12}H_8N_2O$	Ps. aureofaciens	>200 dec; orange; 217, 263, and 388 nm	7,81,112

Table 2 (*continued*)

Compound; CAS Registry No.	Structure; Molecular formula	Microbial sources	mp, °C; Color; λ max	References
1-phenazinol 10-oxide [*14994-67-3*]	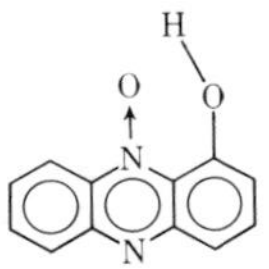 $C_{12}H_8N_2O_2$	*Actinomadura dassonvillei*	165–167; orange; 279, 387, and 468 nm	21–22
1,2,6-tri-methoxy-phenazine [*39039-75-3*]	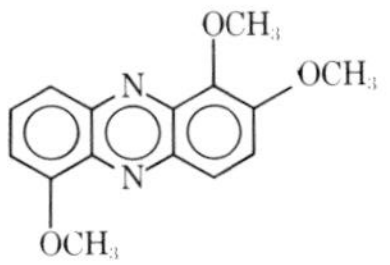 $C_{15}H_{14}N_2O_3$	*S. luteoreticuli*	187–188; orange; 250 and 370 nm	157

Despite its antimicrobial activities, iodinin has not found any direct use as an antibiotic. However, as mentioned earlier, fermentation-produced iodinin is being used as an intermediate for chemical conversion to myxin and copper myxin.

Other Phenazines

In addition to the three compounds already discussed—myxin, lomofungin, and iodinin—there exists another group of phenazine antibiotics that includes griseolutein A and B, griseoluteic acid, hemipyocyanin, pyocyanin, tubermycins A and B, oxychlororaphin and chlororaphin, and aeruginosins A and B. These substances received a great deal of study in the past, and their properties are summarized in Tables 1 and 2. The tables also include additional phenazine intermediates that did not receive trivial names, but were isolated from microorganisms.

BIBLIOGRAPHY

1. Fordos, *Compt. Rend.* **51,** 215 (1860); **56,** 1128 (1863); T. Korzybski and W. Kurylowicz, *Antibiotica,* Gustav Fischer Verlag Jena, Germany, 1961, p. 7; G. A. Swan and D. G. I. Felton, *Phenazines,* Interscience Publishers, a division of John Wiley & Sons, Inc., New York, 1957, p. 190.
2. M. Guignard and N. Sauvageau, *C. R. Soc. Biol.* **46,** 841 (1894).
3. G. R. Clemo and H. McIlwain, *J. Chem. Soc.* 479 (1938).
4. N. N. Gerber and M. P. Lechevalier, *Biochemistry* **4,** 176 (1965).
5. R. B. Herbert and F. G. Holliman, *Proc. Chem. Soc.* 19 (1964).
6. F. G. Holliman, *Chem. Ind.* 1668 (1957).
7. M. E. Levitch and P. Rietz, *Biochemistry* **5,** 689 (1966).
8. J. I. Toohey, C. D. Nelson, and G. Krotkov, *Can. J. Bot.* **43,** 1055 (1965).
9. F. Wrede and E. Strack, *Z. Physiol. Chem.* **140,** 1 (1924); **177,** 177 (1928); *Ber. Dtsch. Chem. Ges.* **62,** 2051 (1929); Ref. 1, pp. 7–11.
10. R. B. Herbert, F. G. Holliman, and P. N. Ibberson, *J. Chem. Soc. Chem. Commun.* 355 (1972).
11. T. Irie, E. Kurosawa, and I. Nagaoka, *Bull. Chem. Soc. Jpn.* **33,** 1057 (1960).
12. M. Podojil and N. N. Gerber, *Biochemistry* **6,** 2701 (1967).
13. O. E. Edwards and D. C. Gillespie, *Tetrahedron Lett.* **40,** 4867 (1966).
14. H. Akabori and M. Nakamura, *J. Antibiot.* **12,** 17 (1959).
15. N. N. Gerber and M. P. Lechevalier, *Biochemistry* **3,** 598 (1964).
16. N. N. Gerber, *J. Org. Chem.* **32,** 4055 (1967).
17. Jpn. Kokai 76 32,790 (Mar. 13, 1976), T. Hasegawa and co-workers (to Takeda Chemical Industries, Ltd).
18. K. Yagishita, *J. Antibiot. Ser. A* **13,** 83 (1960).
19. H. Prauser and K. Eckardt, *Z. Allg. Mikrobiol.* **7,** 409 (1967).
20. H. A. Lechevalier in Z. Vanek and Z. Hosvalek, eds., *Biogenesis of Antibiotic Substances,* Vol. 16, Academic Press, Inc., London, 1965, pp. 227–232.
21. N. N. Gerber, *Biochemistry* **5,** 3824 (1966).
22. N. N. Gerber in A. I. Laskin and H. A. Lechevalier, eds., *Handbook of Microbiology,* Vol. 3, CRC Press Inc., Cleveland, Ohio, 1973, pp. 329–332.
23. N. N. Gerber, *J. Heterocycl. Chem.* **6,** 297 (1969).
24. P. C. Chang and A. C. Blackwood, *Can. J. Biochem.* **46,** 925 (1968).
25. U. Hollstein and L. G. Marshall, *J. Org. Chem.* **37,** 3510 (1972).
26. G. A. Swan and D. G. I. Felton, *Phenazines,* Interscience Publishers, a division of John Wiley & Sons, Inc., New York, 1957.
27. J. C. MacDonald in D. Gottlieb and P. D. Shaw, eds., *Antibiotics,* Vol. 2, Springer Verlag Berlin, Germany, 1967, pp. 52–65.
28. J. M. Ingram and A. C. Blackwood, *Adv. Appl. Microbiol.* **13,** 267 (1970).

29. U.S. Pat. 3,502,774 (Mar. 24, 1970), E. Grunberg (to Hoffmann-La Roche Inc.).

30. U.S. Pat. 3,502,773 (Mar. 24, 1970), E. Grunberg (to Hoffmann-La Roche Inc.).

31. U.S. Pat. 3,495,006 (Feb. 10, 1970), G. R. Wendt and K. W. Ledig (to American Home Products Corporation).

32. U.S. Pat. 3,367,765 (Feb. 6, 1968), C. D. Nelson and J. I. Toohey (to Queen's University, Kingston, Ontario, Canada).

33. Belg. Pat. 669,039 (Jan. 3, 1966), (to Shell Int. Res. M1J).

34. M. T. Huang, A. P. Grollman, and S. B. Horwitz, *Paper 150 presented at the 13th Interscience Conference on Antimicrobial Agents and Chemotherapy, Washington, D.C., Sept. 19–21, 1973.*

35. U.S. Pat. 3,359,165 (Dec. 19, 1967), M. E. Bergy and L. E. Johnson (to The Upjohn Company).

36. M. E. Flood, R. B. Herbert, and F. G. Holliman, *Chem. Commun.,* 1514 (1970).

37. E. A. Kiprianova and co-workers, *Mikrobiol. Zh. (Kiev)* **33**(1), 12 (1971).

38. F. G. Holliman, *J. Chem. Soc.* 2514 (1969).

39. G. S. Hansford, F. G. Holliman, and R. B. Herbert, *J. Chem. Soc. Perkin Trans. 1,* 103 (1972).

40. F. G. Holliman, *S. Afr. Ind. Chem.* **15,** 233 (1961).

41. A. M. LaCoste, S. Labeyrie, and E. Neuzil, *Bull. Soc. Pharm. Bordeaux* **110,** 177 (1971); *Chem. Abstr.* **77,** 31309b; K. P. Mil'chenko, E. A. Kiprianova, and O. I. Boiko, *Mikrobiol. Zh. (Kiev)* **38,** 24 (1976) (in Ukrainian); *Chem. Abstr.* **84,** 130344k (1976).

42. L. Birkofer, *Chem. Ber.* **80,** 212 (1947); **85,** 1023 (1952).

43. F. Sierra and H. A. Veringa, *Nature (London)* **182,** 265 (1958).

44. R. E. Carter and J. H. Richards, *J. Am. Chem. Soc.* **83,** 495 (1961).

45. H. McIlwain, *Nature (London)* **148,** 628 (1941).

46. M. Guignard and N. Sauvageau, *C. R. Soc. Biol.* **46,** 841 (1894); T. Korzybski and W. Kurylowicz, *Antibiotica,* Gustav Fischer Verlag Jena, Germany, 1961, p. 11.

47. S. Nakamura, K. Yagishita, and H. Umezawa, *J. Antibiot. Ser. A.* **14,** 108 (1961).

48. S. R. Challand, R. B. Herbert, and F. G. Holliman, *Chem. Commun.* 1423 (1970).

49. S. Nakamura and co-workers, *J. Antibiot.* **12,** 55 (1959).

50. Y. Ogata, *Jpn. J. Med. Sci. Biol.* **6,** 493 (1953).

51. F. Tausig, F. J. Wolf, and A. K. Miller, *Antimicrob. Agents Chemother.,* 59 (1964).

52. T. Osato, K. Maeda, and H. Umezawa, *J. Antibiot.* **7,** 15 (1954).

53. H. Umezawa and co-workers, *Jpn. Med. J.* **3,** 111 (1950).

54. Y. Ogata, *Jpn. Med. J.* **3,** 213 (1950).

55. S. Nakamura, K. Maeda, and H. Umezawa, *J. Antibiot.* **17,** 33 (1964).

56. S. Nakamura, *Chem. Pharm. Bull.* **6,** 547 (1958).

57. Y. Ogata and co-workers, *J. Antibiot.* **6,** 139 (1953).

58. Y. Ikura, O. Tajima, and T. Fukimbara, *Hakko Kogaku Zasshi* **51,** 840 (1973).

59. R. Schoental, *Br. J. Exp. Pathol.* **22,** 137 (1941); J. L. Stokes, R. L. Peck, and C. R. Woodward, *Proc. Soc. Exp. Biol. Med.* **51,** 126 (1942).

60. G. T. Bottger and A. P. Yerington, *U.S. Dept. Agric. Bur. Entomol. Plant Quarantine,* E-744 (1948).

61. U.S. Pat. 3,663,373 (May 6, 1972), J. Berger, R. H. Epps, E. M. Jenkins, and B. Tabenkin (to Hoffmann-La Roche Inc.).

62. H. McIlwain, *Biochem. J.* **37,** 265 (1943).

63. M. Oda, Y. Sekizawa, and T. Watanabe, *Appl. Microbiol.* **14,** 365 (1966).

64. T. Suzuki, K. Uno, and T. Deguchi, *Agric. Biol. Chem.* **35,** 92 (1971).

65. Jpn. Kokai 72 04,998 (Feb. 12, 1972), K. Tanaka, T. Suzuki, I. Matsubara, and T. Ide (to Kyowa Fermentation Industry Co., Ltd.).

66. I. Tanabe, *Mem. Fac. Agric. Kagoshima Univ.* **8,** 367 (1971); *Chem. Abstr.* **76,** 83442 (1972); I. Tanabe and A. Obayashi, *Mem. Fac. Agric. Kagoshima Univ.* **8,** 373 (1971); *Chem. Abstr.* **76,** 83318c (1972).

67. S. Mann, *Arch. Mikrobiol.* **71,** 304 (1970).

68. M. E. Bergy, *J. Antibiot.* **22,** 126 (1969).

69. L. E. Johnson and A. Dietz, *Appl. Microb.* **17,** 755 (1969).

70. C. D. Tipton and K. L. Rinehart, Jr., *J. Amer. Chem. Soc.* **92,** 1425 (1970).

71. C. D. Tipton, *University Microfilms,* Ann Arbor, Mich., 1971, Order No. 72-7089, 202 pp.

72. C. E. Lewis and L. E. Johnson, The Upjohn Company, private communication.

73. S. M. Lesley and R. M. Behki, *J. Gen. Physiol.* **71,** 195 (1972).

74. I. L. Stevenson, *Can. J. Microbiol.* **15,** 707 (1969).

75. I. L. Stevenson, *Can. J. Microbiol.* **16,** 1249 (1970).

76. M. Weigele and W. Leimgruber, *Tetrahedron Lett.* **8,** 715 (1967).
77. H. P. Sigg and H. Toth, *Helv. Chim. Acta* **50,** 716 (1967).
78. E. Grunberg and co-workers, *Chemotherapia* **12,** 272 (1967).
79. W. Leimgruber and E. Grunberg, *Proceedings of the International Symposium on Drug Research, Montreal, Canada, June 12–14, 1967,* pp. 240–241.
80. E. A. Peterson, *Can. J. Microbiol.* **15,** 133 (1969).
81. F. E. Pansy, W. P. Jambor, and H. H. Gadebusch, *Appl. Microbiol.* **16,** 817 (1968).
82. M. Weigele and co-workers, *10th Interscience Conference on Antimicrobial Agents and Chemotherapy, Washington, D.C., Oct. 18–21, 1970,* pp. 46–49.
83. O. E. Edwards and D. C. Gillespie in Ref. 79, pp. 236–239.
84. U.S. Pat. 3,432,505 (Mar. 11, 1969), W. Rosenbrook, Jr., and A. C. Sinclair (to Abbott Laboratories).
85. R. Kimbrough and T. B. Gaines, *Nature (London)* **211,** 146 (1966).
86. J. A. Zapp, Jr., *Science* **190,** 422 (1975).
87. U.S. Pat. 3,530,130 (Sept. 22, 1970), W. Leimgruber and M. Weigele (to Hoffmann-La Roche Inc.).
88. U.S. Pat. 3,822,265 (July 2, 1974), W. Leimgruber and M. Weigele (to Hoffmann-La Roche Inc.).
89. U.S. Pat. 3,829,423 (Aug. 13, 1974), W. Leimgruber and M. Weigele (to Hoffmann-La Roche Inc.).
90. U.S. Pat. 3,700,679 (Oct. 24, 1972), W. Leimgruber and M. Weigele (to Hoffmann-La Roche Inc.).
91. U.S. Pat. 3,678,051 (July 18, 1972), W. Leimgruber and M. Weigele (to Hoffmann-La Roche Inc.).
92. P. C. Chang and A. C. Blackwood, *Can. J. Microbiol.* **15,** 439 (1969).
93. F. Kögl and B. Tonnis, *Ann. Chem.* **497,** 265 (1932).
94. I. Yoshioka and Y. Kidani, *J. Pharm. Soc. Jpn.* **72,** 847 (1952).
95. Jpn. Pat. 6348 (June 28, 1962), M. Nakamura and G. Akabori (to Sankyo Seiyaku Co.).
96. G. S. Byng and J. M. Turner, *Biochem. Soc. Trans.* **3,** 742 (1975).
97. S. C. Bell and J. M. Turner, *Biochem. Soc. Trans.* **1,** 751 (1973).
98. K. Isono, K. Anzai, and S. Suzuki, *J. Antibiot. Ser. A* **11,** 264 (1958).
99. M. E. Levitch and E. R. Stadtman, *Arch. Biochem. Biophys.* **106,** 194 (1964).
100. T. Higashihara and A. Sato, *Agric. Biol. Chem.* **33,** 1802 (1969); Jpn. Kokai 72 07,957 (Mar. 7, 1972), T. Higashihara and A. Sato (to Japanese Bureau of Industrial Technology); *Chem. Abstr.* **77,** 32703n (1972).
101. J. C. Hill and G. T. Johnson, *Mycologia* **41,** 452 (1969).
102. J. I. Toohey, C. D. Nelson, and G. Krotkov, *Can. J. Bot.* **43,** 1151 (1965).
103. E. A. Kiprianova and A. S. Rabinovich, *Mikrobiologiya* **38,** 224 (1969) (in Russian); *Chem. Abstr.* **71,** 19689u (1969).
104. T. Higashihara and A. Sato, *Hakko Kogaku Zasshi* **48,** 73 (1970).
105. Jpn. Kokai 73 40,994 (June 15, 1973), T. Higashihara (to Agency of Industrial Sciences and Technology); Jpn. Kokai 73 35,089 (Sept. 8, 1973), T. Higashihara (to Agency of Industrial Sciences and Technology).
106. G. Nakamura, *J. Antibiot.* **14,** 86 (1961).
107. F. G. Holliman, M. E. Flood, and R. B. Herbert, *J. Chem. Soc. D* **22,** 1514 (1970).
108. R. C. Millican, *Biochem. Biophys. Acta* **57,** 407 (1962).
109. R. P. Longley and co-workers, *Can. J. Microbiol.* **18,** 1357 (1972); M. Kurachi, *Bull. Inst. Chem. Res. Kyoto Univ.* **37,** 48, 85, 101 (1959).
110. D. H. Calhoun, M. Carson, and R. A. Jensen, *J. Gen. Microbiol.* **72,** 581 (1972).
111. Ref. 36, pp. 1514–1515.
112. M. E. Flood, R. B. Herbert, and F. G. Holliman, *J. Chem. Soc. Perkin Trans. 1,* 622 (1972).
113. U. Hollstein, R. A. Burton, and J. A. White, *Experientia* **4,** 210 (1966).
114. W. M. Ingledew and J. J. R. Campbell, *Can. J. Microb.* **15,** 535 (1969).
115. R. B. Herbert, F. G. Holliman, and J. B. Sheridan, *Tetrahedron Lett.* **48,** 4201 (1974).
116. U. Hollstein and D. A. McCamey, *J. Org. Chem.* **38,** 3415 (1973).
117. G. S. Byng and J. M. Turner, *J. Gen. Microbiol.* **97,** 57 (1976).
118. N. N. Gerber and M. Podojil, *Biochemistry* **9,** 4616 (1970).
119. R. B. Herbert, F. G. Holliman, and P. N. Ibberson, *Tetrahedron Lett.* **2,** 151 (1974).
120. R. Takeda and I. Nakanishi, *Hakko Kogaku Zasshi* **38,** 9 (1959).
121. R. B. Herbert and co-workers, *Tetrahedron Lett.* **8,** 639 (1976).
122. U. Hollstein and co-workers, *Tetrahedron Lett.* **37,** 3267 (1976).
123. M. E. Levitch, *J. Bacteriol.* **103,** 16 (1970).
124. U. Hollstein and R. J. Van Gemert, Jr., *Biochemistry* **10,** 497 (1971).

125. E. A. Peterson, D. C. Gillespie, and F. D. Cook, *Can. J. Microbiol.* **12,** 221 (1966).
126. Can. Pat. 784,213 (Apr. 30, 1968), F. D. Cook, E. A. Peterson, and D. C. Gillespie (to Atomic Energy of Canada, Limited).
127. U.S. Pat. 3,609,153 (Sept. 28, 1971), F. D. Cook, O. E. Edwards, D. C. Gillespie, and E. R. Peterson (to Canadian Patents and Development, Limited).
128. A. I. Rachlin, *Chem. Eng. News* **45,** 32 (1967).
129. A. W. Hanson, *Acta Cryst. Sect. B* **24,** 1084 (1968).
130. U.S. Pat. 3,681,331 (Aug. 1, 1972), W. Leimgruber and M. Weigele (to Hoffmann-La Roche Inc.).
131. U.S. Pat. 3,937,707 (Feb 10, 1976), W. Leimgruber and M. Weigele (to Hoffmann-La Roche Inc.).
132. U.S. Pat. 3,586,674 (June 22, 1971), W. Leimgruber, G. P. Maestrone, M. Mitrovic, and M. Weigele (to Hoffmann-La Roche Inc.).
133. U.S. Pat. 3,852,442 (Dec. 3, 1974), W. Leimgruber, G. P. Maestrone, M. Mitrovic, and M. Weigele (to Hoffmann-La Roche Inc.).
134. G. Maestrone and co-workers, *Am. J. Vet. Res.* **33,** 185 (1972).
135. U.S. Pat. 3,989,830 (Nov. 2, 1976), M. H. Infeld and H. L. Newmark (to Hoffmann-La Roche Inc.).
136. U.S. Pat. 3,966,734 (June 29, 1976), J. D. Surmatis (to Hoffmann-La Roche Inc.).
137. H. Baker and C. Vézina in Ref. 79, pp. 242–243.
138. U.S. Pat. 3,760,075 (Sept. 18, 1973), J. A. Ranucci (to Hoffmann-La Roche Inc.).
139. G. Maestrone and M. Mitrovic, *12th Interscience Conference on Antimicrobial Agents and Chemotherapy, Sept. 29, 1972, Washington, D.C.,* p. 111 of abstracts.
140. W. E. Snyder and R. K. Imhoff, *Vet. Med. Small Anim. Clin.* **70,** 1421 (1975).
141. W. E. Snyder and G. Maestrone, *Vet. Med. Small Anim. Clin.* **71,** 585 (1976).
142. S. M. Lesley, R. M. Behki, and D. C. Gillespie, *Can. J. Microbiol.* **13,** 1251 (1967).
143. S. M. Lesley and R. M. Behki, *J. Bacteriol.* **94,** 1837 (1967).
144. S. M. Lesley and R. M. Behki, *Can. J. Microbiol.* **17,** 1327 (1971).
145. P. E. Hartman, H. Berger, and Z. Hartman, *J. Pharmacol. Exp. Ther.* **186,** 390 (1973).
146. U.S. Pat. 3,929,790 (Dec. 30, 1975), W. Leimgruber and M. Weigele (to Hoffmann-La Roche Inc.).
147. R. S. S. Fraser and J. Creanor, *Biochem. J.* **147,** 401 (1975).
148. R. S. S. Fraser, J. Creanor, and J. M. Mitchison, *Nature (London)* **244,** 222 (1973).
149. F. R. Cano, S.-C. Kuo, and J. O. Lampen, *Antimicrob. Agents Chemother.* **3,** 723 (1973).
150. M. Cannon and A. Jimenez, *Biochem. J.* **142,** 457 (1974).
151. D. Gottlieb and G. Nicolas, *Appl. Microb.* **18,** 35 (1969).
152. M. Cannon, J. E. Davies, and A. Jimenez, *FEBS Lett.* **32,** 277 (1973).
153. S.-C. Kuo, F. R. Cano, and J. O. Lampen, *Antimicrob. Agents Chemother.* **3,** 716 (1973).
154. A. Ruet and co-workers, *Biochemistry* **14,** 4651 (1975).
155. U.S. Pat. 3,764,679 (Oct. 9, 1973), P. H. Jones and P. Somani (to Abbott Laboratories).
156. S. Yamagishi and co-workers, *Yakugaku Zasshi* **91,** 351 (1971).
157. S. Yamanaka, *Chiba Igakkai Zasshi* **48,** 63 (1972); *Chem. Abstr.* **77,** 162986t (1972).

General References

Biological activities of synthetic phenazines

H. B. Anstall, B. List-Young, J. M. Trujillo, and W. O. Russell, *Biochem. Pharmacol.* **15,** 998 (1966).
H. B. Anstall, D. M. Peterson, J. M. Trujillo, and M. L. Samuels, *Cancer Chemother. Rep.* **43,** 43 (1964).
L. R. Duvall, *Cancer Chemother. Rep.* **23,** 63 (1962).
Belg. Pat. 678,404 (Sept. 26, 1966), (to Rhone-Poulenc, France).
M. G. Kelly, N. H. Smith, and J. Leiter, *J. Nat. Cancer Inst.* **20,** 1113 (1958).
K. Katagiri and co-workers, *Ann. Rep. Shionogi Res. Lab.* **17,** 127 (1967).
K. Katagiri and co-workers, *Ann. Rep. Shionogi Res. Lab.* **17,** 133 (1967).
K. Katagiri and co-workers, *Ann. Rep. Shionogi Res. Lab.* **17,** 137 (1967).
K. Katagiri and co-workers, *Ann. Rep. Shionogi Res. Lab.* **16,** 58 (1966).
K. Katagiri and co-workers, *Ann. Rep. Shionogi Res. Lab.* **16,** 52 (1966).
K. Katagiri and co-workers, *Ann. Rep. Shionogi Res. Lab.* **15,** 84 (1965).
Belg. Pat. 669,039 (Jan. 3, 1966), (to Shell Int. Res. M1J).
U.S. Pat. 3,495,006 (Feb. 10, 1970), G. R. Wendt and K. W. Ledig (to American Home Products Corporation).

Copper complex of myxin

U.S. Pat. 3,966,734 (June 29, 1976), J. D. Surmatis (to Hoffmann-La Roche Inc.).

JULIUS BERGER
Hoffmann-La Roche Inc.

POLYENES

The observation in 1950 that *Streptomyces noursei* produced a novel antifungal agent (1) led to the discovery of nystatin, the first of the polyene macrolide antifungal antibiotics. Polyenes named in the text not given in earlier tables are listed on p. 39. Most of the polyenes isolated to date (1977) have been produced from soil actinomycetes, mainly of the genus *Streptomyces*. As a class they are characterized by excellent activity against a variety of dermatophytes and fungi but little or no antibacterial activity; many possess good antiprotozoal activity. The polyenes have a large lactone ring bearing a number of hydroxy substituents and a conjugated polyene chromophore from 3–7 double bonds. The highly characteristic uv spectrum of the polyene chromophore has proved to be the single most widely used physical property for recognizing and classifying these structurally complex natural products. There are a number of excellent reviews covering the isolation and production (2–5), the chemistry (6–11), the biological activity and mode of action (12–23), the therapeutic use (24–25), and the analysis (26) of polyene antifungal antibiotics (see also Fungicides).

Production and Isolation

The majority of polyene macrolides with a few exceptions (27–29) are produced by a variety of *Streptomyces* species of soil microorganisms. They are invariably formed as a complex mixture of both polyenic and nonpolyenic products by submerged aerobic fermentation of suitable cultures at 20–40°C in an aqueous nutrient medium. The fermentations are generally allowed to proceed for 3–4 d. The inorganic salt composition of the medium can affect polyene production (30–31). The bulk of the polyene is contained in the mycelium which is usually separated from the whole broth and extracted with suitable polar solvents such as water-saturated n-butanol (29). After suitable manipulation, a crude polyene complex is obtained as a yellow-orange solid which is insoluble in all but very polar solvents such as aqueous alcohols, dimethylformamide, and dimethyl sulfoxide. The various components of the complex are usually separated by counter-current distribution (32–33), column chromatography (34), or high-pressure liquid chromatography (35). A variety of paper and thin layer chromatographic systems have been developed for determining the identity and checking the homogeneity of the polyenes (26,36). Owing to their lack of solubility, their instability, and their poor chromatographic characteristics, it is often difficult to assess the purity and identity of many polyene samples and consequently some confusion is inevitable in the literature.

The polyenes are classified according to the number of double bonds present in the principal chromophore either as trienes, tetraenes, pentaenes, hexaenes, or heptaenes.

Trienes

Although several trienes have been reported in the literature very little is known at the present time about their chemical structures and some may have to be reclassified in the future. Members of this group of polyenes are listed in Table 1.

Tetraenes

The nystatin complex produced by *Streptomyces noursei* (1) consists of three parts: a major component, nystatin A_1 (1), and two minor components, nystatin A_2

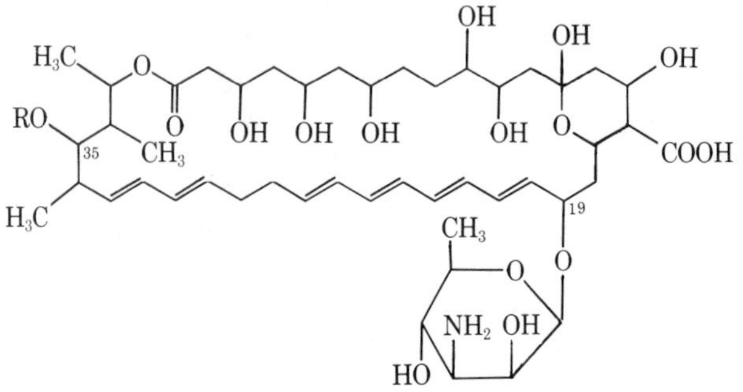

(1)   R = H   nystatin A_1

(2)   R = 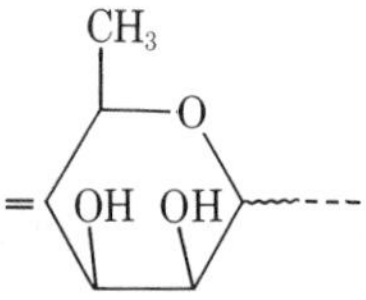   nystatin A_3

Table 1.   Trienes

Compound	Source	General chemical features	References
MM 8	*Streptomyces* sp. ACC 1293	CHNO; mol wt 726; uv; ir; nmr; no carbohydrate	37
mycotrienin [62851-53-0]	*Streptomyces* sp.	CHNO; uv; no carbohydrate	38
trienin [62362-55-4]	*Streptomyces* sp. SC 3725	CHNO; mol wt 1400; uv, ir	39
resistaphylin [12708-08-6]	*Streptomyces antibioticus* No. K869	$C_{24}H_{34}N_2O_7$ mol wt 486; uv; ir; nmr; $[\alpha]_D$	40
triene 141-18	*Actinomyces* sp.	CHNO; uv; ir	41
proticin [12689-28-0]	*Bacillus licheniformis* var. *mesentericus.*	$C_{31}H_{45}O_7P$; mol wt 582; uv; ir; nmr; $[\alpha]_D$	27, 42
A triene	*Actinomyces chromogenes* var. *trienicus* var. nov.	CHNO; uv; ir; alanine isolated	43
A triene	*Actinomyces robefuscus* Krassilnikov.	uv; alanine isolated	44
rapamycin [53123-88-9]	*Streptomyces hygroscopicus* NRRL 5491	CHNO; uv; ir; nmr	45

and nystatin A_3 (2) and is the most widely used polyene in clinical use.

The components have been separated by counter-current distribution (46–47). The structures of the carbohydrate moiety D-mycosamine (48–51) and of the aglycone of nystatin A_1 (52–55) were deduced by chemical degradation. Further chemical studies have led to the elucidation of the structure of nystatin A_1 (56–58). The existence of the hemiketal structure (1) in solution has been demonstrated (59–60). The structure of nystatin A_2 has not yet been determined. Nystatin A_3 (2) (61) differs from (1) by virtue of the glycosidic attachment of D-janose (3) at the C-35 hydroxy group.

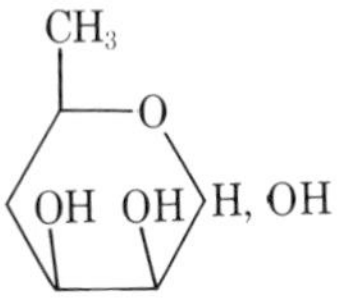

(3)   *D*-janose

Recently (46–47) *Streptomyces noursei* var. *polifungini* ATCC 21581 has been shown to produce nystatin A_1, nystatin A_2, nystatin A_3, and in addition a new tetraene polifungin B whose structure is as yet unknown.

In contrast to the nystatin group, which has a 38-membered macrocyclic lactone, many of the tetraenes have a 26-membered lactone. Pimaricin (natamycin), isolated from *Streptomyces natalensis* (62), has the novel structure (4) (63), necessitating revision of the structures proposed earlier (64–70). Tennecetin, isolated from *Streptomyces chattanoogensis* (71), is thought to be identical with pimaricin (72). The closely related tetraene, lucensomycin, produced by *Streptomyces lucensis* (73), has the structure (5) (74–77) differing only in the nature of the alkyl substituent at C-25. By chemical degradation the absolute stereochemistry of the chiral centers at C-25 in pimaricin (4) and lucensomycin (5) have been shown to have the *R*-configuration (78–79). The biosynthesis of (5) has been studied and the aglycone was shown to be derived from 12 acetate units and 2 propionate units (Fig. 1) (80). In pimaricin the

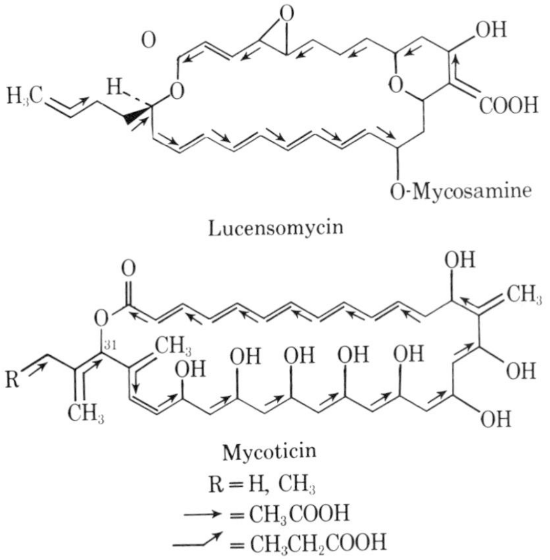

Lucensomycin

Mycoticin

R = H, CH₃

→ = CH₃COOH

↗ = CH₃CH₂COOH

Figure 1. Biosynthetic pathways.

chain development is initiated by an acetyl–coenzyme A unit. Recently, some high mol wt acid degradation products of pimaricin, having the intact lactone ring have been described (81). Spectroscopic studies (59,60,82) have indicated that in solution both (4) and (5) exist as the hemiketal structures.

Tetrin A (6) (58,60,82–84) and tetrin B (7) (58,60,82–83,85) produced by a *Streptomyces* species (86) have many structural features in common with pimaricin (4). The chiral center at C-25 in the tetrins has been shown to have *S* stereochemistry (84–85). Arenomycin B (8) produced by *Actinomyces tumemacerans Krass.*, Kov., 1962, var. *griseoarenicolor* var. nov. (87–88) has many structural features in common with both (5) and (6).

The only remaining tetraene for which a structure has been determined is rimocidin (9), which is produced by *Streptomyces rimosus* (89). Early work (90,91) led to a structure for the aglycone, which was subsequently revised when the complete structure was determined (58,92).

Other tetraene macrolides have been isolated and characterized (Table 2), but little is known about their chemical structures.

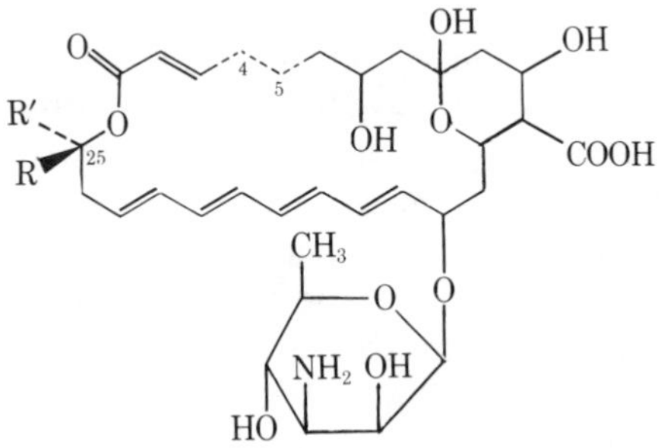

(4) 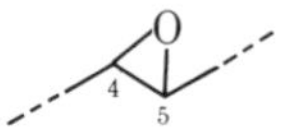   R = CH₃, R′ = H   pimaricin

(5)   R = —(CH₂)₃—CH₃, R′ = H   lucensomycin

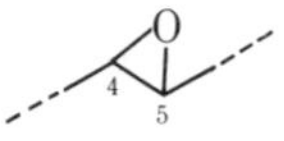

(6)   R = H, R′ = CH₃   tetrin A

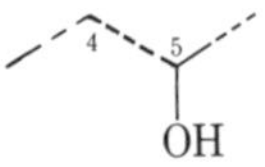

(7)   R = H, R′ = CH₃   tetrin B

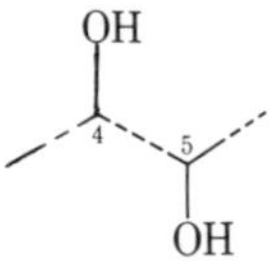

(8)   R or R′ = —(CH₂)₃CH₃, H   arenomycin B

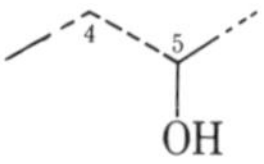

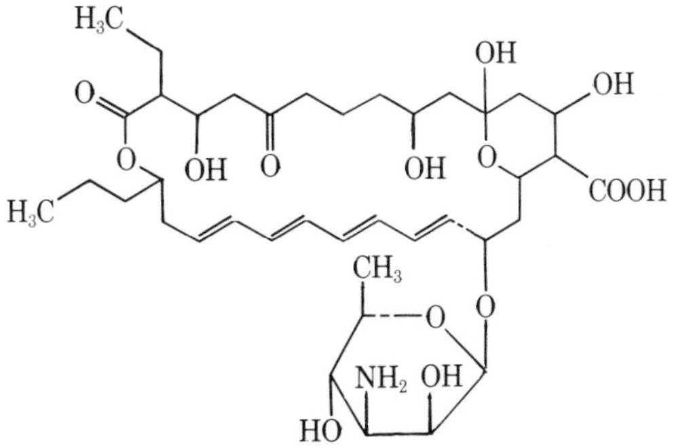

(9)   rimocidin

Pentaenes

The pentaenes may be divided into three subgroups.

Group 1: The first group possess a pentaene chromophore having a terminal methyl substituent and may either be neutral compounds or contain an aminosugar moiety.

Streptomyces filipinensis produces filipin (124), which was initially thought to be a single compound. Chemical (125–128) and mass spectral (129) studies have shown filipin to have structure (10). More recently filipin was demonstrated to be a mixture of 4 components (33) which were separated by column chromatography and designated filipin I, II, III, and IV. The components were characterized by mass spectrometry (130) and the major component, filipin III was found to have the structure (10). The field desorption mass spectrum of (10) has been reported (131). Filipin IV was shown to be isomeric with (10). Filipin II has one less hydroxyl group (probably at C-1' or C-3 (132) and filipin I has two less hydroxyl groups.

Another methyl pentaene whose structure has been elucidated (133) is fungichromin (11), produced by *Streptomyces cellulosae* (134). The absolute stereochemistry at C-26 and C-27 was determined to be S and R, respectively (133). Lagosin, isolated from a different *Streptomyces* species (135), was shown to have the same gross structure (125–126) and the relative stereochemistry of C-26 and C-27 has been shown to be *erythro* (136) as in fungichromin (133). Pentamycin, isolated from *Streptomyces pentaticus* (137) is thought to be identical (138) with lagosin. Moldcidin B produced by *Streptomyces griseofuscus* is considered to be identical to pentamycin (139). Cogomycin, isolated recently from *Streptomyces fradiae* (140) has been shown to have an identical gross structure (11) (140–141). The principal products of autoxidation of filipin and lagosin have been found to be the corresponding diastereomeric 16,17-epoxides (12) and (13), respectively (142).

Chainin (14) a methyl pentaene closely related to filipin III (10), has been isolated from a *Chainia* species (132). It differs from (10) in the nature of the side chain at C-2. All of the above methyl pentaenes have a 28-membered lactone.

Aurenin (15) and homoaurenin (16), methyl pentaenes isolated from *Actinomyces aureorectus* sp. nov. (143), have been assigned rather unusual 26-membered lactone structures (144). Other methyl pentaenes (Group 1) that have been isolated and characterized are listed in Table 3.

Table 2.   Tetraenes

Compound	Source	General chemical features	References
endomycin A (helixin A) [1391-41-9]	Streptomyces endus, Streptomyces hygroscopicus var. enhygrus	CHNO; mol wt 1450; uv; ir; amphoteric	93, 94
antimycoin A (C 381) [642-15-9]	Streptomyces aureus	$C_{28}H_{40}N_2O_9$; uv	95
chromin [1407-01-8]	Streptomyces chromogenes	CHNO; uv; ir	96, 97
PA 86	Streptomyces rimosus	CHNO; uv	98
sistomycosin [1404-63-3]	Streptomyces viridosporus	CHNO; uv; ir; amphoteric	99
amphotericin A [1405-32-9]	Streptomyces nodosus	CHNO; mol wt 915; uv; ir; $[\alpha]_D$	100, 101
A 5283	Streptomyces gilvosporeus A 5283 ATCC 13326	CHNO; uv; ir; $[\alpha]_D$; amphoteric	102
RP 7071	Streptomyces sp.	CHNO; mol wt 859; uv; $[\alpha]_D$	103
protocidin [53597-22-1]	Streptomyces sp. 964A	CHNO; mol wt 615; uv; ir; $[\alpha]_D$; amphoteric	104
J_4 B	Streptomyces sp.	uv	105
PA 166	Streptomyces glaucus ATCC 12730	CHNO; mol wt 708; uv; ir; $[\alpha]_D$; amphoteric	106, 107
akitamycin (toyamycin) [62851-49-4]	Streptomyces akitaensis	CHNO; uv; ir; $[\alpha]_D$	108, 109
unamycin [11006-86-3]	Streptomyces fungicidicus	CHNO; uv; ir, $[\alpha]_D$	110
ornamycin [11006-32-9]	Streptomyces ornatus	uv	111
tetraesin (tetrahexin) [62851-65-4]	Streptomyces sp. 5391	CHNO; uv; amphoteric; also contains a hexaene chromophore	112
Ac₂ 435	Streptomyces sp. Ac₂ 435	CHO; uv; $[\alpha]_D$	113
RP 9971	Streptomyces gascariensis NRRL 2955	CHNO; mol wt 710; uv; $[\alpha]_D$; amphoteric	114
polifungin B [37371-05-4]	Streptomyces noursei var. polifungini	CHNO; uv	46, 47, 115
BH 890 α [37348-98-4] and β [37348-99-5]	Streptomyces sp. NRRL 3609	CHNO; uv; ir; $[\alpha]_D$	116
tetramycin [11076-50-9]	Streptomyces noursei var. jenensis nov. var. JA 3789	$C_{34}H_{53}NO_{14}$; mol wt 715; uv; ir; $[\alpha]_D$; amphoteric	117
tetraenin A [62851-67-6] and B [62851-66-5]	Streptomyces fragmentans HA33 and HA34	uv; amphoteric	118
plumbomycin A [37199-59-0] and B [37199-60-3]	Actinomyces plumbeus sp. nov.	CHNO; uv; ir; $[\alpha]_D$	119
P 42-3	Actinomyces lumemacerans No. P42	uv	120
flavoviridomycin [51668-32-7]	Actinomyces flavoviridis Krass, 1941, var. fungicidicus var. nov.	CHNO; uv; ir; $[\alpha]_D$	121
tetramedin [39300-60-2]	Actinomyces mediocidicus	CHNO; uv, ir	122
abkhazomycin [56092-86-5]	Actinomyces badiocolor var. abhasus var. nov.	CHNO; uv; ir; $[\alpha]_D$	123

Group 2.   The second subgroup of pentaenes is characterized by a conjugated lactone chromophore. The mycoticins produced by *Streptomyces ruber* (171) have been separated into 2 components, mycoticin A (**17**) and mycoticin B (**18**) (172). The

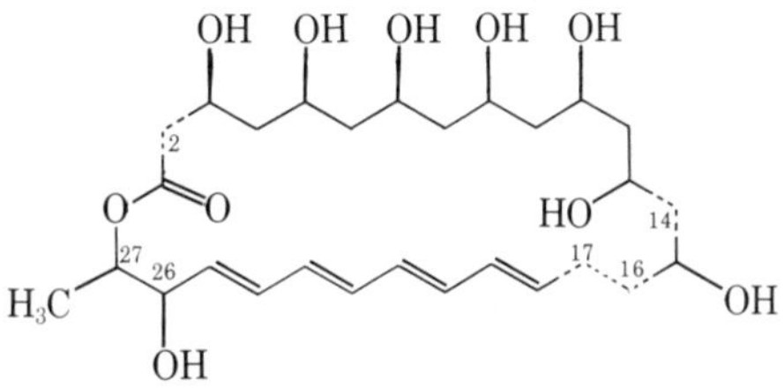

(10) 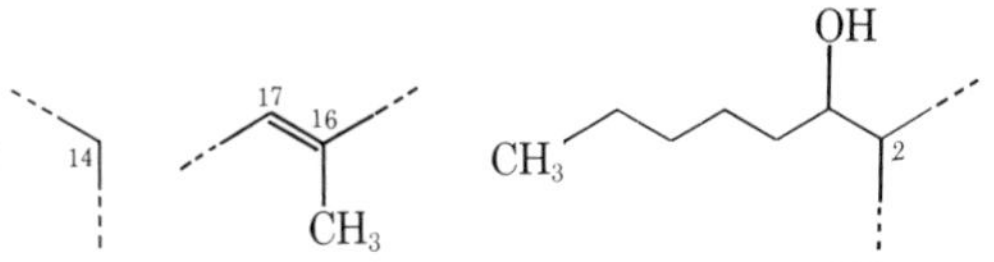 filipin III

(11) 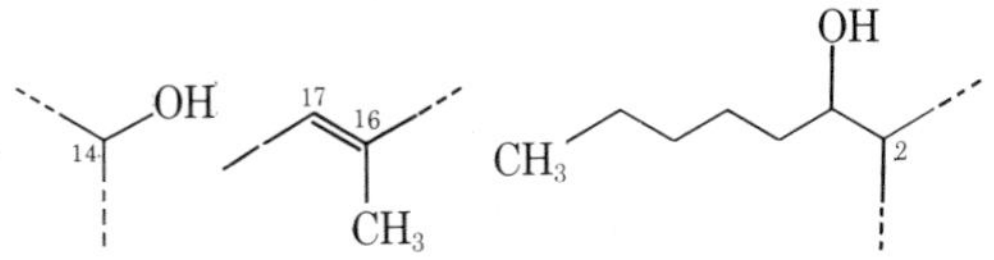 fungichromin

(12) 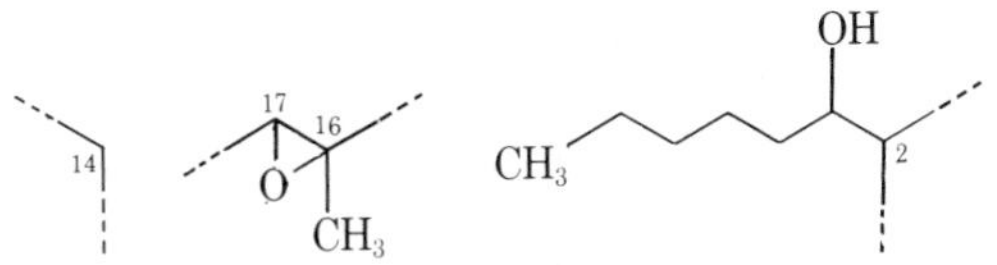 autoxidation product of filipin III

(13) 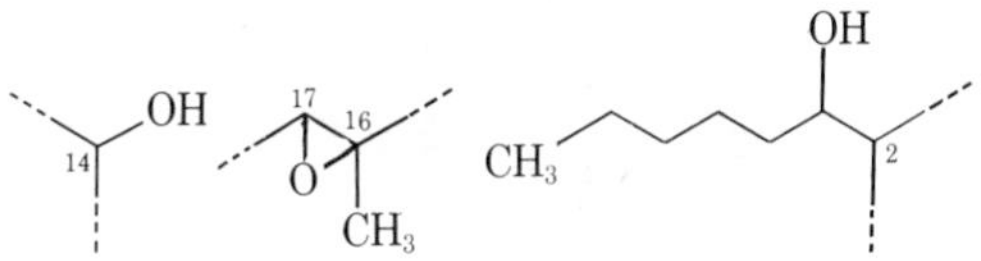 autoxidation product of lagosin

(14) 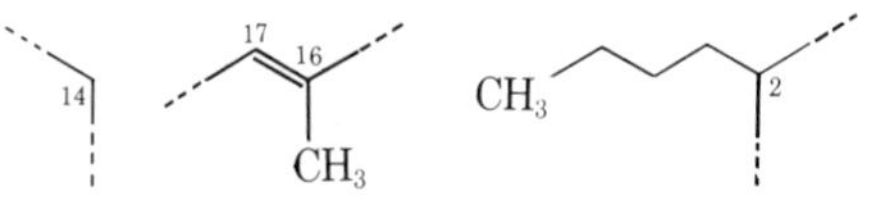 chainin

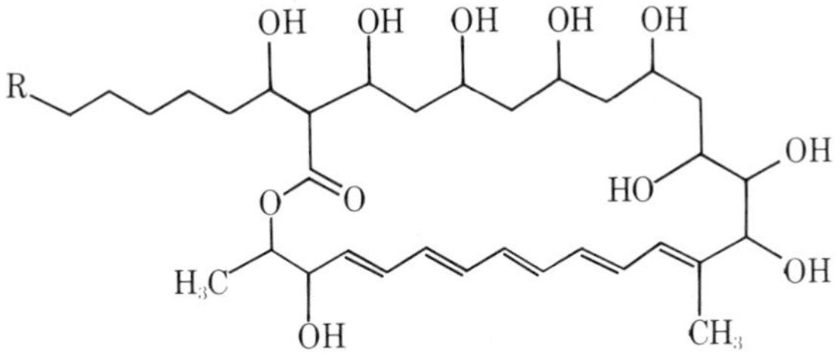

(15) R = |H| aurenin
(16) R = CH₃ homoaurenin

structures of flavofungin A and B, produced by *Streptomyces flavofungini* (173–174), are the same as those of the corresponding mycoticins (175). A partial structure has been proposed for flavomycoin (176) which is produced by *Streptomyces roseflavus* ARA1 1951, var. *jenensis* nov. var. JA 5068 (177) and it has been suggested (175) that it may be identical with the flavofungins and mycoticins, as well as with roseofungin (178). All of the above pentaenes contain a 32-membered macrocyclic lactone. The biosynthetic pathway is summarized in Figure 1 (179).

Table 3. Pentaenes

Compound	Source	General chemical features[a]	References
fungichromatin	Streptomyces sp.	group 1; uv	134
A pentaene	Streptomyces sanguineus	group 1; CHO; uv	145
cabicidin [53123-85-6]	Streptomyces gourgeroti	group 1; $C_{35}H_{60}O_{13}$; mol wt 688; uv; $[\alpha]_D$	146
moldcidin A [62851-55-2]	Streptomyces griseofuscus	group 1; CHNO; mol wt 903; uv; ir; amphoteric	147, 148
onomycin-I [65086-33-1]	Streptomyces sp. J-4	group 1; CHNO; uv; ir; $[\alpha]_D$; amphoteric	149
123	Streptomyces sp.	group 1; CHO; uv	150
neopentaene [62851-44-9]	Streptomyces sp. 2236	group 1; CHO; uv; ir; $[\alpha]_D$	151
xantholycin [52037-72-6]	Streptomyces xantholyticus	group 1; CHO; uv	152
durhamycin [11003-68-2]	Streptomyces durhamensis	group 1; CHO; uv	153
pentacidin [56093-99-3]	Streptomyces hygroscopicus	group 1; $C_{31}H_{50}O_{10}$; mol wt 598; uv; ir; $[\alpha]_D$; ms	154
A pentaene	Actinomyces bruneofungus sp. nov.	group 2; CHO; uv	155
surgumycin [51938-50-2]	Actinomyces surgutus sp. nov.	group 2; CHO; uv; ir; $[\alpha]_D$	156
aliomycin [62851-48-3]	Streptomyces acidomyceticus	group 3; CHNOS; uv	157
A 228a and b	Streptomyces sp.	group 3; CHNOS; uv	158
A petaene	Streptomyces effluvius	group 3; CHNO; uv	159
PA 153	Streptomyces sp.	group 3; CHNO; mol wt 744; uv; ir; $[\alpha]_D$	107
quinquamycin [62851-69-8]	Streptomyces lavendulae E 20–27	group 3; uv	160
capacidin [11002-18-9]	Streptomyces sp. 5913	group 3; CHNO; uv; ir; $[\alpha]_D$; amphoteric	161
2814P	Streptomyces sp. 2814	group 3; CHNO; uv; $[\alpha]_D$; amphoteric	162
58	Streptomyces fasciculus ATCC 12703	group 3; CHNO; uv; ir; $[\alpha]_D$; amphoteric	163
616	Streptomyces parvisporogenes	group 3; CHNO; uv	164
pentafungin [11031-02-0]	Streptomyces antimycoticus	group 3; $C_{41}H_{74}NO_{17}$; uv; $[\alpha]_D$; amphoteric; contains mycosamine	165
gangtokmycin [37220-69-2]	Streptomyces gangtokensis	group 3; CHNO; uv; ir; $[\alpha]_D$	166
HA 106	Streptoverticillium cinnamoneum var. sparsum	group 3; uv	167
HA 135	Streptoverticillium sporiferum	group 3; uv	168
HA 145	Streptoverticillium cinnamoneum var. albosporum	group 3; uv	169
HA 176	Streptoverticillium cinnamoneum var. lanosum	group 3; uv	170
distamycin B [62851-60-9]	Streptomyces distallicus NCIB 8936	$C_{41}H_{66}O_{11}$; uv	168
17–41 B	Actinomyces sp. no. 17–41	uv	169
fumanomycin [50925-98-9]	Actinomyces lavendobrunneus sp. nov.	uv	170

[a] Group 1 = methyl pentaenes; group 2 = conjugated lactones; group 3 = classical pentaenes.

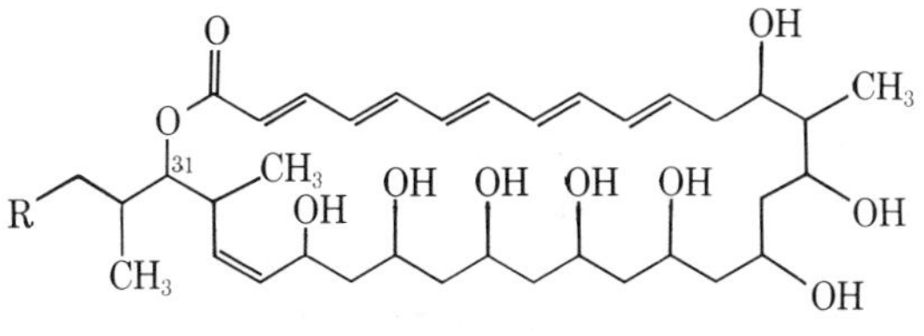

(17)   R = H mycoticin A
(18)   R = CH₃ mycoticin B

Other pentaenes belonging to this subgroup have been isolated (Table 3) but little is known about their chemical structures.

Group 3.   The third subgroup of the pentaenes comprises the classical polyene structure of an unsubstituted, isolated pentaene chromophore. Within this group, partial structures have been proposed for eurocidin A (19) and eurocidin B (20) produced by *Streptomyces albireticuli* (180–181). Both compounds contain (21) but the site of glycosylation has not been determined. The only other member of this subgroup for which a partial structure has been proposed is rectilavendomycin which is produced by *Actinomyces rectilavendulae* var. *pentaenicus* var. nov. (182). The structure (22) has been proposed for the aglycone of rectilavendomycin (183).

A number of pentaenes belonging to this subgroup have been isolated and partially characterized (Table 3), but little is known about their chemical structures. Some of the pentaenes in Table 3 have insufficient data published for reliable classification at present.

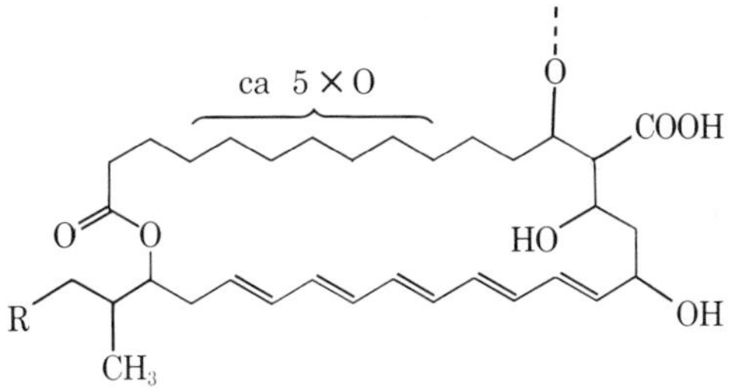

(19)   R = H eurocidin A
(20)   R = CH₃ eurocidin B

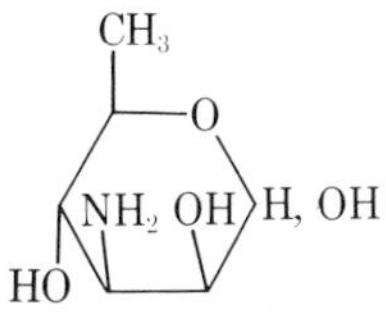

(21)   D-mycosamine

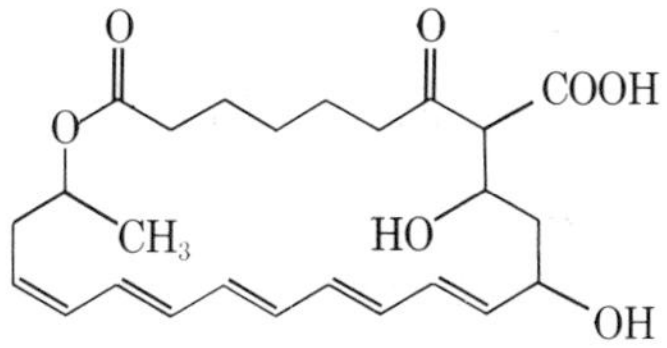

(22)   aglycone of rectilavendomycin

Hexaenes

Very little is known about the chemical structures of this group of polyenes as structures have only been assigned to two hexaenes. *Streptomyces viridogriseus* produces the dermostatins (184,185) and the structures of dermostatin A (**23**) and dermostatin B (**24**) have been determined (186). They possess a novel 36-membered macrocyclic conjugated lactone and their field desorption mass spectra have been reported (131). A number of hexaenes have been isolated and these are described in Table 4.

Heptaenes

The heptaenes have been used in clinical practice to treat systemic fungal infections and may be divided into two groups, namely the nonaromatic and aromatic groups.

Nonaromatic Group. Amphotericin B (**25**) produced by *Streptomyces nodosus* (100–101) is the most widely studied member of the nonaromatic group. Acid hydrolysis of amphotericin B led to the isolation of (**21**) (50,51,198). Chemical studies resulted in a partial structure for amphotericin B (199–205). Subsequently, an x-ray crystallographic study on the *N*-iodoacetyl derivative (206–207) revealed the complete structure of amphotericin B including the absolute stereochemistry. The existence of the hemiketal structure was demonstrated in the crystalline state and also in solution (59–60,206). The x-ray study revealed the β-configuration for the first time for the glycosidic bond between D-mycosamine and the aglycone. Independent chemical studies led to the demonstration of the same gross structure for amphotericin B (208).

The structure of candidin (**26**) produced by *Streptomyces viridoflavus* (209) has

Table 4. **Hexaenes**

Compound	Source	General chemical features	References
fradicin [1403-61-8]	*Streptomyces fradiae*	CHNO; uv; $[\alpha]_D$	187
endomycin B (helixin B) [1391-41-9]	*Streptomyces endus*	uv	93, 188
mycelin [1392-57-0]	*Streptomyces roseoflavus*	CHO; uv	189, 190
flavacid [525-12-2]	*Streptomyces flavus*	$C_{18}H_{22}N_3Cl$; uv	191
mediocidin [1403-95-8]	*Streptomyces mediocidicus*	uv	192, 193
mycelin IMO [62851-52-9]	*Streptomyces diastatochromogenes*	CHNO; mol wt 345; uv; $[\alpha]_D$	194
cryptocidin [62851-62-1]	*Streptomyces* sp.	CHNO; mol wt 983–986; uv; ir	195
hexaenes	*Actinomyces plumbeus* sp. nov.	uv	119
A hexaene	*Actinomyces mediocidicus*	uv	122
candihexin I [54328-23-3] and II [54328-24-4]	*Streptomyces viridoflavus*	CHNO; uv; amphoteric	196, 197

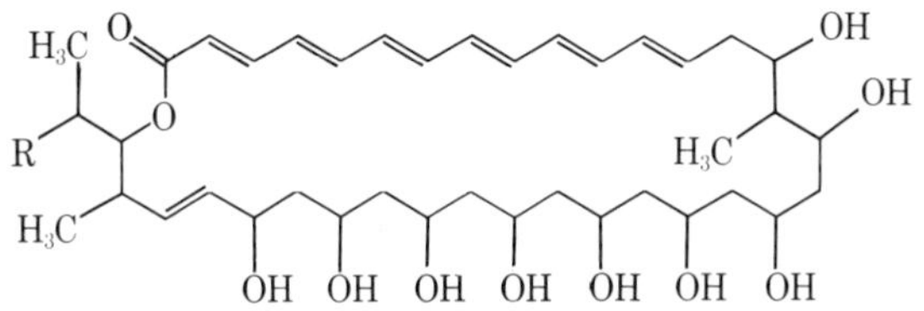

(23)   R = CH₃ dermostatin A
(24)   R = CH₂CH₃ dermostatin B

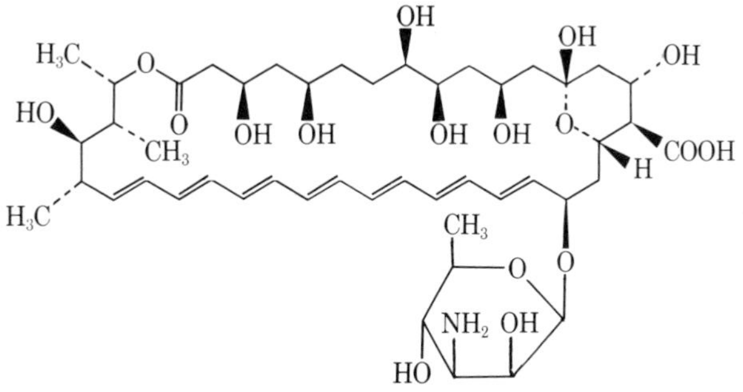

(25)   amphotericin B

been determined (210). Like amphotericin B it also contains a 38-membered lactone and has (21) as the sugar component. However, candidin has a different oxygen sequence with a keto group at C-7 and a vicinal glycol at C-10 and -11. In addition to candidin, the organism also produces two other partially characterized nonaromatic heptaenes named candidinin and candidoin (211,212).

The structure of mycoheptin (27) (213), produced by *Streptomyces netropsis* (214), has been shown to be very similar to that of candidin except that the keto group is at C_5 and the hydroxy group at C_7.

Preliminary chemical studies on aureofungin B, one of four minor components produced by *Streptomyces cinnamomeus* var. *terricola* (215–218), have revealed the partial structure (28) (219), in which the position of one of the keto groups remains to be determined.

Aromatic Group. The heptaenes of the aromatic group give rise on base catalyzed retro-aldol cleavage either to 4-aminoacetophenone or 4-methylaminoacetophenone. In general they are amphoteric and have an aminosugar attached by a glycoside bond to a macrocylic lactone. Several structures have been worked out for this group of heptaenes and partial structures have been proposed for a number of others.

Aureofungin A, the major component produced by *Streptomyces cinnamomeus* var. *terricola* (215–218), has been shown to have the partial structure (29) (219) containing (21) and 4-methylamino-acetophenone. The location of the keto group is uncertain.

The trichomycin complex produced by *Streptomyces hachijoensis* (220) has been separated into a major component trichomycin A, and two minor components, trichomycin B and C, by chromatography on alumina (221). Trichomycin A (33,222–228) contains mycosamine and 4-aminoacetophenone and has been proposed to have a highly unusual partial structure (228) which needs to be reinvestigated.

Streptomyces surinam produces two aromatic heptaenes, DJ-400 B₁ and DJ-400 B₂ (229–230). Both contain mycosamine although its position of attachment to the

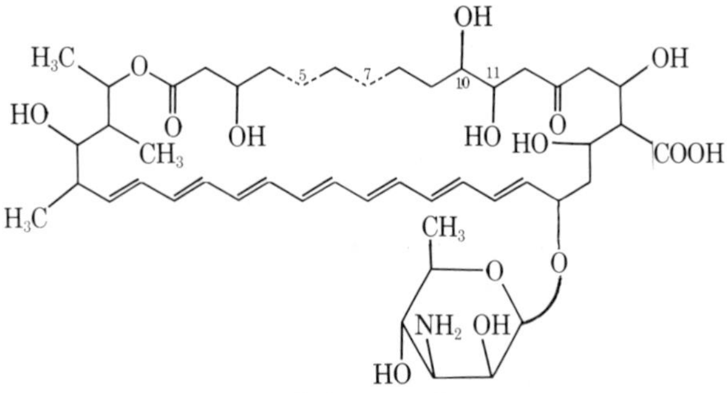

(26) 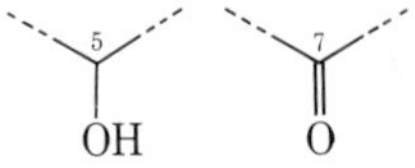 candidin

(27) mycoheptin

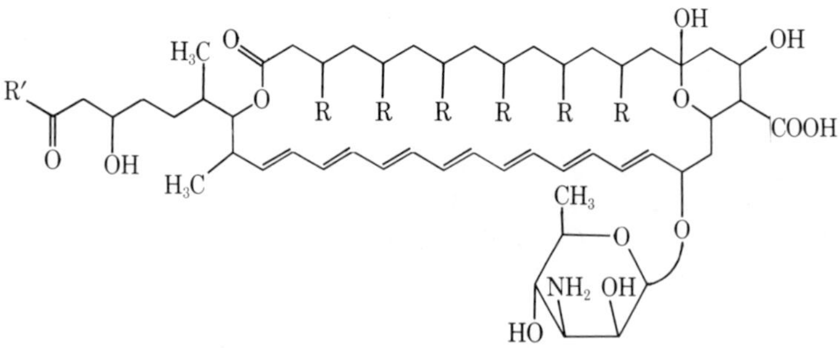

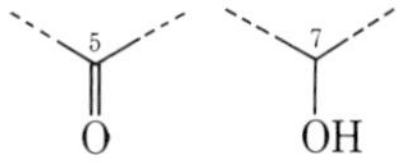

(28) R = 5×—OH 1× =O R′ = H₃C   aureofungin B

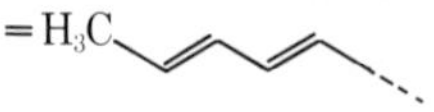

(29) R = 5×—OH 1× =O R′ = 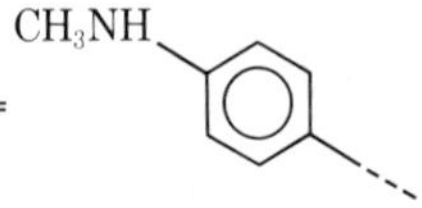   aureofungin A

aglycone is unknown. DJ-400 B$_1$ contains 4-methylaminoacetophenone, and DJ-400 B$_2$ has 4-aminoacetophenone in the molecule. Chemical studies have led to the proposal of structures (30) and (31) for the aglycones of DJ-400 B$_1$ and J-400 B$_2$, respectively (230).

Vacidin A, an aromatic heptaene produced by *Streptomyces aureofaciens*, has been assigned the partial structure (32) (231). The position of closure of the lactone and the location of 2 carbonyl and 5–7 hydroxyl groups have yet to be determined.

Hamycin and hamycin X have been isolated from *Streptomyces pimprina* Thirum (232–237). Alkaline hydrolysis of hamycin was shown to produce 4-aminoacetophenone (236). It has been suggested that hamycin, candicidin, and trichomycin A are very similar (236). Studies using pyrolysis gas chromatography (238) suggest that trichomycin and candicidin are not identical. Recent high-pressure liquid chromatographic (HPLC) comparisons of candicidin, trichomycin, and levorin (239) have shown that the candicidin and levorin complexes are identical, but differ from trichomycin. Previous HPLC studies have demonstrated that hamycin, candicidin, and trichomycin are different (35). Structural studies on hamycin A (240) indicate that it has the structure (33), with many similar structural features to aureofungin A (29)

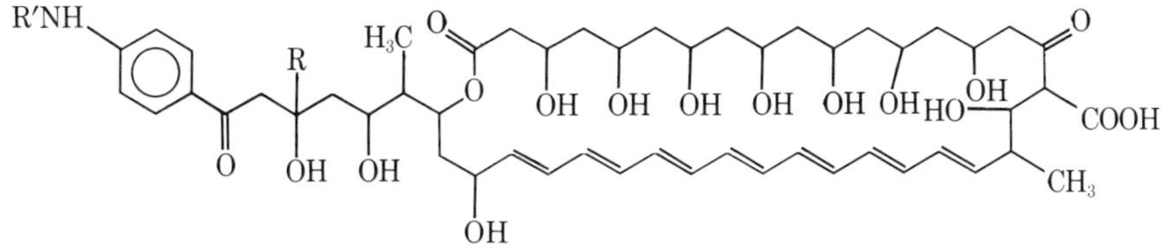

(30) R = 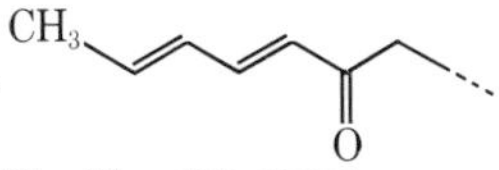   R' = CH₃   DJ-400 B₁

(31) R = R' = H   DJ-400 B₂

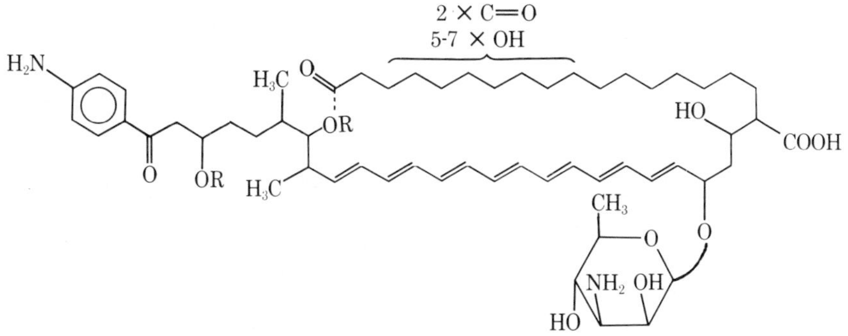

2 × C=O
5-7 × OH

(32)   vacidin A, partial structure

R = H, or lactone junction

and vacidin A (32). Coproduced with hamycin A (33) are three minor components hamycin B, C, and D (240) of unknown structure.

Notable amongst the aromatic group is perimycin (fungimycin, 1968) produced by *Streptomyces coelicolor* var. *aminophilus* (241–242). The major component perimycin A (36) contains the 4-methylaminoacetophenone moiety and a novel aminosugar, perosamine (37) (243,244), which has been shown to be 4-amino-4,6-dideoxy-D-mannose. The structure of perimycin A has recently been determined (245) and it is unique among the heptaenes in that it contains no carboxylic acid function (242). The structures of the minor components (Table 5) have not yet been determined. The synthesis of methyl perosaminide has been reported (246).

A number of aromatic heptaenes have been isolated and partially characterized. In many instances the nature of the aromatic moiety and the identity of the sugar have been determined, but little else is known about their structures (Table 5).

The aromatic heptaenes 67-121 A (34) and 67-121 C (35) have been shown to contain 4-methylaminoacetophenone. In addition (34) contains (21), while (35) contains a novel disaccharide, *O*-β-D-mannopyranosyl-(1 → 4)-D-mycosamine (38) (267).

The optical rotatory dispersion spectra of amphotericin B, mycoheptin, the levorins, cryptomycin, and candidin have been reported (288) to show a complex Cotton effect in the region of absorption of the polyene chromophore.

Biosynthetic studies have shown that the aromatic moieties of candicidin (289) and perimycin (290) are formed from shikimic acid with 4-aminobenzoic acid as the terminal intermediate. The *N*-methyl group in the aromatic moiety of perimycin has been shown to be derived from methionine (290).

Table 5. Heptaenes

Compound	Source	General chemical features	References
ascosin [1402-88-6]	Streptomyces canescus	aromatic group; CHNO; uv; ir; [α]ᴅ; amphoteric; mycosamine; 4-aminoacetophenone	247
candicidin [1403-17-4]	Streptomyces griseus	aromatic group; $C_{63}H_{85}N_{21}O_{19}$; uv; ir; [α]ᴅ; amphoteric; mycosamine; 4-aminoacetophenone	3, 211, 248
candimycin [37217-65-5]	Streptomyces ehimensis	aromatic group; CHNO; uv; 4-methylaminoacetophenone	249
perimycin B [62362-44-1] and C [62362-45-2]	Streptomyces coelicolor var. aminophilus	aromatic group; uv	241–245
heptamycin [12767-57-6]	Streptomyces sp.	aromatic group; acidic; uv	250
ayfactin A [62851-47-2] and B [62851-46-1] (aureofacin)	Streptomyces viridofaciens Streptomyces aureofaciens	aromatic group; CHNO; uv; ir; 4-aminoacetophenone	251, 252
azacolutin (F17-C) [12768-47-7]	Streptomyces cinnamomeus var. azacoluta	aromatic group; uv; ir; amphoteric; 4-aminoacetophenone.	253
2339	Actinomyces levoris 2339	aromatic group; CHNO; uv; mycosamine; 4-aminoacetophenone	254, 255
2789	Actinomyces levoris 2789	aromatic group; CHNO; uv; mycosamine; 4-aminoacetophenone	254, 255
X 63	Streptomyces sp.	aromatic group; uv; ir; 4-methylaminoacetophenone	256
heptafungin A [39405-61-3]	Streptomyces longisporolavendulae	aromatic group; CHNO; uv; mycosamine; 4-aminoacetophenone	257, 258
levorin A[a] [11014-70-3]	Streptomyces levoris	aromatic group; CHNO; mol wt 1180; uv; ir; [α]ᴅ; mycosamine; 4-aminoacetophenone	259–262
levorin B [62851-45-0]	Streptomyces levoris	aromatic group; CHNO; uv; ir; mycosamine; 4-aminoacetophenone	260
cryptomycin [58591-41-6] (6–7 components)	Actinomyces bulgaricus	aromatic group; CHNO; uv; ir; [α]ᴅ; mycosamine; 4-aminoacetophenone and 4-methylaminoacetophenone	263
flavomycin A [57608-58-9]	Actinomyces flavus var geptinicus var. nov.	aromatic group; ca $C_{70}H_{121}N_5O_{40}P$ uv; ir; [α]ᴅ; mycosamine; 4-aminoacetophenone	264, 265
fulvomycin A [57608-60-3] B [57608-61-4] and C [57608-62-5]	Actinomyces fulvoviolaceus var. achromogenes var. nov.	aromatic group; CHNO; uv; ir; [α]ᴅ; amphoteric; mycosamine; 4-aminoacetophenone	266

288

67–121 B[b] [57515-51-2]	*Actinoplanes* sp. NRRL 5325	aromatic group; CHNO; uv; ir; $[\alpha]_D$; mycosamine; 4-aminoacetophenone	29, 267
757	*Streptomyces* sp. No. 757	uv	268
eurotin A [62851-59-6]	*Streptomyces griseus* H-5592	CHNO; uv; ir; amphoteric	269
PA 150	*Streptomyces* sp.	CHNO; uv; ir; $[\alpha]_D$; amphoteric	106, 107
champamycin A [62851-64-3] and B [62851-63-2]	*Streptomyces champavati*	uv	270–272
grubilin [62851-57-4]	*Streptomyces* sp. BA-27	uv	273
4915	*Streptomyces paucisporogenes*	CHNO; uv	274
two heptaenes	*Streptomyces* sp.	uv	275
AE56	*Streptomyces* sp.	uv	276
PA 616	*Streptomyces parvisporogenes* ATCC 12568	CHNO; uv; ir; $[\alpha]_D$; amphoteric	164
2814H	*Streptomyces* sp. 1A 2814	CHNO; $[\alpha]_D$; amphoteric	277
AF 1231	*Streptomyces* sp. 1231	CHNO; uv	278
1645 P$_1$	*Streptomyces* sp. Cepa 1645-IAUR	CHNO; uv	279
takemycin (C 11) [62851-68-7]	*Streptomyces takataensis*	CHNO; uv	280, 281
G 83	*Streptomyces coriofaciens* ATCC 14155	CHNO; uv; ir; $[\alpha]_D$	282
gerobriecin [62851-58-5]	*Streptomyces jujuy* ATCC 13670	CHNO; uv; $[\alpha]_D$	283
monicamycin [62851-54-1]	*Streptoverticillium cinnamomeus* var. *monicae*	CHNO; uv; ir; acidic	284
neophetaene [62851-51-8]	*Streptomyces* sp.	uv	285
hepcin [62851-56-3]	*Actinosporangium griseoroseum*	uv; $[\alpha]_D$	286
partricin [11096-49-4]	*Streptomyces aureofaciens* NRRL 3878	CHNO; uv; ir; amphoteric	287
flavomycin B [57608-59-0]	*Actinomyces flavus* var. *geptinicus* var. nov.	CHNO; uv; ir; $[\alpha]_D$	264

[a] Separated into levorin A$_0$, A$_1$, A$_2$, A$_3$, and A$_4$ (261) where A$_4$ is the major component.
[b] The complex of 67-121 A, B, and C is referred to as SCH 16656 (29).

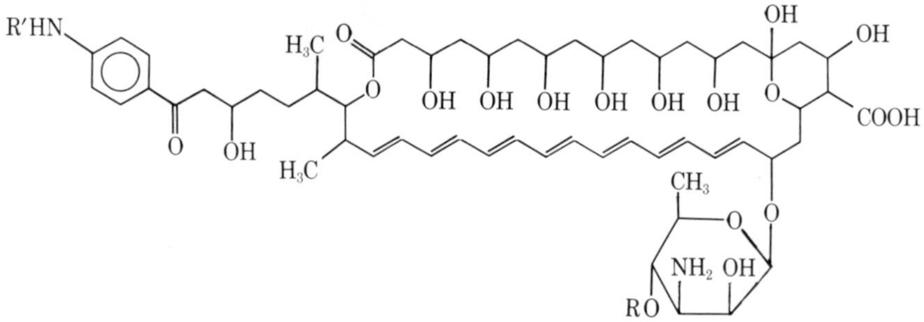

(33) R = R′ = H hamycin A
(34) R = H, R′ = CH₃ 67-121 A
(35) R = O-β-D-mannosyl, R′ = CH₃ 67-121 C

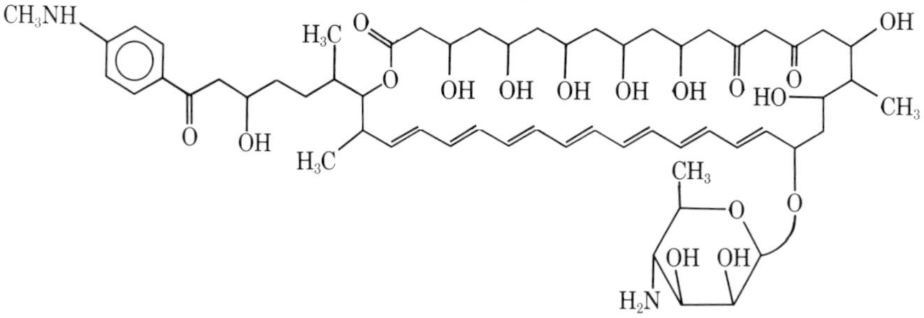

(36)   perimycin A

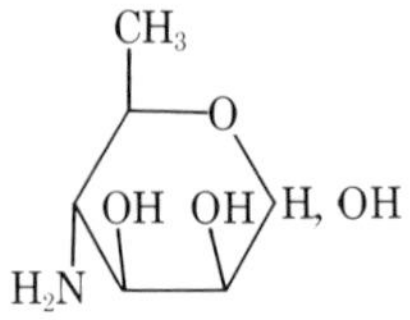

(37)   perosamine

Derivatives of Polyenes

The poor solubility characteristics of the polyene macrolides greatly restrict their parenteral use and consequently a variety of derivatives have been prepared with a view to increasing the solubility in aqueous solutions, while retaining the antifungal activity.

The formation of complexes between polyenes such as amphotericin A and amphotericin B and calcium ions has been reported (291–293). The complexes have enhanced solubility in water and methanol, retain the biological activity of the parent polyene, and have proved to be useful in their industrial purification. The borate complex of amphotericin B has been prepared (294) and shown to be water soluble and to retain the activity of the parent polyene.

The N-acylation of polyene antibiotics such as amphotericin B (212,295–296), nystatin (297), and perimycin (298) with a variety of acyl groups such as acetyl, propionyl, and succinyl has been reported. The N-acyl derivatives are less potent and less toxic than the parent polyenes and their sodium salts are water soluble. The N-acyl derivatives of amphotericin B methyl ester were also reported to be less active than the parent polyene (295).

Nystatin (299) and amphotericin B (300) hydrochloride salts are somewhat more soluble in water and retain the biological activity. Treatment of amphotericin B with one mol of dry hydrogen chloride (301) has been reported to give a water soluble acidic product. At pH 6 a neutral derivative is obtained. Both derivatives retain the biological activity.

The preparation of a variety of N-glycosyl derivatives of several polyenes including amphotericin B has been reported to give derivatives whose water soluble sodium salts show similar activity but have reduced toxicity (302). The derivative formed from amphotericin B and D-glucose has the structure (**39**).

The N-methylglucamine salts of polyenes containing carboxylic acid groups such as amphotericin B have been prepared (303) and shown to be water soluble active derivatives.

The preparation of the methyl ester derivatives of amphotericin B and a number of other polyenes have been reported (295,304–311). The methyl esters have been found to retain the activity of the original polyene (305,311–312) and the hydrochloride salt of amphotericin B methyl ester (295) and also the sodium desoxycholate complex (313) have the advantage of being water soluble. The stability (314) and toxicity (305, 307, 315) of amphotericin B methyl ester hydrochloride have been studied. In general the methyl ester derivatives show reduced toxicity relative to the parent polyenes. The preparation of radioactively labeled amphotericin B methyl ester has been described (313,316) and absorption, distribution, and excretion studies have been carried out (317).

Irradiation of levorin A$_2$ with uv light has been shown to produce a *cis*-isomer, isolevorin A$_2$, which has greater antifungal activity than levorin A$_2$ (318).

Activity

In general the polyene macrolides are essentially devoid of antibacterial activity, but possess excellent activity against a wide range of yeasts and fungi (eg, *Candida, Cryptococcus, Coccidioides, Torulopsis, Blastomyces, Histoplasma, Pityrosporum,*

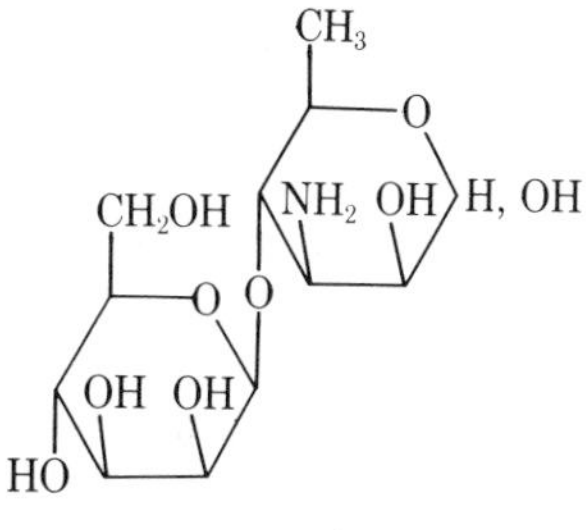

(**38**)   *O*-β-D-mannopyranosyl-(1 → 4)-D-mycosamine

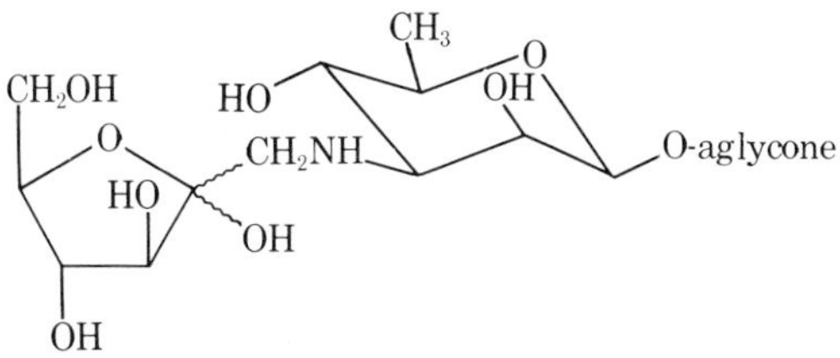

(**39**)   derivative of amphotericin B and D-glucose

Rhodotorula, Saccharomyces, Monosporium species), dermatophytes (eg, *Epidermophyton, Microsporum, Trichophyton* species), and molds (eg, *Aspergillus, Penicillium* species). The *in vitro* activity (minimum inhibitory concentration) of four representative polyenes is given in Table 6 (319). In general the heptaenes of the aromatic group have the greatest antifungal potency. Although some strains of *Candida* that show resistance to polyenes have been grown *in vitro* (320) and isolated reports of clinical resistance to polyenes (321) have appeared, there has been no widespread development of resistance associated with the use of the polyenes.

In addition to their antifungal activity, many of the polyenes exhibit good antiprotozoal activity against organisms such as *Trichomonas vaginalis* (322), *Entamoeba histolytica* (323), and a number of *Leishmania* strains (324). Trienin has also been reported to exhibit antitumor activity (39). Heptaene macrolides have been reported to be useful in treating prostatic hypertrophy (325–328), in reducing cholesterol absorption (17,329–330), and in the oral treatment of acne (331).

The polyene macrolides have a high degree of potential toxicity associated with their use. The magnitude of the toxicity varies according to the route of administration, being greatest when the polyene is administered intravenously or intraperitoneally. Amphotericin B (intravenous) remains the most widely used polyene for the treatment of systemic infections. However, adverse reactions are invariably produced by systemic therapy such as chills, fever, headache, anorexia, nausea, vomiting, and anemia (332). Nephrotoxicity is a major problem with amphotericin B and can only be successfully controlled by minimizing exposure of the kidneys to the drug (332). The aromatic heptaenes exhibit the greatest toxicity. The polyenes show very low toxicity when administered orally due to the lack of absorption during passage through the gastro-intestinal tract. Candicidin and nystatin are used topically to treat vaginal candidiasis. Nystatin is also used in other topical, as well as oral, treatments.

A considerable body of experimental evidence has been published indicating that polyene macrolide antibiotics form complexes with sterols in the plasma membrane of various cells resulting in morphological and permeability changes in the cells (22). It is believed that this produces pore formation (23) resulting in lysis and death of the

Table 6. MIC (mcg/mL) After 72 h Incubation

	Pimaricin	Nystatin	Amphotericin B	Candicidin
Candida albicans Burke	7.5	0.75	0.3	<0.01
Candida albicans Collins	7.5	0.75	0.055	<0.01
Candida albicans Sparks	7.5	0.3	0.3	<0.01
Candida albicans Wisconsin	7.5	0.75	0.055	<0.01
Candida tropicalis	3.0	0.75	0.3	0.3
Candida stellatoidea	<0.01	0.3	<0.01	<0.01
Cryptococcus neoformans	3.0	0.3	0.3	<0.01
Pityrosporum ovale	<0.01	0.3	0.75	0.3
Rhodotorula rubra	7.5	0.3	0.3	<0.01
Torulopsis glabrata	17.5	3.0	0.3	0.055
Trichophyton rubrum	7.5	0.3	0.3	0.3
Microsporum canis	3.0	0.75	0.055	3.0
Microsporum gypseum	>50	0.75	0.3	3.0
Monosporium apiospermum	3.0	3.0	0.3	0.3
Aspergillus niger	>50	>50	>50	>50
Geotrichum candidum	0.75	3.0	>50	>50

cell. This is thought to be the reason for susceptibility of fungi to polyenes, whereas bacteria with no sterols in their cell membranes, are not susceptible.

The biological activity of polyene antibiotics has recently been reviewed (333).

Economic Aspects

The polyene macrolides marketed in the United States are shown in Table 7.

Table 7. Polyene Macrolide Antifungals Marketed in the United States

Polyene macrolide	Trade name	Manufacturer
amphotericin B[a] [1397-89-3]	Fungizone	E.R. Squibb and Sons
candicidin[a] [1403-17-4]	Candeptin	Schmid Laboratories, Inc.
	Vanobid	Merrell-National Laboratories (Div. Richardson-Merrell, Inc.)
nystatin[a] [1400-61-9]	Nilstat	Lederle Laboratories (Div. American Cyanamid Company)
	Mycostatin	E.R. Squibb and Sons
	Korostatin	Holland-Rantos Company, Inc.
	Nystaform	Dome Laboratories (Div. Miles Laboratories, Inc.)
	Terrastatin[b]	Pfizer Laboratories (Div. Pfizer, Inc.)

[a] Produced by fermentation.
[b] In combination with oxytetracycline.

All of the polyenes named in text are listed alphabetically in Table 8.

Table 8. Alphabetical List of Polyenes Named in the Text

Compound	CAS Registry Number	Structure number	Molecular formula
amphotericin	[1397-89-3]	(25)	$C_{47}H_{73}NO_{17}$
amphotericin B, N-iodoacetyl	[34324-38-4]		$C_{49}H_{74}INO_{18}$
antibiotic DJ 400 B$_1$	[65086-28-4]	(30)	$C_{66}H_{96}N_2O_{21}$
antibiotic DJ 400 B$_2$	[65086-29-5]	(31)	$C_{58}H_{86}N_2O_{20}$
antibiotic 67-121 A	[57515-52-3]	(34)	$C_{59}H_{88}N_2O_{19}$
antibiotic 67-121 C	[57515-50-1]	(35)	$C_{65}H_{98}N_2O_{24}$
arenomycin B	[51449-09-3]	(8)	$C_{36}H_{55}NO_{13}$
aurenin	[34820-53-6]	(15)	$C_{33}H_{54}O_{11}$
aureofungin	[8065-41-6]		
aureofungin A	[63278-45-5]	(29)	$C_{59}H_{86}N_2O_{19}$
aureofungin B	[63278-44-4]	(28)	$C_{57}H_{85}NO_{19}$
candidin	[1405-90-9]	(26)	$C_{47}H_{71}NO_{17}$
candidinin	[65776-68-3]		
candidoin	[65776-69-4]		
chainin	[38264-25-4]	(14)	$C_{33}H_{54}O_{10}$
cogomycin	[56389-81-2]	(11)	$C_{35}H_{58}O_{12}$
dermostatin A	[51053-36-2]	(23)	$C_{40}H_{64}O_{11}$
dermostatin B	[51141-40-3]	(24)	$C_{41}H_{66}O_{11}$
eurocidin A	[1403-52-7]	(19)	
eurocidin B	[1403-52-7]	(20)	
filipin I	[38723-93-2]		
filipin II	[38620-77-8]		
filipin III	[480-49-9]	(10)	$C_{35}H_{58}O_{11}$

Table 8 (*continued*)

Compound	CAS Registry Number	Structure number	Molecular formula
filipin IV	[38404-99-8]		$C_{35}H_{58}O_{11}$
flavofungin	[11006-22-7]		
flavofungin A	[29919-25-3]	(17)	$C_{36}H_{58}O_{10}$
flavofungin B	[29843-28-5]	(18)	$C_{37}H_{60}O_{10}$
flavomycoin	[11076-76-9]		
fungichromin	[6834-98-6]	(11)	$C_{35}H_{58}O_{12}$
fungimycin	[11016-07-2]		
hamycin	[1403-71-0]		
hamycin A	[62534-55-8]	(33)	$C_{58}H_{86}N_2O_{19}$
hamycin B	[62534-57-0]		
hamycin C	[65086-27-3]		
hamycin D	[65086-31-9]		
hamycin X	[66120-72-7]		
hemoaurenin	[65776-70-7]	(16)	$C_{34}H_{56}O_{11}$
lagosin	[31981-50-7]	(11)	$C_{35}H_{58}O_{12}$
lucensomycin	[13058-67-8]	(5)	$C_{36}H_{53}NO_{13}$
moldcidin B	[31981-50-7]		
mycoheptin	[12609-89-1]	(27)	$C_{47}H_{71}NO_{17}$
mycoticin A	[29919-25-3]	(17)	$C_{36}H_{58}O_{10}$
mycoticin B	[29843-28-5]	(18)	$C_{37}H_{60}O_{10}$
natamycin	[7681-93-8]	(4)	$C_{33}H_{47}NO_{13}$
nystatin A_1	[34786-70-4]	(1)	$C_{47}H_{75}NO_{17}$
nystatin A_2	[65086-32-0]		
nystatin A_3	[65104-03-2]	(2)	$C_{53}H_{85}NO_{20}$
pentamycin	[31981-50-7]	(11)	$C_{35}H_{58}O_{12}$
perimycin	[11016-07-02]		
perimycin A	[62327-61-1]	(36)	$C_{59}H_{88}N_2O_{17}$
pimaricin	[7681-93-8]	(4)	$C_{33}H_{47}NO_{13}$
rectilavendomycin	[56092-88-7]	(22)	
rimocidin	[1393-12-0]	(9)	$C_{39}H_{61}NO_{14}$
tennecetin	[7681-93-8]	(4)	$C_{33}H_{47}NO_{13}$
tetrin A	[34280-28-9]	(6)	$C_{33}H_{49}NO_{13}$
tetrin B	[34280-27-8]	(7)	$C_{33}H_{49}NO_{14}$
trichomycin complex	[1394-02-1]		
trichomycin A	[12698-99-6]		
trichomycin B	[12699-00-2]		
trichomycin C	[6576-71-8]		
vacidin A	[66120-71-6]	(32)	

BIBLIOGRAPHY

"Polyene Antibiotics" in *ECT* 2nd ed., Vol. 16, pp 133–143, by James D. Dutcher, The Squibb Institute for Medical Research.

1. E. L. Hazen and R. Brown, *Science* **112**, 423 (1950).
2. S. A. Waksman, *Adv. Appl. Microbiol.* **5**, 235 (1963).
3. S. A. Waksman, H. A. Lechevalier, and C. P. Schaffner, *Bull. W. H. O.* **33**, 219 (1965).
4. D. Perlman, *Prog. Ind. Microbiol.* **6**, 3 (1967).
5. J. F. Martin and L. E. McDaniel, *Adv. Appl. Microbiol.* **21**, 1 (1977).
6. A. Neelameghan, *Hind. Antibiot. Bull.* **2**, 131 (1960).
7. L. C. Vining, *Hind. Antibiot. Bull.* **3**, 37 (1960).
8. W. Oroshnik and A. D. Mebane, *Prog. Chem. Org. Nat. Prod.*, **21**, 17 (1963).
9. H. Umezawa, *Recent Advances in Chemistry and Biochemistry of Antibiotics*, Microbial Chemistry Research Foundation, Tokyo, 1964, p. 44.

10. K. K. Rinehart, Jr., and G. E. van Lear, in G. R. Waller, ed., *Antibiotics in Biochemical Applications of Mass Spectrometry,* John Wiley & Sons, Inc., New York, 1972, p. 451.
11. W. Keller-Schierlein, *Prog. Chem. Org. Nat. Prod.,* **30,** 313 (1973).
12. E. Drouhet, *Antibiot. Chemother. (Basel)* **11,** 21 (1962).
13. J. O. Lampen, *Symp. Soc. Gen. Microbiol.* **16,** 111 (1966).
14. J. O. Lampen, in B. A. Newton and P. E. Reynolds, eds., *Biochemical Studies of Antimicrobial Drugs,* Cambridge Univ. Press, London, 1966, p. 111.
15. S. C. Kinsky, in D. Gottlieb and P. D. Shaw, eds., *Antibiotics,* Vol 1, Springer-Verlag, Berlin, 1967, pp. 122, 749.
16. D. Gottlieb and P. D. Shaw, in *Mechanism of Action,* Vol. 1, Springer-Verlag, Berlin, 1967, p. 785.
17. J. O. Lampen, *Amer. J. Clin. Pathol.* **52,** 138 (1969).
18. S. C. Kinsky, *Ann. Rev. Pharmacol.* **10,** 119 (1970).
19. D. Gottlieb and P. D. Shaw, *Ann. Rev. Phytopathol.* **8,** 371 (1970).
20. W. Mechlinski, A. I. Laskin, and H. A. Lechevalier, eds., *Handbook of Microbiology,* Vol. 3, CRC Press, Cleveland, Ohio, 1973, p. 93.
21. J. M. T. Hamilton-Miller, *Bact. Rev.* **37,** 166 (1973).
22. A. W. Norman, A. M. Spielvogel, and R. C. Wong, *Adv. Lipid Res.* **14,** 127 (1976).
23. T. E. Andreoli, *Ann. N. Y. Acad. Sci.* **235,** 448 (1974).
24. E. Drouhet, in G. E. W. Wolstenholme and R. Porter, eds., *Systemic Mycoses, CIBA Foundation Symposium,* J. and A. Churchill Ltd., London, 1968, p. 206.
25. J. P. Utz, in G. E. Wolstenholme and R. Porter, eds., *Systemic Mycoses, CIBA Foundation Symposium,* J. and A. Churchill Ltd., London, 1968, p. 242.
26. A. H. Thomas, *Analyst* **101,** 321 (1976).
27. G. Neseman and co-workers, *Naturwissenschaften* **59,** 81 (1972).
28. K. S. Gopalkrishnan and co-workers, *Nature* **218,** 597 (1968).
29. G. H. Wagman and co-workers, *Antimicrob. Agents Chemother.* **7,** 457 (1975).
30. C. P. Schaffner and co-workers, *Antibiot. Ann.* 869 (1957–1958).
31. M. Musilikova, *Folia Microbiol.* **6,** 175 (1961).
32. L. C. Vining, W. A. Taber, and F. J. Gregory, *Antibiot. Ann.* 980 (1954–1955).
33. K. Hattori and co-workers, *J. Antibiot.* **9A,** 176 (1956).
34. M. E. Bergy and T. E. Eble, *Biochemistry* **7,** 653 (1968).
35. W. Mechlinski and C. P. Schaffner, *J. Chromatogr.* **99,** 619 (1974).
36. G. H. Wagman and M. J. Weinstein, *Journal of Chromatography Library,* Vol. 1, *Chromatography of Antibiotics,* Elsevier, New York, 1973.
37. J. J. Armstrong and co-workers, *Nature* **206,** 399 (1965).
38. C. Coronelli and co-workers, *J. Antibiot.* **20A,** 329 (1967).
39. A. Aszalos and co-workers, *J. Antibiot.* **21,** 611 (1968).
40. S. Aizawa, M. Shibuya, and S. Shirato, *J. Antibiot.* **24,** 393 (1971).
41. V. A. Poltorak and co-workers, *Antibiotiki* **17,** 738 (1972).
42. L. Vertesy, *J. Antibiot.* **25,** 4 (1972).
43. K. A. Vinogradova and co-workers, *Antibiotiki* **18,** 876 (1973).
44. V. A. Poltorak and co-workers, *Antibiotiki* **19,** 99 (1974).
45. U.S. Pat. 3,929,992 (Dec. 30, 1975), S. N. Sehgal, T. M. Blazekovic, and C. Vezina (to Ayerst McKenna and Harrison Ltd.).
46. Y. Shenin, T. Kotienko, and O. Ekzemplarov, *Antibiotiki* **13,** 387 (1968).
47. N. Porowska and co-workers, *Rec. Trav. Chim. Pays-Bas* **91,** 780 (1972).
48. D. R. Walters, J. D. Dutcher, and O. Wintersteiner, *J. Am. Chem. Soc.* **79,** 5076 (1957).
49. M. H. von Saltza and co-workers, *J. Am. Chem. Soc.* **83,** 2785 (1961).
50. J. D. Dutcher, D. R. Walters, and O. Wintersteiner, *J. Org. Chem.* **28,** 995 (1963).
51. M. von Saltza and co-workers, *J. Org. Chem.* **28,** 999 (1963).
52. A. J. Birch and co-workers, *Tetrahedron Lett.* 1485 (1964).
53. A. J. Birch and co-workers, *Tetrahedron Lett.* 1491 (1964).
54. M. Ikeda, M. Suzuki, and C. Djerassi, *Tetrahedron Lett.* 3745 (1967).
55. D. G. Manwaring, R. W. Rickards, and B. T. Golding, *Tetrahedron Lett.* 5319 (1969).
56. C. N. Chong and R. W. Rickards, *Tetrahedron Lett.* 5145 (1970).
57. E. Borowski and co-workers, *Tetrahedron Lett.* 685 (1971).
58. R. C. Pandey and K. L. Rinehart, Jr., *J. Antibiot.* **30,** 146 (1977).
59. C. N. Chong and R. W. Rickards, *Tetrahedron Lett.* 5053 (1972).

60. R. C. Pandey and K. L. Rinehart, Jr., *J. Antibiot.* **29**, 1035 (1976).
61. E. Borowski and co-workers, *8th International Symposium on the Chemistry of Natural Products,* IUPAC, New Dehli, India, 1972, paper F18.
62. A. P. Struyk and co-workers, *Antibiot. Ann.* 878 (1957–1958).
63. B. T. Golding and co-workers, *Tetrahedron Lett.* 3551 (1966).
64. J. B. Patrick and co-workers, *J. Am. Chem. Soc.* **80**, 6688 (1958).
65. J. B. Patrick, R. P. Williams, and J. S. Webb, *J. Am. Chem. Soc.* **80**, 6689 (1958).
66. O. Ceder and co-workers, *Chimia* **17**, 352 (1963).
67. O. Ceder, *Acta Chem. Scand.* **18**, 77, 103, 126 (1964).
68. O. Ceder and co-workers, *Acta Chem. Scand.* **18**, 83 (1964).
69. O. Ceder and co-workers, *Acta Chem. Scand.* **18**, 98 (1964).
70. O. Ceder and co-workers, *Acta Chem. Scand.* **18**, 111 (1964).
71. J. Burns and D. F. Holtman, *Antibiot. Chemother.* **9**, 398 (1959).
72. P. V. Divekar and co-workers, *Antibiot. Chemother.* **11**, 377 (1961).
73. F. Arcamone and co-workers, *G. Microbiol.* **4**, 119 (1957).
74. G. Gaudiano, P. Bravo, and A. Quilico, *Tetrahedron Lett.* 3559 (1966).
75. G. Gaudiano and co-workers, *Tetrahedron Lett.* 3567 (1966).
76. G. Gaudiano, P. Bravo, and A. Quilico, *Gazz. Chim. Ital.* **96**, 1322, 1351 (1966).
77. G. Gaudiano and co-workers, *Gazz. Chim. Ital.* **96**, 1470 (1966).
78. O. Ceder and B. Hansson, *Tetrahedron* **23**, 3753 (1967).
79. G. Gaudiano, P. Bravo, and G. Mauri, *Chem. Ind. (Milan)* **48**, 1327 (1966).
80. D. G. Manwaring and co-workers, *J. Antibiot.* **22**, 545 (1969).
81. H. Brik, *J. Antibiot.* **29**, 632 (1976).
82. K. Dornberger, H. Thrum, and G. Engelhardt, *Tetrahedron Lett.* 4469 (1976).
83. K. L. Rinehart, Jr. and co-workers, *Justus Liebigs Ann. Chem.* **688**, 77 (1963).
84. R. C. Pandey and co-workers, *J. Am. Chem. Soc.* **93**, 3738 (1971).
85. K. L. Rinehart, Jr., W. P. Tucker, and R. C. Pandey, *J. Am. Chem. Soc.* **93**, 3747 (1971).
86. D. Gottlieb and H. L. Pote, *Phytopathology* **50**, 817 (1960).
87. V. A. Tsyganov, Y. D. Shenin, and V. N. Soloviev, *Antibiotiki* **18**, 973 (1973).
88. Y. D. Shenin, V. N. Soloviev, and A. A. Nevinsky, *Antibiotiki* **18**, 872 (1973).
89. J. W. Davisson and co-workers, *Antibiot. Chemother.* **1**, 289 (1951).
90. A. C. Cope and co-workers, *J. Am. Chem. Soc.* **87**, 5452 (1965).
91. A. C. Cope, U. Axen, and E. P. Burrows, *J. Am. Chem. Soc.* **88**, 4221 (1966).
92. L. Falkowski and co-workers, *J. Antibiot.* **29**, 197 (1976).
93. D. Gottlieb and co-workers, *Phytopathology* **41**, 393 (1951).
94. L. C. Vining and W. A. Taber, *Can. J. Chem.* **35**, 1461 (1957).
95. F. Raubitscheck, R. F. Acker, and S. A. Waksman, *Antibiot. Chemother.* **2**, 179 (1952).
96. S. Wakaki and co-workers, *J. Antibiot.* **5B**, 680 (1952).
97. S. Wakaki and co-workers, *J. Antibiot.* **6B**, 247 (1953); **6A**, 145 (1953).
98. Brit. Pat. 719,878 (Dec. 8, 1954) (to Parke-Davis).
99. Brit. Pat. 712,547 (July 28, 1954) (to Parke-Davis).
100. W. Gold and co-workers, *Antibiot. Ann.* 579 (1955–1956).
101. J. Vandeputte, J. L. Wachtel, and E. T. Stiller, *Antibiot. Ann.* 587 (1955–1956).
102. Ger. Pat. 1,056,785 (May 6, 1959), E. J. Backus and M. Dann (to American Cyanamid Co.).
103. R. Despois and co-workers, *G. Microbiol.* **2**, 76 (1956).
104. J. M. J. Sakamoto, *J. Antibiot.* **10A**, 128 (1957).
105. H. Taguchi and A. Nakano, *J. Ferment. Technol.* **35**, 145 (1957).
106. A. R. English and T. J. McBride, *Antibiot. Ann.* 893 (1957–1958).
107. B. K. Koe and co-workers, *Antibiot. Ann.* 897 (1957–1958).
108. M. Soeda and H. Fujita, *J. Antibiot.* **12B**, 293 (1959).
109. H. Fujita, *J. Antibiot.* **12B**, 297 (1959).
110. M. Matsuoka and H. Umezawa, *J. Antibiot.* **13A**, 114 (1960).
111. L. Calot and A. P. Cercos, *Ann. Inst. Pasteur* **105**, 159 (1963).
112. R. Craveri and co-workers, *Ann. Microbiol. Enzimol.* **12**, 155 (1962).
113. A. Pal and P. Nandi, *Experientia* **20**, 321 (1964).
114. Fr. Pat. M2620 (July 24, 1964), L. Ninet, S. Pinnert, and J. Preud'homme (to Rhone-Poulenc S.A.).
115. Ger. Pat. 2,044,004 (Apr. 1, 1971) (to Institute of Antibiotics, Warsaw).

116. Belg. Pat. 82,737 (May 6, 1970), J. H. E. J. Martin and J. N. Porter (to American Cyanamid Co.).
117. K. Dornberger and co-workers, *J. Antibiot.* **24,** 172 (1971).
118. M. J. Thirumalachar, P. Rahalkar, and P. V. Deshmukh, *Hind. Antibiot. Bull.* **13,** 67 (1971).
119. V. A. Tsyganov, N. P. Barashkova, and Y. D. Shenin, *Antibiotiki* **17,** 483 (1972).
120. K. Fukushima and co-workers, *Japan Antibiotics Research Association,* 185th Meeting, Sept. 1972.
121. V. M. Mitskevich and co-workers, *Antibiotiki* **18,** 867 (1973).
122. V. A. Tsyganov, L. O. Bolshakova, and N. P. Barashkova, *Antibiotiki* **18,** 195 (1973).
123. N. P. Barashkova and co-workers, *Antibiotiki* **20,** 195 (1975).
124. G. B. Whitfield and co-workers, *J. Am. Chem. Soc.* **77,** 4799 (1955).
125. M. L. Dhar, V. Thaller, and M. C. Whiting, *Proc. Chem. Soc.* 310 (1960).
126. M. L. Dhar, V. Thaller, and M. C. Whiting, *J. Chem. Soc.* 842 (1964).
127. C. Djerassi and co-workers, *Tetrahedron Lett.* 383 (1961).
128. O. Ceder and R. Ryhage, *Acta Chem. Scand.* **18,** 558 (1964).
129. B. T. Golding, R. W. Rickards, and M. Barber, *Tetrahedron Lett.* 2615 (1964).
130. R. C. Pandey and K. L. Rinehart, Jr., *J. Antibiot.* **23,** 414 (1970).
131. K. L. Rinehart, Jr. and co-workers, *J. Antibiot.* **27,** 1 (1974).
132. R. C. Pandey and co-workers, *J. Am. Chem. Soc.* **94,** 4306 (1972).
133. A. C. Cope and co-workers, *J. Am. Chem. Soc.* **84,** 2170 (1962).
134. A. A. Tytell and co-workers, *Antibiot. Ann.* 716 (1954–1955).
135. S. Ball, C. J. Bessel, and A. Mortimer, *J. Gen. Microbiol.* **17,** 96 (1957).
136. M. P. Berry and M. C. Whiting, *J. Chem. Soc.* 862 (1964).
137. S. Umezawa and co-workers, *J. Antibiot.* **11A,** 26 (1958).
138. A. N. Boyd, *Manuf. Chem.* **32,** 318 (1961).
139. H. Ogawa and co-workers, *J. Antibiot.* **13A,** 353 (1960).
140. V. Pozsgay, J. Tamas, and G. Czira, *Acta Chim. Acad. Sci. Hung.* **85,** 215 (1975).
141. V. Pozsgay and co-workers, *J. Antibiot.* **29,** 472 (1976).
142. R. W. Rickards, R. M. Smith, and B. T. Golding, *J. Antibiot.* **23,** 603 (1970).
143. M. M. Taig, N. K. Solovyeva, and P. S. Braginskaya, *Antibiotiki* **14,** 873 (1969).
144. T. A. Ushakova and co-workers, *Khim. Farm. Zh.* **5,** 18 (1971).
145. Ger. Pat. 1,012,430 (1957), F. Lindner and co-workers.
146. Jpn. Pat. 9,245 (1958), K. Ogata, S. Igarashi, and Y. Nakao.
147. J. M. J. Sakamoto, *J. Antibiot.* **12A** 169 (1959).
148. Jpn. Pat. 1,148 (Mar. 7, 1961), M. Arishima and J. Sakamoto (to Meiji Seika).
149. Jpn. Pat 13,896 (Sept. 21, 1960), H. Taguchi (to Ono Yakuhin).
150. M. A. Gordon and E. Lapa, *N.Y. State Dep. Health, Annu. Rep. Div. Lab. Res.* 70 (1963).
151. D. S. Bhate, W. V. Lavate, and S. P. Acharya, *Hind. Antibiot. Bull.* **6,** 153 (1964).
152. S. N. Soloviev and L. Y. Severinets, *Antibiotiki* **10,** 9 (1965).
153. M. A. Gordon and E. W. Lapa, *Appl. Microbiol.* **14,** 754 (1966).
154. V. I. Frolova and co-workers, *Antibiotiki* **20,** 198 (1975).
155. N. A. Krasilnikov and co-workers, *Antibiotiki* **16,** 197 (1971).
156. L. Y. Severinets and Y. E. Konev, *Antibiotiki* **19,** 291 (1974).
157. M. Igarashi, K. Ogate, and A. Miyake, *J. Antibiot.* **9B,** 101 (1956).
158. Ger. Pat. 942,047 (April 26, 1956), S. Ball (to Glaxo Lab).
159. Ger. Pat. 1,017,329 (Oct. 10, 1957), F. Lindner and co-workers, (to Farbwerke Hoechst A.G.).
160. T. Arai and H. Katoh, *Fuhai Kenkyusho Hokoku* **11,** 56 (1958).
161. R. Brown and E. L. Hazen, *Antibiot. Chemother.* **10,** 702 (1960).
162. H. Thrum, *Naturwissenschaften* **46,** 87 (1959).
163. Brit. Pat. 841,495 (July 13, 1960), (to Chas. Pfizer and Co.).
164. Brit. Pat. 832,391 (June 6, 1960), F. W. Tanner (to Chas. Pfizer and Co.).
165. J. Berdy and I. Horvath, *Abstract of Antibiotics Congress,* Prague, 1964, p. 148.
166. Jpn. Pat. 13,798 (July 2, 1965), M. Shibata and co-workers (to Takeda Chemical Industries, Ltd.).
167. M. J. Thirumalachar and P. W. Rahalkar, *Prog. Antimicrob. Anticancer Ther.* **1,** 70 (1970).
168. Ger. Pat. 1,039,198 (Sept. 19, 1958), F. Arcamore and co-workers (to Soc. Farm. Ital.).
169. V. D. Kuznetsov, N. O. Blinov, and N. W. Vikhrova, *Microbiologia* **31,** 811 (1962).
170. V. A. Tsyganov, N. P. Barashkova, and Y. D. Shenin, *Antibiotiki* **18,** 771 (1973).
171. R. C. Burke and co-workers, *J. Invest. Dermatol.* **23,** 163 (1954).
172. H. H. Wasserman and co-workers, *J. Am. Chem. Soc.* **89,** 1535 (1967).
173. J. Uri and I. Bekesi, *Nature* **181** 908 (1958).

174. R. Bognar and co-workers, *Antibiotiki* **10,** 1059 (1965).

175. R. Bognar and co-workers, *Tetrahedron Lett.* 471 (1970).

176. ʼR. Schlegel and H. Thrum, *J. Antibiot.* **24,** 368 (1971).

177. *Ibid.,* p. 360.

178. L. A. Vetlugina, *Antibiotiki* **13,** 992 (1968).

179. H. W. Wasserman, P. A. Zoretic, and P. S. Mariano, *Chem. Comm.* 1634 (1970).

180. K. Nakazawa, *J. Agric. Chem. Soc. Japan* **29,** 650 (1955).

181. S. Horii, T. Shima, and A. Ouchida, *J. Antibiot.* **23,** 102 (1970).

182. V. M. Mitskevich and co-workers, *Antibiotiki* **20,** 202 (1975).

183. Y. D. Shenin and T. A. Lvovich, *Antibiotiki* **21,** 40 (1976).

184. M. J. Thirumalachar and S. K. Menon, *Hind. Antibiot. Bull.* **4,** 106 (1962).

185. N. Narasimhachari and M. B. Swami, *J. Antibiot.* **23,** 566 (1970).

186. R. C. Pandey and co-workers, *J. Antibiot.* **26,** 475 (1973).

187. E. A. Swart, H. H. Romano, and S. A. Waksman, *Proc. Soc. Exp. Biol. Med.* **73,** 376 (1950).

188. R. R. Smeby and co-workers, *Phytopathology* **42,** 506 (1952).

189. K. Aiso and co-workers, *J. Antibiot.* **5,** 218 (1952).

190. R. Utahara and co-workers, *J. Antibiot.* **12A,** 73 (1959).

191. I. Takahashi, *J. Antibiot.* **6A,** 117 (1953).

192. Y. Okami and co-workers, *J. Antibiot.* **7A,** 98 (1954).

193. R. Utahara and co-workers, *J. Antibiot.* **7A,** 120 (1954).

194. Jpn. Pat. 5,898 (Aug. 3, 1957), K. Ogata and co-workers, (to Takeda Pharmaceutical Industries, Ltd.).

195. J. M. J. Sakamoto, *J. Antibiot.* **12A,** 21 (1959).

196. J. F. Martin and L. E. McDaniel, *J. Antibiot.* **27,** 610 (1974).

197. L. E. McDaniel, *J. Antibiot.* **29,** 195 (1976).

198. J. D. Dutcher and co-workers, *Antibiot. Ann.* 866 (1956–1957).

199. E. Borowski and co-workers, *Tetrahedron Lett.* 473 (1965).

200. L. Falkowski and co-workers, *Rocz. Chem.* **39,** 225 (1965).

201. E. Borowski and co-workers, *Rocz. Chem.* **39,** 400 (1965).

202. W. Mechlinski and co-workers, *Rocz. Chem.* **39,** 497 (1965).

203. E. Borowski and co-workers, *Rocz. Chem.* **39,** 1933 (1965).

204. A. C. Cope and co-workers, *J. Am. Chem. Soc.* **88,** 4228 (1966).

205. E. Borowski and co-workers, *Rocz. Chem.* **41,** 61 (1967).

206. W. Mechlinski and co-workers, *Tetrahedron Lett.* 3873 (1970).

207. P. Ganis and co-workers, *J. Am. Chem. Soc.* **93,** 4560 (1971).

208. E. Borowski and co-workers, *Tetrahedron Lett.* 3909 (1970).

209. W. A. Taber, L. C. Vining, and S. A. Waksman, *Antibiot. Chemother.* **4,** 455 (1953).

210. E. Borowski and co-workers, *Tetrahedron Lett.* 1987 (1971).

211. E. Borowski and C. P. Schaffner, *5th International Congress of Biochemistry, Moscow, 1961,* Pergamon Press, London, 1961, p. 3.

212. C. P. Schaffner and E. Borowski, *Antibiot. Chemother.* **11,** 724 (1961).

213. E. Borowski and co-workers, *8th International Symposium on the Chemistry of Natural Products, IUPAC,* New Dehli, India, 1972, paper F19.

214. E. Borowski and co-workers, *Chemotherapia* **9,** 359 (1964).

215. D. S. Bhate and S. P. Acharya, *Hind. Antibiot. Bull.* **6,** 170 (1964).

216. G. R. Deshpande and N. Narasimhachari, *Hind. Antibiot. Bull.* **9,** 76 (1967).

217. *Ibid.,* p. 163.

218. M. J. Thirumalachar and co-workers, *Hind. Antibiot. Bull.* **6,** 108 (1964).

219. M. D. Lee and K. L. Rinehart, Jr., *16th Interscience Conference on Antimicrobial Agents and Chemotherapy,* Chicago, Ill., 1976, paper 40.

220. S. Hosoya and co-workers, *Japan J. Exp. Med.* **22,** 505 (1952).

221. S. Hosoya, N. Hamamura, and S. Ogata, *J. Antibiot.* **8A,** 48 (1955).

222. K. Hattori and co-workers, *J. Antibiot.* **8B,** 89 (1955).

223. K. Hattori and co-workers, *J. Antibiot.* **8B,** 312 (1955).

224. H. Nakano and co-workers, *J. Antibiot.* **9A,** 172 (1956).

225. H. Nakano, *J. Antibiot.* **14A,** 68 (1961).

226. *Ibid.,* p. 72.

227. K. Hattori, *J. Antibiot.* **15B,** 37 (1962).

228. *Ibid.,* p. 39.

229. F. Bohlmann and co-workers, *Tetrahedron* **26,** 2191 (1970).
230. *Ibid.,* p. 2199.
231. T. Ziminski and K. L. Rinehart, Jr., *15th Interscience Conference on Antimicrobial Agents and Chemotherapy,* Washington D.C., 1975, paper 428.
232. M. J. Thirumalachar, S. K. Menon, and V. V. Bhatt, *Hind. Antibiot. Bull.* **3,** 136 (1961).
233. D. S. Bhate and S. P. Acharya, *Hind. Antibiot. Bull.* **6,** 1 (1963).
234. D. S. Bhate and co-workers, *Hind. Antibiot. Bull.* **3,** 139 (1961).
235. D. S. Bhate and S. P. Acharya, *Hind. Antibiot. Bull.* **5,** 16 (1962).
236. P. V. Divekar, V. C. Vora, and A. W. Khan, *J. Antibiot.* **19,** 63 (1966).
237. G. R. Deshpande, D. R. Kerur, and N. Narasimhachari, *Hind. Antibiot. Bull.* **8,** 185 (1966).
238. D. H. Calam, *J. Chromatogr. Sci.* **12,** 613 (1974).
239. S. H. Hansen and M. Thomsen, *J. Chromatogr.* **123,** 205 (1976).
240. R. C. Pandey and K. L. Rinehart, Jr., *16th Interscience Conference on Antimicrobial Agents and Chemotherapy,* Chicago, Ill., 1976, paper 41.
241. E. J. Oswald, R. J. Reedy, and W. A. Randall, *Antibiot. Ann.* 236 (1955–1956).
242. E. Borowski and co-workers, *Antimicrob. Agents Ann.* 532 (1960).
243. C. H. Lee and C. P. Schaffner, *Tetrahedron Lett.* 5837 (1966).
244. C. H. Lee and C. P. Schaffner, *Tetrahedron* **25,** 2229 (1969).
245. P. Kolodziejczyk and co-workers, *Tetrahedron Lett.* 3603 (1976).
246. C. L. Stevens and co-workers, *J. Am. Chem. Soc.* **92,** 3160 (1970).
247. R. J. Hickey and co-workers, *Antibiot. Chemother.* **2,** 472 (1952).
248. H. Lechevalier and co-workers, *Mycologia* **45,** 155 (1953).
249. M. Shibata and co-workers, *J. Antibiot.* **7B,** 168 (1954).
250. Y. Henis, N. Grossowiez, and M. Aschner, *Bull. Res. Counc. Isr.* **6E,** vii (1957).
251. M. A. Kaplan and co-workers, *Antibiot. Chemother.* **8,** 491 (1958).
252. S. Igarasi, K. Ogata, and A. Miyoke, *J. Antibiot.* **9B,** 79 (1956).
253. R. Craveri and co-workers, *Antibiot. Chemother.* **10,** 430 (1960).
254. A. I. Korenjako, Y. M. Khokhlova, and N. I. Nikitina, *Mikrobiologiya* **30,** 633 (1961).
255. Y. M. Khokhlova, A. V. Puchnina, and N. O. Blinov, *Antibiotiki* **8,** 417 (1963).
256. L. V. Kannan and co-workers, *J. Antibiot.* **20A,** 293 (1967).
257. Hung. Pat. 155,813 (Mar. 24, 1969), H. Kalasz and co-workers (to Gyogyszerkutato Intezet).
258. H. Kalasz and co-workers, *Acta Microbiol. Acad. Sci. Hung.* **19,** 111 (1972).
259. V. A. Tsyganov and co-workers, *Antibiotiki* **4,** 21 (1959).
260. E. Borowski and co-workers, *Chemotherapia* **10,** 176 (1965).
261. A. I. Filippova and Y. D. Shenin, *Antibiotiki* **19,** 32 (1974).
262. Y. E. Konev and co-workers, *Antibiotiki* **18,** 354 (1973).
263. V. A. Tsyganov and co-workers, *Antibiotiki* **17,** 1067 (1972).
264. L. F. Kruglikova and co-workers, *Antibiotiki* **20,** 771 (1975).
265. L. F. Kruglikova and Y. D. Shenin, *Antibiotiki* **21,** 407 (1976).
266. V. A. Tsyganov and co-workers, *Antibiotiki* **20,** 579 (1975).
267. J. J. Wright and co-workers, *J. Chem. Soc. Chem. Commun.* 710 (1977).
268. R. Craveri and G. Giolitti, *Ann. Microbiol. Enzimol.* **7,** 81, (1956).
269. M. Soeda and H. Fujita, *J. Antibiot.* **12B,** 368 (1959).
270. P. L. N. Rao and B. N. Uma, *Nature* **182,** 115 (1958).
271. U. K. Rao and P. L. N. Rao, *Indian J. Exp. Biol.* **5,** 39 (1967).
272. B. N. Uma and P. L. N. Rao, *Indian Inst. Sci. Golden Jubilee Research Volume,* 1909–1959, p. 130.
273. J. Uri, I. Szilagyi, and I. Bekesi, *Symposium on Antibiotics,* Prague, 1959, p. 78.
274. Ger. Pat. 1,053,738 (Mar. 26, 1959), G. Hagemann, G. Nomine, and L. Penasse (to Laboratoire Francaise de Chimotherapie).
275. M. V. Nefelova and I. N. Pozmogova, *Mikrobiologiya* **6,** 856 (1960).
276. S. Thadee and A. Faivre-Amiot, *C. R.* **250,** 1730 (1960).
277. H. Thrum and I. D. Dcho, *Naturwissenschaften* **47,** 474 (1960).
278. Jpn. Pat. 1,147 (Mar. 7, 1961), M. Arishima and J. Sakamoto (to Meiji Seika).
279. F. D. Lyra and co-workers, *Recife* **4,** 19 (1962).
280. K. Iwashita, K. Ueda, and T. Fujimoto, *J. Antibiot.* **15B,** 119 (1962).
281. Fr. Pat. M 1872 (July 22, 1963), (to Chugai Pharm. Co., Ltd.).
282. Ger. Pat. 1,128,083 (April 19, 1962), J. Schmidt-Thome and co-workers (to Farbwerke Hoechst A.G.).

283. U.S. Pat. 3,159,541 (Dec. 1, 1964), M. S. Cataldi, J. Pahn, and O. L. Galmarini (to Olin Mathieson Chemical Corp.).

284. K. C. Gupta, *Antimicrob. Agents Chemother.* 65 (1964).

285. M. J. Thirumalachar and co-workers, *Proceedings of the 9th International Congress on Microbiology,* Moscow, 1966, p. 170.

286. V. A. Tsyganov and co-workers, *Antibiotiki* **15,** 963 (1970).

287. T. Bruzzese and co-workers, *Farmaco Sci.* **29,** 331 (1974).

288. A. F. Morgunova and co-workers, *Antibiotikǐ* **20,** 1059 (1975).

289. C. M. Liu, L. E. McDaniel, and C. P. Schaffner, *J. Antibiot.* **25,** 116 (1972).

290. *Ibid.,* p. 187.

291. U.S. Pat, 2,908,612 (Oct. 13, 1959), J. D. Dutcher and co-workers (to Olin Mathieson Chemical Corp.).

292. U.S. Pat. 3,928,570 (Dec. 23, 1975), J. Metzger (to E.R. Squibb and Sons, Inc.).

293. Ger. Pat. 2,163,274 (July 13, 1972), A. Adorjan and J. Vandeputte (to E.R. Squibb and Sons, Inc.).

294. U.S. Pat. 3,740,424 (June 19, 1973), J. Vandeputte (to E. R. Squibb and Sons, Inc.).

295. W. Mechlinski and C. P. Schaffner, *J. Antibiot.* **25,** 256 (1972).

296. U.S. Pat. 3,965,090 (June 22, 1976), J. Metzger (to E.R. Squibb and Sons, Inc.).

297. H. Lechevalier and co-workers, *Antibiot. Chemother.* **11,** 640 (1961).

298. E. Michalska, *Chemotherapia* **9,** 52 (1964).

299. P. Cocchi and G. Rapi, *Chemotherapia* **6,** 319 (1963).

300. U.S. Pat. 2,908,611 (Oct. 13, 1959), J. D. Dutcher and co-workers (to Olin Mathieson Chemical Corp.).

301. U.S. Pat. 3,914,409 (Oct. 21, 1975), W. J. McGahren and M. P. Kunstmann (to American Cyanamid Co.).

302. L. Falkowski and co-workers, *J. Antibiot.* **28,** 244 (1975).

303. N.L. Pat. 73,513 (Oct. 20, 1975), (to Institute of Antibiotics, Leningrad).

304. C. P. Schaffner and W. Mechlinski, *J. Antibiot.* **25,** 259 (1972).

305. D. P. Bonner, W. Mechlinski, and C. P. Schaffner, *J. Antibiot.* **25,** 261 (1972).

306. T. Bruzzese and co-workers, *Experientia* **28,** 1515 (1972).

307. T. Bruzzese, M. Cambieri, and F. Recusani, *J. Pharm. Sci.* **64,** 462 (1975).

308. U.S. Pat. 3,936,526 (Feb. 3, 1976), T. Bruzzese and R. Ferrari (to Societa Prodotti Antibiotici).

309. U.S. Pat. 3,945,993 (Mar. 23, 1976), C. P. Schaffner and W. Mechlinski (to Rutgers Research and Educational Foundation).

310. U.S. Pat. 3,961,047 (June 1, 1976), T. Bruzzese and G. Ghielmetti (to Societa Prodotti Antibiotici).

311. R. C. Pandey and K. L. Rinehart, Jr., *J. Antibiot.* **30,** 158 (1977).

312. D. P. Bonner and co-workers, *Antimicrob. Agents Chemother.* **7,** 724 (1975).

313. N. Monji, W. Mechlinski, and C. P. Schaffner, *J. Antibiot.* **29,** 438 (1976).

314. D. P. Bonner, W. Mechlinski, and C. P. Schaffner, *J. Antibiot.* **28,** 132 (1975).

315. G. R. Keim, Jr. and co-workers, *Science* **179,** 584 (1973).

316. H. A. B. Linke, W. Mechlinski, and C. P. Schaffner, *J. Antibiot.* **27,** 155 (1974).

317. M. Monji and co-workers, *J. Antibiot.* **28,** 317 (1975).

318. A. I. Filippova and co-workers, *Antibiotiki* **17,** 932 (1972).

319. J. A. Waitz and D. Loebenberg, Schering-Plough Corporation, unpublished observations.

320. M. Athar and H. I. Winner, *J. Gen. Microbiol.* **4,** 505 (1971).

321. J. Bodenhoff, *Odontol. Tidskr.* **76,** 279 (1968).

322. S. Hosoya and co-workers, *J. Antibiot.* **6A,** 92 (1953).

323. H. Seneca, *Antibiot. Ann.* 697 (1955–1956).

324. B. K. Ghosh and A. N. Chatterjee, *Indian J. Microbiol.* **1,** 147 (1961).

325. C. P. Schaffner and H. W. Gordon, *Proc. Nat. Acad. Sci. USA* **61,** 36 (1968).

326. H. W. Gordon and C. P. Schaffner, *Proc. Nat. Acad. Sci. USA* **60,** 1201 (1968).

327. U.S. Pat. 3,584,118 (June 8, 1971), H. W. Gordon (to Julius Schmid, Inc.).

328. U.S. Pat. 3,954,971 (May 4, 1976), H. W. Gordon (to Julius Schmid, Inc.).

329. U.S. Pat. 3,714,348 (Jan. 30, 1973), H. W. Gordon and C. P. Schaffner (to Julius Schmid, Inc.).

330. U.S. Pat. 3,793,448 (Feb. 19, 1974), H. W. Gordon and C. P. Schaffner (to Julius Schmid, Inc.).

331. U.S. Pat. 3,629,403 (Dec. 21, 1971), H. W. Gordon and C. P. Schaffner (to Julius Schmid, Inc.).

332. D. Pappagianis, in P. D. Hoeprich, ed., *Infectious Diseases,* Harper and Row, New York, 1972, p. 405.

333. S. M. Hammond, in G. P. Ellis and G. B. West, eds., *Progress in Medicinal Chemistry*, Vol. 14, North Holland Publishing Co., Amsterdam, 1977, p. 105.

ALAN K. MALLAMS
Schering-Plough Corporation

POLYETHERS

All the known polyether antibiotics are isolated from the *Streptomyces* genus of microorganisms. The two most popular sources have been *S. albus* and *S. hygroscopicus* which account for more than half of the thirty polyether antibiotics reported. The polyethers exhibit good *in vitro* activity against gram-positive and mycobacteria but do not inhibit gram-negative microorganisms. Some of the compounds have been reported active against phytopathogenic bacteria and fungi. Due to the high parenteral toxicity of the polyethers, they have found no use as clinical antibacterial agents, but are playing an increasing role in veterinary medicine as coccidiostats in poultry and growth promotants in ruminants such as cattle and sheep.

These antibiotics are all monocarboxylic acids, but unlike simple acids, eg, acetic acid, they cannot be extracted from organic solvents by aqueous sodium carbonate or bicarbonate. On the contrary, under these conditions the polyether antibiotics extract alkali metal cations like sodium into the organic phase from which the antibiotic salt complexes can be isolated by evaporation and crystallization. For compounds capable of transporting cations into or through a lipophilic environment, Pressman has coined the name ionophore (1). The polyether antibiotics are just one of a large variety of ionophores (see Chelating agents). Others include the synthetic crown ethers and cryptates in addition to antibiotics of the cyclodepsipeptide and macrotetralide type such as valinomycin and nonactin (see Antibiotics, peptides). The polyethers are distinguished from these other ionophores, however, in being acids which yield neutral salt complexes, whereas valinomycin and many of the other naturally occurring ionophores are neutral cyclic structures which yield positively charged cation complexes. The name polyether has become the term of choice to characterize these antibiotics as a result of the multiplicity of cyclic ethers found in all members of this unique group of microbial products (2) (see also Polyethers).

Classification

The polyether antibiotics can be classified by many criteria, but the method used here is based on their ability to transport mono- and divalent cations and the presence (or absence) of a common glycoside moiety found in five distinct polyethers (2). The classes are illustrated in Figures 1–3. Using this method, most polyether antibiotics are classified as monovalent (Table 1) based on their ability to transport monobasic cations into a lipophilic environment more efficiently than dibasic cations. The second class, called monovalent monoglycosides (Table 2) have 2,3,6-trideoxy-4-*O*-methyl-D-erythropyranose [65104-53-2] moieties attached as an α-glycoside in A 204, and as a β-glycoside in the other four antibiotics of the monovalent monoglycoside class. The number of divalent polyether antibiotics (Table 3) is much lower than that belonging to the two classes of monovalent polyethers.

Table 1. Monovalent Polyether Antibiotics

Antibiotic	Structure	Producing *Streptomyces*	Culture collection no.	References
		R	R'	R"			
monesin		CH$_3$ CH(CH$_3$)CO$_2$H C$_2$H$_5$	*S. cinnamonensis*	ATCC 15413, NRRL 11588	3
factor B		CH$_3$ CH(CH$_3$)CO$_2$H CH$_3$			
factor C		CH$_3$ (CH$_2$)$_3$CO$_2$H CH$_3$			
laidlomycin		COCH$_2$CH$_3$ CH(CH$_3$)CO$_2$H CH$_3$	*S. eurocidicus*		4
nigericin [antibiotic X 464, polyetherin A, helixin C, antibiotic K 178, and azolomycin M]	R = OH	*S. violaceoniger*	NRRL B1356	5–10
grisorixin	R = H	*S. griseus*		11

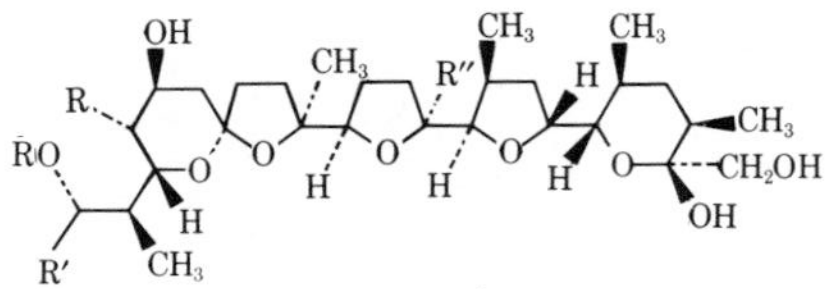

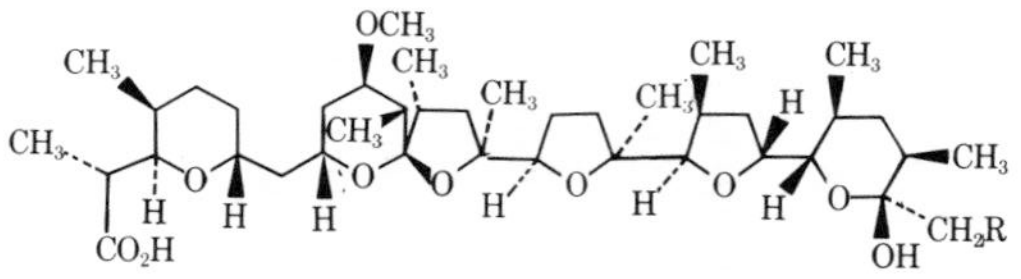

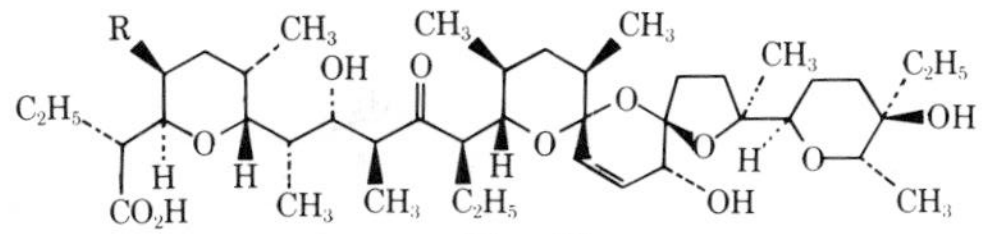

salinomycin
narasin (A28086)

R = H
R = CH$_3$

Ionomycin [58785-63-0]
[antibiotic DE 3936,
emericid, and antibiotic
A 218]

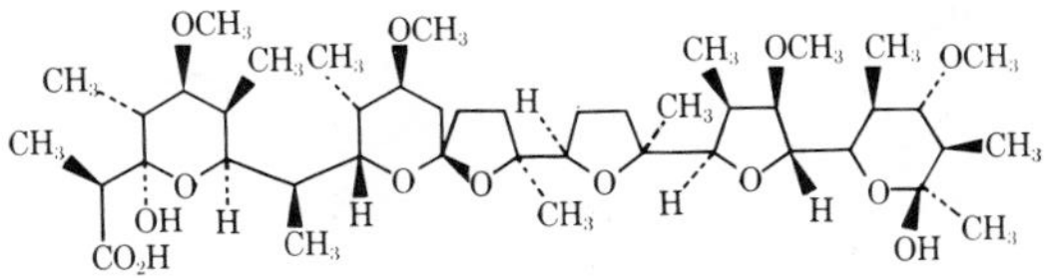

antibiotic X 206
alborixin

	R	R'	R''
	H	H	OH
	CH$_3$	OH	H

S. albus 80614
S. aureofaciens

S. ribocidificus TM

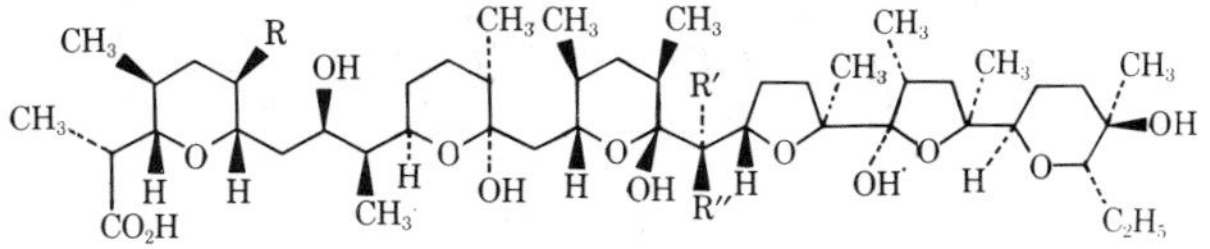

Streptomyces sp X 206
S. albus

ATCC 21838
NRRL 5758,
8092

ATCC 31051

12
13

14

18
19

Table 2. Monovalent Monoglycoside Polyethers

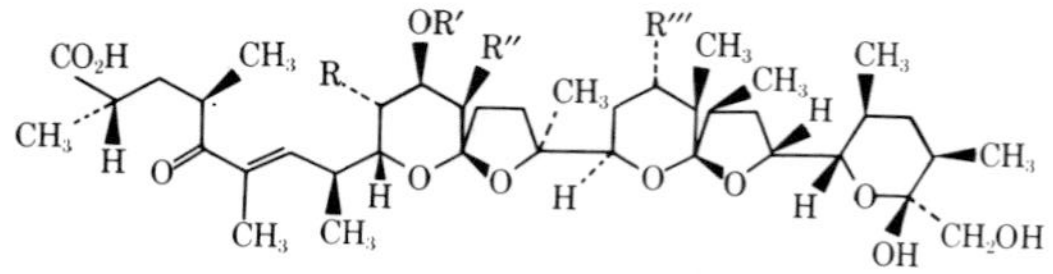

Antibiotic	Structure				Producing *Streptomyces*	Culture collection no.	References
	R	R'	R''	R'''			
dianemycin	CH$_3$	H	H	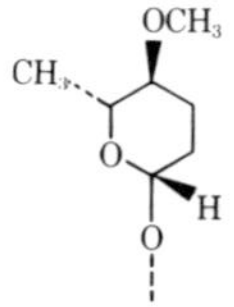	*S. hydroscopicus*	NRRL 3444	20
lenoremycin Ro 21-6150	H	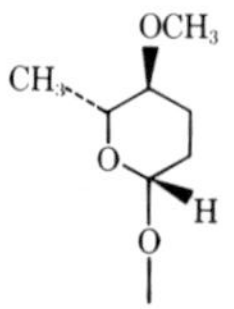	CH$_3$	H	*S. hygroscopicus* X-14563		21

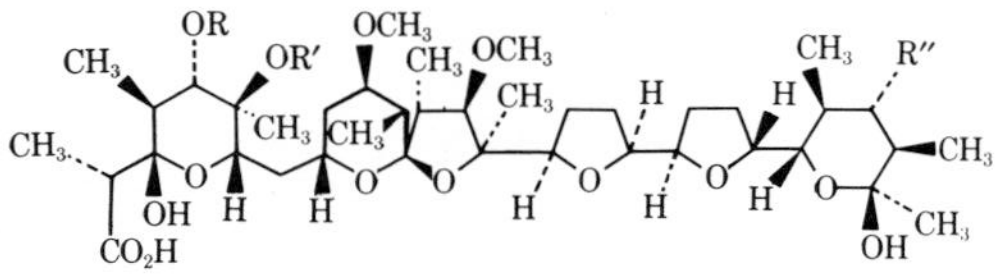

septamycin [*54927-63-8*]
[antibiotic A 28695A]

antibiotic 204A

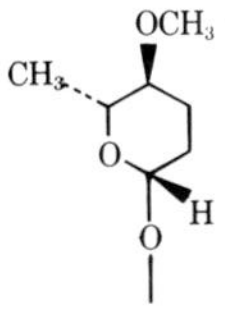

etheromycin
[antibiotic CP 38295]

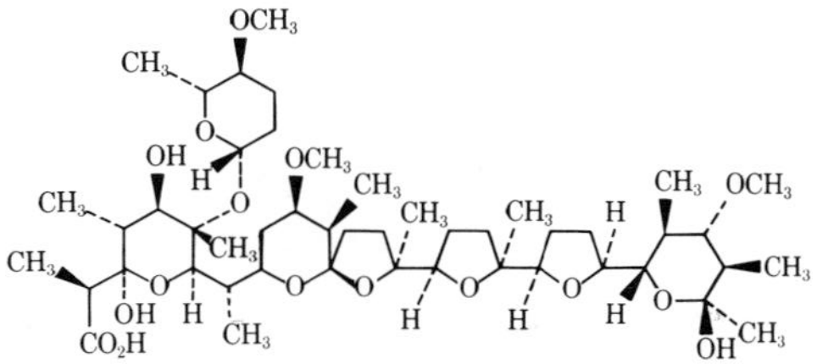

	R	R'	R''
	CH₃		H
		OCH₃	OCH₃

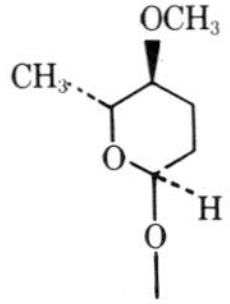

S. hygroscopicus   NRRL 5678   22–23

S. albus   NRRL 3384   24

S. hygroscopicus   ATOC 31050   25–26

Table 3. Divalent Polyether Antibiotics

Antibiotic	Structure	Producing *Streptomyces*	Culture collection no.	References
lasalocid A				27–28
		S. lasaliensis	NRRL 3382, ATCC 31180	29
				29
				29
				29
iso-lasalocid A	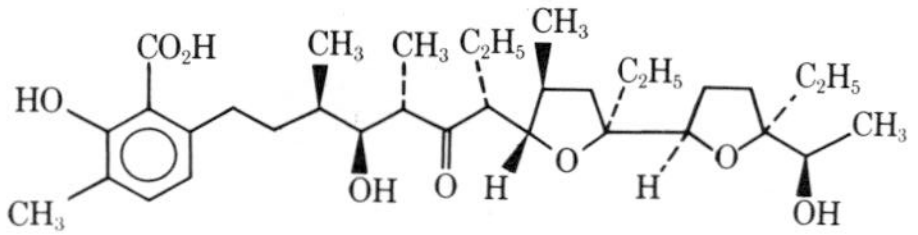	*S. lasaliensis*		30
lysocellin [55898-33-4]		*S. cacaoi var. ascensis*		31
antibiotic A23187		*S. longwoodensis*	ATCC 20251	32
		S. chartreusensis	NRRL 3882	33

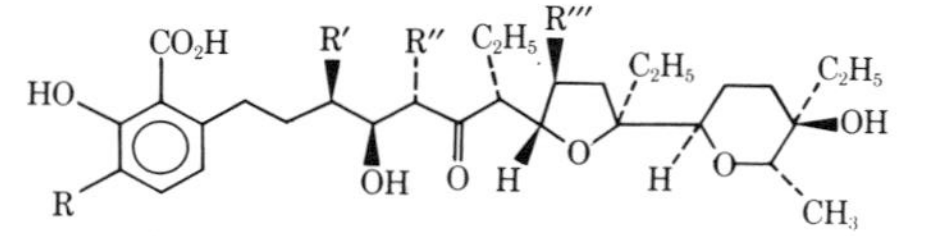

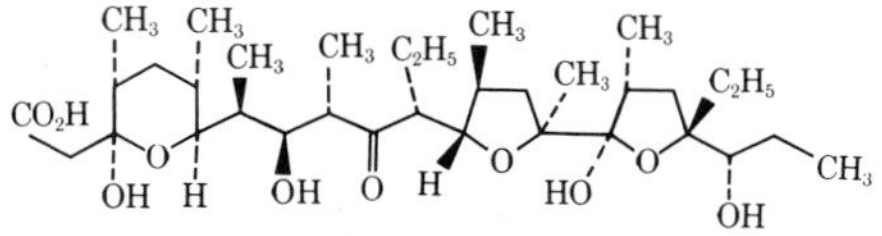

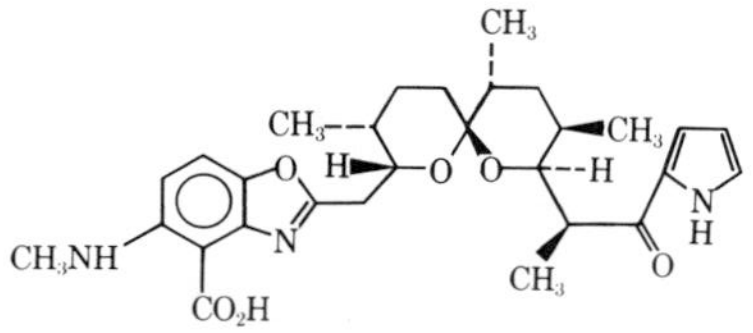

For lasalocid A series:

	R	R'	R''	R'''
A	CH_3	CH_3	CH_3	CH_3
B	C_2H_5	CH_3	CH_3	CH_3
C	CH_3	C_2H_5	CH_3	CH_3
D	CH_3	CH_3	C_2H_5	CH_3
E	CH_3	CH_3	CH_3	C_2H_5

To demonstrate the kind of differences that monovalent and divalent polyethers exhibit in transporting different cations across triply stacked synthetic membrane systems, the results of two different studies on lasalocid (1), a divalent polyether, and salinomycin (34), a monovalent polyether, are summarized in Table 4.

Physical Properties

Selected physical constants of the polyether antibiotics are listed in Table 5.

Although not recognized as polyether antibiotics at the time, the isolations of the first antibiotics of this class were reported in 1951. They consisted of nigericin (5,35), antibiotics X 206, X 464 (later shown to be identical to nigericin), and X 537A (lasalocid). Little interest was stirred by these early results because of the compounds' high parenteral toxicity (mouse LD_{50} of all of them was less than 100 mg/kg intraperitoneal, ip). However, sixteen years later the structure of monensin was published (36) and in 1968, workers at the Eli Lilly Laboratories revealed that monensin, nigericin, dianemycin, and X 206 were orally effective in the control of coccidial infections in poultry (37). Because of the potential market for coccidiostats (20–30 million dollars in the United States alone), this report prompted a number of laboratories to start actively searching for polyethers and by 1976 over thirty distinct compounds of this type had been reported (2).

Twenty-five polyether antibiotics have had their structure elucidated by a combination of x-ray analysis and mass spectrometry. One of the original polyethers isolated in 1951, nigericin, was the second polyether antibiotic to be structurally elucidated by x-ray analysis of a heavy atom salt (8–10,38). The structure of nigericin is similar in several ways to monensin (36). In addition to the C-methyl substitution patterns of the two antibiotics, three features in common are a spiro-ketal group, a methoxy group, and a hydroxymethyl group.

Other polyether antibiotics possessing two of these three features are laidlomycin (39) and grisorixin (11).

The two other antibiotics isolated in 1951 (at Hoffmann-La Roche) were antibiotics X 206 and X 537A (lasalocid). When the structures of these were elucidated, they were found to lack all three of the features common to monensin and nigericin and in particular, both X 206 and lasalocid are devoid of spiro-ketal groups.

Antibiotic X 206 was shown to have the longest carbon backbone (C_{36}) to date (monensin is C_{26} and nigericin C_{30}) and yet the correct structure of this large molecule was solved by x-ray analysis of the free acid monohydrate (18). The carbon backbone or skeleton refers to the longest chain of contiguous carbons between the carboxyl

Table 4. Bulk Phase Transport Capacities[a] of Lasalocid and Salinomycin

Cation	Diameter of cation, nm	Initial transport rates, mol/h	
		Lasalocid	Salinomycin
Na^+	0.190	39	95
Rb^+	0.296	45	105
Cs^+	0.338	118	
Ca^{2+}	0.198	119	6
Ba^{2+}	0.270	89	

[a] For experimental details see Refs. 1 and 34.

Table 5. Physical Constants of the Polyether Antibiotics

Antibiotic	CAS Registry No.	Molecular formula	Molecular weight	Melting point, °C	$[\alpha]_D$ CHCl₃	$[\alpha]_D$ CH₃OH
monensin						
free acid	[17090-79-8]	$C_{36}H_{62}O_{11} \cdot H_2O$	688.9	103–105	+51° [a]	+47.7°
sodium salt	[22373-78-0]	$C_{36}H_{61}O_{11}Na \cdot 2H_2O$	728.9	267–269	+75° [a]	+57.3°
factor B	[30485-16-6]	$C_{35}H_{60}O_{11}$	656.9	227–228		
factor C	[31980-87-7]	$C_{37}H_{64}O_{11}$	684.9	212–214		
factor D	[65208-36-8]	$C_{37}H_{64}O_{11}$	684.9	251–252		
laidlomycin						
free acid	[56283-74-0]	$C_{37}H_{62}O_{12}$	698.9	151–153	+51.3°	
sodium salt	[61489-98-3]	$C_{37}H_{61}O_{12}Na$	720.9	277–279	+78.9°	
nigericin (X 464)						
free acid	[28380-24-7]	$C_{40}H_{68}O_{11}$	725.0	183–185	+35.2°	+9.2°
sodium salt	[33775-57-4]	$C_{40}H_{67}O_{11}Na$	747.0	245–255	+2° [a]	+7.8°
grisorixin						
free acid	[31357-58-1]	$C_{40}H_{68}O_{10}$	709.0	75–78	+16°	
sodium salt	[34052-60-3]	$C_{40}H_{67}O_{10}Na$	731.0	242–246	(acetone)	
salinomycin						
free acid	[53003-10-4]	$C_{42}H_{70}O_{11}$	751.0	113		−63°
sodium salt	[55721-31-8]	$C_{42}H_{69}O_{11}Na$	773.0	140–142		−37°
narasin (A 28086A)						
free acid	[55134-13-9]	$C_{43}H_{72}O_{11}$	765.0	98–100		−54°
sodium salt	[58331-17-2]	$C_{43}H_{71}O_{11}Na$	787.0	114–124[a]		−55° [a]
A-28086B	[58439-49-9]	$C_{43}H_{70}O_{11}$	763.0	150–153		
A-28086D	[58334-78-4]	$C_{44}H_{74}O_{11}$	779.1	96–98		−56°
lonomycin (emericid, DE 3936, A 218)						
sodium salt	[58845-80-0]	$C_{44}H_{75}O_{14}Na$	851.1	188–189	+67°	+47°
X 206						
free acid	[36505-48-3]	$C_{47}H_{82}O_{14} \cdot H_2O$	889.2	133–145	−1.9°	+17.7°
sodium salt	[65104-52-1]	$C_{47}H_{81}O_{14}Na$	893.1	189–190	+21°	+15°
alborixin						
free acid	[57760-36-8]	$C_{48}H_{84}O_{14}$	885.2	100–115	−7°	
potassium salt	[57684-41-0]	$C_{48}H_{83}O_{14}K$	923.3	209–210	(acetone)	
dianemycin						
free acid	[35865-33-9]	$C_{47}H_{78}O_{14} \cdot H_2O$	885.1	156–157		+39.9°
sodium salt	[65101-87-3]	$C_{47}H_{77}O_{14}Na$	889.1	212		+37.1°
lenoremycin (Ro 21-6150)						
free acid	[51257-84-2]	$C_{47}H_{78}O_{13}$	851.1		+71°	+45° [a]
sodium salt	[58399-44-3]	$C_{47}H_{77}O_{13}Na$	873.1	235	+95°	+94° [a]
septamycin (A 28695A)						
sodium salt	[55924-40-8]	$C_{48}H_{81}O_{16}Na$	937.2			+19.1°
A 204A						
free acid	[43110-10-7]	$C_{49}H_{84}O_{17}$	945.2	96–98		+68.1°
sodium salt	[43110-06-1]	$C_{49}H_{83}O_{17}Na \cdot C_3H_6O$	1025.3	144–145		+55°
A 204B						
sodium salt	[65208-37-9]	$C_{50}H_{85}O_{17}Na$	981.2	177–179		+42.3°
etheromycin (CP 38295)						
free acid	[59149-05-2]	$C_{48}H_{82}O_{16}$	915.2	135–138		+38°
sodium salt	[59202-85-6]	$C_{48}H_{81}O_{16}Na$	937.1	197–198		+38°

Table 5 (*continued*)

Antibiotic	CAS Registry No.	Molecular formula	Molecular weight	Melting point, °C	$[\alpha]_D$ CHCl$_3$	CH$_3$OH
lasalocid A (X 537A)						
free acid	[25999-31-9]	C$_{34}$H$_{54}$O$_8$.C$_2$H$_6$O	636.9	100–109	−39.8°	−7.6°
sodium salt	[25999-20-6]	C$_{34}$H$_{53}$O$_8$Na	612.8	168–171	−84.6°	−30°
lasalocid B	[55051-86-0]	C$_{35}$H$_{56}$O$_8$	604.8	85–87	−36.3°	
lasalocid C	[55051-84-8]	C$_{35}$H$_{56}$O$_8$.C$_3$H$_8$O	664.9	97–100	−52.7°	
lasalocid D	[55051-82-6]	C$_{35}$H$_{56}$O$_8$.C$_3$H$_8$O	664.9	102–104	−63.6°	
lasalocid E						
free acid	[55051-80-4]	C$_{35}$H$_{56}$O$_8$	604.8	90	−42.1°	
sodium salt	[57761-60-1]	C$_{35}$H$_{55}$O$_8$Na	626.8	181–182	−79.5°	
iso-lasalocid A						
free acid	[54156-67-1]	C$_{34}$H$_{54}$O$_8$	590.8	203	−39.2°	
sodium salt	[57793-47-2]	C$_{34}$H$_{53}$O$_8$Na	612.8	183–185	−93.9°	
lysocellin						
sodium, hemihydrate	[55898-33-4]	C$_{34}$H$_{59}$O$_{10}$Na.1/2H$_2$O	659.8	158–160	+9.9° [a]	+11.5°
A 23187	[52665-69-7]	C$_{29}$H$_{37}$N$_3$O$_6$	523.6	181–182	−56° [a]	
BL 580α, sodium salt (A 28695A)	[65208-39-1]	C$_{38}$H$_{65}$O$_{12}$Na [b]	711.0	173–175[a]	+16° [a]	+15.6°
BL 580β, sodium salt (A 28695B)	[65208-38-0]	C$_{36}$H$_{57}$O$_{12}$Na [b]	641.0		+1.1°	
ionomycin						
calcium salt	[56092-82-1]	C$_{41}$H$_{70}$O$_9$Ca	746.0	205		
30,504 RP	[57515-31-8]	C$_{48}$H$_{76}$O$_{11}$ [b]	829.0	200		−79°
K 41						
sodium salt	[65208-40-4]	C$_{41}$H$_{69}$O$_{16}$Na	857.0	196–198		+1.9°

[a] New data from the author's laboratory.

[b] Molecular formula calculated from microanalytical data reported in the patent literature.

group and the terminal carbon, and equals twice the number of subunits involved in the biosynthesis of the antibiotic. This observation has been proposed as the basis of a universal numbering system for the polyethers (40) as illustrated for the carbons of lenoremycin (1) and in Figure 1 for the oxygens of antibiotic X 206.

Antibiotic X 206 free acid, hydrate was shown by x-ray analysis to have a cyclic conformation in the crystalline state with the two ends of the molecule held together by a hydrogen bond between the carboxyl oxygen and a terminal hydroxyl at O-14.

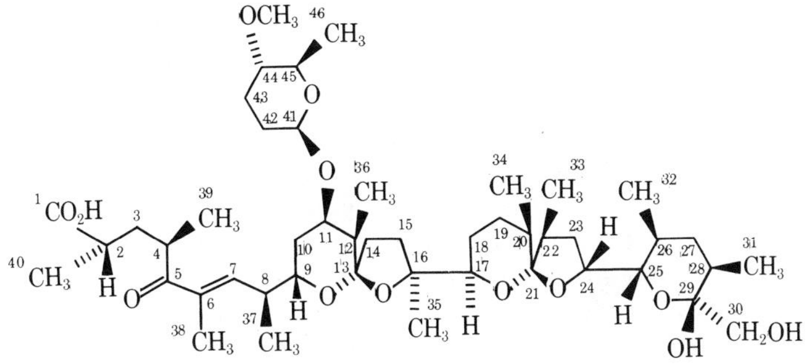

(1)

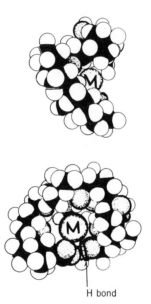

Figure 1. Two views of a CPK (Corey-Pauling-Koltun) model (41) of X 206 from the x-ray analysis of the antibiotic. In the upper picture, the tennis ball seam conformation can be discerned. The lower view accentuates the carboxyl to hydroxyl (O-14) hydrogen bond holding the two ends of the molecule together.

This characteristic cyclic structure has been found in all the polyethers with the exception of salinomycin (where an ester derivative was used for x-ray analysis). In the case of antibiotic X 206, this cyclic structure folds in such a way that the carbon backbone describes a path similar to that of the seam on a tennis ball (18) with the alkali metal cation, M (Fig. 1) or a water molecule held securely in the center.

The structure of lasalocid (Table 3) was determined in 1970 (27–28) and found to have a number of features that had not been previously reported for a polyether antibiotic. The molecular weight (590) was considerably lower than those of the other polyethers which ranged from 700 to 900. Lasalocid was found to contain an aromatic chromophore, which together with three C-ethyl groups (an unprecedented number among natural products) prompted an investigation into the biosynthesis of the antibiotic (42). This study revealed that lasalocid was derived basically from three types of subunit; butyrate, propionate, and acetate via the coenzyme A esters of 2-ethylmalonate, 2-methylmalonate, and malonate, respectively (43–44). These results represented the first illustration of butyrate incorporation to form a C-ethyl group and have since been confirmed in biosynthetic studies of monensin (45) and narasin (7).

The cyclic structure found in X 206 (Fig. 1) is also present in the complexes of lasalocid, but unlike the C_{36} backbone of X 206, the considerably shorter C_{24} backbone of lasalocid does not permit the cyclic structure to fold any further, resulting in two distinct surfaces for the lasalocid complex, one of which is considerably more polar than the other (Fig. 2). This accounts for the dimeric complexes lasalocid forms (as revealed by x-ray analysis), consisting of two monovalent or one divalent cation surrounded by two lasalocid molecules per unit cell (46–47). These dimeric complexes can be thought of as a pair of saucers with polar concave surfaces entrapping the cation while the lipophilic, convex outer surfaces render the lipid membrane permeable to the cation.

The versatility of lasalocid in complexing cations ranging in size and valency from Na^+ to Cs^+ and Ba^{2+} (Table 6) is due to the fact that all the oxygens, except O-3 being available for ligand formation, and the ability to form dimeric complexes gives the antibiotic more flexibility in accommodating different cations by simply adjusting the separation and orientation of the two lasalocid molecules.

With lasalocid, the barium cation, although by far the most strongly complexed, is not the most rapidly transported. There is an optimal binding constant for these salt complexes that allows facile association to occur on the concentrated (cation) side of a membrane but equally facile dissociation to occur at the second lipid–water in-

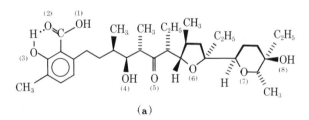

(a)

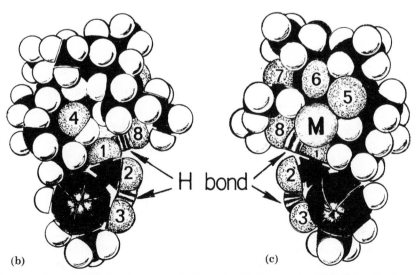

(b)   (c)

Figure 2.   Lasalocid (**a**) showing the numbering system for the oxygens. CPK (Corey-Pauling-Koltun) model of a lasalocid salt showing the conformation in the crystalline state from both the polar (**b**) and lipophilic sides (**c**) of the molecule.

terface where the cation is released in exchange for a proton on the more dilute aqueous side of the membrane (Table 6). This process is known as passive diffusion (48).

The first monovalent monoglycoside to have its structure elucidated was dianemycin, in 1971 (20). Shown to have the 2,3,6-trideoxy-4-O-methyl-D-erythropyranose present as a β-glycoside, the dianemycin molecule also contains an α,β-unsaturated ketone and two spiro-ketal groups. The three polyethers (monensin (49), nigericin, and dianemycin) are found to exhibit similar ion selectivities as summarized in Table 6. However monensin, which is rather specific for sodium, forms a rigid complex and nigericin has the ability to rotate the carboxylate group according to the cation complexed. The most flexible of these three polyethers is dianemycin which can adopt conformations to form almost equally stable complexes with sodium, potassium, rubidium, or cesium (50).

The first reported α-glycoside polyether, in 1973, was antibiotic A 204 (24). Unlike dianemycin, A 204 contains five methoxyl groups and one spiro-ketal (dianemycin has no methoxyls, but two spiro-ketals). Antibiotic A 204 is the most toxic of the polyethers described up to 1976 with oral LD_{50} values in mice of 8–10 mg/kg (51). A similar monovalent monoglycoside polyether with the β-configuration, reported in 1976, is antibiotic CP 38295 (25) (etheromycin (26)) which was shown to contain three methoxyls and one spiro-ketal function.

The aglycone parts of the five polyether glycosides as well as nigericin, grisorixin, laidlomycin, and lonomycin, have C_{30} carbon skeletons. The structure of lonomycin can best be described as the aglycone of a septamycin type (four methoxyls, one spiro-ketal) glycoside. The C_{30} backbone is by far the most frequently occurring carbon skeleton and implies a preference on the part of the *Streptomyces* to biosynthesize polyethers from fifteen subunits.

Some time after the isolation and characterization of salinomycin from *Streptomyces albus* 80614 had been reported by Kaken (12) the same culture (ATTC 21838) was examined by the group at Hoffmann-La Roche (52) who isolated two C-17 epimers of deoxy-(O-8)-salinomycin. The major metabolite described in the later study was epi-17-deoxy-(O-8)-salinomycin (Fig. 3) which was present at three to four times the level of the two other products, salinomycin and deoxy-(O-8)-salinomycin. The change in configuration at just one (C-17) of the forty-two carbons in the two molecules shown

Table 6.   Cation Selectivity[a] of Polyether Antibiotics as Determined by Either Fluorimetric or Two-Phase Distribution Studies[b]

Antibiotic	Mol wt	Cation selectivity
lasalocid	590	$Ba^{2+} \gg Cs^+ > Rb^+, K^+ > Na^+, Ca^{2+}, Mg^{2+} > Li^+$
monensin	671	$Na^+ \gg K^+ > Rb^+ > Li^+ > Cs^+$
nigericin	724	$K^+ > Rb^+ > Na^+ > Cs^+ > Li^+$
salinomycin	750	$K^+ > Na^+ > Cs^+ \gg Ca^{2+}$
dianemycin	866	$Na^+, K^+ > Rb^+, Cs^+ > Li^+$
antibiotic X-206	870	$K^+ > Rb^+ > Na^+ > Cs^+ > Li^+$

[a] Lyotropic series (with ionic radii in nm) are: Cs^+ (0.169) > Rb^+ (0.148) > K^+ (0.133) > Na^+ (0.095) > Li^+ (0.060) and Ba^{2+} (0.135) > Sr^{2+} (0.113) > Ca^{2+} (0.099) > Mg^{2+} (0.065).

[b] Ref. 1.

in Figure 3 results in a profound alteration in conformation from the U-shaped sali-nomycin molecule to the remarkably linear epi-17-deoxy-(O-8)-salinomycin [64129-77-7].

The second tricyclo-spiroketal polyether reported was narasin and the structure was assigned by mass spectral comparison with salinomycin. The only difference be-tween the two antibiotics is an extra C-methyl in the case'of narasin at C-4 (53). A

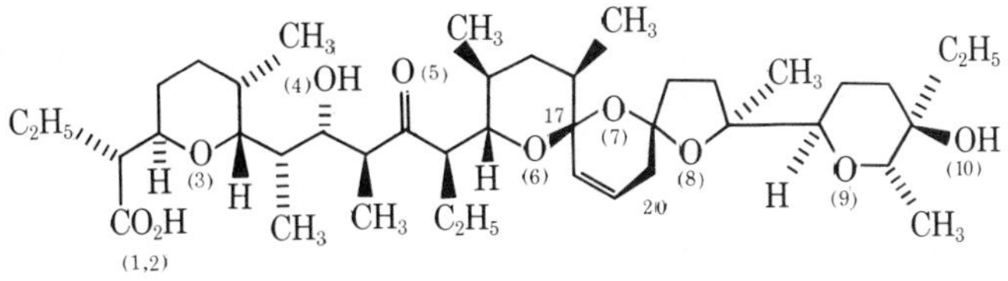

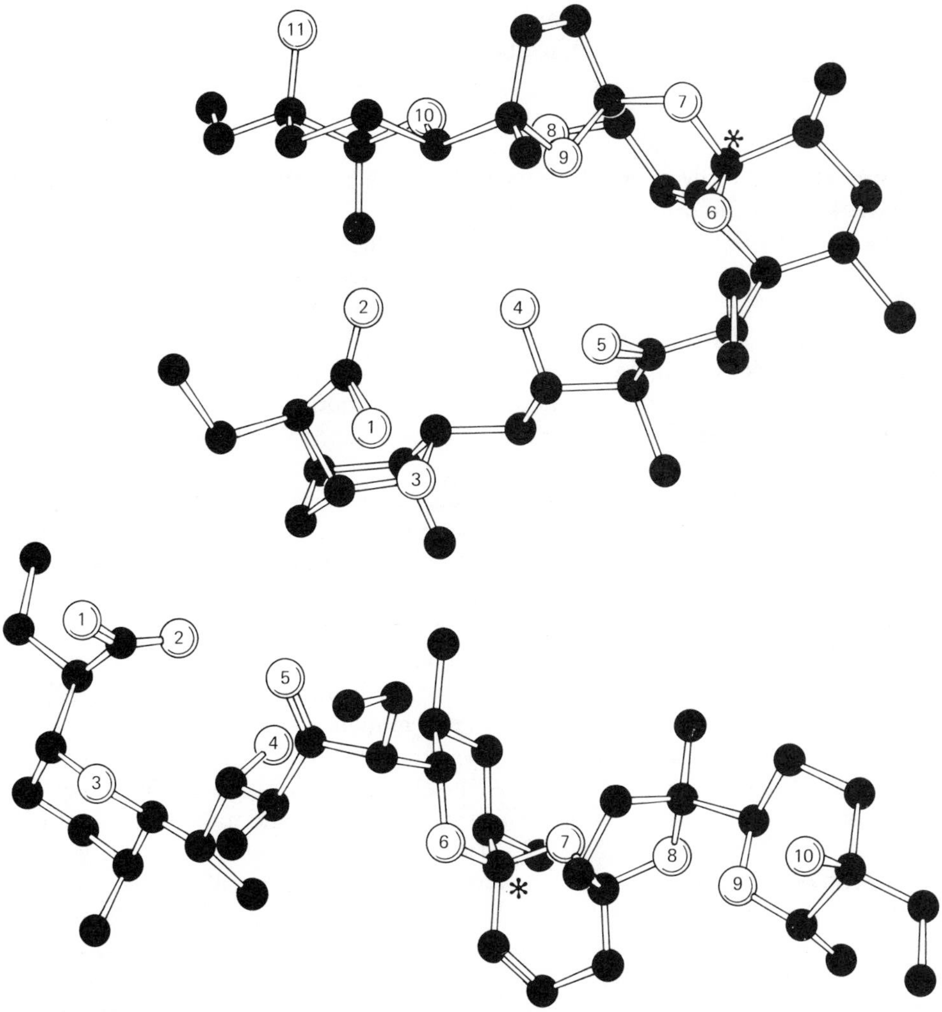

Figure 3. Comparison of the salinomycin (upper) and *epi*-17-deoxy-(O-8)-salinomycin (lower) conformations in the crystalline state with the C-17 carbon labeled with an asterisk.

second component of the narasin complex (A 28086B) has an allylic ketone function in place of the alcohol in narasin. An alternative way of classifying the monovalent polyethers does not rest on the glycoside differences shown in Tables 1 and 2; it has the following breakdown of monovalent polyethers:

no spiro-ketals	alborixin and antibiotic X 206
single spiro-ketals	monensin, nigericin, grisorixin, and laidlomycin
double spiro-ketals	dianemycin and lenoremycin (Ro 21-6150)
trispiro-ketals	salinomycin and narasin
multimethoxyls	lonomycin, septamycin, A 204, and etheromycin

Antibiotic A 23187 (Table 3) is not, strictly speaking, a polyether antibiotic because the molecule contains three nitrogens, but because of the similarity in transporting properties to the divalent polyethers, the antibiotic has been included as the first of the pyrrole-ethers (33,54). Antibiotic A 23187 is the most specific of the divalent antibiotics and shows no affinity for the alkali metals. In comparing the divalent polyethers and A 23187 for their relative affinities as measured in a U-tube transport system with chloroform as the organic phase, the following results were obtained:

(1) Transport of $^{86}Rb^+$: lasalocid, iso-lasalocid, lysocellin $\gg$ A 23187

(2) Transport of $^{45}Ca^{2+}$: lasalocid, A 23187 > lysocellin > iso-lasalocid

Biological Activity

Antimicrobial Activity and Toxicity in Mice. The antimicrobial spectra of the polyethers do not help in resolving the question of classification. The most active antibiotics *in vitro* are nigericin, grisorixin, X 206, lenoremycin (Ro 21-6150), lysocellin, and A 23187 (Table 7). The mechanism of the antimicrobial action is not yet known, but loss of K^+ ions is a possibility, by analogy with valinomycin (55). However, another mechanism must also operate for the A 23187 pyrrole–ether which is very specific for dibasic cations. Some support for the two distinct mechanisms of action comes from a closer study of the spectra in Table 7. The most sensitive microorganism for all the monovalent polyethers is *Bacillus* sp *E,* whereas *Sarcina lutea* is most sensitive to A 23187.

The *in vitro* spectra are of limited value, however, because of the lack of correlation with *in vivo* data. For instance although nigericin is the most active polyether *in vitro,* the two commercially used antibiotics monensin and lasalocid are among the least active *in vitro* according to the results in Table 7.

Toxicity of Polyether Antibiotics. The acute toxicity of the polyether antibiotics in mice (Table 7) ranges from LD_{50} of 1–250 mg/kg (ip) and 8–1000 mg/kg, oral (po). The most toxic of the antibiotics (LD_{50} < 20 mg/kg, ip and < 50 mg/kg, po) are X 206, A 204A, A 23187, lonomycin, salinomycin, and monensin.

Lasalocid, nigericin, and lysocellin have virtually identical LD_{50} at 65 mg/kg (ip) but the least toxic of those reported is iso-lasalocid with an LD_{50} of 250 mg/kg (ip).

In most cases, the drugs are only moderately absorbed and using the ratio of LD_{50} (po)–LD_{50} (ip) as a measure, they fall between 3 and 5:1.

Coccidiostat Activity. *Coccidia,* an order of protozoa of the subphylum *Sporozoa,* are parasitic in the epithelial cells of the internal tract of birds and mammals. Included among the genera found most commonly in the avian species such as poultry are *Eimeria.* Coccidiostats are agents that when mixed with feed at approximately 100 ppm, control infections of *Coccidia* and are particularly important agents to the poultry industry.

Table 7. _In Vitro_ Antimicrobial Activity and Toxicity of the Polyether Antibiotics

Polyether antibiotic	Staph. aureus ATCC No. 6538P	Sarcina lutea 9341	Bacillus sp E 27859	Bacillus subtilis 558[b]	Bacillus megaterium 8011	Bacillus sp TA 27860	Mycobacterium phlei 355	Streptomyces cellulosae 3313	Paecilomyces varioti 26820	Toxicity in mice, LD$_{50}$, mg/kg[c] ip	po
				Minimum inhibitory concentration, μg/mL[a]							
monensin (A3823)	3.1	12.5	0.4	1.6	3.1	1.6	12.5	6.3	d	16.8	43.8[e]
nigericin (X 464)	0.2	0.1	0.004	0.1	0.1	0.02	0.4	0.4	0.8	65	190
grisorixin	0.4	0.2	0.1	0.2	0.1	0.4	0.2	0.2	3.1		
salinomycin	3.1	3.1	0.2	0.8	0.2	0.8	6.3	3.1	3.1	18	50[f]
narasin (A 28086A)	0.8	1.6	0.2	0.9	0.4	0.4	3.1	3.1		12	45
Ionomycin (DE 3936)	1.6	12.5	1.6	3.1	0.8	1.6	12.5	6.3	50	13	45.8[g]
X 206	0.2	0.8	0.02	0.4	0.2	0.2	0.2	0.8	0.8	1.2	17
dianemycin	1.6	3.1	0.2	3.1	3.1	1.6	6.3	6.3	6.3	9	150
lenoremycin (Ro 21-6150)	0.2	0.2	0.02	0.4	0.1	0.4	0.2	1.6	0.8		55
septamycin (A28695A)	0.8	1.6	0.006	1.6	1.6	0.2	1.6	3.1	6.3		41.1[h]
A 204A	3.1	12.5	0.8	6.3	12.5	1.6	12.5	12.5	25		8[i]
CP 38952	12.5	6.3	1.6	6.3	3.1	3.1	3.1	12.5	12.5		
lasalocid (X 537A)	1.6	3.1	0.2	1.6	3.1	1.6	12.5	6.3		64	146
iso-lasalocid	12.6	6.3	1.6	1.6	1.6	3.1	6.3	25	12.5	250	1000
lysocellin	0.8	0.4	0.03	0.2	0.4	0.4	3.1	1.6	1.6	65	350
A 23187	0.2	0.04	0.2	0.1	0.8	0.04	1.6	6.3		10[j]	
BL 580α	0.8	1.6	0.2	0.4	0.4	0.4	3.1	3.1		14	220
ionomycin		12.5	12.5	25	6.3		3.1			12	650

[a] Lowest two-fold dilution giving zone of inhibition in agar-well diffusion assay.
[b] NRRL collection number.
[c] 24 h acute toxicities unless reference is given.
[d] Indicates no activity up to 50 μg/mL.
[e] Ref. 56.
[f] Ref. 57.
[g] Ref. 58.
[h] Ref. 23.
[i] Ref. 51.
[j] Ref. 54.

Production. Some examples of the coccidiostat activity of the polyether antibiotics are given in Table 8. The patent for the use of monensin as a coccidiostat was issued to Haney and co-workers of Eli Lilly in 1970 (56) and under the trade name of Coban was marketed the following year. Since that time, monensin has acquired ca 80% of the coccidiostat market. The utility patent for lasalocid as a coccidiostat by Berger (59) of Hoffmann-La Roche was issued three years after the monensin patent and lasalocid was approved by the FDA in October 1976, when the drug entered the market as Avatec.

Ruminant Growth Promotion. Chemical analysis of the fermentation occurring in the rumen of animals, such as cows, sheep, and goats, has revealed a correlation between improved efficiency of feed utilization by the ruminant and an increase in the amount of propionic acid produced in the rumen. The volatile fatty acids (VFA) are produced in the rumen fermentation by microorganisms which degrade carbohydrate present in the diet to pyruvic acid.

Utilization of the VFA occurs after absorption from the gut of the animal. One of the major inefficiencies in the rumen fermentation is the production of acetate (and hence butyrate) which is accomplished with the sacrifice of one of the pyruvate carbons as methane and loss of the associated energy. Any agent, therefore, which tends to direct the fermentation towards propionate production will also result in more efficient utilization of the cellulose which is the major component in the diet of most ruminants.

Several polyether antibiotics have recently been claimed (60) to exhibit the ability of changing the levels of VFA production in favor of propionate as demonstrated by glc analysis of *in vitro* fermentations of rumen fluid (from steers) treated with these antibiotics. The antibiotics are also claimed to benefit monogastric animals, such as horses, swine, and rabbits, which ferment fibrous vegetable matter in the cecum. Monensin has been used in cattle feed since 1976. High toxicity (1–2 mg/kg) has precluded its use in horses (61) (see Pet and other livestock feeds).

Table 8.   Effect of Polyether Antibiotics on Experimental Infections with *Eimeria tenella* in Chickens[a]

Antibiotic	Level tested in diet, ppm	Mortality, %	Weight gain per survivor
uninfected, nontreated control[b]	0	0	100
monensin	110	0	101
infected control	0	80	60
nigericin	200	0	106
infected control	0	80	68
antibiotic X 206	80	0	102
infected control	0	32	37
dianemycin	40	0	50
	20	20	110
	10	60	127
infected control	0	95	lost weight

[a] Ref. 37.

[b] All values are relative to this control in which the weight gain per survivor is normalized to 100.

Optical Resolution

The ability of the polyether antibiotic lasalocid to transport catecholamines across lipid membranes led to an investigation into the nature of the lasalocid–amine complexes. On finding that the naturally occurring R enantiomer of norepinephrine gave a highly crystalline, equimolar salt with lasalocid, there seemed a possibility that the antibiotic might be able to resolve racemic amines by fractional crystallization as lasalocid salts. As a consequence, several types of amines were successfully resolved, and in one case the resolved complex was analyzed by x-ray crystallography. The results of this analysis provided a possible explanation for the high enantioselectivity displayed by lasalocid on preferential crystallization of salts formed from the antibiotic with racemic amines (62).

BIBLIOGRAPHY

1. B. C. Pressman and de Guzman, *Ann. N. Y. Acad. Sci.* **264,** 373 (1975).
2. J. W. Westley, *Adv. Appl. Microbiol.* (1977).
3. M. Gorman, J. W. Chamberlin, and L. Hamill, *Antimicrob. Agents Chemother.* **1967,** 363 (1968).
4. F. Kitame and N. Ishida, *J. Antibiot.* **29,** 759 (1976).
5. J. Berger and co-workers, *J. Am. Chem. Soc.* **73,** 5295 (1951).
6. T. Kubota and co-workers, *Chem. Commun.* 1541 (1968).
7. D. E. Dorman and co-workers, *Helv. Chim. Acta.* **59,** 2625 (1976).
8. L. K. Steinrauf, M. Pinkerton, and J. W. Chamberlin, *Biochem. Biophys. Res. Commun.* **33,** 29 (1968).
9. L. Horvath, L. Lovrekovich, and J. M. Varga, *Z. Allg. Mikrobiol.* **4,** 236 (1964).
10. Jpn. Pat. 13,791 (1966), H. Okazaki and M. Arai (to Sankyo Co. Ltd.).
11. P. Gachon and co-workers, *Chem. Commun.* 1421 (1970).
12. H. Kinashi, N. Otake, and H. Yonehara, *Tetrahedron Lett.* **49,** 4955 (1973).
13. Belg. Pat. 830,043 (Oct. 12, 1975), D. H. Berg and co-workers (to Eli Lilly & Co.).
14. S. Omura and co-workers, *J. Antibiot.* **29,** 15 (1976).
15. M. Oshima and co-workers, *J. Antibiot.* **29,** 354 (1976).
16. C. Riche and C. Pascard-Billy, *Chem. Commun.* 951 (1975).
17. N. Tsuji and co-workers, *J. Antibiot.* **29,** 10 (1976).
18. J. F. Blount and J. W. Westley, *Chem. Commun.* 533 (1975).
19. M. Alleaume and co-workers, *Chem. Commun.* 411 (1975).
20. E. W. Czerwinski and L. K. Steinrauf, *Biochem. Biophys. Res. Commun.* **45,** 1284 (1971).
21. J. F. Blount and co-workers, *Chem. Commun.* 853 (1975).
22. T. J. Petcher and H. P. Weber, *Chem. Commun.* 697 (1974).
23. U.S. Pat. 3,839,558 (Oct. 1, 1974), R. L. Hamill and M. M. Hoehn (to Eli Lilly & Co.).
24. N. D. Jones and co-workers, *J. Amer. Chem. Soc.* **95,** 3399 (1973).
25. Belg. Pat. 831,947 (Feb. 2, 1976), W. D. Celmer and co-workers (to Chas. Pfizer Inc.).
26. Y. Kusakabe and co-workers, *Abstract, Annual Meeting of the Agricultural Chemistry Society (Japan)* *1975,* p. 83.
27. J. W. Westley and co-workers, *Chem. Commun.* 71 (1970).
28. S. M. Johnson and co-workers, *J. Am. Chem. Soc.* **92,** 4428 (1970).
29. J. W. Westley and co-workers, *J. Antibiot.* **27,** 597 (1974).
30. J. W. Westley and co-workers, *J. Antibiot.* **27,** 744 (1974).
31. N. Otake and co-workers, *Chem. Commun.* 92 (1975).
32. B. T. La Prosser and N. J. Palleroni, *Intern. J. System. Bact.* **26,** 319 (1976).
33. M. O. Chaney and co-workers, *J. Am. Chem. Soc.* **96,** 1932 (1974).
34. Y. Miyazaki and co-workers, *Agri. Biol. Chem.* **40,** 1963 (1976).
35. R. L. Harned and co-workers, *Antibiot. Chemother.* **1,** 594 (1951).
36. A. Agtarap and co-workers, *J. Am. Chem. Soc.* **89,** 5737 (1967).
37. R. F. Shumard and M. E. Callender, *Antimicrob. Agents Chemother.* **1967,** 359 (1968).
38. R. R. Smeby and co-workers, *Phytopathology* **42,** 506 (1952).

39. F. Kitame and N. Ishida, *J. Antibiot.* **29,** 759 (1976).
40. J. W. Westley, *J. Antibiot.* **29,** 584 (1976).
41. U.S. Pat. 3,170,246 (Feb. 23, 1965), W. L. Koltun (to U.S. Department of Health, Education and Welfare).
42. J. W. Westley and co-workers, *Chem. Commun.* 1467 (1970).
43. J. W. Westley, D. L. Pruess, and R. G. Pitcher, *Chem. Commun.* 161 (1972).
44. J. W. Westley and co-workers, *J. Antibiot.* **27,** 288 (1974).
45. L. E. Day and co-workers, *Antimicrob. Agents Chemother.* **1972,** 410 (1973).
46. C. A. Maier and I. C. Paul, *Chem. Commun.* 181 (1971).
47. E. C. Bissell and I. C. Paul, *Chem. Commun.* 967 (1972).
48. B. C. Pressman, *Ann. Rev. Biochem.* **45,** 501 (1976).
49. W. K. Lutz, F. K. Winkler, and J. D. Dunitz, *Helv. Chim. Acta.* **54,** 1103 (1971).
50. E. W. Cerwinski and L. K. Steinrauf, *Biochem. Biophys. Res. Commun.* **45,** 1284 (1971).
51. H. M. Worth and co-workers, *Antimicrob. Agents Chemother.* **1970,** 357 (1971).
52. J. W. Westley and co-workers, *J. Antibiot.* **30,** 610 (1977).
53. J. L. Occolowitz and co-workers, *Biomed. Mass Spectrosc.* **3,** 272 (1976).
54. U.S. Pat. 3,923,823 (Dec. 2, 1975), R. M. Gale, C. E. Higgins, and M. M. Hoehn (to Eli Lilly & Co.).
55. F. M. Harold and J. R. Baarda, *J. Bacteriol.* **94,** 53 (1967).
56. U.S. Pat. 3,501,568 (March 17, 1970), M. E. Haney, M. M. Hoehn, and J. M. McGuire (to Eli Lilly & Co.).
57. Y. Miyazaki and co-workers, *J. Antibiot.* **27,** 814 (1974).
58. M. Oshima and co-workers, unpublished.
59. U.S. Pat. 3,719,753 (Mar. 6, 1973), J. Berger (to Hoffmann-La Roche Inc.); M. Mitrovic and E. G. Schildknecht, *Poultr. Sci.* **54,** 750 (1975).
60. U.S. Pat. 3,937,836 (Feb. 10, 1976) A. P. Raun (to Eli Lilly & Co.).
61. T. Matsuoka, *J. Am. Vet. Med. Assoc.* **169,** 1098 (1976).
62. J. W. Westley, R. H. Evans, and J. F. Blount, *J. Am. Chem. Soc.* **99,** 6057 (1977).

JOHN W. WESTLEY
Hoffmann-La Roche Inc.

TETRACYCLINES

The tetracyclines are a group of antibiotics having an identical 4-ring carbocyclic structure as a basic skeleton and differing from each other chemically only by substituent variation. The very large number of prescriptions written for tetracyclines is proof of their importance to modern medicine. Certain of these antibiotics have been used in large quantities as additives to the food of meat-producing animals where they improve the efficiency of converting animal feeds to meat protein (see Pet and livestock feeds).

In Figure 1 are names (generic and chemical) and structural formulas of the principal tetracycline derivatives now used commercially.

The first tetracycline discovered, produced by a soil organism, *Streptomyces aureofaciens*, now known as chlortetracycline, was marketed by Lederle Laboratories

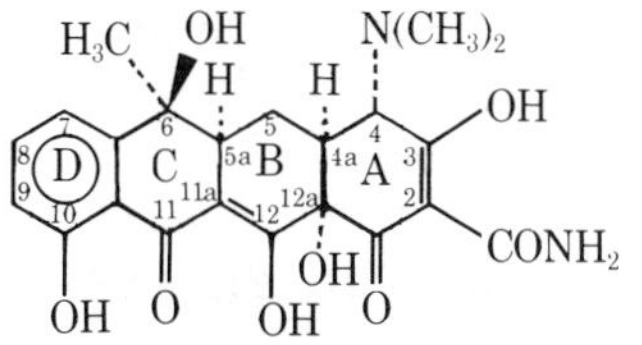

(1)

Tetracycline
[60-54-8]

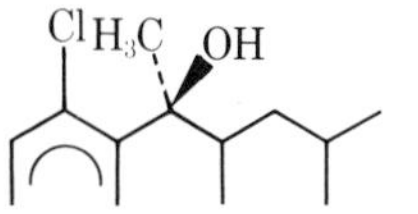

(2)

Chlortetracycline [57-62-5],
7-chlorotetracycline

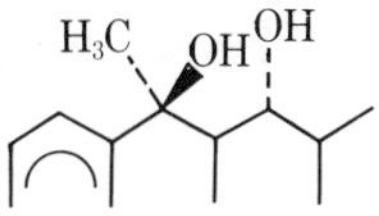

(3)

Oxytetracycline [79-57-2],
5-hydroxytetracycline

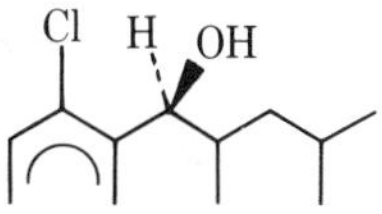

(4)

Demeclocycline [127-33-3],
6-demethyl-7-chlorotetracycline

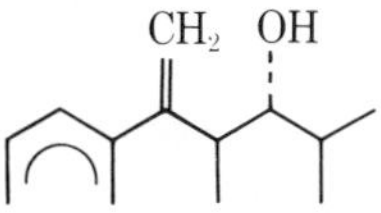

(5)

Methacycline [914-00-1],
6-demethyl-6-deoxy-
5-hydroxy-6-methyl-
enetetracycline

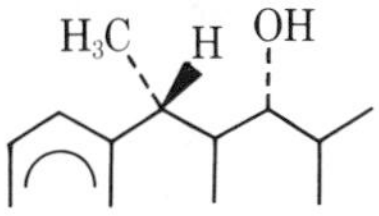

(6)

Doxycycline [564-25-0],
6α-deoxy-5-
hydroxytetracycline

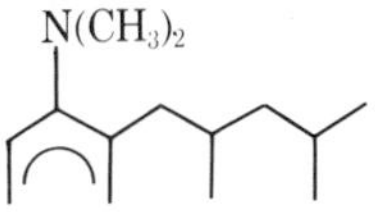

(7)

Minocycline [10118-90-8],
6-demethyl-6-deoxy-
7-dimethylamino
tetracycline

Figure 1.   Principal tetracycline derivatives.

in 1948 (1). This compound ushered in a new era in antibacterial chemotherapy since it was not only effective orally but was also effective against a much wider range of gram-positive and gram-negative bacteria. It was joined by the second member of the family, oxytetracycline, produced by another actinomycete, *Streptomyces rimosus,* and was marketed by Chas. Pfizer & Co. in 1950 (2). Tetracycline (1) was discovered in 1953. It lacks the 7-chloro of chlortetracycline (2) and the 5-hydroxyl group of oxytetracycline (3), and was produced either by reductive dechlorination of (2) (3–4) or by a direct fermentation (5). 6-Demethylchlortetracycline (4) was discovered (6) as a metabolite of a mutant strain of the original *Streptomyces aureofaciens,* and was introduced in 1958.

During this period of development, chemists were seeking to produce better tetracycline antibiotics by chemically modifying the naturally occurring ones (semisynthesis) and by synthesizing them completely. It is significant that the three tetracyclines most recently marketed were made by a semisynthetic pathway. The first of these was methacycline (5), 6-methylene oxytetracycline (7), and its reduction product doxycycline (6) (7–8). The latter compound is a potent antibiotic which is well absorbed and slowly excreted thus allowing small and infrequent (once or twice a day) dosage schedules. Finally, the most recent addition to the commercial tetracyclines is minocycline (7), 7-dimethylamino-6-demethyl-6-deoxytetracycline (9), which is well absorbed and slowly excreted. It protects mice against staphylococcal infections which are resistant to most tetracyclines, penicillins, and many other antibiotics. In addition, it shows a marked superiority over other tetracyclines when tested against large numbers of randomly occurring, hospital-isolated gram-positive bacteria (10).

During the early years (1948–1952) considerable research was devoted to determining the structures of these compounds. The gross structure (3) was determined by a combination of degradation sequences and application of uv and ir spectral studies by Pfizer chemists in collaboration with Woodward (11). Very soon thereafter this same group published the structure (2) (12); simultaneously, a nearly complete structure was arrived at by different degradative pathways by a group of Lederle chemists (13). The more subtle points of structure, such as the stereochemical configurations, were later determined by x-ray methods (14), and the absolute configuration by degradation. The structures of those tetracyclines developed since 1952 were easily arrived at by relating them to the known structures.

Physical Properties

In general, the tetracyclines are yellow crystalline compounds with amphoteric properties. They are soluble in both aqueous acid and aqueous base. The acid salts tend to be soluble in organic solvents such as 1-butanol, dioxane and 2-ethoxyethanol. In fact, 1-butanol is used to extract the salts from aqueous solution.

Each tetracycline possesses a characteristic uv absorption spectrum and this property was used extensively in the structure elucidation (12–13). This spectrum results from the contribution of two chromophores, the BCD ring system and the A ring; the former gives a λ max at approximately 350 nm and the latter gives a λ max at approximately 265 nm. Some representative examples are given below.

Antibiotic	Solvent	λ max, nm	Log ϵ
tetracycline (1)	methanol	268, 363	4.27, 4.17
chlorotetracycline (2)	ethanol	270, 355	4.2, 4.0
oxytetracycline (3)	ethanol	267, 357	4.32, 4.10

During the original structure and chemical modification work, paper chromatography was used to monitor the reactions to determine the composition of the reaction mixture (13,15–16). The tetracyclines are usually detected by uv fluorescence on the paper strip or by bioautography. This latter method uses the antibacterial properties of the tetracyclines by determining what areas on the paper strip inhibit the growth of the microorganism. The transference of paper chromatography solvent systems to column chromatography has been accomplished (43). Recently, high-speed liquid chromatography has been used with excellent success (18).

In the ir spectra, a variety of carbonyl bands are found in the 6.0 μm region. Only when new absorption bands (below 6.0 μm) are generated do the ir spectra become useful.

Mass spectral analysis (19) and nmr (9) have become useful tools for tetracycline structure determinations.

Semisynthetic Modifications

The tetracycline molecule (1) presents a special challenge to the organic chemist who is interested in the study of structure–activity relationships. The difficulty has been to devise chemical pathways that would bring about the necessary transformation, yet preserve the BCD ring chromophore and its antibacterial properties. The lability of the 6-hydroxy group to acid and base degradation (12–13), plus the ease of epimerization (20) at the carbon atom at position 4 contributed to chemical instability under many reaction conditions.

Under acidic conditions, dehydration to an anhydrotetracycline [20154-34-1] (8) occurs, and with base ring C opens to an isotetracycline [3811-31-2] (9). Epimerization (20–22) at C-4 is somewhat more troublesome because it occurs in a variety of solvents within the pH range 2–6, particularly in acetic acid (21). A number of anions (23) facilitate this epimerization. The reverse process, epitetracycline [79-85-6] to tetracycline, is promoted by ions that can chelate such as calcium (24).

Conversion of the C-2 amide to a biologically inactive nitrile (25) has been accomplished using an arylsulfonyl chloride in pyridine as the dehydrating agent. A Ritter reaction on the nitrile (25) yields the corresponding alkylated amide. When the 6-hydroxyl derivatives were used, dehydration occurred at this step to give the anhydro amide. Substituting an N-hydroxymethylimide for isobutylene in the Ritter reaction yields the acylaminomethyl derivative (26). Hydrolysis affords an aminomethyl compound.

Numerous examples (27–31) have been reported of the conversion of a C-2 amide to active Mannich adducts. It should be emphasized that these adducts are extremely labile compounds and easily undergo hydrolysis to the parent tetracycline. This reverse reaction probably accounts for their antibacterial activity.

A considerable effort has been devoted to reactions at the C-4 carbon atom. With the exception of (3), reaction with methyl iodide (32–33) converts the 4-amino group to a quaternary amine with a concomitant loss of antibacterial activity. Treatment of this quaternary derivative with zinc in acetic acid results in a selective removal of the 4-dimethylamino grouping (32). It has been shown (34) that this deamination can be accomplished by photolysis of a tetracycline in methanol for several hours. In this case the stereochemical requirements are more strictly defined since the 4-epitetracyclines will not undergo the photoelimination.

A transformation (15) involving the C-4 position has resulted in the synthesis of 4-hydroxy-6-methylpretetramid [2011-31-6], an important precursor (35) in the biosynthesis of tetracycline.

Another unusual reaction (36–37) involving the C-4 carbon atom has yielded the 4,6-hemiketals. Reactions of (1) or 6-demethyltetracycline [987-02-0] (10) with positive halogens, or cupric or mercuric acetates yields the corresponding 4,6-hemiketals (11) and (12).

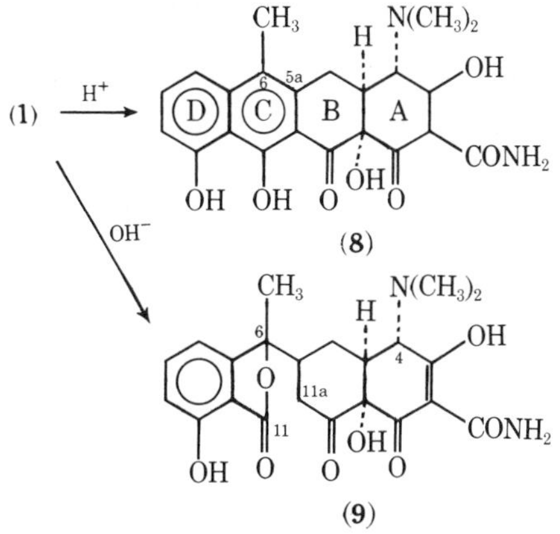

The hemiketal products (11) and (12) have been converted to the corresponding oximes, hydrazones, and substituted amines (36–37). Although many of these derivatives exhibit substantial antibacterial activity, they are generally less active than the parent tetracyclines. Reactions at the C-5 position of the tetracycline molecule have been limited to the introduction of an alkoxy group (38) and the acetylation of the hydroxyl group (39) in 5-hydroxytetracycline. Neither of these modifications improved the biological activity of the molecule.

The original investigations (12–13) on structures (2) and (3) correctly demonstrated the important role played by the C-6 hydroxyl group in the degradative reactions of the molecule. Acid catalyzed dehydration yields (8) and base treatment affords (9). The isoderivatives are biologically inactive; however, the anhydrotetracyclines appear to exhibit a mode of antibacterial action unlike that of tetracycline (40).

The isolation of the 6-deoxytetracyclines (41) permitted substantial progress in the field of chemical modification of (1). 6β-Deoxytetracycline [6746-03-8] (13) was prepared by catalytic hydrogenolysis of tetracycline (1). This reaction results in an inversion (42) of the configuration at the C-6 position with retention of antibacterial activity. Catalytic reduction (7–8) of the 6-methylene derivative (14) yields both the 6α-methyl (15) and 6β-methyl compound (13). The product (15) is also obtained by a free radical addition of a mercaptan to the 6-methylene double bond, followed by desulfurization with Raney Nickel (8). The 6α-isomer (15) is reported (7,42) to be more active than the 6β-isomer (13). The α-isomer (6), doxycycline, is an example of a semisynthetic tetracycline that has become commercial.

The 6-methylene derivatives, (5) and (14), used in the preparation of the 6α-methyl derivatives are prepared (7) from the 11a-halotetracyclines (16) and (17), respectively, followed by dehydration in hydrogen fluoride. The material (5) or (14) is then deblocked by a mild reducing agent, such as sodium hydrosulfite, or by catalytic hydrogenation.

In contrast, the reaction of 11a-chloro-6-demethyltetracycline [22920-22-5] (18) in liquid hydrogen fluoride (17) yielded a mixture of two 6-fluorostereoisomers, (19) and (20). Mild catalytic reduction of either of these compounds yielded the corresponding 6-fluoro derivatives (21) and (22).

The 6-fluoro isomers, (21) and (22), showed relatively high *in vitro* and *in vivo* biological activities compared to the parent tetracyclines.

The increased chemical stability of the 6-deoxytetracyclines helped to address the problem of chemical modification with retention of biological activity by electrophilic substitutions at C-7 and C-9 under strongly acidic conditions (43–50). Reactions of 6-deoxy-6-demethyltetracycline (23) with electrophiles, such as nitrate ion (46), bromomium ion (43–44) (from *N*-bromosuccinimide), or *N*-hydroxymethylphthalimide (50), in strong acid yielded 7-substituted tetracyclines, (24). In the case of the nitration reaction, both the 7- and 9-nitro isomers, (25) and (26), were obtained. A similar series of reactions could be carried out in the 6-methyl series, (13) and (15). Catalytic reduction afforded the amino compounds, ie, (27). These could then be

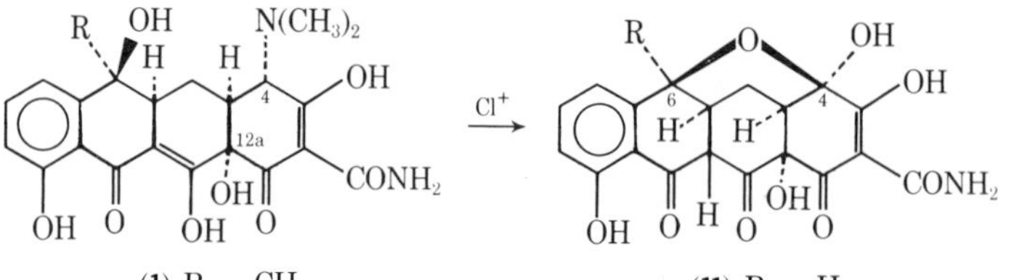

(1) R = CH$_3$
(10) R = H

(11) R = H
(12) R = CH$_3$

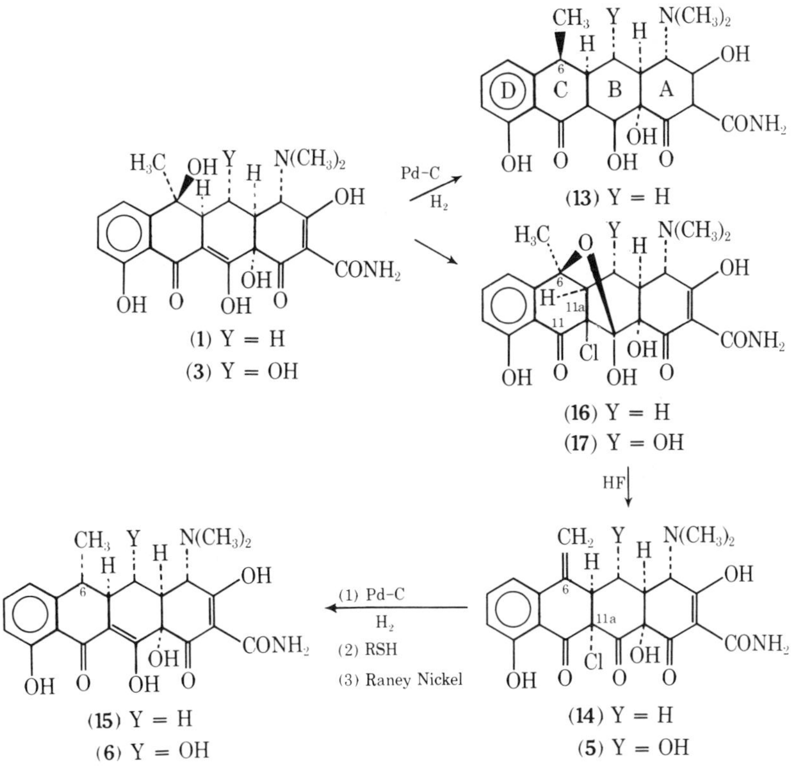

CH$_3$ Y H N(CH$_3$)$_2$
H   H   OH
D   C   B   A
CONH$_2$
OH   OH O   OH   O
(13) Y = H

H$_3$C OH Y H N(CH$_3$)$_2$
H   H   OH
CONH$_2$
OH   ÖH O   OH   O
(1) Y = H
(3) Y = OH

Pd–C
H$_2$

H$_3$C   O Y H N(CH$_3$)$_2$
6   OH
H 11a
11
CONH$_2$
OH   O   Cl OH   O
(16) Y = H
(17) Y = OH

HF

CH$_3$ Y H N(CH$_3$)$_2$
H   H   OH
6
CONH$_2$
OH O   OH   O
(15) Y = H
(6) Y = OH

(1) Pd–C
H$_2$
(2) RSH
(3) Raney Nickel

CH$_2$ Y H N(CH$_3$)$_2$
H   H   OH
6
11a
CONH$_2$
OH O   Cl OH   O
(14) Y = H
(5) Y = OH

converted to the alkyl–amino derivative (7) by reductive alkylation or to the diazonium compound (28) with butyl nitrite (9). Displacement of the diazonium group with azide, fluoride, hydroxyl, or xanthate yielded (29–32).

Disubstituted products (48) (C-7 and C-9) could also be obtained by the proper combination of reactions, ie, bromination followed by nitration.

Recently, the 7- and 9-methyl tetracyclines were prepared and reported to retain biological activity (51).

Convincing evidence (46) for the exact assignment of the incoming groups at the 7-position was obtained by carrying out the electrophilic substitution on a tetracycline labeled with tritium in the 7-position. Replacement of the tritium provided proof for the structural assignment.

Many of the new tetracycline derivatives (Table 1) showed useful *in vivo* activity against a wide spectrum of pathogenic organisms. However, few of them showed significant improvement in overall activity when compared to tetracycline. The exception is (7) (9) which exhibits superior activity against tetracycline-sensitive organisms and many tetracycline-resistant strains of gram-positive bacteria.

A rather novel use of a radioactive tetracycline molecule has been described (52). Utilizing the property that tetracycline localizes in tumor tissue, radioactive 7-iodo-6-demethyl-6-deoxytetracycline was administered to dogs with well-developed mammory tumors. The level of radioactivity was determined in different areas by external scanning. As was expected, the liver, kidney, spleen, and blood contained the highest level of radioactivity. However, the tumors contained twice as much radioactivity as adjacent healthy tissue.

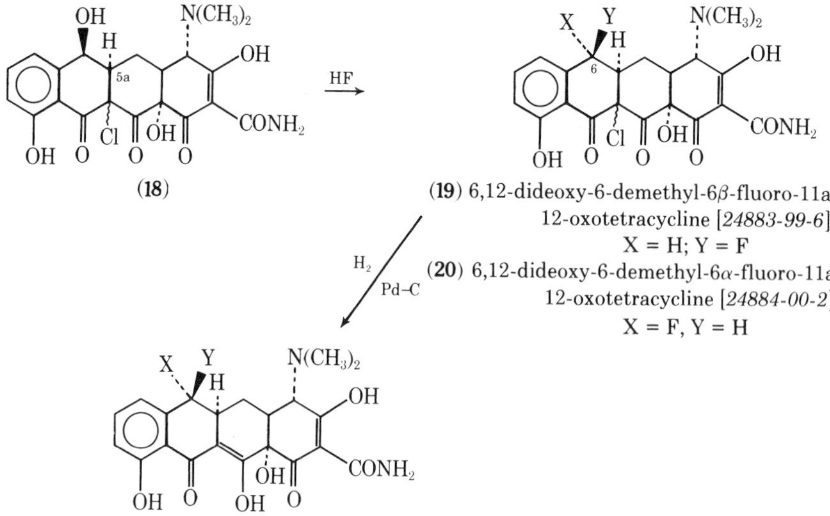

(18)

(19) 6,12-dideoxy-6-demethyl-6β-fluoro-11a-chloro-
12-oxotetracycline [24883-99-6]
X = H; Y = F

(20) 6,12-dideoxy-6-demethyl-6α-fluoro-11a-chloro-
12-oxotetracycline [24884-00-2]
X = F, Y = H

(21) 6-deoxy-6-demethyl-6β-fluorotetracycline [24333-20-8]
X = H; Y = F
(22) 6-deoxy-6-demethyl-6α-fluorotetracycline [24333-21-9]
X = F; Y = H

Structure–Activity Correlations

Any structure variation of the C-11 to C-12 β-ketone system results in loss of activity. Since this portion of the molecule is involved in its exceptional chelating ability (54–56) this affords an insight into the possible mode of action at the receptor site. In addition, structure modification at the C-5, C-6, C-7, and C-9 centers can increase the biological potency of the parent molecule (see Table 1).

There appears to be some correlation between the type of group at positions C-7 and C-9 and their effect on *in vitro* biological activity. The introduction of a strong electron withdrawing group, such as NO$_2$ at C-7, increases the *in vitro* activity. However an electron-donating group, such as an amino, decreases the *in vitro* potency with the reverse being true at C-9. There is not enough *in vivo* testing data on all the modifications at these centers to carry over this correlation to *in vivo* activity. In particular, the 7-dimethylamino group, an electron donating center, imparts unique *in vivo* activity to the tetracycline molecule.

Factors other than electronic contribute to the *in vivo* activity requirements of the molecule, eg, hydrophilicity, ease of metabolism to inactive compounds, and the pH environment at the reaction site. Efforts have been made to correlate electronic structure and biological activity in the tetracycline series by the use of the square of the Hammet substituent index (σ^2) (57) or perturbation energy (ΔEi) (58). In both cases, the predicted activities are of the same order as observed *in vitro* activities with some exceptions. For example, (27) is one of the less active tetracyclines both *in vivo* and *in vitro* although it appears to be one of the more active tetracyclines in these calculations. The most serious drawback to these calculations is the lack of carry-over

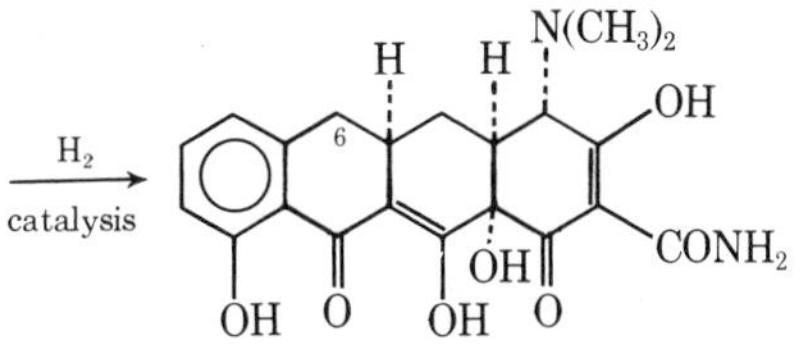

(23)

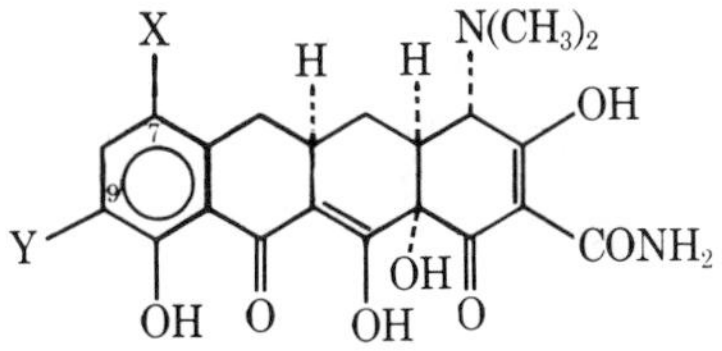

(24) X = Br; Y = H
(25) X = NO₂; Y = H
(26) X = H; Y = NO₂
(27) X = NH₂; Y = H
(28) X = N≡N; Y = H
(29) X = F; Y = H
(30) X = N₃; Y = H
(31) X = OH; Y = H
(32) X = SCOC₂H₅; Y = H

to *in vivo* antibacterial activity. Thus (26) has a high *in vitro* activity coefficient in these calculations but has mediocre *in vivo* biological activity (59).

Attempts have also been made (60) to correlate partition coefficients and antibacterial activity of the tetracyclines. The stereochemical requirements are somewhat better defined. Thus, 4-epitetracycline [79-85-6] and 5a-epitetracycline [65517-29-5] are inactive (61). The 6-epi compound [19369-52-9] (8) on the other hand is about one-half as active as the 6α (or natural) configuration.

The unexpected biological activities of tetracyclines (37) such as 5a-epi-6-epi-tetracycline [19543-88-5] and 7-chloro-5a,11a-dehydro-6-epitetracycline [22688-60-4] make predicting structure–activity relationships difficult. Aside from the C-2 amide Mannich-base derivatives, variation at other centers in the molecule (ie, C-4, 4a, 5a, 12a) decreases the biological activity.

Total Synthesis

In the late 1950s and early 1960s three groups published descriptions of the synthesis of compounds containing the four carbocyclic rings of a tetracycline having at least some of the proper stereoconfiguration and containing most but not all of the functional groups of the compound produced by microorganisms.

The synthesis of two such compounds, dedimethylamino-12a-deoxyanhydro-6-demethyltetracycline [64939-48-6] and dedimethylamino-6,12a-dideoxy-6-demethyltetracycline [64939-49-7], were described by Fields and co-workers (62–66).

Muxfeldt and co-workers, first at Braunschweig and later at Wisconsin, synthe-

Table 1.   *In Vitro* Activities of Tetracycline Derivatives Compared to Tetracycline[a]

Name	CAS Registry Number	Activity, %	Ref.
tetracycline (1)	[60-54-8]	100	
6α-deoxytetracycline (15)	[6746-03-8]	140	7
6β-deoxytetracycline hydrochloride[b]	[51025-87-7]	70	47
6-demethyl-6-deoxytetracycline hydrochloride (23)	[6625-20-3]	160	45
7-bromo-6-demethyl-6-deoxytetracycline (24)	[31642-30-5]	200	43
7-iodo-6-demethyl-6-deoxytetracycline	[27743-50-6]	120	43
9-amino-6-deoxytetracycline	[17781-63-4]	60	43
7-amino-6-demethyl-6-deoxytetracycline (27)	[5679-00-5]	40	47
9-amino-6-demethyl-6-deoxytetracycline hydrochloride	[4198-34-2]	160	47
6-demethyl-6-deoxytetracycline-7-diazonium sulfate hydrochloride (28)	[61665-02-9]	20	43
7-azido-6-demethyl-6-deoxytetracycline sulfate (30)	[61618-23-3]	90	43
9-azido-6-demethyl-6-deoxytetracycline hydrochloride	[61618-24-4]	90	43
7-ethoxythiocarbonylthio-6-demethyl-6-deoxytetracycline (32)	[61618-25-5]	50	43
6-demethyl-6-deoxy-7-nitrotetracycline (25)	[5585-59-1]	640	47
6-demethyl-6-deoxy-9-nitrotetracycline (26)	[4199-35-3]	12	47
6-demethyl-6-deoxy-7,9-dinitrotetracycline	[21754-14-3]	60	48
7-chloro-6-demethyl-6-deoxy-9-nitrotetracycline	[17781-56-5]	21	48
7-bromo-6-demethyl-6-deoxy-9-nitrotetracycline	[17781-51-0]	15	48
9-amino-7-chloro-6-demethyl-6-deoxytetracycline	[17781-57-6]	525	48
9-amino-7-bromo-6-demethyl-6-deoxytetracycline	[17781-55-4]	320	48
9-amino-6-demethyl-6-deoxy-7-nitrotetracycline	[17781-59-8]	275	48
9-amino-7-bromo-6-deoxytetracycline	[17845-09-9]	140	48
7-isopropylamino-6-demethyl-6-deoxytetracycline	[4708-97-8]	100	48
7-dimethylamino-6-demethyl-6-deoxytetracycline (7)	[10118-90-8]	220	9
7-fluoro-6-demethyl-6-deoxytetracycline (29)	[61618-26-6]	220	17
7-hydroxy-6-demethyl-6-deoxytetracycline (31)	[61650-68-8]	23	45

[a] Activities were measured turbidimetrically against *Staphylococcus aureus* (53).

[b] All other 6-deoxy derivatives listed in this table are in the 6β-series.

sized several tetracyclic compounds also lacking in certain functional groups, eg, dedimethylamino-6,12a-dideoxydecarboxamido-7-chlorotetracycline [64939-50-0] (67–69) and dedimethylamino-7-chloroanhydrotetracycline [4572-57-0] (69–70).

Conover and others of the Pfizer group, in cooperation with Woodward (71–73), described the synthesis of the first tetracycline having full biological activity, 6-demethyl-6-deoxytetracycline (23). This compound contained the important and difficult to obtain 4-dimethylamino group, but still lacked the 6-hydroxyl.

An alternative total synthesis of (23) was devised by Muxfeldt and co-workers in 1965 (74) using for the first time methods that could lead to the synthesis of tetracyclines in large quantities and in good yields. The key step in this synthesis is the reaction of the azlactone (33) with the acetone–dicarboxylic acid derivative (34) to form the last two rings in one step and in 82% yield.

In 1967, the Russian group under Shemyakin (75) synthesized 12a-deoxyanhydrotetracycline [64939-51-1] using the quinone juglone as a starting material.

The only total synthesis of a fermentation-produced tetracycline was carried out by Muxfeldt and co-workers. The end product was the compound (3) with 6-asymmetric centers (76).

Many other laboratories have contributed partial syntheses of these compounds.

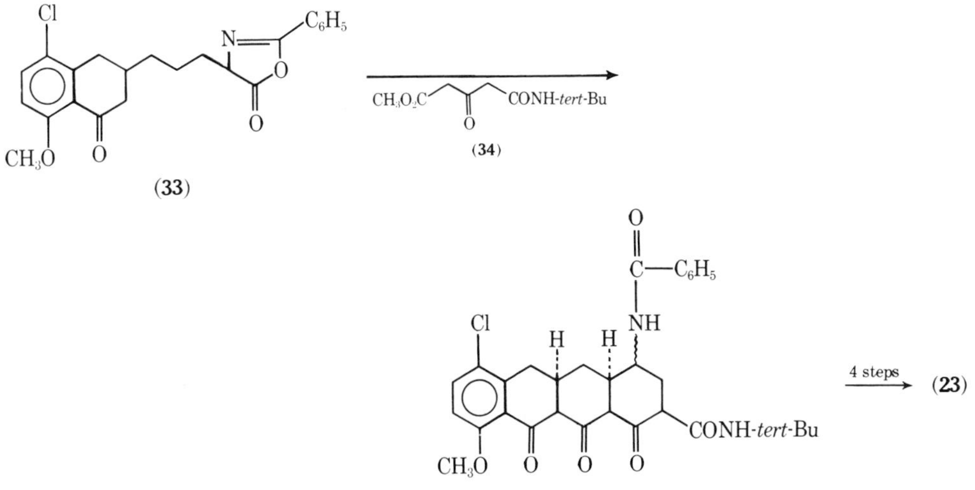

(33)   (34)

4 steps (23)

Preeminent among these contributors are D. H. R. Barton and co-workers, who published 10 papers on the subject in 1971 (77).

Manufacture

Most of the fermentation and isolation processes for manufacture of the tetracyclines are described in patents rather than in journals. Rather than citing individual patents in the bibliography, two compilations of patents are suggested which are so organized that specific compounds and processes can be located rather easily. These are *The Technology of the Tetracyclines* (78) a collection of excerpts (especially the examples) of 65 key patents through 1967, and *Tetracycline Manufacturing Processes* (79) a collection of photocopies of 196 patents on the subject.

The manufacture of tetracyclines begins with the cultivated growth of certain selected strains of *Streptomyces* in a chosen medium that produces optimum growth and maximum production of the antibiotic. Some clinically useful tetracyclines (2–4) are produced directly in these fermentations; others (5–7) are produced by subjecting the fermentation products to one or more chemical alterations.

The choice of the strain of microorganism is one of the important variables in the process. The strains to be used in manufacture are mutants of the original producer, which are chosen as the result of a planned program of mutant selection. Sometimes a spontaneous mutation occurs; usually, it is induced by mutagenic agents or irradiation of various sorts. The choice of the best strain depends on its ability to produce large amounts of the proper antibiotic in a reasonable time from ingredients that are economically feasible.

Chemical modification of the tetracyclines is responsible for the production of three medically used members of the class (5–7). The purified antibiotic produced by fermentation is used as the starting material for a series of chemical transformations.

All steps of manufacture are monitored for antibiotic potency, purity, stability, and bioavailability by quality control methods. In addition, each batch of bulk powder and each lot of finished pharmaceutical dosage form must be certified by the FDA. During all stages of manufacture the FDA requires compliance with specified standards of manufacture.

Economic Aspects

The total United States antibiotic market for 1975 was about 790 million dollars (manufacturers selling price), 20% of that was the cost of tetracyclines. Since tetracyclines are, in general, inexpensive, they account for about one-third of the patient-days of therapy. During the 1950s and early 1960s the tetracyclines accounted for a larger share of the market, but the development of the semisynthetic β-lactam antibiotics has steadily reversed this position (see Antibiotics, β-lactams). The U.S. International Trade Commission reports that production of tetracycline and its derivatives for the year 1974 was about 2.4 kt.

In the United States, the manufacturers of fermentation-derived tetracyclines (1–3) are the Lederle Laboratories, Division of American Cyanamid, Charles Pfizer, Bristol Laboratories, and Rachelle Laboratories. There are also several manufacturers abroad. Tetracycline is now sold generically by many companies. Pfizer's doxycycline (6) and Lederle's minocycline (7), which are more recently developed, semisynthetic tetracyclines, are the only members of the group whose sales continue to increase.

Biosynthesis

The prediction that the biosynthesis of tetracyclines occurs via acetate condensation (80) was proved by equal incorporation of ^{14}C-1 acetate and ^{14}C-2 acetate into 7-chlorotetracycline (2) (81–82). Portions of the biosynthetic pathway have been elucidated by McCormick and co-workers (83–88) and is shown in Figure 2.

Biological Aspects

The evaluation of biological activities of the various tetracyclines usually begins in the laboratory with an *in vitro* turbidimetric assay (89) against the organism, *Staphylococcus aureus*. The assay is a modification of existing penicillin techniques (90). Graded concentrations of the test samples are diluted with buffer, inoculated with *Staphylococcus aureus* and incubated for 3 h. These samples are compared to an equivalent number of tetracycline reference solutions. The turbidity, ie, amount of bacterial growth, is measured in a photoelectric cell.

The agar diffusion method (91) for measuring the *in vitro* potency of antibiotics is also available. However, it is less precise than the turbidimetric method.

The *in vivo* evaluation in mice is usually against a wide range of bacterial infections (92), eg, staphylococci, streptococci, and pneumococci. The drug is administered either in the diet or as a single oral dose.

The ED_{50} (effective dose which prevents death in 50% of test animals) and LD_{50} are determined in mice following oral, intraperitoneal, and intravenous doses.

Investigations (93–94) into the mode of action of the tetracyclines support previous observations (95–97) that the tetracyclines inhibit the protein synthesis of sensitive bacteria. This inhibition is reported to interfere with a variety of biochemical systems: cell wall synthesis (98), biosynthesis of bacterial respiratory systems (99), and similar systems (100).

The genetic code for a specific protein is translated to the ribosome site via messenger ribonucleic acid (RNA), where it acts as a programmed tape for protein synthesis. The site then received amino–acyl transfer RNA units which transfer their amino acids to a growing peptide chain according to the code in the messenger RNA.

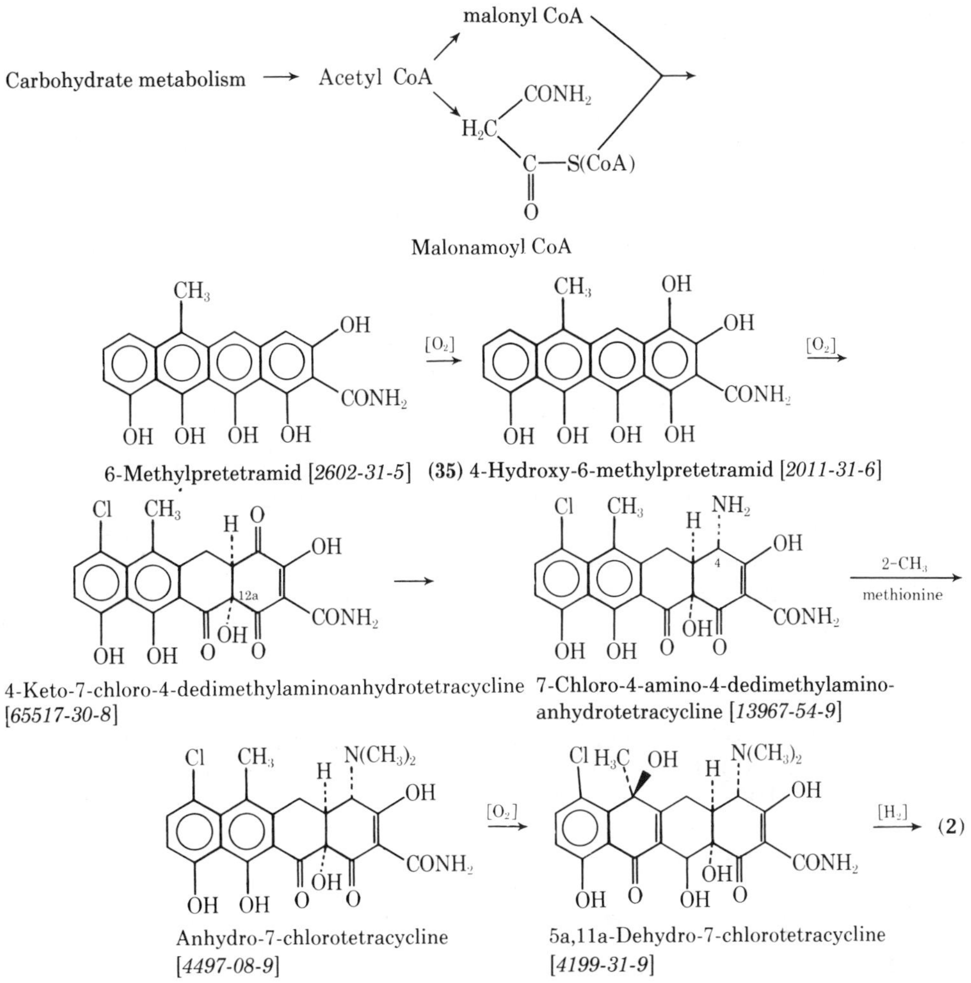

Figure 2.   Biosynthesis of tetracyclines.

Addition of a tetracycline molecule to this system prevents the approach of the aminoacyl tRNA to the ribosome site with a resultant break in the normal protein synthesis of a pathogenic organism (101–102). Possibly this interference with protein synthesis is the primary mechanism of tetracycline antibacterial action (103), but there are other unrelated reactions that are affected by the presence of a tetracycline molecule. The process (104) by which peptides are released from the tRNA after synthesis is completed appears to be inhibited by the tetracyclines. Tetracyclines block the exchange reaction between ribosomal subunits (105).

During the early studies on the chemotherapeutic approach, it was learned that many bacteria are able to adapt to their environment. Some investigators (106) advocated the single massive dose approach in order to lessen the possibility of the development of bacterial resistance to drugs. Finland (107) found strains of group A streptococci developing resistance to sulfadiazine during World War II. With the advent of the general use of penicillin, resistant staphylococcal infections began to spread through public institutions and hospitals (108–109). Since the introduction of tetracyclines into clinical practice, a number of microorganisms have developed a resistance to these drugs (110–112). The changes leading to this resistance probably result from spontaneously occurring mutations leading to modified biochemical processes in the resistant microorganisms. This genetic change once acquired is a stable property of the organism and is hereditary. It appears that this resistance (113) involves a change in the permeability of the cells to the tetracycline, ie, a decreasing ability of the resistant strain to concentrate tetracyclines intracellularly. The ability of sensitive bacteria to effect this intracellular antibiotic concentration accounts for the difference in tetracycline toxicity in bacterial cells versus the nontoxicity in mammalian cells.

Studies with *Escherichia coli* (114) show a change in the tetracycline transport mechanism as resistance develops. It still is not known whether this change is due to a decrease in the concentration of some enzyme or an increase in the concentration of some inhibitor. Some recent studies on multiple drug resistance (115) in bacteria have shown that the drug resistance may be transferred from one bacterial strain to another by a resistance transfer factor. Some genetic properties of this factor and the kinetics of its transfer have been defined; however, the origin of this transfer factor is still unknown.

Minocycline has been shown to be effective orally against tetracycline-resistant staphylococcal infections in mice (92). These infections fail to respond to large dosages of tetracycline.

BIBLIOGRAPHY

"Tetracyclines" in *ECT* 1st ed., Vol. 13, pp. 771–810, by Peter P. Regna, Chas. Pfizer & Co., Inc. (Oxytetracycline, Tetracycline), C. H. Demos and L. M. Preuss, Lederle Laboratories, American Cyanamid Company (Chlortetracycline); "Tetracyclines" in *ECT* 2nd ed., Vol. 20, pp. 1–33, by Robert K. Blackwood, Chas. Pfizer & Co., Inc.

1. R. W. Broschard and co-workers, *Science* **109**, 199 (1949); B. M. Duggar, *Ann. N. Y. Acad. Sci.* **51**, 177 (1948).
2. A. C. Finlay and co-workers, *Science* **111**, 85 (1950); P. P. Regna and co-workers, *J. Am. Chem. Soc.* **73**, 4211 (1951).
3. J. H. Boothe and co-workers, *J. Am. Chem. Soc.* **75**, 4621 (1953).
4. L. H. Conover and co-workers, *J. Am. Chem. Soc.* **75**, 4622 (1953).
5. P. P. Minieri and co-workers, *Antibiot. Ann.* **1953–1954**, 81.
6. J. R. D. McCormick and co-workers, *J. Am. Chem. Soc.* **79**, 4561 (1957).
7. R. K. Blackwood and co-workers, *J. Am. Chem. Soc.* **85**, 3943 (1963).
8. C. R. Stephens and co-workers, *J. Am. Chem. Soc.* **85**, 2643 (1963).
9. M. J. Martell, Jr., and J. H. Boothe, *J. Med. Chem.* **10**, 44 (1967); G. S. Redin, in G. L. Hobby, ed., *Antimicrobial Agents and Chemotherapy*, Williams & Wilkins, Baltimore, Md., 1966, p. 371.
10. N. H. Steigbigel, C. W. Reid, and M. Finland, *Am. J. Med. Sci.* **255**, 179 (1968).
11. F. A. Hochstein and co-workers, *J. Am. Chem. Soc.* **75**, 5455 (1953).
12. C. R. Stephens and co-workers, *J. Am. Chem. Soc.* **76**, 3658 (1954); **74**, 4976 (1952).
13. C. W. Waller and co-workers, *J. Am. Chem. Soc.* **74**, 4981 (1952).
14. S. Hirokawa and co-workers, *Z. Kristallogr. Kristallgeom. Kristallphys. Kristallchem.* **112**, 439 (1959); J. Donohue and co-workers, *J. Am. Chem. Soc.* **85**, 851 (1963).
15. J. J. Hlavka and P. Bitha, *J. Am. Chem. Soc.* **87**, 1795 (1965).
16. J. J. Hlavka, P. Bitha, and J. H. Boothe, *J. Am. Chem. Soc.* **87**, 1795 (1965); **90**, 1034 (1968).
17. P. Bitha, J. Hlavka, and J. H. Boothe, *J. Med. Chem.* **13**, 89 (1970).
18. K. Tsuyi, J. Robertson, and W. Beyer, *Anal. Chem.* **46**, 539 (1974).
19. D. Hoffman, *J. Org. Chem.* **31**, 792 (1966).
20. J. R. D. McCormick and co-workers, *J. Am. Chem. Soc.* **79**, 2849 (1957).
21. C. R. Stephens and co-workers, *J. Am. Chem. Soc.* **78**, 1515 (1956).
22. A. P. Doerschuk, B. A. Bitler, and J. R. D. McCormick, *J. Am. Chem. Soc.* **77**, 4687 (1955).

23. E. G. Remers, G. Steiger, and A. Doerschuk, *J. Pharm. Sci.* **52**, 753 (1963).
24. U.S. Pat. 3,009,956 (Nov. 21, 1961), M. Noseworthy (to Chas. Pfizer & Co.).
25. C. R. Stephens and co-workers, *J. Am. Chem. Soc.* **85**, 2643 (1963); U.S. Pat. 3,028,409 (Apr. 3, 1962), C. R. Stephens (to Chas. Pfizer & Co.).
26. M. J. Martell, Jr., A. S. Ross, and J. H. Boothe, *J. Med. Chem.* **10**, 485 (1967).
27. G. C. Barrett, *J. Pharm. Sci.* **52**, 309 (1963).
28. A. Brunzell, *Acta. Chem. Scand.* **16**, 245 (1962).
29. R. Hultenrauch and J. Keiner, *Naturwissenschaften* **53**, 552 (1966).
30. W. J. Gottstein, W. F. Minor, and L. C. Cheney, *J. Am. Chem. Soc.* **81**, 1198 (1959).
31. W. Seidel, A. Soder, and F. Linder, *Munch. Med. Wschr.* **17**, 661 (1958); S. Afr. Pat. Spec. 57/3169 (1957).
32. J. H. Boothe and co-workers, *J. Am. Chem. Soc.* **80**, 1654 (1958).
33. L. H. Conover, *Symposium Antibiotics of Mold Metabolites, Spec. Publ. No. 5*, The Chemical Society, London, 1956.
34. J. J. Hlavka and P. Bitha, *Tetrahedron Lett.* **32**, 3843 (1966).
35. J. R. McCormick and co-workers, *J. Am. Chem. Soc.* **87**, 1793 (1965).
36. R. C. Esse and co-workers, *J. Am. Chem. Soc.* **86**, 3874, 3875 (1964); S. Afr. Pat. Appl. 63/4791 (1963), (to American Cyanamid Co.); J. H. Van Den Hende, *J. Am. Chem. Soc.* **87**, 929 (1965).
37. R. K. Blackwood and C. R. Stephens, *J. Am. Chem. Soc.* **86**, 2736 (1964); *Can. J. Chem.* **43**, 1382 (1965).
38. M. Schach von Wittenau, F. Hochstein, and C. Stephens, *J. Org. Chem.* **28**, 2454 (1963).
39. M. Kolosov and co-workers, *Chemistry of Antibiotics*, Vol. 1, U.S.S.R. Academy of Science, Moscow, p. 180.
40. K. Koschel and co-workers, *Biochem. Z.* **344**, 76 (1966).
41. J. McCormick and co-workers, *J. Am. Chem. Soc.* **82**, 3331 (1960); S. Afr. Pat. Appl. 58/513 (May 13, 1958), (to American Cyanamid Co.).
42. M. Schach von Wittenau and co-workers, *J. Am. Chem. Soc.* **84**, 2645 (1962).
43. J. J. Hlavka and co-workers, *J. Am. Chem. Soc.* **84**, 1426 (1962).
44. J. J. Hlavka and H. M. Krazinski, *J. Org. Chem.* **28**, 1422 (1963).
45. J. J. Hlavka, H. M. Krazinski, and J. H. Boothe, *J. Org. Chem.* **27**, 3674 (1962).
46. J. H. Boothe and co-workers, *J. Am. Chem. Soc.* **82**, 1253 (1960).
47. J. Petisi and co-workers, *J. Med. Pharm. Chem.* **5**, 538 (1962).
48. J. L. Spencer and co-workers, *J. Med. Chem.* **6**, 405 (1963).
49. J. J. Beereboom and co-workers, *J. Am. Chem. Soc.* **82**, 1003 (1960).
50. M. J. Martell, Jr., A. S. Ross, and J. H. Boothe, *J. Med. Chem.* **10**, 359 (1967).
51. L. Bernardi and co-workers, *Il Farmaco Ed. Sc.* **30**, 1025 (1975).
52. J. Hlavka and D. Buyske, *Nature (London)* **186**, 1064 (1960).
53. E. Pelcak and A. Dornbush, *Ann. N. Y. Acad. Sci.* **51**, 218 (1948).
54. M. Burstall, *Manuf. Chem.* **31**, 474 (1960).
55. J. Doluisio and A. Martin, *J. Med. Chem.* **6**, 16 (1963).
56. P. Brown, Ph.D. Dissertation, Syracuse University, Syracuse, N. Y., June 1965.
57. A. Cammarata and co-workers, *Mol. Pharmacol.* **6**, 61 (1970).
58. F. Peradejordi, A. Martin, and A. Cammarata, *J. Pharm. Sci.* **60**, 577 (1971).
59. G. Redin, American Cyanamid Co., private communication.
60. J. Colaizzi and P. Klink, *J. Pharm. Sci.* **58**, 1185 (1969); M. Schach von Wittenau, *Chemotherapy (Basel)* **13**, 41 (1968).
61. J. R. D. McCormick and co-workers, *J. Am. Chem. Soc.* **80**, 5572 (1958).
62. J. H. Boothe and co-workers, *J. Am. Chem. Soc.* **81**, 1006 (1959).
63. T. L. Fields, A. S. Kende, and J. H. Boothe, *J. Am. Chem. Soc.* **82**, 1250 (1960).
64. R. G. Wilkinson, T. L. Fields, and J. H. Boothe, *J. Org. Chem.* **26**, 637 (1961).
65. A. S. Kende and co-workers, *J. Am. Chem. Soc.* **83**, 439 (1961).
66. T. L. Fields, A. S. Kende, and J. H. Boothe, *J. Am. Chem. Soc.* **83**, 4612 (1961).
67. H. Muxfeldt, *Chem. Ber.* **92**, 3122 (1959).
68. H. Muxfeldt, H. Rogalsky, and K. Striegler, *Angew. Chem.* **72**, 170 (1960).
69. H. Muxfeldt, *Angew. Chem. Int. Ed. Engl.* **1**, 372 (1962).
70. H. Muxfeldt and A. Kreutzer, *Chem. Ber.* **94**, 881 (1961).
71. L. H. Conover and co-workers, *J. Am. Chem. Soc.* **84**, 3222 (1962).
72. R. B. Woodward, *Pure Appl. Chem.* **6**, 561 (1963).
73. J. J. Korst and co-workers, *J. Am. Chem. Soc.* **90**, 439 (1968).

74. H. Muxfeldt and W. Rogalsky, *J. Am. Chem. Soc.* **87,** 933 (1965).

75. A. I. Gurevich and co-workers, *Tetrahedron Lett.* 131 (1967).

76. H. Muxfeldt and co-workers, *J. Am. Chem. Soc.* **90,** 6534 (1968).

77. D. H. R. Barton and co-workers, *J. Chem. Soc.,* 2164 (1971).

78. R. C. Evans, *The Technology of the Tetracyclines,* Quadrangle Press, New York, 1968.

79. *Tetracycline Manufacturing Processes,* Noyes Development Corp., Park Ridge, N. J., 1969.

80. R. Robinson, *Structural Relations of Natural Products,* Oxford University Press, London, 1955, p. 58.

81. J. F. Snell, R. Wagner, and F. A. Hochstein, *Proc. Int. Conf. Peaceful Uses At. Energy* **12,** 431 (1955).

82. P. A. Miller, J. R. D. McCormick, and A. P. Doerschuk, *Science* **123,** 1030 (1956).

83. J. R. D. McCormick in D. Gottlieb and P. D. Shaw, eds., *Antibiotics,* Vol. 2, Springer-Verlag, Berlin, Ger., 1967.

84. J. R. D. McCormick, *Genetics and Breeding of Streptomyces,* Yugoslav Academy of Arts and Sciences, Zagreb, Yugoslavia, 1969.

85. J. R. D. McCormick and co-workers, *J. Am. Chem. Soc.* **84,** 3023 (1962); J. R. D. McCormick, *The Biogenesis of Antibiotic Substances,* Academic Press, Inc., New York, 1965, p. 83; L. A. Mitscher, *J. Pharm. Sci.* **57,** 1633 (1968); J. R. D. McCormick and co-workers, *J. Am. Chem. Soc.* **90,** 2201 (1968); J. R. D. McCormick and E. R. Jensen, *J. Am. Chem. Soc.* **90,** 7126 (1968); J. R. D. McCormick, S. Johnson, and N. O. Sjolander, *J. Am. Chem. Soc.* **85,** 1692 (1963).

86. J. R. D. McCormick and co-workers, *J. Am. Chem. Soc.* **87,** 1793 (1965).

87. J. R. D. McCormick and E. R. Jensen, *J. Am. Chem. Soc.* **91,** 206 (1969).

88. J. R. D. McCormick and co-workers, *J. Am. Chem. Soc.* **80,** 5572 (1958).

89. A. Dornbush and E. Pelcak, *Ann. N. Y. Acad. Sci.* **51,** 218 (1948).

90. J. R. McMahon, *J. Biol. Chem.* **153,** 249 (1944).

91. S. Waksman and S. Reilly, *Ind. Eng. Chem.* **17,** 556 (1945).

92. G. S. Redin, *Antimicrob. Agents Chemother.* 371 (1966).

93. G. Suarez and D. Nathans, *Biochem. Biophys. Res. Commun.* **18,** 743 (1965).

94. A. Cammarata and co-workers, *Mol. Pharmacol.* **6,** 61 (1970).

95. R. Rendi and S. Ochoa, *J. Biol. Chem.* **237,** 3711 (1962); *Science* **133,** 1367 (1961).

96. T. J. Franklin, *Biochem. J.* **87,** 449 (1963); **84,** 110P (1962).

97. T. Akiba and T. Yokota, *Igaku To Seibutsugaku* **64,** 34, 39 (1962).

98. J. Park, *Biochem. J.* **70,** 2P (1958).

99. A. I. Laskin, *Antibiotics, Mechanism of Action I,* Springer-Verlag, New York, 1967, p. 331.

100. J. Snell and L. Cheng, *Dev. Ind. Microbiol.* **2,** 107 (1961).

101. G. Suarez and D. Nathans, *Biochem. Biophys. Res. Commun.* **18,** 743 (1965).

102. R. Connamacher and H. Mandel, *Biochim. Biophys. Acta* **166,** 475 (1968).

103. A. Larkin and J. Laro, *Antibiot. Chemother.* **17,** 1 (1971).

104. Z. Vogel, *Biochemistry* **8,** 5161 (1969).

105. R. Kaempfer, *Proc. Nat. Acad. Sci. U.S.A.* **61,** 106 (1968).

106. M. Barker and L. Garrod, *Antibiotics and Chemotherapy,* 4th ed., E & S Livingstone Ltd., Edinburg, Eng., 1973.

107. M. Finland, *N. Engl. J. Med.* **253,** 909 (1955).

108. J. Dexter and H. Bates, *Minn. Med.* **53,** 205 (1970).

109. O. Jessen and K. Rosendal, *N. Engl. J. Med.* **281,** 627 (1969).

110. R. McCormack, R. Kaye, and E. Hook, *N. Engl. J. Med.* **267,** 323 (1969).

111. A. R. Ragsdale and J. Sanford, *Antimicrob. Agents Chemother.* 164 (1964).

112. A. Percival and E. Armstrong, *Lancet* **1,** 998 (1969).

113. T. J. Franklin, *Symposia of the Society for General Microbiology,* Number XVI (1966).

114. T. J. Franklin and A. Godfrey, *Biochem. J.* **94,** 54 (1965).

115. S. Mitsuhashi, *J. Infect. Dis.* **119,** 89 (1969).

JAMES H. BOOTHE

JOSEPH J. HLAVKA

Lederle Laboratories Division, American Cyanamid Company

CHEMOTHERAPEUTICS

ANTHELMINTIC

Anthelmintic drugs are used to relieve disease caused by parasitic flatworms or roundworms. Flatworms that infect humans are of two major types: flukes, which have the shape of a simple lanceolate leaf, and tapeworms, which are ribbonlike, made up of serially repeated sections behind a neck and an attachment organ called the scolex. All roundworms have a basic cylindrical shape, with major variations in proportions, in size, and in structure. There is a group of drugs for treatment of blood flukes, another for flukes that live in the lungs, the liver, or the intestine, a third for tapeworms, another for intestinal roundworms, and one for roundworms of blood and tissues. However, this classification of drug use is not rigidly exclusive, and a drug that has its greatest effectiveness against one class of worm may also have effects against some species of another class; also a drug that is very effective against one species may be fairly effective against another species of the same class.

The drugs considered in this article, and the worms against which they are effective, are presented in Table 1. The term drug of choice is avoided because the true drug of choice is sure to change with time. Drugs discussed are specific chemotherapeutic agents. Anthelmintics are used to injure or destroy worm parasites, or to facilitate their removal from the body, or to interfere in some way with their protective mechanisms against the natural defenses of the host.

Frequently, helminthic disease will require medication in addition to the chemotherapeutic agent itself. Allergic conditions are common when there is tissue invasion by worms, so that antihistamines and corticosteroids may be necessary adjuncts to therapy. In fact, some allergic responses can be seriously aggravated by successful anthelmintic therapy. Anemia, indigestion, and secondary bacterial infections may be associated with the presence of worms, and under these conditions hematinics and suitable antibiotics are needed. Some practitioners use cathartics to help remove certain helminths from the digestive tract, after the worms have been temporarily incapacitated by a specific drug (see Gastrointestinal agents).

Drugs that have been found safe and effective in other parts of the world may not be available in the United States by prescription because the market is too small for a manufacturer to undertake the cost of approval through FDA procedures (24–25). However, physicians can obtain such drugs (3), (6), (7), and (12) for their patients, and information about their use, from the Parasitic Diseases Drug Service, Center for Disease Control. U.S. Public Health Service (USPHS), Atlanta, Ga. In an emergency the Service can be reached by telephone (404-633-3311). In Table 1 these drugs are referred to as available from the USPHS.

The danger of infection must be balanced against the hazards of drug use. The situation is not as serious as it was in the 1940s when the anthelmintic armamentarium included some of the most dangerous drugs then available.

Table 1. Anthelmintics: Uses and Properties

Drug and structure no.	CAS Registry No.	Trade names	Physical properties	Solubility	Disease (organism)	Refs.
antimony potassium tartrate USP (1)	[28300-74-5]	Tartar emetic	colorless crystals or white powder, mp 100°C- $\frac{1}{2}$ H$_2$O and 210°C - 1 H$_2$O	1 g in 12 mL water; insoluble in ethanol	oriental blood fluke disease (*Schistosoma japonicum*)	1–2
bephenium hydroxynaphthoate USP (15)	[3818-50-6]	Alcopar(a), Befenio, Lecibis, Nemex	crystals or yellow powder, mp ca 170°C	insoluble in water; soluble in hot ethanol	hookworm disease (*Ancylostoma duodenale*)	3–4
bithionol (7)[a]	[97-18-7]	Actamer, Bithin, Lorothidol	crystals or gray–white powder, mp 188°C	insoluble in water; soluble in acetone and 4% NaOH	lung fluke disease (*Paragonimus westermani*)	5–6
chloroquine USP (10)	[54-05-7]	Aralen, Artrichin, Bemophate, Bipiquin, Nivaquine B, Résoquine, Reumachlor, Sanoquin, Tankan	slightly yellowish crystalline powder, mp 87–92°C	very slightly soluble in water; soluble in dilute acids, in CHCl$_3$ and in ether	Chinese liver fluke disease (*Clonorchis sinensis*)	7
dichlorophen BAN (14)	[97-23-4]	Antiphen, Dicestal, Didroxane, Di-phentahane-70, Hyosan, Parabis, Plath-Lyse, Preventol G-D, Teniathane, Teniatol	cream-colored powder with slight phenolic odor, mp 174–178°C	almost insoluble in water; freely soluble in 95% ethanol and in ether	dwarf tapeworm disease (*Hymenolepis nana*)	8
diethylcarbamazine citrate USP (21)	[1642-54-2]	Dirocide, Filazine, Franocide, Longicid, Loxuran	white crystalline powder, mp 141–143°C	soluble in water and hot ethanol; insoluble in acetone	elephantiasis and other filariases (*Wuchereria bancrofti*, *Loa loa*, and other filaria)	9
hexylresorcinol NF (8)	[136-77-6]	Caprocol, Crystoids, Gelovermin, Sucrets	yellow–white, needle-shaped crystals turning brownish-pink on exposure, mp ca 68°C	1 g in 2000 mL water; freely soluble in ethanol and acetone	roundworm disease (mixed intestinal nematodes)	10

334

No.	Compound	CAS Registry Number	Trade/Other Names	Physical Properties	Solubility	Disease/Use
11	hycanthone mesylate (5) (hycanthone base)	[23255-93-8] [3105-97-3]		hycanthone base is a yellow–orange crystalline powder, mp ca 68°C	base is soluble in water	intestinal blood fluke disease, urinary tract blood fluke disease (*Schistosoma mansoni* and *Schistosoma haematobium*)
12	lucanthone hydrochloride (4)	[548-57-2]	Miracil D, Miracol, Nilodin, Tixantone	yellow crystals or yellow–orange powder, mp ca 195°C, water solution is orange and stains the skin	1 g in 110 mL water; 1 g in 85 mL ethanol	urinary tract blood fluke disease (*Schistosoma haematobium*)
13	mebendazole (19)	[31431-39-7]	Pantelmin, Telmin, Vermox	crystals or yellow amorphous powder, mp ca 289°C	very slightly soluble in water and most organic solvents	whipworm disease (*Trichuris trichiura*)
14	niclosamide (12)[a]	[50-65-7]	Bayer 2353, Cestocid, Fenesal, Lintex, Mansonil, Nasemo, Sulqui, Tredemine, Vermitid, Yomesan	pale yellow crystals, or yellow–white powder, mp 225–230°C	insoluble in water; sparingly soluble in ethanol	tapeworm disease (*T. saginata, T. solium, D. latum,* and *H. nana*)
15	niridazole (6)[a]	[61-57-4]	Ambilhar	yellow crystalline powder, mp ca 261°C	sparingly soluble in water and most organic solvents	urinary tract blood fluke disease, guineaworm disease (*S. haematobium,* and *D. medenensis*)
16	piperazine citrate USP (16)	[144-29-6]	Antepar, Arpezine, Exelmin, Exopin, Helmazine, Multifuge, Nematidal, Oxucide, Oxyzin, Parazine, Pinozan, Pinrou, Piperaverm, Pipazan Citrate, Pipracid, Piptelate, Rhomex, Uvilon	white crystalline powder, mp ca 185°C (dec)	freely soluble in water; insoluble in ethanol	large roundworm disease (*Ascaris lumbricoides*)
17	pyrantel pamoate (17)	[22204-24-6]	Antiminth, Cobrantil, Combrantin, Helmix, Piranver	white or yellow or tan crystalline powder, melts and decomposes, mp ca 250°C	insoluble in water and nearly so in ethanol	pinworm disease and large roundworm disease (*Enterobius vermicularis,* and *Ascaris lumbricoides*)

Table 1 (*continued*)

Drug and structure no.	CAS Registry No.	Trade names	Physical properties	Solubility	Disease (organism)	Refs.
pyrvinium pamoate USP (**18**)	[3546-41-6]	Alnoxin, Altolat, Molevac, Neo-Oxypaat, Pamovin, Povan, Povanyl, Pyrcon, Tolapin, Tru, Vanquil, Vanquin	orange, red, or darker crystalline powder stains skin, textiles and stool red, softens ca 190°C, melts ca 210°C	insoluble in water; very slightly soluble in ethanol	pinworm disease and threadworm disease (*Enterobius vermicularis*, and *Strongyloides stercoralis*)	18
quinacrine hydrochloride (**13**)	[69-05-6]	Acrichine, Acriquine, Atabrin(e), Chinacrin, Erion, Italchin, Metoquin, Palacrin	yellow crystals, mp ca 250°C	1 g in 35 mL water; slightly soluble in ethanol	beef tapeworm and broad fish tapeworm (*Taenia saginata* and *Diphyllobothrium latum*)	19
stibocaptate (**3**)[a]	[3064-61-7]	Astiban	white to yellow–green crystalline powder	soluble in water and unstable in solution at RT	intestinal blood fluke disease (*Schistosoma mansoni*)	20
stibophen (**2**)	[15489-16-4]	Corystibin, Fantorin, Fouadin, Fuadin, Neoantimosan, Pyrostib, Repodral, Sodium Antimosan, Trimon	white to slightly yellow or pink crystals, mp >300°C, chars 300°C	soluble in water; solns oxidize and turn yellow; insoluble in ethanol	blood fluke disease (*Schistosoma mansoni*, and *S. haematobium*)	21
tetrachloroethylene USP (**9**)	[127-18-4]	Ankilostin, Didakene, Nema, Perclene, Tetracap, Tetropil	colorless, nonflammable fluid with ethereal odor, deteriorates in warm climates, bp 121°C	soluble 1:10,000 in water; miscible with ethanol	hookworm disease (*Necator americanus*)	22
thiabendazole USP (**20**)	[148-79-8]	Bovisole, Eprofil, Equizole, Lombristop, Mertect, Mintezol, Minzolum, Nemapan, Omnizole, Polival, Thiaben, Thiabenzole	white crystals, mp ca 300°C	almost insoluble in water, but readily soluble in dilute acids or alkalis; slightly soluble in ethanol	threadworm disease, larva migrans (*Strongyloides stercoralis*, *Toxacariss A. braziliensis*)	23

[a] Available from USPHS.

336

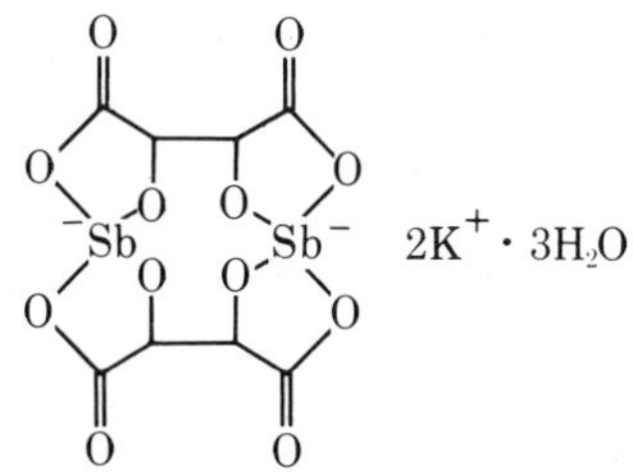

Figure 1.   Drugs effective against schistosomes.

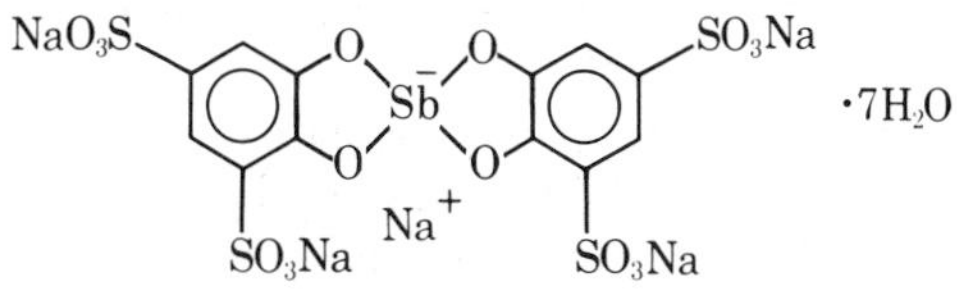

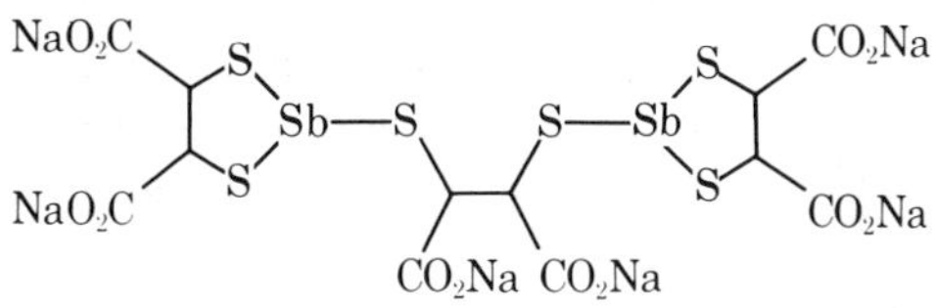

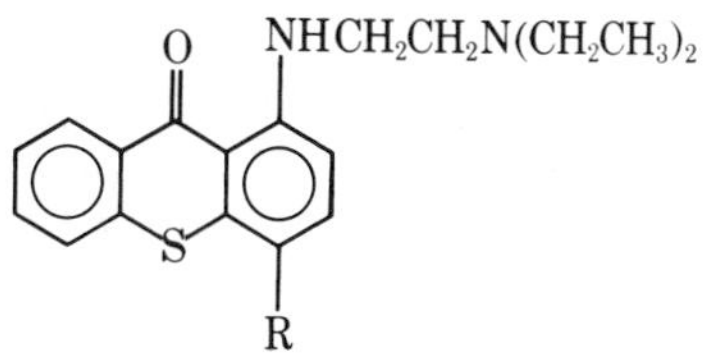

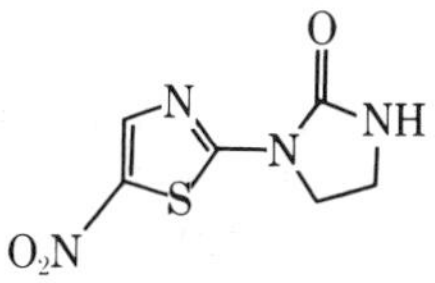

Treatment of Blood Fluke Disease (Schistosomiasis)

Antimony potassium tartrate (1) (Fig. 1) is used against *Schistosoma japonicum*, stibophen (2) against *S. haematobium,* and stibocaptate (3) against *S. mansoni.* Each of these antimonial anthelmintics can be employed to treat any one of the three infections, but it is most successful against the species mentioned.

These compounds traditionally have been called trivalent antimonials: antimony potassium tartrate (1) (tartar emetic) was used first with a regimen for administration of many intravenous injections over a period of a month or more. Stibophen (2) can be given in fewer doses by intramuscular administration over a shorter period and it is stable in solution.

Stibocaptate (3) is the newest of these compounds. The antimony in this drug is bound to sulfur atoms rather than to oxygen atoms as with the others, so that stibocaptate has a higher degree of stability (26). The antimony is less easily dissociated because it is bound tightly to dimercaptosuccinate, which resembles BAL (British Anti-Lewisite, dimercaprol, $HOCH_2CH(SH)CH_2SH$) (27). Stibocaptate is given intramuscularly; fewer doses are needed than (1) or (2). These three drugs are essentially specialties for human schistosomiasis, although (1) and (2) are used in veterinary medicine; and (1) has unrelated uses as mordant in the textile and leather industries.

All antischistosomal antimonials are presumed to have the same mechanism of action. They inhibit phosphofructokinase, an enzyme involved in the anaerobic metabolism of glucose (28). The drugs arrest the conversion of fructose-6-phosphate to fructose-1,6-diphosphate by a reversible inhibition that reduces the rate of glycolysis;

and this causes the worms to lose their energy supply. Schistosomes normally hold their position in the blood vessel by use of suckers, but when treatment with antimonials is started they lose their hold and are swept away to be destroyed, in time, through the action of white cells.

Because the enzyme in schistosomes is much more sensitive than is the corresponding enzyme of human tissues, the Embden-Meyerhof-Parnas scheme of glycolysis (by which glucose is metabolized to lactic acid) is disrupted in schistosomes, but not in man. This selectively toxic effect on schistosome phosphofructokinases is accomplished at low levels of concentration of the drug. In higher concentrations, antimonials can inhibit the activity of glutamic–pyruvic transaminase, and as drug concentration is increased further, many enzyme systems of both parasite and man are affected, probably by union of the antimony with sulfhydryl groups. Therefore, as drug concentration rises in the host, the important effects cease to be therapeutic and become toxic.

Adverse effects from these drugs are legion, thus they are not satisfactory chemotherapeutic agents. Tartar emetic is the most toxic, but all tend to cause the same problems: abdominal pain and diarrhea, nausea and vomiting; fall in blood pressure and a tendency toward fainting; coughing and difficulty in breathing; electrocardiographic changes; headache and joint pain; liver damage; kidney damage; hemolytic anemia; drug rash; exacerbation of concurrent diseases; and other effects. Because of these toxic effects, the search has continued for different, nonmetallic antischistosomal agents.

Lucanthone (4) and hycanthone (5) (thioxanthones) represented a new direction in the development of drugs for schistosomiasis. Lucanthone was introduced first, but hycanthone, which is an hydroxymethyl analogue, was recognized as the active metabolic product in humans (29). Lucanthone, which had been synthesized as one of a series of drugs starting from quinacrine (see below), is important because it was the first oral drug for a schistosomal disease, and the first one that did not contain a metal. Hycanthone worked by intramuscular injection in a single large dose and was used in mass population treatment before it was withdrawn because of hepatotoxicity. The initial effect of this drug on the worms was to cause a decline in egg production. The mechanism of action may have been through shifts in the tissue distribution of 5-hydroxytryptamine (serotonin), which acts as a neurotransmitter in schistosomes (see Neuroregulators).

A more successful line of drug development produced the nitrothiazole derivative niridazole (6). This is given orally twice a day for a week to hospitalized patients infected with *S. haematobium* or *S. mansoni*; and is also effective in treating the guinea worm (*Dracunculus medinensis*). It is active against amoebae but too toxic for that use as compared to other drugs.

Niridazole (6) arrests egg shell formation (30). In the female worm the ovary degenerates; and in the male, spermatogenesis is arrested. Schistosomes feed on blood sugar, and on red blood cells, from which they digest the globin. Normally they absorb glucose through their body surface as well as by way of their intestines, but (6) inhibits uptake of glucose, accelerates the breakdown of glycogen in the parasites, and is suspected of interference with the activity of hexokinase and of phosphorylase phosphatase. Selective toxicity is related to drug concentrations which are three to four times as high in the portal blood, where the worms are found, as compared to the concentration in the general circulation (because the drug is largely metabolized on first pass through the liver).

Among the adverse effects niridazole may cause are abdominal cramps, vomiting, dizziness, agitation, confusion, hallucinations, and convulsions. Liver disease predisposes to toxicity. Persons with glucose-6-phosphate dehydrogenase deficiency may suffer hemolytic anemia. In various laboratory models the drug has been carcinogenic, mutagenic, immunosuppressive, and inhibited cell-mediated hypersensitivity. It may have adverse effects on T lymphocytes.

The efficacy and toxicity of drugs used in the treatment of schistosomiases leaves something to be desired. A number of other compounds are known to have antischistosomal effects, and there has been extensive clinical experience with some of these in limited geographical areas (31).

The influence of antischistosomal drugs on the disease depends upon the decrease or arrest of egg production, since it is the movement of eggs through tissues that produces the pathology. Adult worms about 2 cm long occur as mating pairs within venules, but at intervals the female travels as far as possible toward the capillary bed to lay eggs that break out of the blood vessel and do extensive damage. The number of pairs of worms in a patient varies from a few to hundreds, and in untreated patients the worms may survive for 5 yr, or sometimes for decades.

Treatment of Fluke (Trematode) Infections in the Lungs, Intestines, and Liver

Bithionol (7) (Fig. 2) is used to treat persons infected with *Paragonimus* (lung fluke) or with *Fasciola* (sheep liver fluke). It is a phenolic compound similar to hexachlorophene (see Disinfectants). Both have been used as veterinary anthelmintics (see Veterinary drugs). In the past, bithionol was incorporated for its antibacterial effects in at least 20 medicated skin cleansers manufactured in the United States but such use had to be discontinued when the compound was discovered to be the cause of skin irritations.

Bithionol (7) interferes with the neuromuscular physiology of helminths, impairs egg formation, and may cause the protective cuticle covering the worm to become defective. At the biochemical level, oxidative phosphorylation is inhibited, and the bithionol molecule can chelate iron so that it may inactivate iron-containing enzyme systems.

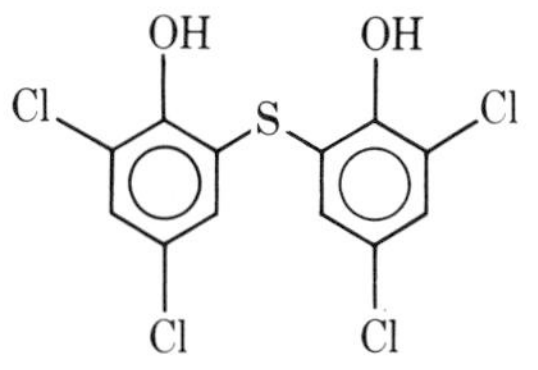

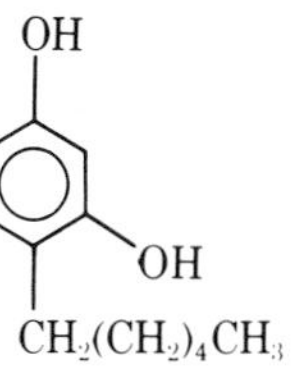

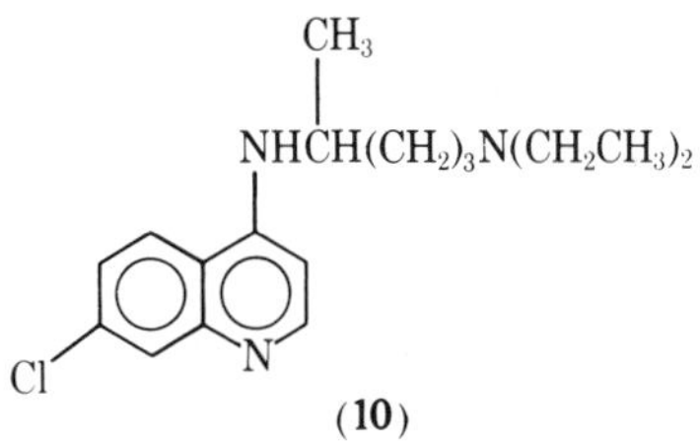

Figure 2.   Drugs effective against trematode infections.

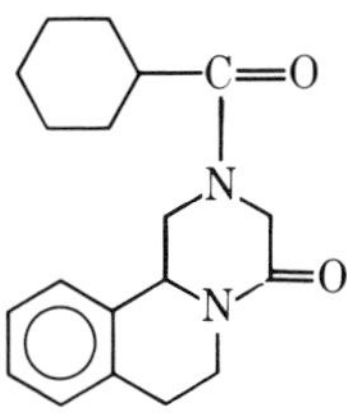

(11)

Paragonimus about 1 cm long are normally in the lungs where a population of 20–50 worms will cause chest pain and shortness of breath; but worms may occur in viscera or the brain causing tumor-like symptoms. *Fasciola* about 3 cm long, after extensive migration, invade the bile ducts where heavy infections result in changes of the bile duct wall and surrounding tissue, and cirrhosis; or as a result of incomplete migrations the worms may arrive at other locations and cause intense tissue reactions. A 10-d oral regimen of bithionol may resolve the pathology of lung disease in about 3 mo, but improvement in cerebral paragonimiasis and in sheep liver fluke infections is variable. Untreated adult worms of both species live more than 5 yr. Adverse effects in patients taking oral bithionol commonly include abdominal pain, diarrhea, vomiting, rashes and photosensitivity.

Hexylresorcinol (8) is another phenolic anthelmintic. It is effective in a single oral dose against trematodes in the intestinal tract, and is used in persons infected with the giant intestinal fluke *Fasciolopsis buski*. It was an important anthelmintic in the 1940s through the 1960s when it was used against intestinal nematodes and the dwarf tapeworm. The drug, which was originally introduced as a stainless antiseptic (ST 37), continues to be used that way, and as an anthelmintic in veterinary medicine.

Hexylresorcinol (8) produces blisters and cuts in the surface of the parasites, presumably because it is a phenolic compound (32). It burns and kills superficial tissues of the body wall, precipitates superficial cell protein, and alters permeability as phosphorus compounds leak from the parasites. Perhaps as a consequence of these effects, it paralyzes the muscles of intestinal nematodes.

The selective toxicity of (8) presumably derives from the natural coatings of the human gastrointestinal tract, but the worms are unprotected. When (8) is administered by mouth as in crystalline form enclosed in hard gelatin-coated pills, it is not readily absorbed by the human intestine (ie, there is little or no systemic toxicity). However, the drug can burn unprotected mucous membranes of the mouth and upper esophagus if it comes into contact with these surfaces by eructation.

Fasciolopsis buski grows to 8 cm long and lives attached to the wall of the small intestine where a population of thousands may cause inflammatory ulceration and toxemia with danger of death in children. Treatment is oral medication with hexylresorcinol or tetrachloroethylene.

Tetrachloroethylene (9) also has a broad anthelmintic spectrum, and it can be used to eradicate either of the two tiny intestinal flukes *Heterophyes heterophyes* and *Metagonimus yokogawai*. It is effective against the hookworm *Necator* (see below in the section on intestinal nematodes). The compound's other uses are as a solvent for dry cleaning (qv) and for degreasing metals (see Chlorocarbons).

As an anthelmintic, (9) replaced carbon tetrachloride, which if absorbed, could destroy the liver. The mechanism by which (9) works is not established but some workers believe the halogenated hydrocarbon dissolves in the lipid of cells of the helmintic neuromuscular system and interferes with their function. Investigators do not agree on the anthelmintic action of tetrachlorethylene or the basic pharmacology of the drug.

For use against either flukes or the hookworm *Necator,* a single oral dose is given on an empty stomach after a day of low-fat diet, because fat in the gastrointestinal tract may increase absorption of the drug. This drug is popular in veterinary medicine (in the United States only the veterinary-type of drug preparation can be obtained) (33).

Adverse effects can be a burning sensation in the stomach, nausea and vomiting, and headache, giddiness, dizziness, inebriation, and loss of consciousness. For these reasons patients are kept quiet and restricted, perhaps in bed, for 4 h after treatment, and are not permitted alcoholic beverages. In those exposed to the liquid and its vapors a defatting action on the skin can lead to dermatitis.

The flukes *Heterophyes* and *Metagonimus* are 2.5 mm or less in length, on or in the wall of the small intestine, and the resulting condition is frequently symptomless; rarely, eggs may enter the circulatory system to be carried to heart and brain and damage those areas. Niclosamide (see structure (12)) used mainly for tapeworms, is also effective against these small flukes.

Chloroquine (10) will reduce the egg output of the Chinese liver fluke (*Clonorchis sinensis*). The primary uses of chloroquine are for malaria and amebiasis, in which situations it is essentially nontoxic (see Chemotherapeutics, antiprotozoal). It has also been used in collagen diseases, such as lupus erythematosus, and for rheumatoid arthritis, but is toxic in large doses for long times as used in those conditions. Chloroquine is a 4-aminoquinoline that bears the same alkyl side chain as the acridine dye quinacrine (see Dyes). Chloroquine, like quinacrine, intercalates with deoxyribonucleic acid (DNA) and this upsets the role of DNA as a template in replication and transcription. It inhibits DNA- and ribonucleic acid, RNA-polymerase activity. Chloroquine accumulates in the liver cells, in red cells parasitized with malaria, and binds to melanin (eg, in the retina). It is more toxic to some tissues than others and one of the factors that makes tissues sensitive to the drug may be cell reproduction and growth, as in the helmintic egg production process. Short term administration of chloroquine is relatively harmless. Patients may have nausea, vomiting and loss of appetite, skin rashes and itch, headaches, and visual difficulty. Long term high dose administration as formerly used for collagen diseases led to blindness and other serious toxicities. The drug may be teratogenetic.

Clonorchis adults grow up to 2 cm long and live in the biliary tree where they cause inflammation. The presence of 20–200 individuals is common but the number can be over 20,000; infection is the consequence of a diet of raw fish. Untreated worms can live for 25 yr. Treatment is chloroquine diphosphate by mouth daily for 3 wk to a year; but results are unsatisfactory because, although egg count decreases, most adult worms are not killed (34).

Treatment of Tapeworm (Cestode) Infections

Niclosamide (12) (Fig. 3) is a convenient, effective drug for treatment of persons who have tapeworm infections. More than 80% of the patients are cured by this orally administered drug, and adjunctive therapy is not required when it is used against the beef tapeworm (*Taenia saginata*), the dwarf tapeworm (*Hymenolepis nana*) or the broad fish tapeworm of man (*Diphyllobothrium latum*). In connection with therapy for the pork tapeworm (*Taenia solium*), a laxative may be used afterward. Other helminthic infections have also been successfully treated with this drug, including small intestinal flukes and the whipworm. Additionally, niclosamide ethanolamine salt is used as a snail control agent against the intermediate host of *Schistosoma mansoni*.

Modes of action for niclosamide (12) are interference with respiration and blocking

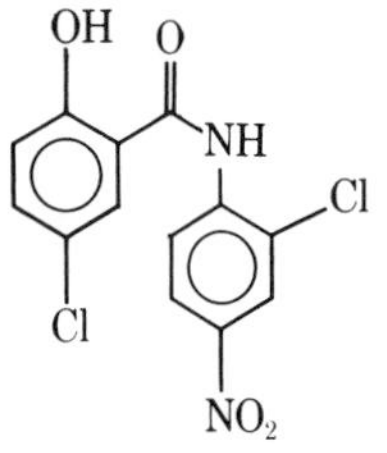

Figure 3. Drugs effective against cestode infections.

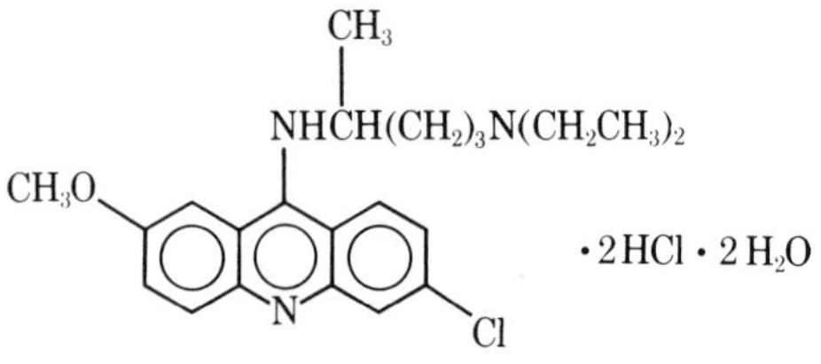

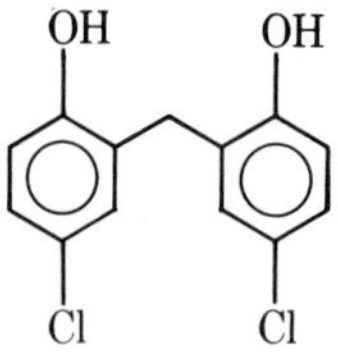

of glucose uptake. This drug uncouples oxidative phosphorylation in both mammalian and taenioid mitochondria (35–36) inhibiting the anaerobic incorporation of inorganic phosphate into ATP. Tapeworms are very sensitive to (12) because they depend on anaerobic metabolism of carbohydrate as their major source of energy. The selective toxicity for the parasites as compared to the host is that very little (12) is absorbed from the gastrointestinal tract (37). Adverse effects are nausea, abdominal pain and malaise in 10% of the patients; a few become lightheaded.

A single dose of niclosamide is used for the large tapeworms. Niclosamide causes the tapeworm head to disengage from the intestinal wall of the host, and the body wall of the parasite disintegrates. Some investigators believe the drug sensitizes the wall of the worm to the action of proteolytic enzymes. When infection by a dwarf tapeworm is treated, the drug taken the first day disposes of the worms that are in the intestinal cavity; however, there are also developing stages in the tissue of the intestinal wall, and these are unharmed. Therefore, dosage must be repeated for 5–7 d to destroy these worms as they finish their development and reenter the intestinal lumen.

There have never been any drugs that are effective against tissue inhabiting stages of cestodes in main; however praziquantel [55268-74-1] (11) (Droncit) is being used against intermediate tissue stages of tapeworms in veterinary medicine.

Quinacrine hydrochloride (13) is an older drug that is effective against tapeworms (38). It is a second choice drug for infections with the beef tapeworm (*T. saginata*) and the large fish tapeworm (*D. latum*), but it is less successful against the dwarf tapeworm (*H. nana*) and some workers advise against its use to treat infection with the pork tapeworm (*T. solium*). It concentrates in the scolex and causes the muscles needed for holding to relax. Worms are stained yellow and pass from the body, still alive. Quinacrine can intercalate with DNA and inhibit nucleic acid synthesis. Quinacrine creates fluorescent bands in deoxyadenylate–deoxythymidylate-rich regions of DNA and has been used as a stain in the study of human genetics.

The selective toxicity of this drug is unexplained except for accumulation in the head of the tapeworm. The drug is readily absorbed from the gastrointestinal tract and may persist in human tissues for 2 mo after administration. Prolonged treatment with the large dose used in helminthiases may cause yellow discoloration of skin. An anthelminthic dose may commonly cause vomiting in one out of four patients and possible regurgitation of *T. solium* eggs into the stomach, with the subsequent possibility of producing an autoinfection of incurable cysticercosis. Quinacrine (13) is more toxic than niclosamide (12) without being more efficacious and is troublesome to administer.

Dichlorophen (14) was used for many years in veterinary medicine before it was introduced for human disease. This is an oral drug available in Europe but not in the United States, and is used against intestinal tapeworms. The drug is still employed in veterinary medicine, and as a germicide in soaps and shampoos, and as a fungicide in agriculture (39) (see Fungicides). Some authors regard dichlorophen as structurally similar to niclosamide (12) and bithionol (7), considering them as halogenated derivatives of diphenylmethane, and related substances (40). The tapeworm detaches under the influence of dichlorophen, dies, and is digested, and does not come out of the host in a recognizable state. Adverse effects are gastrointestinal disturbance, lassitude and depression, and hives. The drug itself is laxative.

Paromomycin [7542-37-2] (Humatin) is a broad-spectrum antibiotic that has been employed for treatment of *H. nana* and *T. saginata*, and for amoebiasis, as well as for its antibacterial effects in diarrheas and dysenteries (see Antibiotics, aminoglycosides).

The broad fish tapeworm grows to a length of 10 m with 4000 proglottides that tend to remain attached and discharge eggs which appear with the feces. Besides absorbing host foodstuffs, this worm avidly sequesters vitamin B_{12} and folic acid . The nearer to the stomach that it is attached in the small intestine, the more vitamin it takes up. This may so deplete the supplies available to the host that pernicious anemia can develop with associated neurological symptoms. There is usually only one worm in a patient and it can survive for 10 yr.

The beef tapeworm is of worldwide distribution in people who eat rare beef. Worms are often 5–10 m long with about 1000 proglottides, and usually a patient carries only one worm. Cases are frequently asymptomatic; however, detached sections of worm 0.5 cm × 2 cm may creep out of the end of the digestive tract.

Both the adult and the larval bladderworm of the pork tapeworm are able to live in man, the parasite being sporadic in occurrence wherever uncooked pork is eaten. The adult is 5 m long and untreated adult worms may survive for 25 yr.

The dwarf tapeworm is only 2–4 cm long, and is of universal distribution in mice and man in temperature zones, where children, especially those in institutions, are the group most frequently infected. Often symptomless, this tapeworm can cause abdominal discomfort and diarrhea if infection is heavy.

Treatment of Intestinal Roundworm (Nematode) Infections

Bephenium hydroxynaphthoate (15) (Fig. 4) is effective against the hookworm *Ancylostoma duodenale* and a one-day oral treatment cures up to 100% of infections (41). The drug can also be used in patients with *Necator* and *Ascaris* but is less effective and may fail against resistant strains of *Necator*. It is used in veterinary medicine.

Bephenium [7181-73-9] is a quaternary ammonium compound with a structure similar to that of acetylcholine, and is more potent than acetylcholine in causing contraction of isolated roundworm muscle strips, an action that can be blocked by *d*-tubocurarine (see Alkaloids). Hookworms become discoordinated under treatment with bephenium, lose their hold on the intestinal mucosa and are carried along in a contracted state with the fecal stream. The selective toxicity for intestinal roundworms may be dependent in part on the fact that it goes essentially unabsorbed through the digestive tract. This is not a dangerous drug but the taste is so bitter that administration can cause nausea and vomiting.

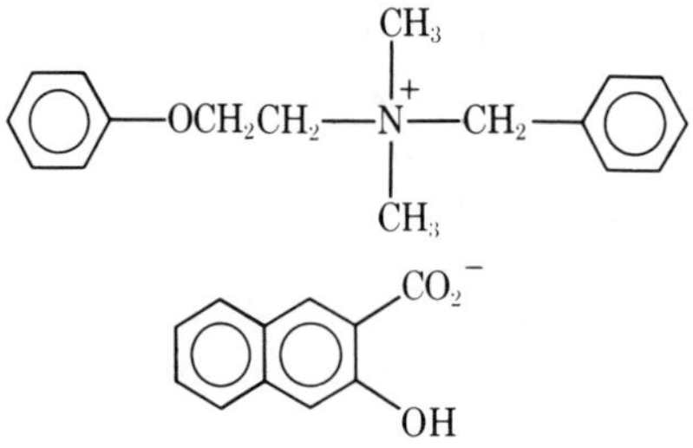

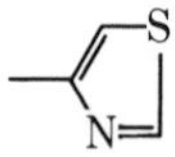

Figure 4. Drugs effective against nematode infections.

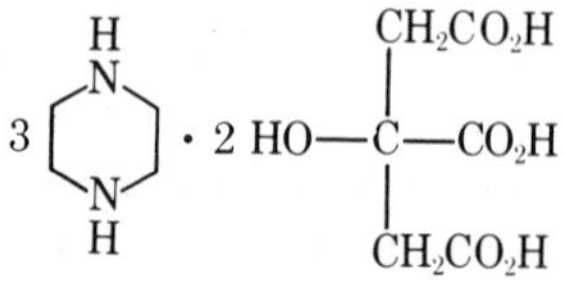

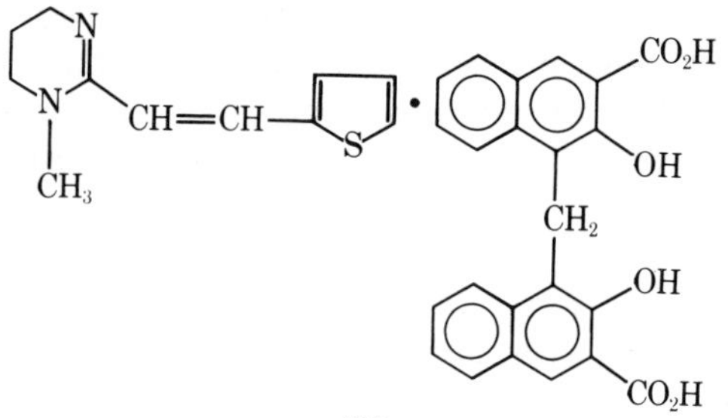

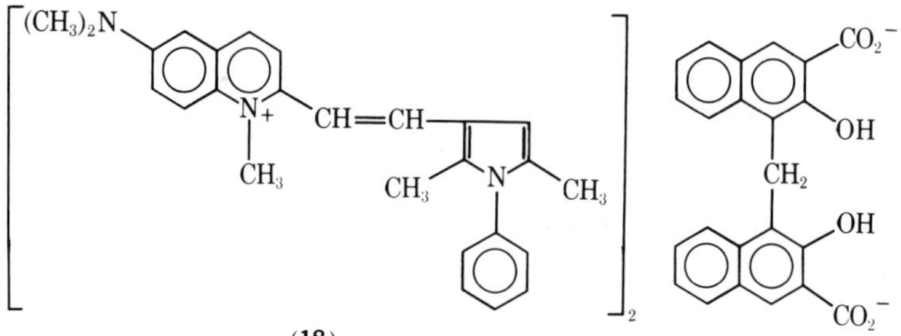

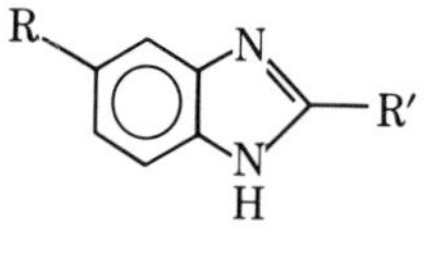

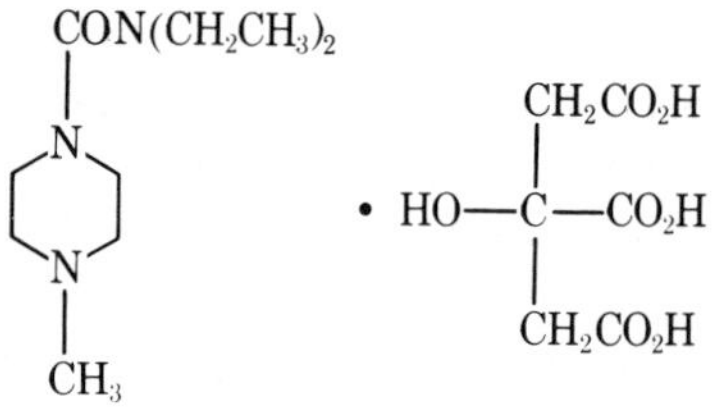

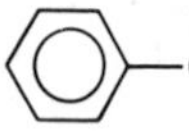

A. duodenale adults are about 1 cm long and live throughout the small intestine holding onto a mouthful of mucosa and draining blood from the capillary circulation. A patient may harbor 1000 worms, and one worm may pump out 2/3 mL blood/d; thus hookworm anemia is caused by blood loss and the severity is related to the number of worms. Untreated worms may survive in the intestine 1–15 yr.

Piperazine (16) (see Amines, cyclic) is taken orally by nonfasting subjects, one dose a day on two consecutive days for large roundworms (Ascaris), and reports continue to indicate that it will cure about 90% of cases treated (42–44). This drug can be used for the human pinworm (Enterobius) with a 7-d course of treatment and it is used in veterinary medicine.

Piperazine causes flaccid paralysis of Ascaris by blocking the ability of the worm to respond to acetylcholine and they lose their position in the digestive tract, and are carried out, still alive. In the helminth, acetylcholine may be a modulating neuro-hormone rather than a chemotransmitter. The drug is well absorbed from the human intestine and the reason for its selective toxicity is uncertain.

Occasional side effects from piperazine include abdominal cramps, nausea, vomiting, and diarrhea. Rarely patients may have headache, vertigo, and tremors, or they may feel weak and have difficulty focusing. Red patches can appear on the skin, sometimes with the flat, elevated, itching welts of urticaria.

Female worms of Ascaris lumbricoides are about 30 cm × 0.5 cm, and as adults they live and feed in the small intestine where they hold their position by taking the shape of a simple spring. Sometimes they cause abdominal discomfort or pain; but frequently light infections are symptomless. Adult worms can migrate in response to disease or surgery when they may penetrate suture lines, perforate the intestinal wall, or travel up ducts. Untreated adult worms may live for a year and a half before they disappear.

Pyrantel pamoate (17) in a single oral dose cures pinworm infections, and is close to 100% effective against Ascaris (45–46). It may be repeated in a month if the worms return. This is also a principal drug for treating hookworm infections of both species, thus it is useful in patients with mixed infections. For hookworms, treatment is continued 3 d. In roundworms, muscle is persistently activated resulting in spastic paralysis. The drug was introduced in veterinary medicine and then applied to clinical medicine.

Since about 90% of the administered dose passes out in the feces of the patient, the selective toxicity of the drug can be attributed primarily to poor absorption. Abdominal pain, nausea, vomiting, diarrhea, and lack of appetite may occur. Patients may have headache and feel dizzy or drowsy. Skin rashes can develop. In the blood chemistry, SGOT (Serum Glutamic Oxaloacetic Transaminase) levels may be elevated.

The pinworm (Enterobius vermicularis) is of worldwide distribution in temperate zones, including cities, where it is frequently a disease of households or institutions. Female worms are about 1 cm long. While growing to maturity, they live in the gut lumen holding on by their mouths to the intestinal mucosa. A symptom is an itchy perianal region, because the mature female migrates out the anus and discharges eggs with itchy secretions. A usual intestinal population is less than 100 worms; however, more than 5000 have been recovered from a single patient. Eggs also get into the household dust and are resistant to drying and may even be inhaled and swallowed, leading to very light infections with very few worms in adult relatives of infected children.

Pyrvinium pamoate (18) is an oral drug used in a single dose against pinworm and repeated in a week. When the drug is used for treatment of threadworm (*Strongyloides*), one dose a day is given for seven days.

Pyrvinium (18) is the salt of an asymmetrical cyanine dye with a resonating amidinium system in the molecule (47). In anaerobic worms, such as pinworm and threadworm, it irreversibly interferes with the absorption of glucose. This causes relative failure of muscular activity, then reduced motility. As adenosine triphosphate (ATP) levels steadily fall within the worms, they eventually die. (In some other aerobic parasitic worms that are not parasites of man, pyrvinium causes respiratory inhibition, thus decreasing oxygen uptake.)

Tetrachloroethylene (9) can be used for hookworm infections that have been diagnosed as caused by *Necator americanus*, in which a single oral dose will cure more than half of the cases treated, and reduce worm burdens and egg production in the rest. (The other hookworm, *Ancylostoma duodenale*, is less responsive to this medication.) Under the influence of tetrachloroethylene the worms detach from the mucosa and do not reattach. They move along with the fecal stream to appear in the stool alive and motile; this effect has been interpreted as reversible paralysis of the worms.

Mebendazole (19), by oral administration repeated 3 or 4 d in a row, is most effective against whipworm (*Trichuris trichiura*). In addition, a single dose usually cures infection of the pinworm, and the drug is effective against hookworms and *Ascaris*, and partially effective against threadworms (*Strongyloides*) and taenioid tapeworms. This benzimidazole derivative is a broad-spectrum anthelmintic (48), and is used in veterinary medicine as well as in clinical practice. It belongs to the same series of drugs as thiabendazole (20), and they are closely related to fungicides (qv) such as benomyl [17804-35-2].

Mebendazole (19) interferes with the glucose metabolism of helminths, irreversibly inhibiting glucose uptake. Thereafter glycogen stores in the worms are depleted, and then ATP supplies fail. The worms are slowly immobilized, die, and are lost from the body over a period of three days. In developing *Trichuris* eggs, larvae fail to form normally. Part of the selective toxicity may be that mebendazole has an antimicrotubule action on the intestinal cells of nematodes but not mammals. Furthermore, relatively little is absorbed from the gastrointestinal tract. Adverse effects that may occur in patients under treatment are abdominal pain and diarrhea.

The adult female whipworm (*Trichuris trichiura*) is 5 cm long, and these worms lie with the thin anterior whip ends buried in the mucosa of the intestine, where they feed on tissue juice and small amounts of blood. Infections of several hundred worms may cause irritation and inflammation of the mucosa with abdominal pain, diarrhea, and gas. Untreated adult worms live for years.

Treatment of Tissue Roundworm (Nematode) Infections

Thiabendazole (20) is an effective oral drug against many roundworms that are affected by other anthelmintics, and also works against some nematode tissue parasites that are not successfully treated with other agents. The threadworm (*Strongyloides stercoralis*) that lives embedded in the intestinal wall was a therapeutic problem until the effectiveness of thiabendazole was discovered; and it was the first drug reported to have a beneficial influence on trichinosis, the disease in which *Trichinella spiralis* larvae migrate through skeletal muscle. This drug is prophylactic against trichinosis in persons known to have just eaten infected pork. It can be used in persons with guineaworm (*Dracunculus medinensis*), or for treating cutaneous larva migrans (*Ancylostoma braziliense*) and visceral larva migrans (*Toxocara*). Among the intestinal nematodes, it works against pinworm (*Enterobius*); and somewhat against hookworms, roundworm, and whipworm; the drug can be given to persons with multiple infection of the intestine (47). Extensively used in veterinary medicine, thiabendazole was the first broad-spectrum benzimidazole anthelmintic.

The mechanism by which nematodes are killed is unknown; however, one of the biochemical effects of thiabendazole is to inhibit fumarate reductase, an enzyme that generates ATP as it converts fumarate to succinate in the mitochondria of helminths. The selective toxicity may be caused by differences between enzymes of parasite and host, since the drug is rapidly absorbed, with 90% of a dose passed in the urine in the first day (mostly as metabolic products, one of which may give urine and sweat a distinctive odor).

One ppm of thiabendazole (20) will prevent *Ascaris* eggs from maturing and, in therapeutic topical concentrations, it is used to prevent development of dog and cat hookworm larvae that have invaded human skin to cause cutaneous larva migrans. In laboratory animals thiabendazole is antipyretic, analgesic, and antiinflammatory, as well as anthelmintic. Probably this is also true in humans and may account for the symptomatic improvement in persons with early systemic trichinosis.

Among the adverse effects are digestive disturbances, neurological symptoms, and manifestations of allergic responses. As many as half the patients are incapacitated for several hours after taking the drug. Overall, effects are dose related and transient.

Niridazole (6), already discussed with drugs used for schistosomaisis, is employed in the treatment of infection with the guineaworm (*Dracunculus medinensis*), as is metronidazole [443-48-1] (Flagyl), the broad-spectrum antiprotozoal agent (see Chemotherapeutics, antiprotozoal). Stringlike worms about 1 m long but less than 2 mm dia can be seen and felt below the skin surface, with the head of the worm usually exposed in an ulcer on the foot. The far end of the worm is hooked, so that although it is possible to grasp the front end and pull, the worm does not slide out easily and is apt to break with infectious, allergic, and toxic consequences as the remainder under the skin dies and deteriorates. The treatment is to give niridazole (6) orally two or three times a day for 7 d. With the effect of the drug, either the worm comes out or it can be pulled easily without danger. If left untreated, within a month the worm may come out naturally, or withdraw from the opening and be resorbed.

Diethylcarbamazine (21) has been successfully employed for decades by oral administration to cure infection with the species that causes elephantiasis, and to treat the other filariases (50). It kills microfilariae of the filarial worms: *Wuchereria bancrofti*, *Brugia malayi*, *Loa loa*, *Mansonella ozzardi*, *Dipetalonema streptocerca*, *D. perstans*, and *Onchocerca volvulus* (however, onchocerciasis recurs after therapy). There is a disease condition called eosinophilic lung, or tropical eosinophilia, the symptoms of which can be relieved by diethylcarbamazine. This drug is one of the anthelmintics that may have pharmacological effects that enhance immunological response. Another such anthelmintic drug is levamisole [14769-73-4, 53631-68-8] (22). Diethylcarbamazine is used in veterinary medicine.

(22)

This derivative of piperazine affects microfilariae so that they become susceptible to phagocytosis by fixed macrophages of the reticulo–endothelial system. Adult *Wuchereria* and *Loa* are killed. Why this drug is selectively toxic is not known. It is well absorbed and widely distributed, and does not cumulate in parasites, neither microfilariae nor adults. Adults of *Wuchereria bancrofti*, the filarial worm that causes elephantiasis, are coiled in the lymph system where females attain a length of 10 cm. Over the years, tissue reactions result in obstruction to lymph return while lymph nodes, lymph vessels, and the spleen may enlarge. Elephantiasis is a late and unusual complication when dependent parts of the body become edematous, enlarge, and then in time become firm and covered with a rough nodular skin. Untreated adult worms live for 5–10 yr.

Loa loa females are about 6 cm long and migrate constantly through connective tissues. The disease caused is Calabar swellings, which are local responses to worms and/or their products that last two or three days and then regress. A worm may get into the anterior chamber of the eye and the patient may be able to see it, or sometimes one eye is puffed shut when a worm is in the vicinity; because of these effects *Loa* is called the eye worm. The untreated worms will live as long as 10 yr. The seriousness of other filarial infections varies all the way from symptomless with *Mansonella* to cosmetic disfiguration and blindness with *Onchocerca*. The regimen for diethylcarbamazine varies with the condition being treated.

Adverse effects of nausea, fever, headache, and dizziness may occur during diethylcarbamazine therapy and simultaneous administration of corticosteroids and antihistamines is intended to reduce the probability of rash, itch, edema, and other more severe allergic responses to the disintegration of worms. Care must be exercised in the management of patients infected with *Onchocerca*. They have a violent reaction within the first day, and toxicity and fever can last as long as a week. Supplementary treatment with Suramin [129-46-4] (an antitrypanosomal drug) is required to rid patients of adult *Onchocerca* (51).

BIBLIOGRAPHY

"Parasitic Infections, Chemotherapy" in *ECT* 2nd ed., Vol. 14, pp. 532–551, by Helmut Mrozik, Merck & Co., Inc.

1. U.S. Pat. 2,335,585 (Nov. 30, 1943), N. A. Davies (to American Cream Tartar).
2. U.S. Pat. 2,391,297 (Dec. 18, 1945), N. A. Davies (to Stauffer Chemical Co.).
3. U.S. Pat. 2,918,401 (Sept. 9, 1959), F. C. Copp (to Burroughs Wellcome).
4. Ger. Pat. 1,117,600 (Nov. 23, 1961), F. C. Copp (to Wellcome Foundation).
5. Ger. Pat. 583,055 (Aug. 28, 1933), F. Muth (to I. G. Farbenind A.G.).
6. U.S. Pat. 2,849,494 (Aug. 26, 1958), R. H. Cooper and K. Goldberg (to Monsanto).
7. U.S. Pat. 2,232,970 (Mar. 4, 1941), H. Ardersag, S. Breitner, and H. Jung (to Winthrop Chemical Co.).
8. U.S. Pat. 2,334,408 (Nov. 16, 1944), W. S. Gump and M. Luthy (to Burton T. Bush).
9. U.S. Pat. 2,467,893; 2,467,894; 2,467,895 (Apr. 19, 1949), S. Kushner and L. Brancone (to American Cyanamid).
10. U.S. Pat. 1,717,101 (June 11, 1929), H. Hirzel (to Sharp & Dohme).
11. U.S. Pat. 3,294,598 (Apr. 4, 1967), G. P. Rosi and D. Peruzzotti (to Sterling Drug).
12. W. Kikuth and R. Gönnert, *Ann. Trop. Med. Parisitol.* **42**, 256 (1948).
13. U.S. Pat. 3,657,267 (Feb. 18, 1971), J. C. H. Van Gelder (to Janssen).
14. U.S. Pat. 3,079,297 (Feb. 26, 1963), E. Schraufstraller and R. Gonnert (to Bayer).
15. Belg. Pat. 632,989 (Nov. 29, 1963) (to Ciba Ltd.).
16. U.S. Pat. 2,901,482 (Aug. 25, 1959), G. F. MacKenzie and K. L. Turbin (to The Dow Chemical Co.).

17. S. Afr. Pat. 68 00516 (June 27, 1968), R. V. Kasubrick and J. W. McFarland (to Chas. Pfizer and Co.).
18. U.S. Pat. 2,952,419 (Feb. 6, 1960), E. F. Elslager and D. F. Worth (to Parke, Davis).
19. U.S. Pat. 2,113,357 (Apr. 15, 1939), F. Mietzsch and H. Mauss (to Winthrop Chemical Co.).
20. U.S. Pat. 2,880,222 (Mar. 31, 1959), E. A. H. Friedheim.
21. U.S. Pat. 1,549,154 (Aug. 11, 1925); 1,873,668 (Aug. 23, 1932), H. Schmidt (to Winthrop Chemical Co.).
22. U.S. Pat. 3,040,109 (June 9, 1959), R. E. Feathers and R. H. Rogerson (to Pittsburgh Plate Glass).
23. U.S. Pat. 3,017,415 (June 16, 1962), L. Sarett (to Merck & Co.).
24. H. Most, *N. Engl. J. Med.* **287,** 495 (1972).
25. *Ibid.,* p. 698.
26. *The Roche Vademecum 1976,* F. Hoffmann-LaRoche & Co. Limited, Basle, Switz., 1976, pp. 31–33.
27. *Informational Material for Physicians Sodium Antimony Dimercaptosuccinate (Astiban),* Parasitic Diseases Branch, Center for Disease Control, Atlanta, Ga., 1968, pp. 1–15.
28. H. J. Saz and E. Bueding, *Pharmacol. Rev.* **18,** 871 (1966).
29. S. Archer and A. Yarinsky, *Progr. Drug Res.* **16,** 11 (1972).
30. *Informational Material for Physicians Niridazole (Ambilhar),* Parasitic Diseases Branch, Center for Disease Control, Atlanta, Ga., 1976, pp. 1–11.
31. N. Katz, *Adv. Pharmacol. Chemother.* **14,** 1 (1977).
32. G. J. Frayha, *Leban. Med. J.* **25,** 507 (1972).
33. U. K. Sheth, *Prog. Drug Res.* **19,** 147 (1975).
34. M. Katz, *Drugs* **13,** 124 (1977).
35. J. Putter, *Z. Parasitenk.* **34,** 23 (1970).
36. J. Putter and P. Andrews, *Conference of the German Society for Parasitology, Wuppertal, Apr. 9–11, 1970.*
37. *Informational Material Yomesan (Niclosamide),* Parasitic Diseases Branch, Center for Disease Control, Atlanta, Ga., 1976, pp. 1–7.
38. J. S. Swartzwelder, *J. La. State Med. Soc.* **111,** 394 (1959).
39. R. B. Burrows, *Progr. Drug Res.* **17,** 108 (1973).
40. G. Gras, *Med. Afr. Noire* **21,** 11 (1974).
41. D. A. Ogunmekan, *West Afr. Med. J.* **22,** 47 (1973).
42. H. S. Pond and co-workers, *South. Med. J.* **63,** 599 (1970).
43. M. A. Haleem, F. A. Lari, and R. J. Rahimtoola, *J. Pak. Med. Assoc.* **22,** 276 (1972).
44. W. Hatchuel, M. Isaacson, and D. J. de Villiers, *South Afr. Med. J.* **47,** 91 (1973).
45. W. J. Bell and S. Nassif, *Am. J. Trop. Med. Hyg.* **20,** 584 (1971).
46. T. Ishizaki and M. Yokogawa, *Yonsei Rep. Trop. Med.* **4,** 159 (1973).
47. E. Bueding and C. Swartzwelder, *Pharmacol. Rev.* **9,** 329 (1957).
48. J. W. McFarland, *Prog. Drug Res.* **16,** 157 (1972).
49. E. Barrett-Connor, *Am. J. Gastroenterol.* **63,** 105 (1975).
50. J. F. Maldonado and co-workers, *P. R. J. Public Health and Trop. Med.* **25,** 291 (1950).
51. *Informational Material for Physicians Suramin (Bayer 205),* Parasitic Diseases Branch, Center for Disease Control, Atlanta, Ga., 1966, pp. 1–11.

General References

American Medical Association Department of Drugs, "Anthelmintics" in *AMA Drug Evaluations,* 3rd ed., Publishing Sciences Group, Inc., Littleton, Mass., 1977, pp. 862–876.

C. L. Bailey and J. D. Shoft, eds., *APhA Drug Names,* American Pharmaceutical Association, Washington, D.C., 1976.

R. Berkow, ed., "Diseases Caused by Worms" in *The Merck Manual,* 13th ed., Merck Sharp & Dohme Laboratories, Rahway, N. J., 1977, pp. 166–177.

D. R. Botero, "Chemotherapy of Human Intestinal Parasitic Diseases" in *Annu. Rev. Pharmacol. Toxicol.* **18,** 1 (1978).

L. A. Bulla, Jr., and T. C. Cheng, eds., "Pathobiology of Invertebrate Vectors of Disease" in *Ann. N.Y. Acad. Sci.* **266,** 332 (1975).

W. C. Campbell and H. Mrozik, "Antiparasitic Agents" in *Annu. Rep. Med. Chem.* **9,** 115 (1974).

L. L. Corrigan, ed., *Evaluations of Drug Interactions,* 2nd ed., American Pharmaceutical Association, Washington, D.C., 1976, 476 pp.

E. C. Faust, P. F. Russell, and R. C. Jung, "Helminths and Helminthic Infections" in *Craig and Faust's Clinical Parasitology,* 8th ed., Lea & Febiger, Philadelphia, Pa., 1970, pp. 251–570.

F. C. Goble and B. G. Maegraith, eds., "The Pharmacological and Chemotherapeutic Properties of Niridazole and other Antischistosomal Compounds" in *Ann. N.Y. Acad. Sci.* **160,** 423 (1969).

A. Goth, "Anthelmintic Drugs" in *Medical Pharmacology* 8th ed., C.V. Mosby, St. Louis, Mo., 1976, pp. 625–635.

G. W. Hunter, III, J. C. Swartzwelder, and D. F. Clyde, "Helminthic Diseases" in *Tropical Medicine,* 5th ed., W. B. Saunders, Philadelphia, Pa., 1976, pp. 451–621.

B. H. Kean and D. W. Hoskins, "Drugs for Intestinal Parasitism" in W. Modell, ed., *Drugs of Choice 1976–77,* C.V. Mosby, St. Louis, Inc., 1976, pp. 356–369.

B. H. Kean, K. E. Mott, and A. J. Russell, *Tropical Medicine and Parasitology, Classic Investigations,* Vols. I and II, Cornell University Press, Ithaca, N. Y. 1978, 678 pp.

A. Korolkovas and J. H. Burckhalter, "Anthelmintic Agents" in *Essentials of Medicinal Chemistry,* John Wiley & Sons., Inc., New York, 1976, pp. 387–402.

K. MacDonald, "Hookworm Disease" in F. H. Top, Sr., and P. F. Wehrel, eds., *Communicable and Infectious Diseases,* 8th ed., C.V. Mosby, St. Louis, Mo., 1976, pp. 359–361.

K. MacDonald, "Larva Migrans, Visceral and Cutaneous" in F. H. Top, Sr., and P. F. Wehrle, eds., *Communicable and Infectious Diseases,* 8th ed., C.V. Mosby, St. Louis, Mo., 1976, pp. 379–383.

E. K. Markell and M. Voge, *Medical Parasitology,* 14th ed., W.B. Saunders, Philadelphia, Pa., 1976, pp. 167–304.

P. D. Marsden and K. S. Warren, "Helminthic Disease" in P. B. Beeson and W. McDermott, eds., *Textbook of Medicine,* 14th ed., W.B. Saunders, Philadelphia, Pa., 1975, pp. 506–539.

E. J. Martin, "Antiparasitic Agents" in *Annu. Rep. Med. Chem.* **11,** 121 (1976).

E. J. Martin, "Antiparasitic Agents" in *Annu. Rep. Med. Chem.* **10,** 154 (1975).

A. W. Mathies, Jr., and K. MacDonald, *Trichinosis* in F. H. Top, Sr., and P. F. Wehrle, eds., *Communicable and Infectious Diseases,* 8th ed., C.V. Mosby, St. Louis, Mo., 1976, pp. 719–723.

J. J. Plorde, I. L. Bennett, Jr., and R. G. Petersdorf, "Diseases Caused by Worms" in W. M. Wintrobe and co-eds., *Harrison's Principles of Internal Medicine* 7th ed., Mack Publishing Co., Easton, Pa., 1974, pp. 1035–1058.

W. B. Pratt, "Chemotherapy of Helminthic Diseases" in *Chemotherapy of Infection,* Oxford University Press, New York, 1977, pp. 373–407.

I. M. Rollo, "Drugs Used in the Chemotherapy of Helminthiasis" in L. S. Goodman and A. Gilman, eds., *The Pharmacological Basis of Therapeutics,* 5th ed., MacMillan, New York, 1975, pp. 1018–1044.

I. S. Rossoff, *Handbook of Veterinary Drugs,* Springer Publishing Company, New York, 1974, 730 pp.

E. A. Swinyard, "Parasiticides Anthelmintics" in A. Osol and J. W. Hoover, eds., *Remington's Pharmaceutical Sciences,* 15th ed., Mack Publishing Company, Easton, Pa., 1975, pp. 1172–1178.

J. H. Thompson, "Drugs Used in the Treatment of Helminthiasis" in J. A. Bevan, ed., *Essentials of Pharmacology,* 2nd ed., Harper & Row, Hagerstown, Md., 1976, pp. 512–518.

A. Wade, ed., *Martindale, The Extra Pharmacopeia,* 27th ed., The Pharmaceutical Press, London, Eng., 1977, pp. 98–115, 1370–1379.

C. C. Wang and M. H. Fisher, "Antiparasitic Agents" in *Annu. Rep. Med. Chem.* **12,** 140 (1977).

C. Wilcocks and P. E. C. Manson-Bahr, "Diseases Caused by Helminths" in *Manson's Tropical Diseases,* 17th ed., Williams & Wilkins Co., Baltimore, Md., 1972, pp. 192–354.

M. Windholz, ed., *The Merck Index,* 9th ed., Merck & Co., Inc., Rahway, N.J., 1976, 9856 pp.

JAMES W. INGALLS
Arnold & Marie Schwartz College of Pharmacy and Health Sciences

ANTIMITOTIC

Cancer is still one of the scourges of man, but encouraging results with various types of treatment offer hope for continuing advances in the fight against this disease. The most frequently used treatments at present are surgery, radiation (including radioactive isotopes), and chemotherapy, with future possibilities' for immunotherapy.

The earliest reference to the chemical treatment of cancer describes the use of arsenic paste in ancient Egypt; later, caustic pastes were used by Hippocrates (1). Little progress was made until the 19th century, when potassium arsenite [10124-50-2], the first systemically effective antitumor agent, was for a time the treatment of choice for leukemia (2), and toxins were used to treat malignancies (3). Subsequently, a great variety of local and systemic agents were used for antineoplastic therapy with varying degrees of success. Hormones (qv) represented the next chemotherapeutic advance, with the first reports of the use of sex hormones in breast cancer in 1896 (4) and in prostatic cancer in 1941 (5). The modern era in cancer chemotherapy, however, began with the introduction of the polyfunctional alkylating agents, such as nitrogen mustard [555-77-1] in malignant lymphoma, in the early 1940s (6–8). Soon after, the folic acid antagonist aminopterin [54-62-6] was found to induce remission in acute lymphocytic leukemia in children (9). By 1950 useful agents had begun to appear in rapid succession (10–12); since then, whole classes of antitumor drugs have become available. With the establishment of a national development program in 1955, the chemical treatment of cancer has joined surgery and radiation therapy as a standard approach.

Although most current antineoplastic drugs were discovered empirically, considerable insight has been gained into the mechanisms by which many of these compounds affect cell growth, and this has allowed a more rational therapeutic application of these agents. This insight has also led to the development of new drugs designed to kill the cancer cell either directly or by depleting its essential growth elements. In addition to the discovery of new experimental compounds, chemotherapy research has been directed toward alteration in dosimetry and employment of various drug combinations to enhance tumoricidal effects and decrease toxicity. Palliative benefits are definitely attainable and include prolongation of useful survival as well as subjective and objective remission of physical and emotional disability. Decreases in tumor mass and metastatic involvement may be obtained with chemotherapy alone. Moreover, it has proved to be a valuable adjunct to surgical and irradiation procedures. Today, several neoplastic diseases (Burkitt's lymphoma, choriocarcinoma, acute leukemia, etc) can be associated with a normal life expectancy after drug treatment, alone or in combination with other types of therapy.

Drug Classification

Many compounds have been investigated in experimental animals, and a few have proven sufficiently useful in the clinical treatment of human neoplasms, at acceptable levels of toxicity, to deserve the designation of chemotherapeutic agents. The drugs currently used in the chemotherapy of malignant diseases may be divided into several classes according to their general pharmacologic activity: alkylating agents; antimetabolites; antibiotics; plant alkaloids; miscellaneous agents; and hormones.

Agents that do not fit any of the other categories are discussed as a separate miscellaneous group. This classification serves as a convenient framework for describing the various types of agents. In addition, functional classification becomes increasingly important as investigators attempt to use this information to design rational chemotherapeutic regimens.

The compounds discussed here all fall under the jurisdiction of the FDA and are, for the most part, those with long and successful clinical use, although a few have been included either because they illustrate special circumstances or because they represent newer developments. Excluded are several compounds whose structural variations offer no particular advantage over existing drugs or that need additional investigation.

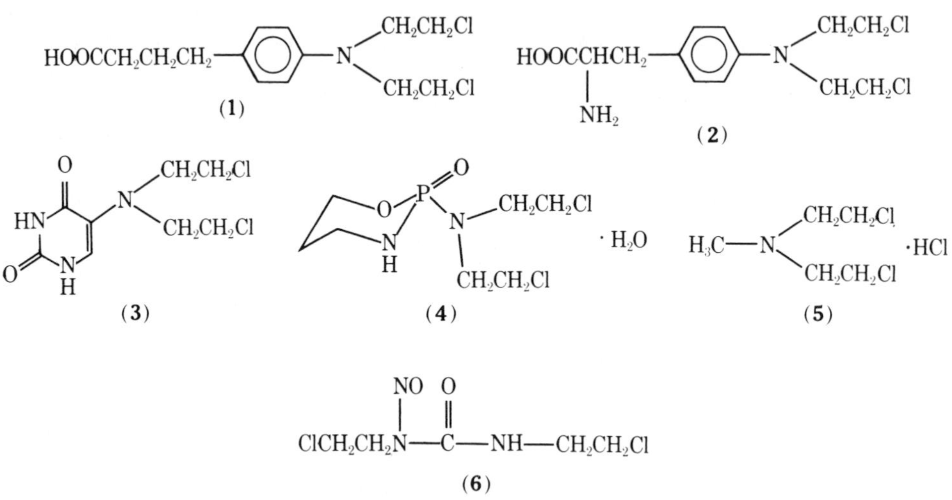

Figure 1. Alkylating agents.

Table 1.   Alkylating Agents

Drug, trade name	CAS Registry No.	mp, °C	Dosage form and dosage
(1) chlorambucil USP, Leukeran	[305-03-3]	64–66	tablet: 2 mg oral initial: 0.1–0.2 mg/(kg·d) for 3–6 wk maintenance: 2–4 mg/d
(2) melphalan USP, Alkeran	[148-82-3]	182–183 (dec)	tablet: 2 mg oral initial: 6 mg once a d for 2–3 wk maintenance: 2–4 mg once a d
(3) uracil mustard NF, Uracil Mustard	[66-75-1]	206 (dec)	capsule: 1 mg oral: 1–2 mg/d for 3 wk, repeat after 1 wk interval or 3–5 mg/d for 7 d, then 1 mg/d for 3 wk

Also excluded are hormones, which are not specific oncolytic agents but act by altering the hormonal environment of endocrine-dependent cancers.

Dosage schedules (which depend on such factors as the clinical indication, drug toxicity, and the patient's nutritional and functional status, and vary more widely than indicated in this survey), available sizes, toxicity (not a comprehensive review), and the clinical indications for use (not an exhaustive listing), are shown under the individual drugs. The proprietary names of the drug are given wherever possible.

Alkylating Agents. These agents (Fig. 1, Table 1) include a diverse group of chemicals (nitrogen mustards (1–6), nitrosoureas (7–8), triazenes (10), etc) that have

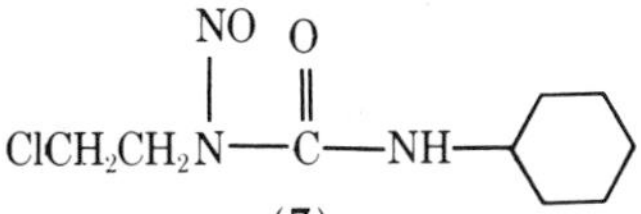

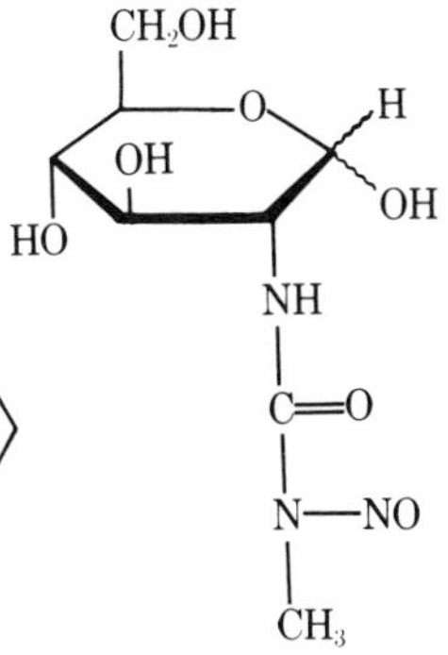

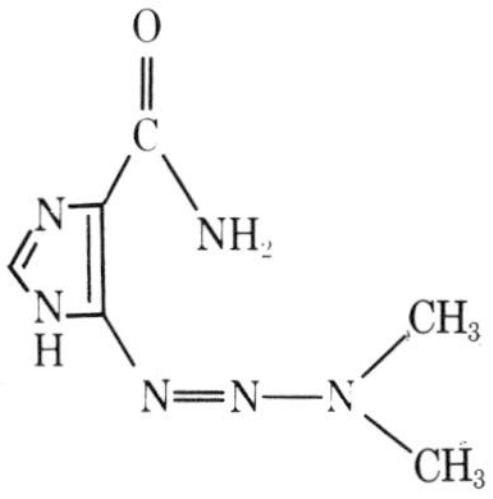

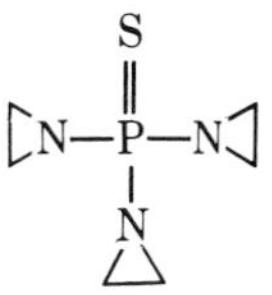

Fig. 1. (*continued*)

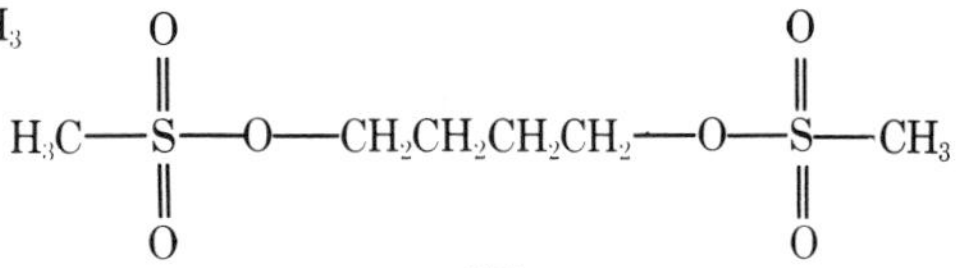

Disease	Toxic effects	Manufacturer
chronic lymphocytic leukemia; cancer of ovary, breast, testis; Hodgkin's disease; non-Hodgkin's lymphomas	bone-marrow depression; nausea; vomiting	Burroughs Wellcome
multiple myeloma; plasmacytic myeloma; cancer of breast and ovary	bone-marrow depression; nausea; vomiting; anorexia	Burroughs Wellcome
Hodgkin's disease; non-Hodgkin's lymphomas; cancer of ovary; chronic lymphocytic leukemia; primary thrombocytosis	bone-marrow depression; dermatitis; diarrhea; nausea; vomiting	Upjohn

Table 1. (*continued*)

Drug, trade name	CAS Registry No.	mp, °C	Dosage form and dosage

(4) Cyclophosphamide USP, Cytoxan	[6055-19-2]	41–45	vials: 100, 200, 500 mg
			tablets: 25, 50 mg
			intravenous (iv), initial:
			  10–20 mg/kg
			  once a d for 2–5 d
			maintenance: 10–15 mg/kg
			  every 7–10 d or
			  3–5 mg/kg two times a
			  wk
			oral: 1–5 mg/kg once a d

(5) mechlorethamine hydrochloride USP, Mustargen hydrochloride	[55-86-7]	108–111	vial: 10 mg
			iv: 0.4 mg/kg as a single
			  dose or 0.1 mg/kg once
			  a d for 4 d
			intraperitoneal (ip) or
			  intrapleural: 0.2–0.4
			  mg/kg as a single dose

(6) carmustine, BCNU	[154-93-8]	30–32	vial: 100 mg
			iv: 100–200 mg/m^2 once a d
			  for 1–2 d; do not repeat
			  for at least 6 wk

(7) lomustine, CCNU	[13010-47-4]	89	capsules: 10, 40, 100 mg
			oral: 100–130 mg/m^2 as
			  a single dose every 6
			  wk or 75 mg/m^2 as a
			  single dose every 3 wk

(8) streptozocin, investigational drug	[18883-66-4]	115 (dec)	investigational drug iv, intraarterial: 1 g/m^2 once a wk for 4 wk

(9) thiotepa NF, Thiotepa	[52-24-4]	52–57	vial: 15 mg
			iv, intramuscular (im):
			  0.2 mg/(kg·d) or
			  10–30 mg once a wk
			intracavitary: 45–60 mg/wk
			  or 0.6–0.8 mg/kg
			  once a wk every 1–4 wk
			bladder instillation: 60 mg
			  once a wk for 4 wk

(10) dacarbazine, DTIC	[4342-03-4]	204–207	vials: 100, 200 mg
			iv: 2.0–4.5 mg/(kg·d) for 10
			  d, repeat every 28 d or
			  250 mg/(m^2·d) for 5 d,
			  repeat every 21 d

(11) busulfan USP, Myleran	[55-98-1]	114–118	tablet: 2 mg
			oral
			initial: 2–8 mg once a d
			  for 2–3 wk
			maintenance: 1–3 mg
			  once a d

Disease	Toxic effects	Manufacturer
acute and chronic lymphocytic leukemia; lung cancer; rhabdomyosarcoma; neuroblastoma; ovarian and mammary carcinoma; multiple myeloma; lymphosarcoma; Burkitt's lymphoma; Hodgkin's disease; retinoblastoma; mycosis fungoides	bone-marrow depression; hepatic toxicity; cystitis; alopecia; nausea; vomiting	Mead Johnson (division of Bristol-Meyers)
Hodgkin's disease; non-Hodgkin's lymphomas; lymphosarcoma; cancer of breast, ovary, lung; neoplastic effusion	bone-marrow depression; nausea; vomiting; anorexia; diarrhea; local irritation	Merck, Sharp, and Dohme
Hodgkin's disease; non-Hodgkin's lymphomas; meningeal leukemia; brain tumor; malignant melanoma; GI cancer; renal cell cancer; breast cancer; lung cancer	bone-marrow depression; hepatic toxicity; nausea; vomiting	Bristol Labs (division of Bristol-Meyers)
malignant brain tumors; Hodgkin's disease; non-Hodgkin's lymphomas; malignant melanoma; multiple myeloma; cancer of lung, GI tract, breast, renal cell	bone-marrow depression; hepatic toxicity	Bristol Labs (division of Bristol-Meyers)
malignant pancreatic islet-cell tumors; malignant carcinoid	bone-marrow depression; renal and hepatic toxicity; nausea; vomiting	
cancer of breast, ovary, lung, bladder; Hodgkin's disease; non-Hodgkin's lymphomas; retinoblastoma; neoplastic effusion	bone-marrow depression; amenorrhea; anorexia; nausea; vomiting	Lederle (division of American Cyanamid)
malignant melanoma; Hodgkin's disease; soft-tissue sarcomas	bone-marrow depression; flu-like syndrome; alopecia; nausea; vomiting; anorexia	Dome (division of Miles Laboratories)
chronic granulocytic leukemia; other myeloproliferative disorders	bone-marrow depression; hyperuricemia; gynecomastia; amenorrhea; skin pigmentation; nausea; vomiting; diarrhea	Burroughs Wellcome

in common the ability to form covalent linkages with various substances, including such important moieties as phosphate, amino, sulfhydryl, hydroxyl, carboxyl, and imidazole groups, in biologically vital macromolecules (see Biopolymers). The key biological compound affected is the purine base, guanine, in the nucleic acids of deoxyribonucleic acid (DNA), in which an alkyl group is substituted for the hydrogen on the N-7 (alkylation). However, less extensive alkylation of the other DNA bases, or of an amino group, or of a sulfhydryl radical of a cell protein, may also occur. These reactions usually lead to gene miscoding, serious damage to the DNA molecule, or major disruption in nucleic acid function, any of which could explain both the mutagenic and cytotoxic effects of alkylating agents. In addition, inhibition of a wide variety of other cell functions, such as glycolysis and respiration, can lead to equally harmful effects on cell viability. The reactions result in the rapid disruption or destruction of

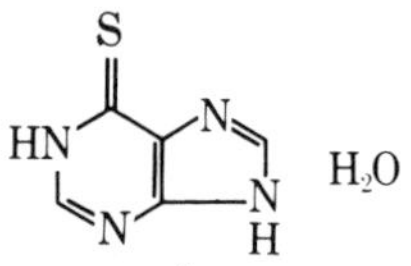

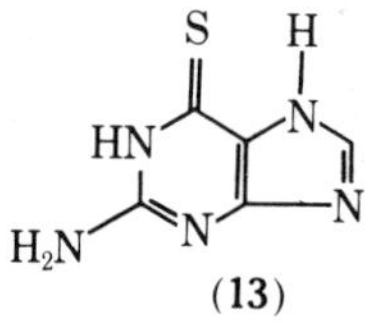

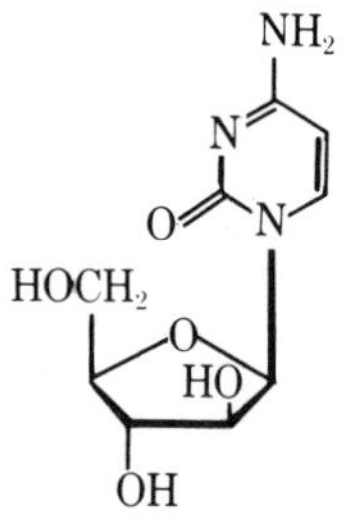

Figure 2.   Antimetabolites.

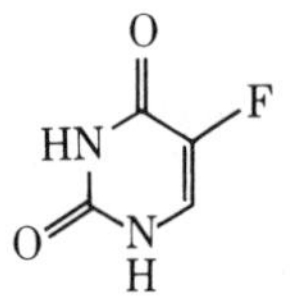

Table 2.   Antimetabolites

Drug, trade name	CAS Registry No.	mp, °C	Dosage form and dosage
(12) mercaptopurine USP, Purinethol	[6112-76-1]	308 (dec)	tablet: 50 mg oral: 2.5–5.0 mg/kg once a d
(13) thioguanine USP, Thioguanine	[154-42-7]	>360	tablet: 40 mg oral: 2 mg/kg once a d for 4 wk; if no improvement, increase to 3 mg/kg once a d
(14) cytarabine USP, Cytosar	[147-94-4]	212–213	vials: 100, 500 mg initial iv: 2 mg/kg once a d for 10 d, then 4 mg/kg once a d iv infusion: 0.5–1.0 mg/kg once a d over a period of 1–24 h for 10 d, then 2 mg/kg once a d maintenance sc: 1 mg/kg once or twice a wk

the fundamental mechanisms concerned with cell division, growth, differentiation, and function. Tumor shrinkage can occur in 1 or 2 days with intravenous drug administration. With few drug exceptions, if one alkylator is ineffective in an individual patient, so are others. All of these agents are potentially mutagenic, teratogenic, and carcinogenic themselves. The toxicity of the alkylating agents for cell functions related and unrelated to cell proliferation explains the antineoplastic activity of these agents throughout the mitotic cycle (cell-cycle independent).

Antimetabolites. This group of antineoplastic drugs (Fig. 2, Table 2) is antagonistic to normal metabolites essential for the synthesis of DNA. These compounds compete with and displace the substrate of specific enzymes involved in DNA synthesis. The reaction between the antimetabolite and the enzyme interferes with the synthesis of nucleic acid for DNA production and therefore inhibits cell reproduction. Antimetabolites can be classified according to their specific inhibitory action (antagonists of purine, pyrimidine, glutamine, etc). These drugs act considerably slower than the alkylating agents, with tumor shrinkage observed only after 4–8 wk of treatment; their cytotoxicity is cell-cycle dependent.

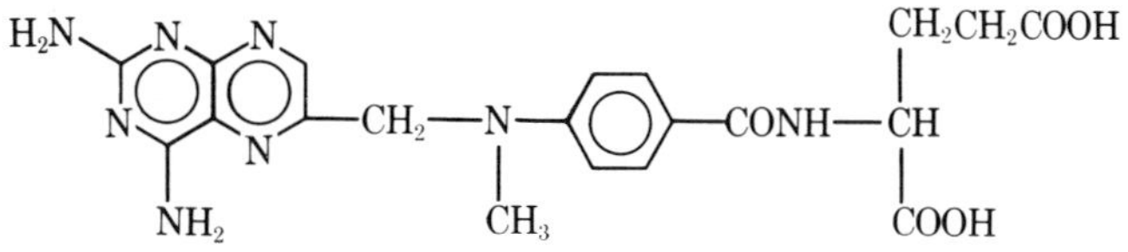

(16)

Fig. 2. (*continued*)

Disease	Toxic effects	Manufacturer
acute leukemia (more effective in children than in adults); chronic granulocytic leukemia	bone-marrow depression; hepatic toxicity; anemia; gastrointestinal (GI) ulceration; nausea; vomiting	Burroughs Wellcome
acute leukemia; chronic granulocytic leukemia	bone-marrow depression; stomatitis; anorexia; nausea; vomiting	Burroughs Wellcome
acute granulocytic leukemia (adults); acute lymphocytic leukemia (children); Hodgkin's disease	bone-marrow depression; hepatic toxicity; megaloblastosis; nausea; vomiting; diarrhea	Upjohn

Table 2. (*continued*)

Drug, trade name	CAS Registry No.	mp, °C	Dosage form and dosage
(15) fluorouracil USP, Fluorouracil	[51-21-8]	282–283 (dec)	vial: 500 mg iv initial: 12 mg/kg once a d for 4 d, then 6 mg/kg every other d for 4 doses maintenance: repeat initial dose once a month or 10–15 mg/kg, not exceeding 1 g, once a wk as a single dose
(16) methotrexate USP, Methotrexate	[59-05-2]	185–204 (dec)	tablet: 2.5 mg vials: 5, 50 mg oral: 2.5–30.0 mg/d iv, im: 2.5–30.0 mg/d intraarterial: 50 mg/d plus leucovorin im 6–9 mg/4–6 h intrathecal: 0.2–0.5 mg/kg every 2–5 d

Antibiotics. These compounds (Fig. 3, Table 3), which are chemical substances produced by certain microorganisms (actinomycetes, fungi, bacteria), suppress the growth of or destroy other microorganisms, and are also being used as antagonists of tumor cells. The mechanisms of their antineoplastic, bactericidal, and bacteriostatic actions are similar (see Antibiotics, peptides). In general, these agents bind to DNA, thus inhibiting DNA-dependent ribonucleic acid (RNA) synthesis and consequently the synthesis of proteins required by the cell. The apparent mechanism of action of one antibiotic, bleomycin (21), is unique. Its cytotoxicity seems most likely to be related to its ability to cause chain scission, nicking, and fragmentation of DNA molecules.

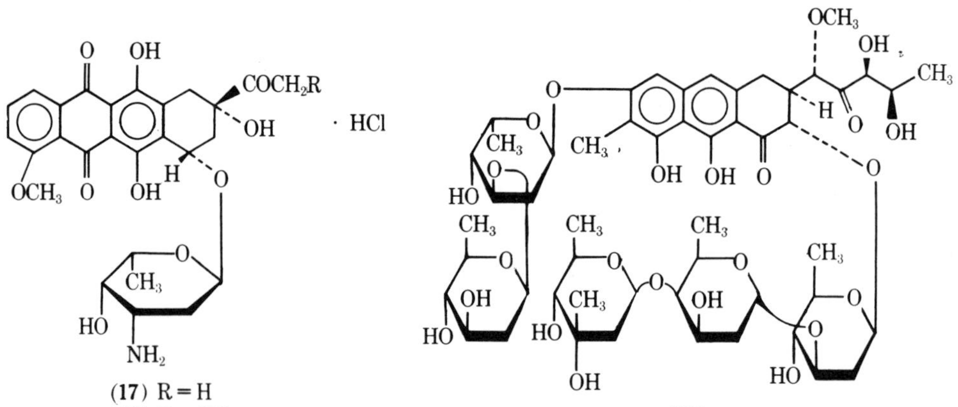

(17) R = H
(18) R = OH

(19)

Figure 3. Antibiotics.

Disease	Toxic effects	Manufacturer
cancer of breast, colon, stomach, pancreas, liver, ovary, prostate, esophagus, bladder, rectum	bone-marrow depression; dermatitis; alopecia; nausea; vomiting; diarrhea; stomatitis; anorexia; GI ulcers; skin pigmentation	Roche
acute lymphocytic leukemia; meningeal leukemia; choriocarcinoma; chorioadenoma destruens; lymphosarcoma; osteogenic sarcoma; cancer of lung, neck, head, cervix; mycosis fungoides; hydatidiform mole	bone-marrow depression; renal and hepatic toxicity; enteritis; stomatitis; alopecia; abdominal distress; erythematous rash; oral and GI ulceration; diarrhea; nausea; vomiting	Lederle (division of American Cyanamid)

In addition, repair of scission is inhibited by this antibiotic, leading to progressive fragmentation of the DNA chain. The bleomycin now used clinically is a mixture consisting mainly of the A_2 [11116-32-8] and B_2 [9060-10-0] forms. Daunorubicin (**17**) and doxorubicin (**18**) are representatives of an extensive series of anthracycline antibiotics being investigated in antimitotic chemotherapy. Antibiotics are not as frequently used as are alkylators and antimetabolites. Their cytotoxicity is cell-cycle dependent.

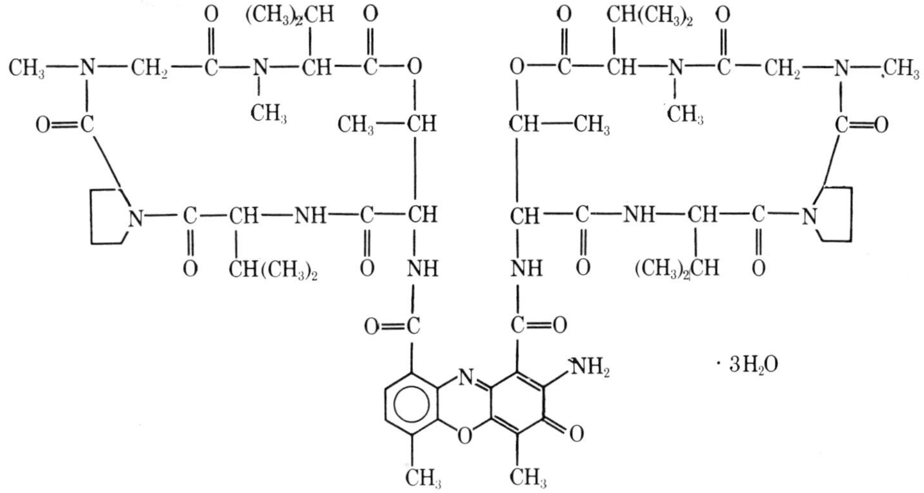

(**20**)

Fig. 3. (*continued*)

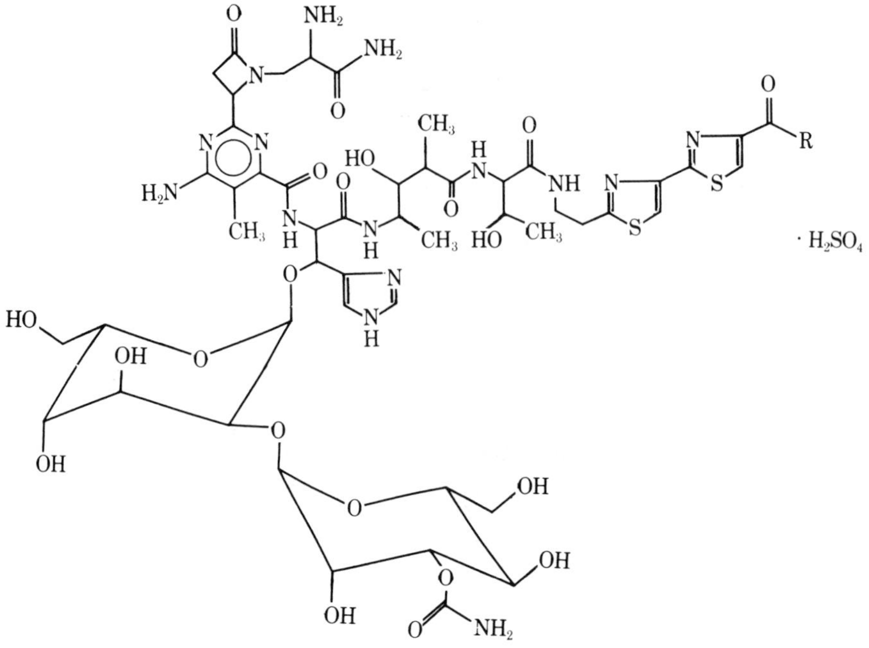

Fig. 3. (*continued*)

Table 3. Antibiotics

Drug, trade name	CAS Registry No.	mp, °C	Dosage form and dosage
(**17**) daunorubicin, investigational drug	[*20830-81-3*]	188–190 (dec)	vial: 20 mg iv: 30–60 mg/(m²·d) for 3 d or once a wk or 0.8–1.0 mg/(kg·d) for 3–6 d
(**18**) doxorubicin, Adriamycin	[*23214-92-8*]	204–205	vials: 10, 50 mg iv: 60–75 mg/m² as a single dose every 21 d or 20–30 mg/m² d for 3 d, repeated every 28 d
(**19**) mithramycin USP, Mithracin	[*18378-89-7*]	180–183	vial: 2.5 mg iv infusion: 0.025–0.030 mg/kg over a period of 4–6 h once a day for 8–10 d
(**20**) dactinomycin USP, Cosmegen	[*50-76-0*]	241–243 (dec)	vial: 0.5 mg iv: 0.5 mg once a day for 5 d or 0.015 mg/(kg·d) for 5 d; if tolerated, repeat at 2–4 wk intervals

Bleomycin A$_2$, R = NHCH$_2$CH$_2$CH$_2$—S$^+$$\overset{CH_3}{\underset{CH_3}{<}}$

Bleomycin B$_2$, R = NHCH$_2$CH$_2$CH$_2$CH$_2$NHC$\overset{NH}{\underset{NH_2}{<}}$

(**21**)

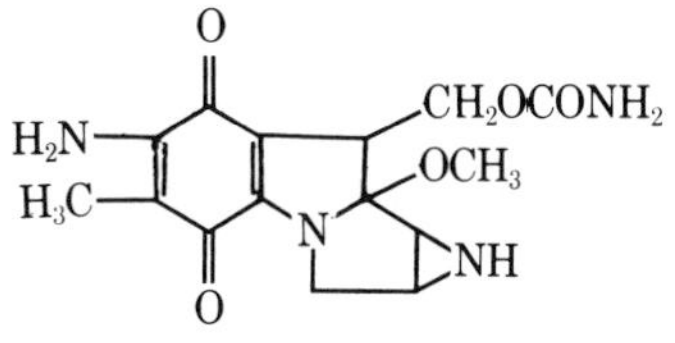

(**22**)

Fig. 3 (*continued*)

Disease	Toxic effects	Manufacturer
acute lymphocytic and granulocytic leukemia; lymphomas; solid tumors (children)	bone-marrow depression; cardiac toxicity; alopecia; stomatitis; GI disturbance	
soft-tissue and osteogenic sarcomas; Hodgkin's disease; non-Hodgkin's lymphomas; acute leukemia; cancer of thyroid, breast, lung, genitourinary (GU) tract; Wilm's tumor; neuroblastoma	bone-marrow depression; cardiac toxicity; alopecia; stomatitis; GI disturbance	Adria
testicular tumors; hypercalcemia and hypercalciuria associated with advanced malignancies	bone-marrow depression; hepatic and renal toxicity; hypocalcemia; hemorrhage; stomatitis; nausea; vomiting; anorexia; diarrhea	Pfizer
Wilm's tumor; Ewing's tumor; choriocarcinoma; testicular carcinoma; rhabdomyosarcoma; neuroblastoma; melanoma; soft-tissue and osteogenic sarcomas	bone-marrow depression; renal and hepatic toxicity; alopecia; mental depression; stomatitis; nausea; vomiting; diarrhea; anorexia; local irritation	Merck, Sharp, 'and Dohme

Table 3. (*continued*)

Drug, trade name	CAS Registry No.	mp, °C	Dosage form and dosage
(21) bleomycin sulfate, Blenoxane	[*11056-06-7*]	196 (dec)	vial: 15 units iv, im, subcutaneous (sc): 0.25–0.50 units/kg (10–20 units/m^2) weekly or twice weekly; total doses exceeding 400 units should be given with great caution
(22) mitomycin, Mutamycin	[*50-07-7*]	>360	vial: 5 mg iv infusion: 10–20 mg/m^2 as a single dose iv: 2 mg/(m^2·d) for 5 d, 2 d rest, then repeat dose for 5 d; not recommended for use as a single agent for primary therapy; use only in combination with other drugs

Plant Alkaloids. The two clinically useful alkaloids (**23–24**) (Fig. 4, Table 4) are derived from the periwinkle plant, *Vinca rosea*, a species of myrtle. These substances interfere with mitosis by aborting it in the metaphase portion of the cycle (metaphase arrest), binding with the protein (tubulin) associated with the formation of the mitotic structure (spindle) used by the dividing cell. These alkaloids may also affect other

Table 4.   Plant Alkaloids

Drug, trade name	CAS Registry No.	mp, °C	Dosage form and dosage
(23) vinblastine sulfate USP, Velban	[*143-67-9*]	284–285	vial: 10 mg iv: 3–10 mg/m^2 once a wk or every 2 wk or 0.1–0.5 mg/kg in weekly increments of 0.05 mg/kg once a wk or every 2 wk
(24) vincristine sulfate USP, Oncovin	[*2068-78-2*]	273–281	vials: 1, 5 mg iv: 1–2 mg/m^2 once a wk or 0.02–0.15 mg/kg once a wk

Disease	Toxic effects	Manufacturer
squamous cell carcinoma of head, neck, esophagus, skin, GU tract; testicular tumor; Hodgkin's disease; non-Hodgkin's lymphomas	pulmonary fibrosis; skin reactions; alopecia; nausea; vomiting; anorexia; fever; stomatitis	Bristol Labs (division of Bristol-Meyers)
chronic myelogenous leukemia; reticulum cell sarcoma; Hodgkin's disease; non-Hodgkin's lymphomas; cancer of stomach, pancreas, lung; epithelial tumors	bone-marrow depression; renal toxicity; alopecia; stomatitis; anorexia; nausea; vomiting	Bristol Labs (division of Bristol-Meyers)

cellular functions associated with tubulin, such as cellular movement and phagocytosis. Other cytologic effects involve aberrations of the cell nucleus (abnormal cleavage, condensation, etc). The cytotoxic effects, which are similar to that of older antimitotic agents such as colchicine [64-86-8] and podophyllotoxin [518-28-5], result in tumor cell death during replication, so that these agents are cell-cycle dependent (see Al-

Disease	Toxic effects	Manufacturer
Hodgkin's disease; lymphosarcoma, reticulum-cell sarcoma; neuroblastoma; choriocarcinoma; carcinoma of breast, lung, oral cavity, testis, bladder; acute and chronic leukemia; histiocytosis; mycosis fungoides	leukopenia; neurological toxicity (paresthesias, mental depression, loss of deep tendon reflexes, etc); dysfunction of autonomic nervous system (ileus, constipation, urinary retention, etc); alopecia; stomatitis; anorexia; diarrhea; nausea; vomiting; local irritation	Lilly
acute leukemia in children; lymphocytic leukemia; Hodgkin's disease; non-Hodgkin's lymphomas; Wilm's tumor; neuroblastoma; rhabdomyosarcoma; reticulum-cell sarcoma	neurological toxicity (paresthesias, foot drop, double vision, etc); constipation; ileus; alopecia; leukopenia (occasional); hyponatremia	Lilly

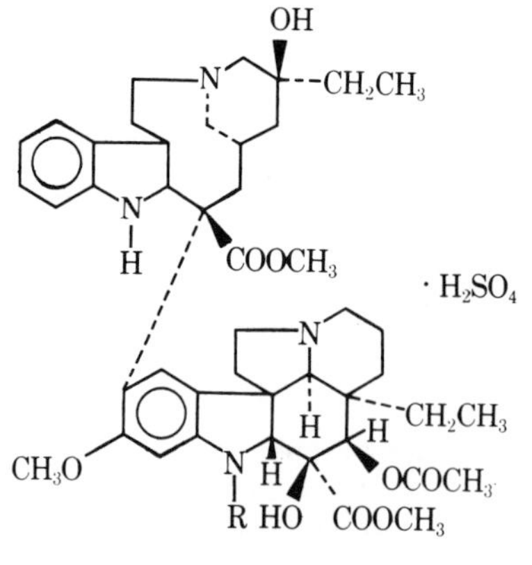

(23) R = CH₃
(24) R = CHO

Figure 4. Plant alkaloids.

kaloids). The two alkaloids differ notably in their potency, clinical use, and toxicity, and this may be caused by variation in their ability to enter specific types of cells. The relatively low toxicity of vincristine (24) for normal cells makes it unusual among antineoplastic drugs and useful in the presence of impaired bone-marrow function.

Miscellaneous Agents.   The following agents, which do not fit any of the preceding categories, are shown in Figure 5 and listed in Table 5.

Table 5. Miscellaneous Agents

Drug, trade name	CAS Registry No.	mp, °C	Dosage form and dosage
(25) asparaginase, Elspar	[9015-68-3]		vial: 10,000 IU iv: 200 IU/(kg·d) for 28 d or 1000 IU/(kg·d) for no more than 10 d
(26) hydroxyurea USP, Hydrea	[127-07-1]	133–136	capsule: 500 mg oral: 80 mg/kg as a single dose every 3 d or 20–30 mg/kg once a d
(27) Mitotane USP, Lysodren	[53-19-0]	75–81	tablet: 500 mg oral: 8–10 g/d in 3 or 4 divided doses or 3 g three or four times a d
(28) procarbazine hydrochloride USP, Matulane	[366-70-1]	223–226	capsule: 50 mg oral initial: 100–200 mg once a d for 1 wk, then 300 mg once a d until maximum response obtained maintenance: 50–100 mg once a d

$$\text{mol wt} = (133 \pm 5) \times 10^3$$

an enzyme

(25)

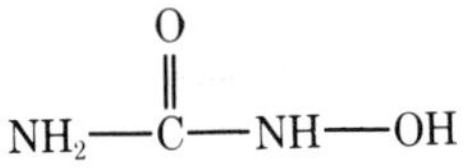

O
‖
NH_2—C—NH—OH

(26)

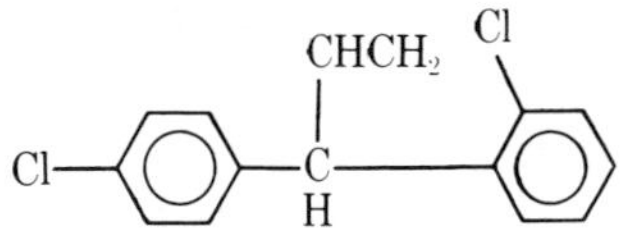

CHCH₂ Cl
|
Cl—⟨⟩—C—⟨⟩
|
H

(27)

O
‖
$(CH_3)_2CHNH$—C—⟨⟩—$CH_2NHNHCH_3$ · HCl

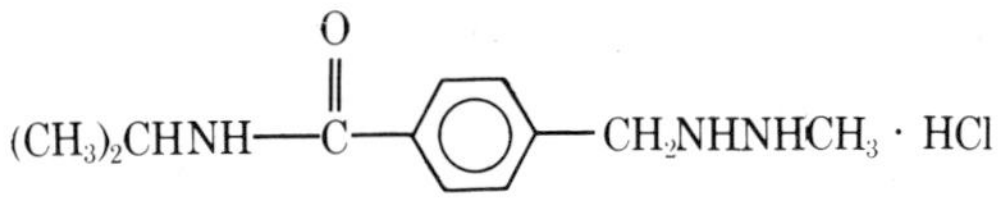

(28)

Figure 5.   Miscellaneous agents.

Enzymes as antitumor agents are at present represented by only one compound, L-asparaginase **(25)**. The amino acid L-asparagine is an essential growth factor for certain malignant cells, including the leukemic cell, since it cannot be synthesized by these cells and must be supplied to them. Most normal cells, including lymphocytes, synthesize their own asparagine. The enzyme, by catalyzing the hydrolysis of asparagine to L-aspartate and ammonia, deprives the malignant cell of an essential amino acid used in protein synthesis, thus producing tumor cell death without similarly damaging normal tissues. This compound was originally thought to represent the first antineoplastic agent to utilize a qualitative biochemical difference between normal cells and certain tumor cells. However, it is now known that several functions of some

Disease	Toxic effects	Manufacturer
acute lymphocytic leukemia	hepatic, renal, and pancreatic toxicity; neurological effects; hypersensitivity reactions; clotting abnormalities; nausea; vomiting; anorexia; fever	Merck, Sharp, and Dohme
chronic granulocytic leukemia; melanoma; cancer of ovary, head, neck	bone-marrow depression; anorexia; nausea; vomiting; diarrhea	Squibb
only in palliative treatment of inoperable adrenal cortical carcinoma	skin toxicity; dizziness; vertigo; lethargy; somnolence; anorexia; nausea; vomiting; diarrhea	Calbio
Hodgkin's disease; non-Hodgkin's lymphomas; lung cancer	bone-marrow depression; neurological and dermatological toxicity; nausea; vomiting	Roche

normal cells, such as the synthesis of specific proteins (plasma albumin, insulin, etc), are also sensitive to L-asparaginase and may be inhibited by this enzyme. Among the complications encountered with its use are rapid drug resistance as leukemic cells utilize alternative metabolic pathways with glutamine instead of asparagine, poor tissue permeability owing to the large molecular weight, and severe hypersensitivity reactions, including anaphylaxis, since it is a large, foreign protein and therefore antigenic. Unfortunately, tumor remissions with L-asparaginase appear to be transient.

Hydroxyurea (26) is representative of a group of compounds (substituted urea, guanazole, thiosemicarbazones, etc) that have as their mechanism of antitumor action the inhibition of the enzyme ribonucleoside diphosphate reductase. This enzyme catalyzes the conversion of ribonucleotides to deoxyribonucleotides, a critical step in the biosynthesis of DNA. Enzyme inhibition presumably occurs through chelation or complexing of the nonheme iron component of the enzyme.

Mitotane (27), a compound chemically related to the insecticides DDT and DDD, is an adrenocortical suppressant which acts selectively on cells of the adrenal cortex, normal and neoplastic. Administration of mitotane causes a rapid reduction in blood and urinary levels of adrenocorticosteroids and their metabolites as the drug suppresses the adrenal tumor.

Antineoplastic effects have been reported with several methylhydrazine derivatives, including procarbazine (28), through inhibition of DNA, RNA, and protein synthesis. The conversion of hydrogen peroxide (formed by auto-oxidation of the drug) to hydroxyl radicals may be responsible for the degradation of DNA. Also, production of formaldehyde and its derivatives may play an important role in cytotoxicity.

Hormones.   These agents, including estrogens, androgens, progestins, and adrenocorticosteroids, are not specific oncolytic agents but are employed to manipulate the hormonal environment of endocrine-dependent cancers such as those of the breast, ovary, and prostate. By changing this environment and thus depriving the tumors of the required hormonal growth factor, it is possible to alter, to some degree, the neoplastic process (see Hormones).

Progestational agents, which have been found useful in the management of endometrial carcinoma previously treated with surgery and radiotherapy, were tried initially because of the concept that endometrial carcinoma results from the prolonged, unopposed overstimulation by estrogen. Progesterone [57-83-0], it was thought, would correct this situation because of its physiological effect in producing maturation and secretory activity of the normal endometrium. Apparently, a proportion of neoplastic cells arising from this tissue is still influenced by normal hormonal controls. Because of their lympholytic effects and their ability to suppress mitosis in lymphocytes, leading to atrophy of lymphoid tissue and reduction in lymphocytes, the greatest value of the adrenocorticosteroids (usually prednisone [53-03-2]) is in the treatment of acute lymphocytic leukemia in children, and malignant lymphomas. In acute leukemia of childhood, these steroids may produce prompt clinical improvement and objective hematological remissions of variable duration (2 wk to 9 mo), unfortunately with invariable relapse and eventual drug resistance. Corticosteroids are therefore usually employed in conjunction with other agents. Estrogens and androgens are of value in the treatment of certain neoplastic diseases because the organs that are often the site of malignant growth, notably the prostate and the mammary gland, are dependent upon hormones for their continuing viability. Carcinomas arising from these organs often retain some of the normal hormonal requirements for varying periods of time. Thus, androgen administration in breast cancer represents an attempt to block estrogen stimulation of the tumor cells. Similarly, androgen control by estrogens produces clinical improvement in prostatic carcinoma, even though relapse eventually occurs. Although chemical cytotoxic agents are associated with untoward and damaging side effects, the anabolic effects of many steroidal agents may be of benefit to the patient (see Steroids).

Combination Therapy

The current philosophy of cancer treatment emphasizes the more aggressive use of combined treatment methods. So far, the combined method that has shown the most effectiveness is adjuvant chemotherapy. Chemotherapy as an adjunct to radiation therapy and/or surgery has improved the curability of two childhood solid tumors, Wilm's tumor and Ewing's sarcoma. The concomitant use of drugs, mainly methotrexate (16) or bleomycin (21), with other treatment has also been reported to improve survival in head and neck cancer, and fluorouracil (15) is useful in conjunction with surgery in colorectal cancer. It is possible that chemotherapy may be most effective when small numbers of tumor cells remain following surgery or radiation. Some drugs that are apparently ineffective against the presurgical tumor cells may cure metastatic disease if given shortly after surgery. As with drug combinations, the use of drugs along with another type of treatment may minimize additive host toxicity and drug resistance.

Multidrug Treatment

The entire population of neoplastic cells must be destroyed in order to obtain optimum results with chemotherapy or with any other treatment. To achieve this, several chemicals, acting as a synergistic combination, are used simultaneously or sequentially. Because different classes of chemotherapeutic agents have different mechanisms of action, they are effective in different phases of the cell cycle. Also, since tumors may differ in biochemical, cytokinetic, or chromosomal characteristics, multitargeted treatment is rational and further explains why combination drug therapies may work when single agents fail. Thus certain tumors, usually slow-growing with only a small fraction of dividing cells, will respond to initial treatment with drugs such as the alkylating agents that can kill cells at any stage of their cycle, even if they are not engaged in DNA synthesis (cycle-independent agents). The cells that survive are the rapidly dividing ones more vulnerable to subsequent attack by cycle-dependent agents (antimetabolites, etc). These agents, representing many of the most cytotoxic drugs, act at specific phases of the cell cycle by inhibiting DNA synthesis and therefore are active only against dividing cells. Accordingly, the human malignancies that are currently most susceptible to single-agent therapy are those with a high percentage of tumor cells in the process of division. In addition, combination chemotherapy using drugs with different modes of action may suppress or delay the emergence of drug-resistant cell lines. There is always the possibility, of course, that one antitumor agent may interfere with the activity of another because of a conflict in their mechanisms of action. Finally, if equally effective drugs with different mechanisms of toxicity are combined (cyclophosphamide (4) with bone-marrow toxicity plus vincristine (24) with neurotoxicity), additive cell-kill may be obtained without additive toxicity, and the patient can tolerate anticancer doses that would be fatal with either drug alone. Multiple-drug programs, therefore, rather than dependence on one agent, are the rule and have been developed for most responsive human tumors. Examples are cyclophosphamide and doxorubicin (18) in breast cancer, cytarabine (14) and thioguanine (13) in acute myelocytic leukemia, and cyclophosphamide, vincristine, methotrexate (16), and cytarabine in diffuse histiocytic lymphoma.

Immunology

The immunological system may be involved in the treatment of cancer, either as the target for the action of a drug or as the focus for its adverse effects.

Immunologic techniques for the treatment of malignant disease (immunotherapy) are undergoing extensive evaluation, all having the fundamental aim of manipulating the patient's defense (immune) mechanisms to combat the neoplastic process. Immunotherapy involves the administration of bacteria, bacterial adjuvants, or other materials, as antigens to amplify cellular or humoral immune responses and activate macrophages. The aim is to enhance the body's natural ability to suppress tumor growth, produce regression of nodules, and prevent metastases. The ultimate aim is to prolong remission and reduce recurrence of the neoplastic process. The most widely tested therapeutic materials to intensify immune responses and increase resistance include BCG (Bacillus-Calmette-Guérin), a live attenuated strain of mycobacteria commonly used for vaccination against tuberculosis, BCG derivatives such as MER (methanol extraction residue) and Ribi vaccine (BCG wall skeleton on oil droplets), the bacillus *Corynebacterium parvum*, tumor cells or antigens from patients or from tissue culture, lymphocytes, antitumor antiserum, purified immunoglobulin derived from antiserum, and levamisole [14769-73-4] (an imidazole compound). From a theoretical point of view and from experience so far, immunotherapy, like chemotherapy, may be most effective when small numbers of tumor cells remain following surgery or radiation which has removed or killed the bulk of cells. The cells most likely to respond to immune effects are those in operable solid tumors that don't metastasize; disseminated cells that cause cancer recurrence rarely respond to immunologic antitumor therapy. Among the neoplasms thus far reported to benefit most from the use of immunological agents, alone or combined with other treatment, are acute myelogenous leukemia, malignant melanoma, soft-tissue sarcomas, colon cancer, lung cancer, and breast cancer. As with any antigenic materials, severe or even fatal adverse hypersensitivity reactions, including asthma and anaphylaxis, may occur. Antitumor immunotherapy cannot yet be recommended as routine cancer therapy.

Many antineoplastic agents have a destructive effect on lymphocytes and thus have the potential to produce profound suppression of the immunological system (immunosuppression), including inhibition of such immune responses as antibody synthesis, delayed hypersensitivity, and graft rejection. It is this very property of immunosuppression that is the basis for the use of some of these agents (cyclophosphamide (4), etc) to block rejection of surgical transplants and to treat autoimmune diseases. However, in cancer chemotherapy inhibition of the body's defense mechanisms is considered an undesirable side effect since some immune responses are thought to play an important role in the natural host resistance to malignant tumors. Immunosuppression may be additionally deleterious in being among the factors responsible for the increased susceptibility of chemically-treated cancer patients to infections. Increased infection may also be a threat when corticosteroids are used as immunosuppressants to treat leukemia and lymphoma.

Since cytotoxic agents can selectively suppress or enhance the immune responses, depending upon dosages or administration schedules, antineoplastic chemotherapy may cause marked alterations of the delicate balance between the patient and his tumor or microbial population. It is essential then, that chemotherapy be carefully designed and monitored to consider the subtle interactions between these drugs and the immunological defenses so as not to critically compromise the patient's ability to withstand either infection by microorganisms or recurrence of the neoplastic process. Examples of such considerations are the observations that small, repeated doses of drugs are far more immunosuppressive than larger, intermittent ones, and that estrogens and androgens appear to stimulate the host defense mechanism.

Drug Toxicity

Anticancer drugs are potent substances and may be expected to have severe adverse effects. For example, normal tissues that proliferate rapidly (bone-marrow, gastrointestinal epithelium, hair follicles) are often subject to damage by some of the cycle-dependent antineoplastic drugs, since these agents do not confine their effects to tumor cells. This toxicity, sometimes severe as with many other potent drugs which have only moderate selectivity, often limits drug utility. Therapeutic usefulness is obtained by careful balancing of dosage so that maximum cytotoxicity is obtained against the proliferating cancer cells with minimum effect against dividing normal ones. Wherever possible, intermittent courses of chemotherapy are used to allow restoration of any normal cells whose numbers may have been reduced by treatment. Certain drugs are toxic because they reduce body levels of essential metabolites, but their adverse effects can be decreased by concomitant administration of the normal metabolite. For example, leucovorin [58-05-9] (citrovorum factor, folinic acid) can ameliorate the toxicity of methotrexate (16) by protecting normal cells against the lethal effects of the drug and also hastening their recovery (leucovorin rescue). The toxicity of anticancer drugs may be markedly increased if liver, kidney, or bone-marrow function has been impaired by previous treatment or disease.

Various aspects of the problem of selective cytotoxicity are being analyzed through the study of cell kinetics (biokinetics of cell growth) and pharmacokinetics (drug metabolism, distribution, and uptake by the cell) (see Pharmacodynamics). In addition, research into cell kinetics is helping to clarify such concepts of carcinogenesis as the role of viruses and immunology, and the biochemical development of the cancer cell. It is now believed, eg, that there is no single cause of cancer. Exposure to a carcinogenic agent such as a chemical or virus is deemed insufficient to induce cancer without other predisposing factors or determinants, such as the immune responses of the host to certain viruses.

Radiation Therapy

Radiation therapy is the primary treatment for some types of malignancy, such as Hodgkin's disease, and can also be useful, in combination with surgery and drugs, against a wide variety of other malignancies. Radiation (α, β, γ) from radioactive isotopes (^{32}P, ^{131}I, ^{198}Au) or electromagnetic sources (x-ray) interacts with atoms and molecules and leads to their excitation and ionization. In irradiated tissue, a variety of chemical radicals are formed from water; these can further interact with altered irradiated proteins and nucleic acids and lead to cell damage, often first expressed at cell division. The value of radiation rests on its capacity to destroy certain types of malignant growth *in situ* without simultaneously destroying the normal tissue in which the tumor is growing. Growths so destroyed must be relatively sensitive to this treatment. Radiation is thus a selectively cytotoxic agent and is not a refined form of cautery. This selectivity is the basis for the following concepts formulated to explain the successful empirical treatment of patients: the lethal dose of radiation to a tumor, the tolerance of normal tissue to radiation, and the ratio between the two (therapeutic ratio) (see Radioactive drugs; Radioisotopes; X-ray techniques).

BIBLIOGRAPHY

"Cancer Chemotherapy" in *ECT* 2nd ed., Suppl. Vol., pp. 81–90, by Charles J. Masur, Lederle Laboratories.

1. S. Perry, "Cancer Chemotherapy: A Broad Overview" in *Proceedings of the Seventh National Cancer Conference,* J. B. Lippincott Co., Philadelphia, Pa., 1973, p. 103.
2. M. B. Shimkin, "Cancer Research" in *Cancer, Diagnosis, Treatment and Prognosis,* 4th ed., C. V. Mosby Co., St. Louis, Mo., 1970, p. 28.
3. W. B. Coley, *Am. J. Med. Sci.* **105,** 487 (1893).
4. G. T. Beatson, *Lancet ii,* 104, 162 (1896).
5. W. P. Herbst, *Trans. Am. Assoc. Genito-Urin. Surg.* **34,** 195 (1941).
6. L. S. Goodman and co-workers, *J. Am. Med. Assoc.* **132,** 126 (1946).
7. A. Gilman, *Am. J. Surg.* **105,** 574 (1963).
8. C. P. Rhoads, *J. Am. Med. Assoc.* **131,** 656 (1946).
9. S. Farber and co-workers, *N. Eng. J. Med.* **238,** 787 (1948).
10. O. H. Pearson and co-workers, *Cancer* **2,** 943 (1949).
11. J. H. Burchenal and co-workers, *Blood* **8,** 965 (1953).
12. A. Haddon and G. M. Timmis, *Lancet i,* 207 (1953).

General References

J. R. Bertino, "Recent Developments in Chemotherapy of Malignancy," *Can. J. Otolaryngol.* **4,** 12 (1975).

J. F. Holland and E. Frei, III, eds., *Cancer Medicine,* Lea and Febiger, Philadelphia, Pa., 1973.

I. Brodsky, S. B. Kahn, and J. H. Moyer, eds., *Cancer Chemotherapy II,* Grune and Stratton Inc., New York, 1972.

A. C. Sartorelli and D. G. Johns, eds., *Antineoplastic and Immunosuppressive Agents,* Part II, Springer Verlag, Berlin, 1975.

B. A. Stoll, ed., *Endocrine Therapy in Malignant Disease,* W. B. Saunders Co., Philadelphia, Pa., 1972.

S. K. Carter and M. Slavik, "Chemotherapy of Cancer," *Annu. Rev. Pharmacol.* **14,** 157 (1974).

E. S. Greenwald, *Cancer Chemotherapy,* Medical Examination Publishing Co., Inc., Flushing, New York, 1973.

R. B. Livingston and S. K. Carter, *Single Agents in Chemotherapy,* IFI/Plenum, New York, 1970.

P. Calabresi and R. E. Parks, Jr., "Chemotherapy of Neoplastic Diseases" in L. S. Goodman and A. Gilman, eds., *The Pharmacological Basis of Therapeutics,* 5th ed., Macmillan Publishing Co., Inc., New York, 1975, pp. 1254–1307.

V. T. DeVita, R. C. Young, and G. P. Canellos, "Combination Versus Single Agent Chemotherapy: A Review of the Basis for Selection of Drug Treatment of Cancer," *Cancer* **35**, 98 (1975).

J. Q. Matthias, "Advances in Oncology," *Practitioner* **211**, 465 (1973).

C. G. Zubrod, "Present Status of Cancer Chemotherapy," *Life Sci.* **14**, 809 (1974).

L. H. Einhorn, "Cancer Chemotherapy," *J. Indiana State Med. Assoc.* **66**, 235 (1973).

CHARLES J. MASUR
WILLIAM PEARL
Lederle Laboratories
American Cyanamid Company

ANTIMYCOTIC AND ANTIRICKETTSIAL

MYCOTIC INFECTIONS

Fungi adversely affect the health and well being of mankind in numerous ways. The most direct of these include a variety of disease processes discussed in this article. Others, perhaps less direct or apparent but in some ways more deleterious, include the adverse economic and societal effects of plant diseases; occasional incidents of severe illness and even deaths associated with ingestion of toxic mushrooms; myco-toxicoses in animals and humans including potential adverse genetic effects resulting from ingestion of fungal toxins such as ergot in contaminated foodstuffs; and atopic allergic manifestations such as hay fever, asthma and rhinitis from repeated exposure to fungal spores and metabolites (see Fungicides).

Fungi are distinct from other microbial pathogens. Like plants and animals, they are eukaryotic organisms with organized nuclei within a nuclear membrane and possess cytoplasmic structures and biosynthetic pathways similar to mammalian cells. They lack the photosynthetic pigments of plants and, as a result, are heterotrophic organisms requiring preformed energy sources.

Morphologically, fungi can exist in a variety of different forms of varying complexity. Yeast cells represent the least complex form. These are several μm in diameter and reproduce either by asexual budding (formation of blastospores) or by a sexual process leading to the formation of ascospores (see Yeasts). Molds are filamentous fungi that form elongated tubelike structures called hyphae. These structures are 2–10 μm dia and usually are separated by crosswalls or septa into individual cellular elements. One class of filamentous fungi, the *Phycomycetes*, lack such crosswalls and are characterized by common, multinucleated cytoplasmic volumes.

The medically important fungi include some 50 species out of a total of 40,000–50,000 different fungi. The infections produced by these fungi can be grouped into 2 major categories: superficial mycoses and systemic or generalized mycoses. In terms of absolute numbers of infections, the superficial mycoses, which involve infections of skin, hair, and nails, are the most important. The systemic mycoses are the most important in terms of pathology or severity of disease, including mortality.

Superficial Mycoses

Dermatophytic infections of the superficial mycoses (Table 1) are infections of keratinized tissues including skin, hair, and nails. They are the most common of the human mycoses and the only fungal infections capable of direct host-to-host transmission. They include six different clinical manifestations depending upon the anatomical site involved. The three genera of the *Deuteromycetes* causing ringworm infections differ in terms of the types of tissues invaded. *Trichophyton* (21 species) can invade hair, skin and nails; *Microsporum* (15 species) usually invade only hair and skin and *Epidermophyton floccosum* invades only skin and nails.

An important distinction between the different dermatophytic fungi involves sources in infection. Certain species are transmitted primarily between humans. These are called the anthropophilic species and are capable of causing epidemics of ringworm infection, particularly in institutionalized children. Anthropophilic species are associated with mild, chronic infections. Other dermatophytes are acquired either from infected animals (zoophilic species) or contaminated soil (geophilic species). Infections in humans caused by these latter organisms generally are more acute than those caused by the anthropophilic species.

Table 1.   Superficial and Cutaneous Mycoses

Infection	Etiologic agents	Principal pathology or symptoms
tinea (pityriasis) versicolor	*Pityrosporum orbiculare*	superficial asymptomatic infection of smooth skin only; characterized by brownish, discolored and elevated scaly patches
piedras (black and white piedra)	*Piedraia hortai* (black) *Trichosporon beigelii* (white)	infection of hair only, characterized by hard nodules along hair shafts
tinea nigra palmaris	*Cladosporium werneckii*	asymptomatic fungus infection of the palmar surfaces of the hand characterized by brown to black patches
dermatophytoses	*Epidermophyton floccosum* *Microsporum* sp. *Trichophyton* sp.	ringworm infections of skin, nails, and hair; infected skin may become macerated (tinea pedis) or scaly (tinea corporis); scalp infections may become inflamed (tinea capitis) with broken hairs; infected nails become brittle and discolored (tinea unguium)
candidiasis (see Table 2)	*Candida albicans* and other *Candida sp.*	mucocutaneous infections of mouth, vagina, etc, characterized by white, adherent patches; skin infections characterized by red, weeping lesions with vesicles

Other superficial fungal infections include tinea versicolor, the piedras and tinea nigra palmaris (Table 1). These are totally asymptomatic infections and are important only for cosmetic reasons. In tinea versicolor, characteristic, irregular, diffuse patches develop on the trunk, arms, neck, and face. These patches often are associated with failure of the skin to tan evenly which may be the chief complaint. The piedras can be best described as nuisance infections in that they are limited to hair shafts of the scalp and beard and are characterized by hard concretions which are gritty feeling when palpated. Tinea nigra palmaris, a totally asymptomatic infection of the palmar surface of the hand, is characterized by superficial, brownish to black patches which may be either discrete or confluent.

Correct diagnosis of a superficial fungus infection, and particularly of a dermatophytic infection, is essential for effective chemotherapy. Such diagnosis can be made on the basis of microscopic examination of infected skin, nails, or hair as well as on the basis of cultural studies. Microscopic examination is usually done with the aid of a 10 or 20% KOH soln which acts as a digestant for cellular debris. In skin and nail specimens, infecting dermatophytic fungi appear as branching hyphae. In hairs, sheaths or rows of spores are seen either along the shaft (ectothrix) or within it (endothrix). Hairs infected by certain zoophilic or geophilic species of *Microsporum* will fluoresce when examined under ultraviolet light.

Systemic and Generalized Mycoses

The deep mycoses include two distinct groups of life-threatening fungal infections of humans (Table 2). First, there are the systemic fungal infections caused by pathogenic fungi in normal hosts. Second, there are the opportunistic infections caused by fungi of low virulence in individuals with compromised resistance factors.

The systemic fungal pathogens share certain common features. Being true pathogens they are capable of causing infections in normal hosts. However, in most instances such infections are usually recognized only by x-ray examination or immunological testing. Some of these organisms, such as *Coccidioides immitis*, are found in nature in highly specific geographic regions, some of which overlap and most of which occur in the Americas. Infections caused by some of these organisms such as *Coccidioides immitis*, *Cryptococcus neoformans*, and *Histoplasma capsulatum* show highly specific patterns of organ involvement, as well as sex, age and racial predilections. Most of the systemic mycoses primarily infect the lungs by inhalation of infective spores. Other infections are acquired by traumatic implantation of contaminated plant materials. Most of the truly pathogenic fungi have two distinct forms depending upon such conditions as temperature, carbon dioxide pressure, presence or absence of sulfhydryl groups and local oxidation–reduction potential.

The opportunistic infections also share common features. Aspergillosis and cryptococcosis occur primarily in individuals with altered resistance owing to leukemia or lymphomas, immunosuppression and corticosteroid therapy. Phycomycosis occurs in diabetics, burn victims and patients with leukemia, lymphomas, or other chronic illnesses. Candidiasis occurs in the same situations as well as with indwelling catheters and broad-spectrum antibiotic treatment. In nearly all instances, these opportunistic invaders are either normal flora of the host or from the environment.

Diagnosis of the deep mycoses is based upon one or more of four factors: epidemiologic fact-finding; demonstration of fungal pathogens in tissue or other specimens;

Table 2. Systemic and Generalized Mycoses

Infection	Etiologic agent	Principal pathology or symptoms
Systemic		
blastomycosis	*Blastomyces dermatitidis*	chronic, granulomatous disease either limited to skin and lungs or widely disseminated; often fatal
chromomycosis	*Phialophora* sp.; *Cladosporium* sp.	chronic, granulomatous infection of skin and lymphatics developing slowly over months or years; rarely fatal
cladosporiosis	*Cladosporium trichoides; Phialophora* sp.	(1) brain abscess; usually fatal (2) small, asymptomatic subcutaneous cysts, rarely fatal
coccidioidomycosis	*Coccidioides immitis*	(1) acute, but benign, self-limiting primary, pulmonary infection (2) progressive, multiorgan, disseminated infection involving skin, viscera and bones (less than 1%)
cryptococcosis	*Cryptococcus neoformans*	slowly developing chronic meningitis; often with remissions and relapses; universally fatal if untreated
histoplasmosis	*Histoplasma capsulatum*	(1) asymptomatic pulmonary infection with granulomatous foci (2) clinical pneumonia with protracted illness but self-limiting (3) disseminated infection with multiple organ involvement, particularly of the reticuloendothelial system with enlarged spleen and liver and focal areas of necrosis and granulomas in multiple organs; often fatal
lobomycosis	*Loboa loboi*	chronic, cutaneous infection with formation of fibrous tumorlike or keloidlike nodules; no inflammatory reaction and nonfatal
maduromycosis (mycetoma)	*Allescheria boydii; Madurella* sp.	slowly progressive and highly destructive infection of subcutaneous tissues of foot or hand; characterized by deep-seated abscesses and chronic, draining sinuses; infection involves both muscle and bone causing malformities and loss of function; rarely fatal

Table 2. (*continued*)

Infection	Etiologic agent	Principal pathology or symptoms
paracoccidioidomycosis	*Paracoccidioides brasiliensis*	chronic, granulomatous disease of skin, mucous membranes, lymph nodes, and internal organs; often fatal
sporotrichosis	*Sporothrix schenckii*	local abscess or ulcer at site of implantation of contaminated thorn or splinter followed by multiple subcutaneous abscesses involving the local lymphatics; may disseminate to produce secondary infections of bones and joints
Opportunistic aspergillosis	*Aspergillus fumigatus* *Aspergillus* sp.	(*1*) necrotizing bronchopneumonia with obstruction of blood vessels and production of local infarcts of lung tissue (*2*) granuloma (aspergilloma) (*3*) obstructive but noninvasive fungus ball
candidiasis (see Table 1)	*Candida albicans* and other *Candida* sp.	systemic infection of lungs, urinary tract, heart, etc, with no specific symptoms; often fatal
mucormycosis (phycomycosis)	*Mucor* sp. *Absidia* sp. *Rhizopus* sp.	(*1*) acute infection of paranasal sinuses characterized by inflammation, vascular obstruction and local necrosis; may ultimately invade brain with subsequent infarction; frequently fatal (*2*) subcutaneous infection of tissues, thorax, abdomen and limbs

isolation, recovery, and identification of the responsible pathogen; and serologic techniques. Epidemiologic fact-finding involves development of a history to include travel in areas endemic for fungal infections; predisposing health factors; and possible occupational exposure to certain fungal pathogens. Demonstration of fungal pathogens in tissues or other pathologic materials includes direct examination of body fluids, staining of pathologic materials, and histological preparations of infected tissues. In some instances, such as cryptococcal meningitis, demonstration of a fungus in pathologic materials may be the only justification required for initiating specific antifungal chemotherapy. Isolation and identification of the responsible pathogen is difficult in some instances as certain of the pathogenic fungi are slow to grow under laboratory conditions. In other situations, such as candidiasis, the significance of the presence of the responsible fungus is a matter of clinical judgement since these organisms are frequently encountered in specimens such as sputa or urines. A variety of serologic techniques now are available for diagnosis of fungal infections. Some have only diagnostic value, others provide both diagnostic and prognostic information. These techniques include agglutination tests, immunodiffusion tests for either antibody or antigen, complement fixation tests, and, most recently, counterimmunoelectrophoresis tests for either antibody or antigen.

Antifungal Agents

Antifungal chemotherapy is limited both in the number of available agents and in therapeutic applications. They can be divided into two categories: antibiotics (secondary metabolites) with antifungal properties, and synthetic compounds. Unlike the current trend in antibacterial chemotherapy (see Antibiotics), there is little emphasis upon development of semisynthetic modifications of antifungal antibiotics. Therapeutic applications include intravenous medication in treatment of the progressive or disseminated cases of systemic mycoses and oral and topical medication in treatment of dermatophytic infections and certain yeast infections. Effective modes of therapy are lacking for most cases of pulmonary aspergillosis, phycomycosis, chromomycosis and maduromycosis. An alphabetical list of compounds mentioned in the text and their CAS Registry Numbers is provided at the end of the article.

The majority of antifungal antibiotics are polyenes produced by different species of *Streptomyces,* a genus of aerobic actinomycetic bacteria (1). In spite of the large number of such antibiotics which have been discovered and characterized, only a few are used in clinical medicine and even fewer have important chemotherapeutic roles (2).

The Polyene Antibiotics. The most important group of antifungal antibiotics are the polyenes (see Antibiotics, polyenes). These are high molecular weight, polyhydroxy compounds belonging to the macrolides but differing from them in possessing conjugated chains of chromophoric double bonds in the macrolactone ring (see Antibiotics, macrolides). Properties of the polyenes include chemical instability; poor solubility in water; strong, characteristic uv absorption spectra; and poor stability to light and temperature. Biologically, the polyenes have potent antifungal activity, some antiprotozoal activity but little or no antibacterial activity. The antifungal mode of action of the polyenes is related to their ability to produce profound changes in cell membrane permeability. This results from binding of the compounds to sterols located in the cell membranes.

Both toxicity and efficacy of the polyenes is determined by the degree of binding and by the specificity and avidity of certain polyenes for specific sterols. For example, the principal sterol in membranes of fungi is ergosterol to which amphotericin B, one clinically useful polyene, binds specifically. A similar sterol, cholesterol, is found in membranes of mammalian cells (see Hormones; Steroids). Amphotericin B also binds to this sterol but to a significantly lesser degree. However, sufficient binding does occur to account for some of the clinical toxicity associated with this compound.

Nystatin. Nystatin (1) (Mycostatin) was the first of the polyene antifungals to become clinically important. Discovered in 1949, nystatin had a major impact in clinical medicine in that it provided the first antibiotic useful in the topical treatment of superficial infections caused by *Candida albicans* (3).

Nystatin is an amphoteric tetraene soluble in dimethyl sulfoxide (DMSO), dimethyl formamide (DMF) and short chain alcohols. It is inactivated by heat, light, and acid or alkali. Its absorption maxima are 235, 291, 304, and 318 nm. It is produced by *Streptomyces noursei.*

Biologically, (1) is active *in vitro* at concentrations of 1–10 μg/mL against most pathogenic fungi including yeasts, filamentous pathogens and dermatophytic fungi. However, its activity against the latter group of organisms is not sufficient to be clinically useful. It has no antibacterial or antiviral properties. Nystatin is highly toxic when given to experimental animals via the intravenous or intraperitoneal routes, LD_{50} values are 3 and 45 mg/kg, respectively. Fortunately, it is not absorbed in significant amounts when given orally [LD_{50} in mice per os (orally), >8000 mg/kg] nor is it absorbed percutaneously.

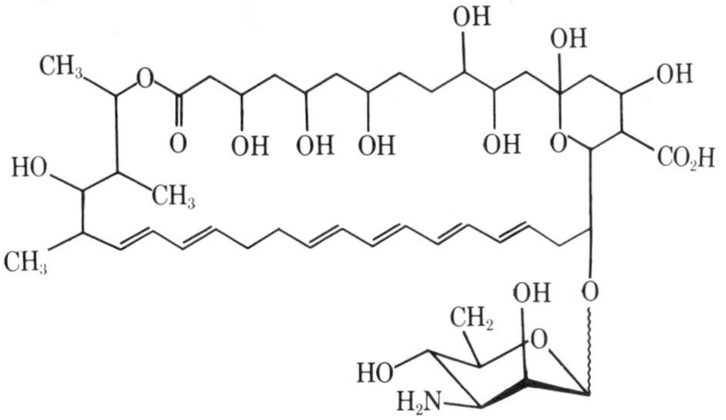

(1)

The parenteral toxicity and lack of oral absorption of nystatin limited the clinical usefulness of this drug to topical applications. Other medicinal uses of nystatin include veterinary medicine where it is used in treatment of yeast infection in poultry, swine, and cattle. Laboratory applications include use in tissue culture media to suppress yeast overgrowth and in the clinical laboratory for isolation of bacteria from specimens heavily contaminated with fungi.

Amphotericin B. Just as nystatin had a major impact on treatment of superficial *Candida* infections, amphotericin B (2) had its impact on the treatment of systemic fungal infections. It was the first effective agent to be used in the treatment of such life-threatening infections as coccidioidomycosis and cryptococcosis.

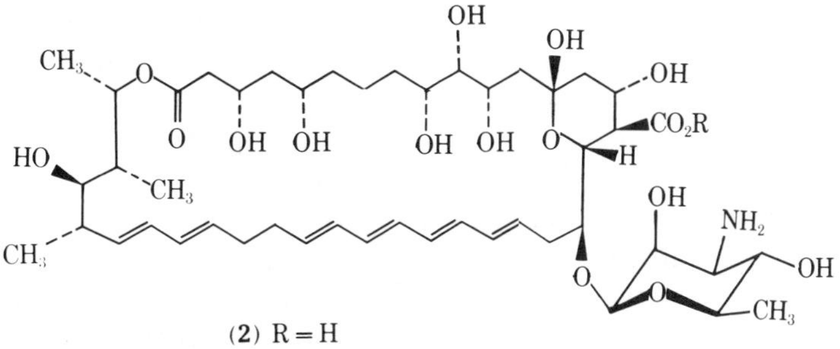

(2) R = H
(3) R = CH_3
(4) tentative formula: $C_{63}H_{85}N_2O_{19}$

Amphotericin B is an amphoteric heptaene with a sugar (mycosamine) moiety. It is insoluble in water except at extreme pH (0.1 mg/mL at pH 2 or 11) and partially soluble in DMF (2–4 mg/mL) and DMSO (30–40 mg/mL). The intravenous preparation contains sodium desoxycholate to provide a dispersible colloidal suspension. Its absorption maxima are 345, 363, 382, and 406 nm. Amphotericin B is part of a complex produced by *Streptomyces nodosus* consisting of amphotericins A and B (1).

Biologically, (2) is active *in vitro* against pathogenic yeasts and dimorphic fungi at concentrations of 0.01–2 μg/mL (4). Its activity against opportunistic, subcutaneous and dermatophytic pathogens is less, 3.12–30 μg/mL. It is even less active against the etiological agents of chromomycosis and maduromycoses (5). Amphotericin B is less toxic than nystatin for laboratory animals. The intravenous LD_{50} is 4–6 mg/kg and the oral LD_{50} is >8000 mg/kg. Unlike (1), (2) is absorbed from the gut both in animals and in humans and a dose of 5 mg/kg given orally to mice is protective against some pathogenic fungi. Unfortunately, the gastrointestinal absorption of the drug in humans is not predictable and oral use of amphotericin B in treatment of systemic fungal infections has not been fully successful (6). Therefore, the clinical application of the drug is limited to the intravenous and topical routes, although oral amphotericin B is available in some countries. Use of intravenous amphotericin B is indicated in the systemic mycoses, opportunistic infections and subcutaneous infections caused by susceptible organisms (7). Some cases of invasive pulmonary aspergillosis, disseminated sporotrichosis and most cases of mycetoma and chromoblastomycosis are clinically resistant to the drug (2).

Amphotericin B normally is administered intravenously at dosages of 1.0–1.5 mg/kg after starting at an initial dose of 0.25 mg/kg (7). It is administered in intravenous glucose over a 2–6-h period. The intravenous preparation consists of 50 mg of active drug, 41 mg of sodium desoxycholate and 25.2 mg of sodium phosphate buffer (Amphotericin B, USP, Fungizone). When prepared for infusion in 5% dextrose, the final concentration is 0.1 mg/mL. Serum levels of the drug range from ca 0.2–4 μg/mL but corresponding spinal fluid levels rarely exceed 0.1 μg/mL. The drug is bound to serum lypoproteins and is slowly excreted in urine over a prolonged period (8).

Amphotericin B is a highly toxic substance when given parenterally. The lesser side effects include fever, headache, nausea, vomiting, and malaise. The most important reaction is nephrotoxicity. Some impairment of renal function is seen in all patients regardless of dosage given. This is evidenced by increases in blood urea (BUN) and creatinine levels. Not infrequently, treatment will be stopped until these parameters return to acceptable levels. Efforts to reduce the nephrotoxicity include concurrent infusion of mannitol, alternate-day treatment, and use of serum drug levels as therapeutic guides. Other toxic reactions associated with amphotericin B include anemia, thrombocytopenia, liver function abnormalities, and thrombophlebitis.

Amphotericin B also has been used with varying degrees of success in certain other clinical indications using other routes of administration. Oral (2) (Fungillin) is used in some countries for treatment of superficial and intestinal *Candida* infections. Serious meningeal fungal infections such as cryptococcal and coccidioidal meningitis may respond only to intraventricular or intrathecal therapy.

Amphotericin B, methyl ester.   The water-soluble methyl ester of amphotericin B (3) has *in vitro* antifungal properties comparable to the parent compound, but reduced acute *in vivo* toxicity (9). Although (3) is less nephrotoxic in animals, it also appears to be less active *in vivo* than the parent compound (10). *In vitro*, (3) is nearly as active as (2) against pathogenic fungi and also appears to be active against certain viruses such as herpes simplex, vaccinia, simbis, and vesicular stomatitis virus (11–12). *In vivo*, (3) is effective in treatment of experimental infections in mice caused by a variety of fungal pathogens such as *C. neoformans*, *B. dermatitidis*, and *C. immitis* but to a lesser degree than (2) (10,13).

Limited clinical and pharmacologic data are available regarding use of (3) in humans. In one study, alternate day intravenous dosages of 5.0 mg/kg using an ascorbate preparation resulted in peak serum levels of 15–30 µg/mL and trough levels of 0.5–2.5 µg/mL (14). Adverse reactions were said to be qualitatively similar to those of (2) but less severe (14). The exact clinical role for (3) has not yet been defined.

Candicidin. Candicidin (4) is a heptaene complex produced by *Streptomyces griseus* (15). Its chemical structure is not fully characterized. Two forms exist: Complex A with maxima at 340, 360, 380, and 403 nm, and Complex B with maxima at 340, 362, 381, and 404 nm. Candicidin is more active *in vitro* than (1) or (2) against pathogenic yeasts. However, its *in vivo* toxicity is greater than either (2) or (1): oral LD_{50} 98–400 mg/kg, intraperitoneal 2–7 mg/kg. The medical indications for (4) are restricted to topical treatment of vaginal and mucocutaneous candidiasis. It is available in the form of ointments (0.06%), vaginal tablets (0.3%) or capsules (Candicidin, NF; Cadeptin). These are used topically twice daily for 2 wk.

Pimaricin. Pimaricin (5) (Natamycin) a tetraene polyene, is produced by *Streptomyces natalensis* (16). It is soluble in propylene glycol (2%). It is thermostable. Its absorption maxima are 279, 290, 303, and 318 nm (17). Pimaricin is inhibitory for fungi at concentrations of from 1–15 µg/mL (18). It is toxic with intraperitoneal and intravenous LD_{50} values of 250 and 5–10 mg/kg, respectively; the oral LD_{50} is 1500 mg/kg. Therapeutic use of (5) is limited to topical treatment of fungus infections with a 5% ointment. The principal value of (5) appears to be in treatment of mycotic keratitis such as the very destructive ocular infections caused by *Fusarium* and *Cephalosporium* species. It is not an approved drug in the United States [Pimafuncin (Brit. Pharm)]. There appears to be no toxicity associated with topical application (19).

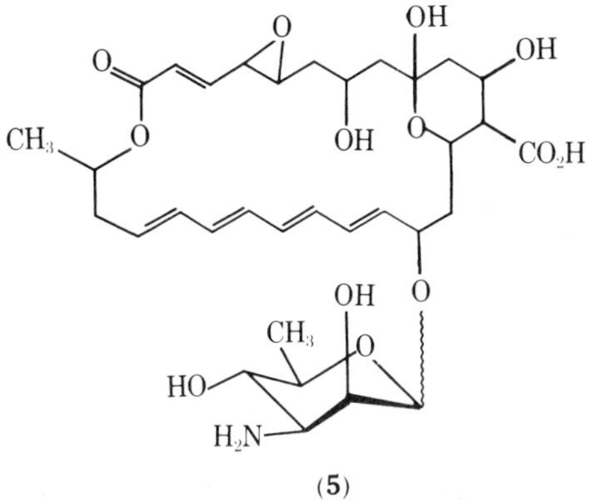

(5)

Nonpolyene Antifungal Antibiotics. The number of nonpolyene antifungal antibiotics is limited and only five are discussed here. These include griseofulvin (6), the only one produced by a fungus; sinefungin (7) (20) and cycloheximide (8), both produced by *Streptomyces* species; and pyrrolnitrin (9) which is produced by a bacterium. The fifth compound, ambruticin (10), which is produced by a myxobacterium, has been only recently described and is of unknown clinical potential (21–22).

Griseofulvin. Griseofulvin (6) is a phenolic, benzofuran cyclohexane produced by several species of *Penicillium* including *Penicillium griseofulvum*, *Penicillium patulum*, and *Penicillium janczewskii*. It is insoluble in water and petroleum ether and only slightly soluble in such solvents as DMF, DMSO, ethanol, benzene, and chloroform. It is thermostable and uv absorption maxima occur at 324, 291, 252, and

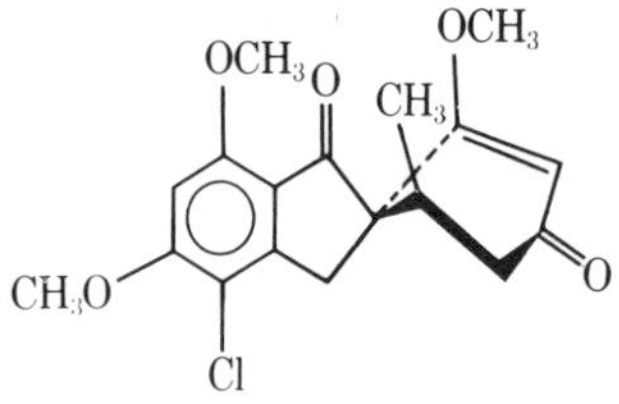

(6)

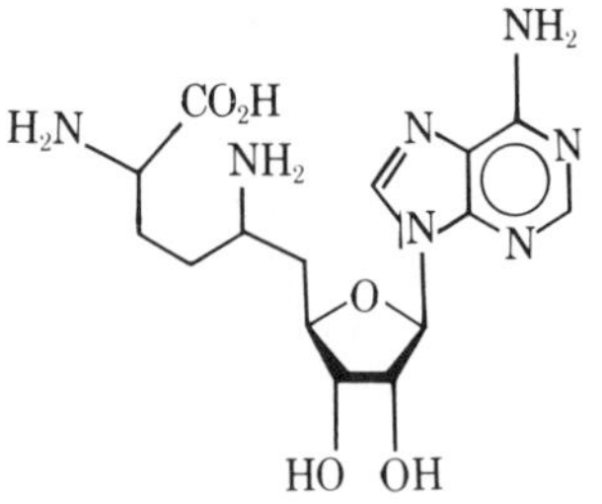

(7)

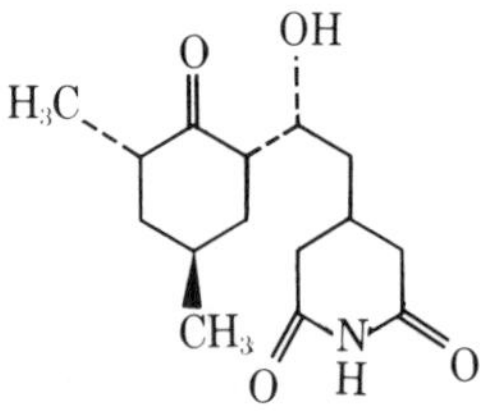

(8)

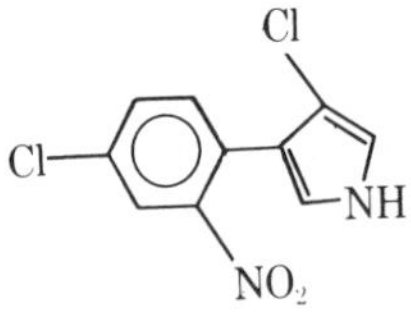

(9)

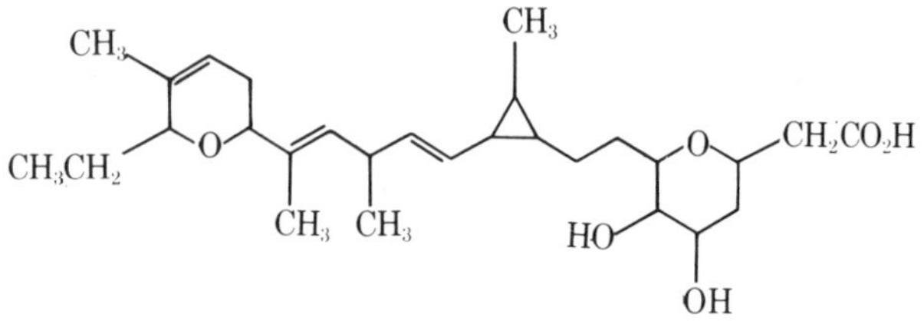

(10)

236 nm. Its antifungal activity is restricted to the dermatophytic species; MIC (min inhibiting conc) values range from 0.14–2.5 μg/mL (18). Griseofulvin has no activity against other filamentous fungi or against yeastlike organisms or bacteria.

The initial uses of (6) were in protection of plants against fungal infections when it was shown in 1951 that (6) introduced into soil was taken up by the roots and transported to the leaves. It was not until 1958 that (6) was shown to be orally effective in guinea pigs experimentally infected with the dermatophytes *Microsporum canis* and *Trichophyton mentagrophytes* (23–24). This revelation was immediately followed by clinical demonstrations of the efficacy of the drug in treatment of human dermatophytic infection (25–26).

The pharmacology and mode of action of griseofulvin are unique. When administered orally in animals, the drug is widely distributed in body fluids and also is deposited in an active form in keratinized tissues (27). Absorption from the gastrointestinal tract generally is poor with as much as 20% remaining unabsorbed (28). Poor absorption, and excretion in the urine in the form of inactive metabolites, accounts for low serum levels. Other factors affecting serum levels include particle size, fat intake, dosage schedule, and dissolution rate. In attempts to obtain higher serum and skin levels micronized formulations of reduced particle size have been used (28).

The mode of action of (6) in fungi is not clearly established. Early studies showed the drug to have a profound effect on cell wall formation (29), mitosis, inhibition of nucleic acid synthesis and alterations in cytoplasmic microtubules (30). All of these suggest that in fungi (6) acts by specific inhibition of mitotic spindle formation.

Although early *in vivo* studies with griseofulvin showed it to be active topically in experimental infections against *Trichophyton mentagrophytes*, similar topical activity rarely has been seen in human infections. Thus, administration is limited to the oral route. A variety of oral preparations are available (Fulvicin, Grifulvin, Grisactin, Gris-Peg, etc). The majority of these are so-called microsize preparations which have replaced the older particulate form of the drug. The average daily dosage of the microsize preparation in adults is 0.5 g/d although 1.0 g daily dosages may be required in certain chronic or severe infections. Generally, the time required for treatment of ringworm infections with griseofulvin is dependent upon the site of infection and the time required for total replacement of infected tissues by normal tissues. *In vivo*, the drug is fungistatic only and thus infections will relapse if all infected tissues are not replaced. This means that 2–4 wk of medication will be required in most infections. Treatment of infections involving the soles of the feet or nails will require more time, at least 1 yr in the case of toenail infections.

Griseofulvin is relatively free of toxicity, even in patients receiving large dosages over prolonged periods (31). Occasionally, a patient will complain of gastrointestinal upset, and hypersensitivity reactions as well as photosensitivity rashes have been reported. The drug is contraindicated in patients with porphyria or liver failure. An etiological diagnosis should be obtained before using the drug.

Cycloheximide.   This antibiotic (8), produced by *Streptomyces griseus*, was used in treatment of cryptococcal infections before the development of (2) (32). Its current use is limited to laboratory and agricultural applications. Cycloheximide (8) (Acti-dione) is a white powder slightly soluble in chloroform, alcohols and other organic solvents. Its activity is mainly against nonpathogenic fungi. It is used in laboratory media as a selective agent to permit isolation of pathogenic fungi from specimens such as sputa and feces which may be contaminated by other fungi. One important exception is that it is active against *C. neoformans* (MIC <0.2 μg/mL). Agricultural use is limited because of phytotoxicity to topical control of downy mildew of onions and shoot blight of larch (33). The mode of action of (8) is at the level of polypeptide formation and nucleic acid synthesis (34).

Other antifungal agents.   Pyrrolnitrin (9) is a potent antifungal metabolite produced from tryptophan by certain species of *Pseudomonas* (35). Chemically, it is slightly soluble in water and petroleum ether and soluble in ethanol and methanol. Pyrrolnitrin is unstable in presence of acid and is bound by serum. The *in vitro* spectrum of (9) includes *T. mentagrophytes* (MIC of 0.78–6.25 μg/mL), *Trichophyton rubrum* (MIC of 1.56–3.12 μg/mL), *Candida albicans* (MIC of 25–50 μg/mL), and systemic fungal pathogens such as *C. immitis*, *C. neoformans*, and *Sporothrix schenckii* (MIC 0.78 μg/mL). Topically, (9) is effective in guinea pigs experimentally infected with *T. mentagrophytes* when applied in 1–2% formulations. The medical use of (9) is limited to topical treatment of dermatophytic infections since it is inactive orally, toxic if given by parenteral routes, and inactivated by serum. It is not an approved drug in the U.S. but is marketed elsewhere.

Sinefugin (7), A9145, is produced by *Streptomyces griseolus* (36,37). Sinefungin is active against *Candida albicans* both *in vitro* (MIC of 0.06–1.0 μg/mL) and *in vivo* (10 mg/(kg·d). Peak blood levels of 64 μg/mL are obtained in mice with subcutaneous dosages of 100 mg/kg (38). The LD_{50} for mice is 185 mg/kg (37). The mode of action of (7) involves inhibition of S-adenosylmethionine-mediated transmethylation, particularly histamine N-methyltransferase (39). The clinical role for (7) has not yet been defined.

Ambruticin (10), W7783, is of a new class of cyclopropyl–pyran antibiotic. Produced by the myxobacterium *Polyangium cellulosum* var. *fulvum* (40). It is active *in vitro* at concentrations as low as 0.025 μg/mL against systemic and dermatophytic fungal pathogens (41–42). *In vivo*, (10) is active topically and orally against *T. mentagrophytes* and orally against *H. capsulatum* and *C. immitis* (43–45). It is both protective and curative in mice infected with *C. immitis* at oral dosages of 25 and 50 mg/kg. Ambruticin is orally absorbed in laboratory animals with peak serum levels of 40 μg/mL attainable one h following a single 50 mg/kg dose (41); it is well distributed throughout the body in a biologically active form (41). Although the exact clinical role of (10) is yet to be defined, both its spectrum as well as its topical and oral activity suggest a role in management of both systemic and superficial mycoses.

Synthetic Antifungal Agents. *Nonspecific Topical Medications.* Use of specific, synthetic antifungal agents is only a recent development in antifungal chemotherapy. This is particularly true for chemotherapy of the systemic mycoses. Earlier forms of therapy were concerned primarily with the superficial mycoses and depended extensively upon the use of nonspecific topical fungicides, drying agents, and keratolytics. Benzoic and salicylic acids combined, 6 and 12%, respectively, in petrolatum and known as Whitfield's ointment is the best example of such preparations. Salicylic acid acts as a keratolytic or desquamating agent, softening and loosening the infected cornified epithelium, and the benzoic acid acts as a fungistat in preventing reinfection of newly formed epithelium. Whitfield's ointment was used in treatment of smooth skin infections only, and because of the fungistatic nature of the ointment, prolonged therapy of several weeks to months was required (46).

Treatment of tinea unguium or fungal nail infections often was accomplished by either close filing of the nail or surgical removal followed by daily soaks in solutions of potassium permanganate (1:4000). After soaking, the infected nails were painted with a fungicide such as a 10% solution of salicylic acid. Potassium permanganate also was used topically (1:5000) and vaginally (1:1500) for treatment of cutaneous and mucocutaneous candidiasis (47).

Gentian or crystal violet (11) (hexamethyl-*p*-rosaniline) is both bacteriostatic and fungicidal and, at one time, was used extensively in topical treatment of superficial fungus infections at concentrations of 0.02–1.0%. Gentian violet solutions also were used in treatment of oral and vaginal candidiasis and in local treatment of ringworm infections of the groin; disadvantages included staining of skin and clothing (48).

Undecylenic acid (12) (10-undecenoic acid) is a fungistatic fatty acid. It and various salts, such as zinc undecylenate, have been used for many years in topical treatment of smooth skin ringworm infections. One popular preparation, Desenex, containing 5% of the acid and 20% of the zinc salt, is available in several forms. The zinc salt acts both as a fungistatic agent and as an astringent which also aids in reduction of inflammation. Preparations of (12) are of value primarily in treatment of ringworm infections of the foot and have no role in treatment of hair or nail infections (49).

Other fatty acids or their derivations also have been used in treatment of superficial fungal infections. They include calcium propionate [4075-81-4] (Sopronol) and sodium propionate [137-40-6] (see Carboxylic acids).

Sulfur-containing compounds that once played an important role in treatment of superficial fungal infections include: sulfur-salicylic ointment; sodium thiosulfate [7772-98-7] (25%) and salicylic acid (1.0%) in isopropyl alcohol and propylene glycol (Tinver) is still highly effective for treatment of tinea versicolor; and selenium sulfide [7488-56-4] for treatment of dandruff, seborrheic dermatitis and tinea versicolor. Both preparations are used once or twice weekly as a shampoo or lotion. Selenium sulfide is less toxic than water soluble selenium salts; its oral LD_{50} in rats in 138 mg/kg (50).

Iodochlorhydroxyquin (13) (5-chloro-7-iodo-8-quinolinol, Vioform) is used

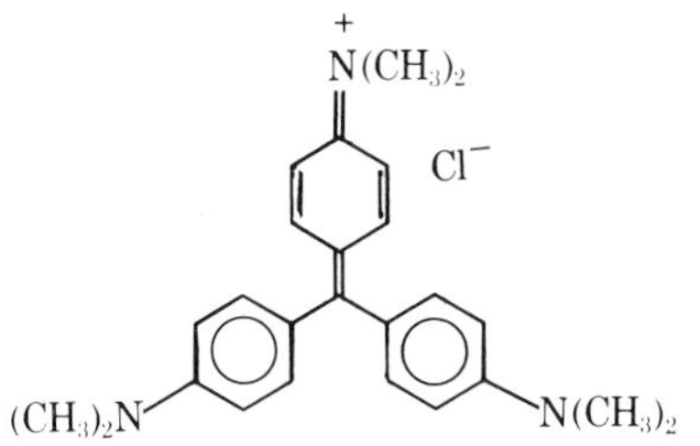

(11)

$CH_2=CH(CH_2)_8CO_2H$

(12)

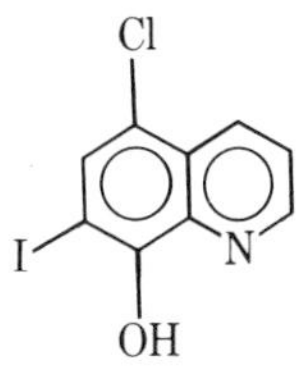

(13)

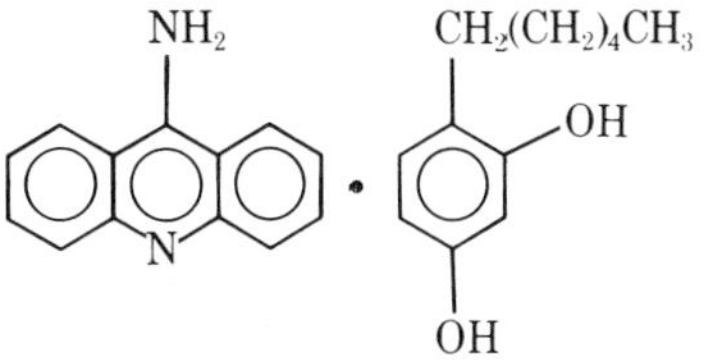

(14)

topically in treatment of the dermatophytic infections and *Candida* vaginal infections. Since (13) is water insoluble and poorly absorbed from the gastrointestinal tract, it is used topically in the form of a 3% suppository or cream in treatment of vaginal trichomoniasis or candidiasis. Side effects are rare but include pruritis and mild iodine reactions (51). Iodochlorhydroxyquin is available in a variety of preparations including topical creams and ointments with and without hydrocortisone and antibiotics, as well as suppositories and oral tablets.

Acrisorcin (14) (9-aminoacridine-4-hexylresorcinolate) is a broad-spectrum nonspecific acridine dye active against bacteria, fungi, and protozoa. It is "cidal" for most such organisms at concentrations of 1–78 μg/mL. Used topically as a 2% cream (Akrinol), (14) is effective only in treatment of tinea versicolor; relapses following treatment are not uncommon. Toxicity includes hives, blisters, erythematous vesicles and photoinduced pruritis (50).

Nonspecific Systemic Medications.   The first systemic antifungal chemotherapeutics were the iodides. Local, cutaneous sporotrichosis is readily treated orally with a saturated solution of potassium iodide given three times daily with water or milk for as long as 6 wk. Side reactions include indigestion, rashes, lacrimation, and cardiac problems. The mode of action is unknown; potassium iodide is not inhibitory for *Sporothrix schenckii in vitro*. Oral iodides are still the drug of choice in nondisseminated cases of sporotrichosis (52).

Various sulfonamides have been employed in treatment of the human mycoses. In cases of blastomycosis, some success was obtained with sulfadiazine (15) but only after prolonged treatment (53). Cases of South American blastomycosis, a disease distinct from that seen in the United States and caused by *Paracoccidioides brasiliensis*, responded dramatically to sulfonamides but, again, effective therapy required long periods of treatment (54). Sulfonamide therapy was not effective in cases of coccidioidomycosis. Today the principal antifungal indication for the sulfonamides is in treatment of paracoccidioidomycosis, or South American blastomycosis, where (15) and other sulfonamides have, at best, only a suppressive effect bringing about clinical improvement but not a true cure (55).

The use of aromatic diamines in the treatment of blastomycosis was first reported in 1950 (56). The first compound so used was stilbamidine (16) which proved effective in patients with disseminated disease when given intravenously at dosages of up to 200 mg/d for up to 30 d. However, this drug also proved to be excessively toxic and was associated with a high rate of relapsing infections. Toxic reactions included breathlessness, tachycardia, dizzyness, and depressed blood pressure. The most serious side effect seen with stilbamidine was a peripheral neuropathy involving facial nerves. Stilbamidine was replaced by 2-hydroxystilbamidine isethionate (17) which also proved partially effective but which was not associated with neuropathic toxicity. 2-Hydroxystilbamidine (18) did produce some toxic reactions including malaise, nausea and headache as well as changes in liver function. Hydroxystilbamidine isethionate (17) was administered intravenously in saline at dosages of 225 mg/d with a maximum dose of 8 g (57). The drug was light-sensitive and infusions had to be shielded. Apart from being concentrated in the liver, little is known about the pharmacology of the drug. With the advent of amphotericin B (2), the use of (18) has been limited to treatment of less severe, primary pulmonary infections (58).

$$H_2N-SO_2NH-\text{(pyrazine ring)}$$

(15)

$$\underset{NH_2}{\overset{NH}{C}}-\text{(benzene ring)}-CH=CH-\text{(benzene ring with R)}-\underset{NH_2}{\overset{NH}{C}}$$

(16) R = H
(17) R = OH · 2HOCH$_2$CH$_2$SO$_3$H
(18) R = OH

5-Fluorocytosine. 5-Fluorocytosine (19) (Flucytosine, 5-FC) was originally developed in 1957 as an antimetabolite for use in treatment of leukemia but, although devoid of anticancer activity (59), it was found to have antifungal activity *in vivo* (60). It is a white powder decomposing at 295°C and partially soluble in water (15 gm/L). It is nontoxic to experimental animals (LD$_{50}$ for mice, >2000 mg/kg, either orally or subcutaneously) and is readily absorbed from the gastrointestinal tract of humans and animals, thus permitting oral medication. In humans, tissue and fluid penetration is good with fungistatic serum and cerebrospinal fluid concentrations of 10–40 μg/mL persisting for 6–10 h after ingestion of a single 2 g dose (61).

The *in vitro* spectrum of (19) includes most isolates of *Cryptococcus neoformans*, many but not all isolates of *Candida albicans* and other species of pathogenic *Candida* strains as well as some isolates of *Aspergillus* species and of dematiaceous fungi such as *Cladosporium trichoides*. Most susceptible organisms are inhibited and killed at concentrations of 0.2–12.5 μg/mL (62); (19) appears to be only fungistatic and not fungicidal for filamentous fungi (63). There is evidence that the hematopoietic toxicity associated with (19) in patients with impaired renal function may be due to 5-fluorouracil (20) (5-FU) (64).

Currently, the therapeutic use of (19) (Ancobon) is limited to treatment of yeast infections caused by organisms of known susceptibity (65).

The mode of action of (19) involves, in part, conversion (deamination) to (20) and subsequent incorporation of (20) into RNA leading to miscoded protein synthesis (66). There is some evidence that inhibition of DNA synthesis by the metabolite 5-fluoro-2'-deoxyuridine-5'-monophosphate (21) also may be involved (67–68). At least four enzymatic actions are involved: permeation, deamination, uptake of (20) as 5-fluorouridine (22) (5-FUR) and incorporation of (22) into RNA. Resistance through mutational changes in enzyme function can result. Mutants with altered permeases are partially susceptible to (19) and mutation at any other site confers total resistance (69).

5-Fluorocytosine has been used with varying degrees of success in a variety of mycotic infections. It has provided a less toxic alternative to amphotericin B (2) in treatment of cryptococcal meningitis, pulmonary cryptococcosis and in pulmonary, urinary and disseminated candidiasis. Unfortunately, the emergence of resistant organisms during therapy has been a major problem in all such infections, particularly in inadequately treated patients with cryptococcosis (70).

Resistance to (19) most commonly involves changes in permease activity. Organisms with altered permeases are still susceptible to the drug if the permeability barrier can be overcome, as with combination therapy of (2) and (19). Some clinicians feel that this is the therapy of choice in patients with cryptococcal meningitis (71). In such patients, the dosage of (2) is reduced to 0.3–0.5 mg/(kg·d) and (19) is given at its full oral dosage of 150 mg/(kg·d). This regimen has proven effective in providing effective cures, reducing toxicity of (2) and preventing the development of (19)-resistant organisms (71).

Toxic reactions observed with (19) include hypersensitivity skin rashes, gastrointestinal disturbances, anemia and liver enlargement (72). The most serious side reactions involve hematopoietic toxicity. These include bone marrow depression and fatal aplastic anemia as well as anemia, neutropenia and thrombocytopenia. Many of these reactions have occurred in patients either previously treated with (2) or receiving combined treatment with the two drugs. Thus it is recommended that all patients receiving (19) be monitored in terms of both renal and marrow functions (73).

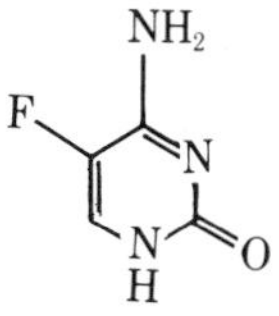

(19)

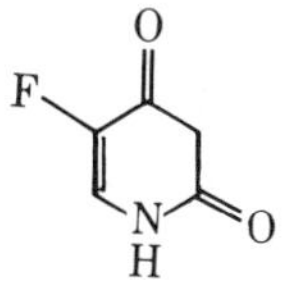

(20)

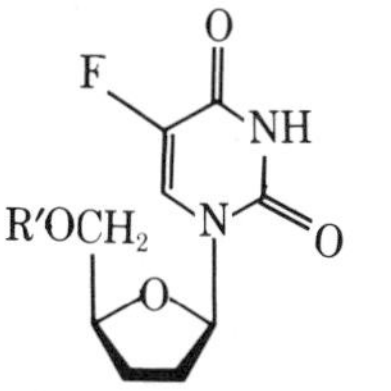

(21) R = H, R′ = PO₃H₂
(22) R = OH, R′ = H

Imidazole Compounds. The imidazoles represent the most versatile, and perhaps, most valuable source of antifungal compounds. As a group, they have a uniquely broad spectrum of activity which includes bacteria, fungi as well as protozoa, helminths and nematodes (74). Specific activity and spectra of individual compounds is highly dependent upon structure. The first of the antifungal imidazoles was 1-chlorobenzyl-2-methylbenzimidazole (23) (Myco-Polycid) which has some topical activity against *Candida* and dermatophytes (75). Subsequently, thiabendazole (24) (Mintezol) was introduced as an oral antihelminthic for medical and veterinary use in treatment of roundworm infections. Thiabendazole also has antifungal properties (76), but they have not been exploited extensively.

Clotrimazole (25) was first described in 1970 as a broad-spectrum orally-active imidazole (77), and active *in vitro* against a variety of fungal pathogens at concentrations as low as 0.1 μg/mL (74,78). Some reports showed (25) is active *in vivo* against both pathogenic yeasts and dermatophytic pathogens and others revealed hepatic enzymatic inactivation both in animals and humans (79–80) which appears to have restricted applications to topical use.

Most isolates of *Candida albicans* are inhibited by concentrations of 0.1–0.5 μg/mL; dermatophytic organisms are inhibited by 0.5–2 μg/mL. *In vivo*, (**25**) has low toxicity in animals when given by the oral route (LD$_{50}$ of 500–2000 mg/kg) and produces peak serum levels of 10–20 μg/mL (77). Oral dosages of (**25**) at 100 mg/kg are protective in acute animal experiments (77) but hepatic enzymatic inactivation of the drug nullifies the antifungal action of the drug in tests with chronic experiments (79,81). Thus the principal medical use of (**25**) appears to be in topical treatment of *Candida* and dermatophytic infections. Vaginal *Candida* infections, including those clinically resistant to (**1**), as well as *Candida* skin infections respond well to topical treatment with either a 1% clotrimazole cream or ointment (Lotrimin) as well as a vaginal tablet preparation (Gyne-Lotrimin). Topical (**25**) appears to be as active as topical (**1**) or Whitfield's ointment for treating cutaneous *Candida* infections (82). Gastrointestinal intolerance was observed in many patients receiving the oral medication.

Miconazole (**26**) also has important broad spectrum antifungal activity. Available both as a base (R 18,134) and as the nitrate (**27**) (R 14,889), (**26**) is a white, crystalline substance insoluble in water (0.03%) but soluble in organic solvents such as DMSO (83). *In vitro*, miconazole is fungistatic toward many pathogenic fungi at concentrations of ≤ 5 μg/mL (74,84). The *in vitro* activity of (**26**) is antagonized by complex culture media (85). There appears to be no difference in the *in vitro* activities of (**26**) and (**27**) (84).

Studies in animals revealed oral (**26**) to be relatively nontoxic with LD$_{50}$ values ranging from >160 mg/kg in dogs to >640 mg/kg in rats. There was no systemic absorption following topical application (86).

In humans, a 522 mg dose of intravenous (**26**) gives peak plasma levels of 2–9 μg/mL in individuals with normal renal function; the half-life was 0.38 h (87). Penetration of (**26**) from serum into cerebrospinal fluid is negligible (88–89). Miconazole is active both orally and topically in experimental animals infected with dermatophytic fungi, yeasts, and systemic pathogens such as *Coccidioides immitis* (83,90).

Topical miconazole cream (2% miconazole nitrate, Monistat) is highly effective in treatment of vaginal candidiasis with cure rates of 80–99% being reported (91). These results include patients who failed on therapy with other agents such as (**1**), (**2**), and (**4**). The relapse rate in such patients is approximately 5%. The usual course of therapy with miconazole cream for vaginal candidiasis is 5 to 6 g once daily for 14 d.

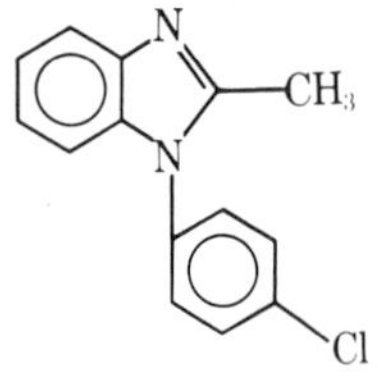

(**23**)

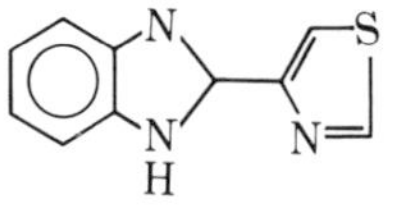

(**24**)

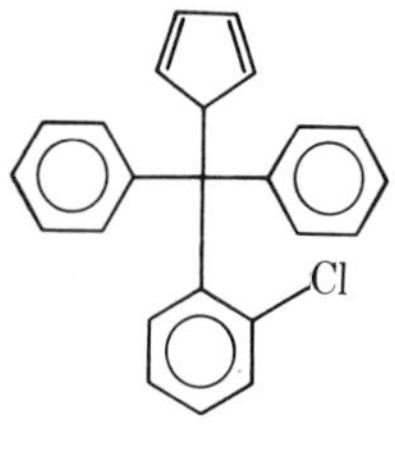

(**25**)

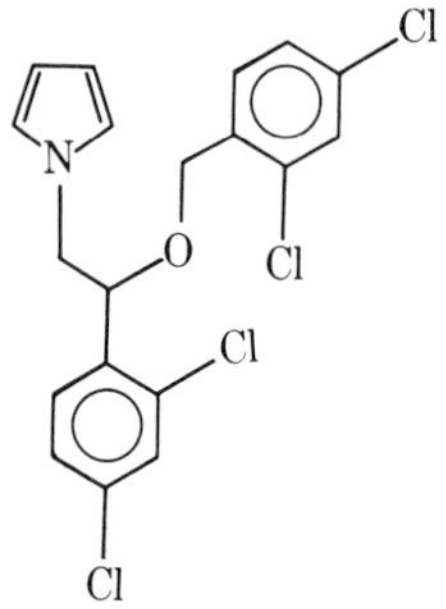

((**26**) • HNO$_3$)
(**27**)

(**26**)

Topical miconazole ointments (2% miconazole nitrate, Micatin) are effective in treatment of fungal skin infections including both dermatophytic and *Candida* infections (91). Cure rates ranged from 63% in cases of tinea corporis to 100% in cases of tinea pedis and tinea cruris. Cure rates of 80–90% also have been reported for a (26) varnish in treatment of nail infections (91).

The role of oral, intravenous, and intrathecal miconazole in systemic fungal infections is difficult to assess. Responses of 35–67%, in cases of coccidioidomycosis, depending upon the site of infection, have been reported (92). The most favorable responses were in patients with chronic pulmonary disease; the least favorable in patients with meningitis. The relapse rate was high: 36% in cases of pulmonary disease, and 63% in patients with meningitis. Similar results were obtained in patients with paracoccidioidomycosis. In another study a recovery rate of 59% in 54 patients with proven systemic fungal infection was observed; cultural examinations of 16 of the 35 patients in this study during posttreatment were still mycologically positive for the infecting organism (93).

Topical miconazole preparations are essentially devoid of toxicity although burning, itching, and irritation have been reported (94). Intravenous medication has been associated with a variety of adverse reactions including vision changes, itching, hyperlipidemia, erythrocyte aggregation, and thrombophlebitis. Some of these reactions have been attributed to the vehicle used for the intravenous preparation (95).

At present, the approved therapeutic uses of miconazole in the United States are limited to topical treatment of cutaneous and mucocutaneous infections by dermatophytes and *C. albicans*. Miconazole is available elsewhere as an oral preparation which has been reported valuable for treatment of oral and gastrointestinal candidiasis (96).

Tolnaftate. Tolnaftate (28) was first described in 1962 as a result of a series of studies on the relationship between chemical structures and selective toxicity of aryl thiocarbamoylthiocarbonates. It is soluble in organic solvents but not water. One of three naphthiocarbamates with antifungal activity (MIC of 0.0125 to 0.025 μg/mL for *Trichophyton* sp.) (28) has low toxicity for animals and is curative in experimental infections with *Trichophyton mentagrophytes*. It is inactive toward bacteria and *C. albicans*. Topical 1% tolnaftate is as effective as oral (6) (10 mg per animal) in treatment of experimental infections. It is highly effective as a topical agent for treating human dermatophytic infections and it is virtually nontoxic and nonsensitizing. Tolnaftate is used topically against smooth skin dermatophyte infections caused by species of *Epidermophyton*, *Microsporum*, and *Trichophyton*. It is not effective for infections of the scalp or nails. Preparations include 1% cream, ointment and powder (86).

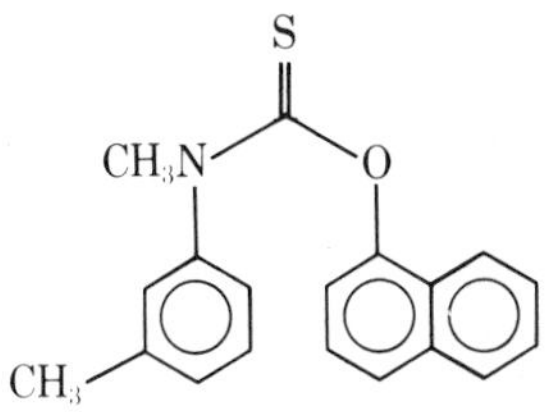

(28) 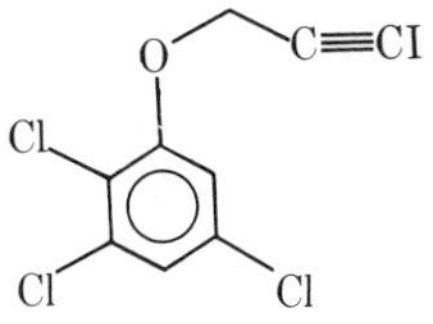   (29)   (30)

Haloprogin. Haloprogin (29) is an analogue of the antibiotic lenamycin (30). It is a white powder soluble in alcohols and slightly soluble in water. The *in vitro* activity of haloprogin includes pathogenic yeasts, gram-positive cocci, *Mycobacterium tuberculosis* and many species of dermatophytic fungi (MIC values of 0.25 μg/mL or less). It is orally nontoxic for animals (LD_{50} for mice = 1000 mg/kg) and sparingly toxic parenterally (LD_{50} for mice intraperitoneally = 510 mg/kg). Haloprogin is used topically in treatment of superficial fungus infections caused by dermatophytes or *C. Albicans.* It is not effective in treatment of scalp or nail infections. Topical (29), as a 1% cream or solution, is not without adverse reactions. These include local irritation, burning sensation and vesicle formation with increased pruritis and exacerbation of preexisting lesions (97).

Agricultural Use of Antifungal Agents

In addition to their use in human and veterinary medicine, antifungal agents also have an important role in control of fungal plant pathogens (phytopathogens), particularly in Japan where government regulations preclude the use of organic fungicides and pesticides containing mercury (see Fungicides).

Griseofulvin (6) is fungistatic for most phytopathogenic fungi and is readily absorbed by roots and transported systemically within treated plants. Its agricultural use includes treatment for powdery mildews, *Fusarium* wilt of melon and apple blossom blight (33). However, the high cost of the drug precludes large-scale applications. Pimaricin (5) is used as a dip to prevent fungal growth in skins of harvested apples. Cycloheximide (8) has a limited application in treatment of downy mildew of onions and shoot blight of Japanese larch.

Four antifungal antibiotics not used in medicine are extensively used for agricultural purposes. These include kasugamycin, blasticidin S, polyoxin D, and validamycin A (98) (see Antibiotics, aminoglycosides and nucleosides).

Economic Aspects of Antifungal Agents

Antifungal agents represent a significant component of the antiinfective drug market, especially the sales of vaginal and topical preparations. In 1975 sales of antifungal products in the United States amounted to 87.6 million dollars including 23 million dollars for vaginal preparations, 64 million dollars for antidermatophytic drugs, including both topical preparations and griseofulvum, and 0.6 million dollars for antisystemic antifungal agents. The international sales figure for the same year was approximately 300 million dollars. The insignificant contribution of antisystemic agents to the above figures is reflected in invoice price data for 1976 for (2) and (19); they were $490,000 and $89,000, respectively.

Agricultural use of antifungal agents represents a lucrative market particularly in the Orient (33,98). For example, in 1968 6.8% of the pesticides produced in Japan were antibiotics (33). These consisted primarily of kasugamycin, 17,565 metric tons; blasticidin-S, 7030 t; and polyoxin D, 3470 t. In 1975, sales for these same antibiotics in Japan totaled 9800 t and the net sales of all agricultural antibiotics was ca 17 million dollars.

RICKETTSIAL INFECTIONS

Infections caused by *Rickettsia* occur worldwide. Although the causative organisms have characteristics of both viruses and bacteria, they are more similar to the
latter. Like bacteria, they have cell walls and contain muramic acid, they have metabolic enzymes and are capable of independent respiratory activity, and their growth
is inhibited by antibiotics. The only characteristic they share with viruses is their inability to propagate (except for *Rickettsia quintana*) outside of living host cells. The
Rickettsia were named in honor of H. T. Ricketts who died of typhus fever in 1910
while studying the etiology of rickettsial infections. All rickettsial infections except
Q fever are transmitted to humans by bloodsucking arthropod vectors including lice,
fleas, ticks and mites. Rickettsial infections are ordinarily classified into five categories:
(*1*) typhus group, (*2*) spotted fever group, (*3*) scrub typhus, (*4*) Q fever, and (*5*) trench
fever. Those that occur in the United States are Rocky Mountain spotted fever, murine
typhus, Brill-Zinsser disease, rickettsialpox, and Q fever. All rickettsial infections are
characterized clinically by fever, headache, and (except Q fever) rash. A summary of
the epidemiologic characteristics of Rickettsial diseases and their prophylaxes are
shown in Table 3.

Treatment of Rickettsial Infections

Miticidal chemicals and the antibiotics used in treatment of rickettsial infections
are shown in structures (**31–37**).

All rickettsial infections respond to treatment with chloramphenicol (**35**) or
tetracycline (**36**). The latter is usually the drug of choice. In rare cases, (**35**) may cause
aplastic anemia due to destruction of bone marrow cells; this untoward reaction has
a high mortality. *Para*-aminobenzoic acid was the first antimicrobial agent available
for therapy of rickettsial infections. It has been used to treat epidemic typhus (99)
and Rocky Mountain spotted fever (100). However, it is less effective than tetracycline
and chloramphenicol and has greater toxicity, including suppression of the white blood
cell count and formation of crystals in the urine with resultant kidney damage.

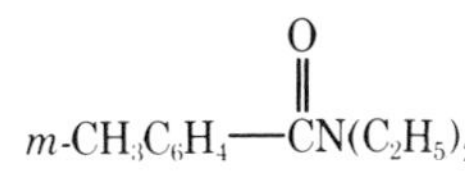

$$m\text{-}CH_3C_6H_4\text{—}\overset{\overset{\displaystyle O}{\|}}{C}N(C_2H_5)_2$$

N,N-diethyl-*m*-toluamide

(**31**)

$$o\text{-}C_6H_4(CO_2R)_2$$

(**32**) dimethyl phthalate R = CH_3
(**33**) dibutyl phthalate R = *n*-Bu

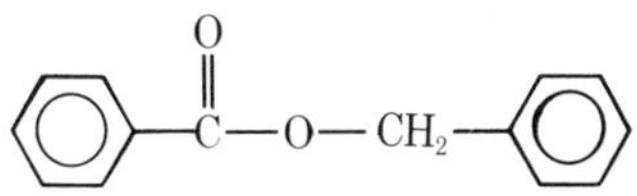

benzyl benzoate

(**34**)

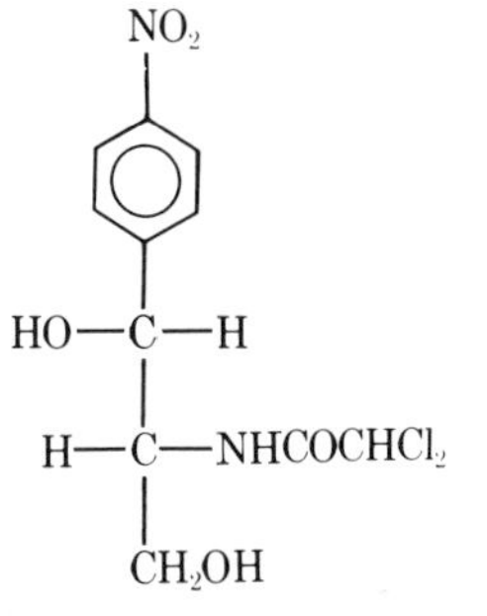

(**35**)

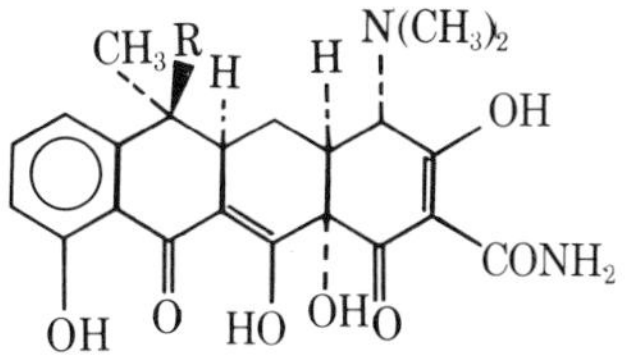

(**36**) R = OH
(**37**) R = H

Table 3. Characterics of Rickettsial Diseases

Disease	Geographic occurrence	Organism	Vector	Reservoir	Control and prophylaxis	Usual incubation period, d
Typhus group						
epidemic typhus	worldwide	*Rickettsia prowazekii*	human body louse	humans	appropriate insecticides[a]	10–14
Brill-Zinsser disease[b]	worldwide	*R. prowazekii*	body louse	humans	appropriate insecticides[a]	7–11
endemic typhus[c]	worldwide	*R. mooseri*	rat flea	rats and mice	appropriate insecticides[a]	6–4
Spotted fever group						
Rocky Mountain spotted fever	eastern and northwestern U.S.	*R. rickettsii*	wood tick, dog tick	wild rodents	vaccination of humans[d], application of (31) and (32) or appropriate insecticides[a]	2–6
tick-borne rickettsioses of eastern hemisphere	Africa; North Asia; Australia	*R. conorii; R. sibirica; R. australis*		wild rodents		5–7
rickettsialpox	U.S. and U.S.S.R., especially urban areas thereof	*R. akari*	mouse mite	house mice	appropriate insecticides[a]	7–10
Scrub typhus	Asiatic–Pacific area	*R. tsutsugamushi*	chigger	mites, rodents	appropriate insecticides[a]; application of (32–34) to clothes; and (35)	6–21
Q fever	worldwide	*Coxiella burnetii*	ticks between animals; to humans via dust or aerosols	mammals	strict hygienic measures	14–28
trench fever	western Europe	*R. quintana*	body louse	humans	appropriate insecticides[a]	10–30

[a] See Insect control technology.
[b] Refs. 99 and 100.
[c] Ref. 101.
[d] Vaccine Technology and ref. 102.

Table 4.   Alphabetical List of Compounds Referred to in the Text

Compound	CAS Registry No.
acrisorcin (14)	[7527-91-5]
ambruticin (10)	[58857-02-6]
amphotericin B (2)	[1397-89-3]
amphotericin B, methyl ester (3)	[36148-89-7]
benzyl benzoate (34)	[120-51-4]
blasticidin S	[2079-00-7]
candicidin (4)	[1403-17-4]
chloramphenicol (35)	[56-75-7]
1-chlorobenzyl-2-methylbenzimidazole (23)	[3689-76-7]
clotrimazole (25)	[23953-75-1]
cycloheximide (8)	[66-81-9]
dibutyl phthalate (33)	[84-74-2]
N,N-diethyl-m-toluamide (31)	[134-62-3]
dimethyl phthalate (32)	[131-11-3]
doxycycline (37)	[564-25-0]
5-fluoro-2'-deoxyuridine-5'-monophosphate (21)	[134-46-3]
5-fluorocytosine (19)	[2022-85-7]
5-fluorouracil (20)	[51-21-8]
5-fluorouridine (22)	[316-46-1]
gentian violet (11)	[548-62-9]
griseofulvin (6)	[126-07-8]
haloprogin (29)	[777-11-7]
2-hydroxystilbamidine (18)	[495-99-5]
2-hydroxystilbamidine isethionate (17)	[533-22-2]
iodochlorhydroxyquin (13)	[130-26-7]
kasugamycin	[6980-18-3]
lenamycin (30)	[543-21-5]
miconazole (26)	[22916-47-8]
miconazole nitrate (27)	[22832-87-7]
nystatin (1)	[1400-61-9]
pimaricin (5)	[7681-93-8]
polyoxin D	[22976-86-9]
pyrrolnitrin (9)	[1018-71-9]
sinefungin (7)	[58944-73-3]
stilbamidine (16)	[122-06-5]
sulfadiazine (15)	[68-35-9]
tetracycline (36)	[60-54-8]
thiabendazole (24)	[148-79-8]
tolnaftate (28)	[2398-96-1]
10-undecenoic acid (12)	[112-38-9]
validamycin A	[37248-47-8]

Although (36) is usually the drug of first choice for rickettsial infections, it may not be the first choice for treatment of children less than eight years of age. In individuals of this age group (36) may cause a brownish discoloration of the permanent teeth. Both (35) and (36) are well absorbed orally and should be given by that route unless the patient has nausea and vomiting or is unconscious. In patients too ill to take the medications orally, both may be given by the intravenous route. Treatment should be initiated as early as possible in the illness. Tetracycline (36) is given in a dose of 500 mg orally every six h for adults or in children at a dose of 25 mg/kg body wt per day divided into equal portions given at six hourly intervals. Chloramphenicol (35) should be given orally in a dose of 50 mg/kg body wt per day divided into four equal doses. Intravenous therapy with (36) is started with 1 gm followed by 500 mg every 6 h. Therapy with (35) is begun with 1 gm and then given in a dose of 500 mg every 4–6 h. When the patient has improved to the point where intravenous therapy is no longer needed, treatment should be switched to the oral route (see Antibiotics, chloramphenical and tetracyclines).

Treatment should be continued until the patient has been without fever for two or three days. Therapy needs to be given for a few days past the termination of the illness to prevent relapse. This is due to the fact that both (35) and (36) are rickettsiostatic and not rickettsiocidal. The antibiotics hold the growth of rickettsiae in check until the body's immune system can erradicate them. Another effective tetracycline antibiotic in the treatment of rickettsial infections is doxycycline (37). Several investigators have found that it is effective in the treatment of epidemic typhus when given in a single oral dose of 100–200 mg (101–103). The penicillin-antibiotics and streptomycin are inactive against rickettsiae. The combination of trimethoprim and sulfamethoxazole (co-trimoxazole) has been found to be ineffective when given to patients with rickettsial infections and are contraindicated (see Antibacterial agents, sulfonamides).

Of course, prevention is attained by elimination of lice, mites, ticks, rodents, and use of the appropriate insecticides (see Insect control technology).

An alphabetical list of compounds referred to in the text is shown in Table 4.

BIBLIOGRAPHY

"Bacterial, Rickettsial, and Mycotic Infections, Chemotherapy" in *ECT* 2nd ed., Vol. 3, pp. 1–36, by Morris Solotorovsky, Rutgers University, and Gordon Kemp, American Cyanamid Company.

1. W. Mechlinski in A. I. Laskin and H. A. Lechevalier, eds., *Handbook of Microbiology, Vol. III*, CRC Press, Cleveland, Ohio, 1973, pp. 93–107.
2. C. W. Emmons and co-workers, *Medical Mycology*, Lea and Febiger, Philadelphia, Pa., 1977, p. 74.
3. E. L. Hazen and R. Brown, *Proc. Soc. Exp. Biol. Med.* **76,** 93 (1951).
4. W. Mechlinski in ref. 1, p. 104.
5. S. Shadomy and A. Espinel-Ingroff in E. H. Lennette, E. H. Spaulding, and J. P. Truant, eds., *Manual of Clinical Microbiology,* 2nd ed., American Society for Microbiology, Washington, D.C., 1974, p. 571.
6. C. Halde and co-workers, *J. Invest. Dermatol.* **28,** 217 (1957).
7. A. Kucers and N. M. Bennett, *The Use of Antibiotics,* 2nd ed., Wm. Heinemann Medical Books, London, Eng., 1975, p. 561.
8. J. E. Bennett. *N. Engl. J. Med.* **290,** 30, 320 (1974).
9. W. Mechlinski and C. P. Schaffner, *J. Antibiot.* **25,** 256 (1972).
10. H. H. Gadebusch and co-workers, *J. Infect. Dis.* **134,** 423 (1976).
11. N. M. Stevens and co-workers, *Arch. Virol.* **48,** 391 (1975).
12. G. W. Jordan and E. C. Seet, *Antimicrob. Agents Chemother.* **13,** 199 (1978).
13. D. P. Bonner and co-workers, *Antimicrob. Agents Chemother.* **7,** 724 (1975).
14. P. D. Hoeprich, L. K. Henth, and R. M. Lawrence, *Abstr. 16th Intersci. Conf. Antimicrob. Agents Chemother.* abst. **306** (1976).
15. H. Lechevalier and co-workers, *Antibiot. Chemother.* **11,** 640 (1961).
16. E. Drouhet in ref. 1, p. 693.
17. W. Mechlinski in ref. 1, p. 101.
18. W. Mechlinski in ref. 1, p. 104.
19. Ref. 7, p. 604.
20. D. R. Berry and B. J. Abbott, *J. Antibiot.* **31,** 185 (1978).
21. S. M. Ringel and co-workers, *J. Antibiot.* **30,** 371 (1977).
22. H. B. Levine, S. M. Ringel, and J. M. Cobb, *Chest* **73,** 202 (1978).

23. J. C. Gentles, *Nature (London)* **183,** 476 (1958).
24. A. R. Martin, *Vet. Rec.* **70,** 1232 (1958).
25. H. Blank and F. J. Roth, Jr., *AMA Arch. Dermatol.* **79,** 259 (1959).
26. D. I. Williams, R. H. Martin, and I. Sarkany, *Lancet ii,* 1212 (1958).
27. G. Hildick-Smith, H. Blank, and I. Sarkany, *Fungus Diseases and Their Treatment,* Little, Brown and Co., Boston, Mass., 1964, p. 438.
28. C. Lin and S. Symchowicz, *Drug Metab. Rev.* **4,** 79 (1975).
29. P. W. Brian, *Ann. Bot. (London)* **13,** 59 (1949).
30. G. Evans and N. H. White, *J. Exp. Bot.* **18,** 465 (1967).
31. Ref. 7, p. 598.
32. A. J. Whiffen, *J. Bacteriol.* **56,** 283 (1948).
33. J. Dekker, *World Rev. Pest Control* **10,** 9 (1971).
34. M. R. Siegel and H. D. Sisler, *Biochim. Biophys. Acta* **87,** 70 (1964).
35. R. S. Gordee and T. R. Mathews, *Antimicrob Agents Chemotherapy-1967,* American Society for Microbiology, Ann Arbor, Mich., 1968, p. 378.
36. L. D. Boeck and co-workers, *Antimicrob. Agents Chemother.* **11,** 49 (1973).
37. R. Hamill and M. M. Hoehn, *J. Antibiot. (Tokyo)* **26,** 463 (1973).
38. R. S. Gordee and T. F. Butler, *J. Antibiot. (Tokyo)* **26,** 466 (1973).
39. J. R. Turner and co-workers, *Abst. 17th Intersci. Conf. Antimicrob. Agents Chemother. abst* **49,** (1977).
40. S. M. Ringel and co-workers, *J. Antibiot. (Tokyo)* **30,** 371 (1977).
41. S. M. Ringel, *Antimicrob. Agents Chemother.* **13,** 762 (1978).
42. S. Shadomy and co-workers, *Antimicrob. Agents Chemother.* **14,** 99 (1978).
43. H. B. Levine and S. M. Ringel in L. Ajello, ed., *Coccidioidomycosis: Current Clinical Diagnostic Status,* Symposia Specialists Publishers, Miami, Fl., 1977, p. 319.
44. H. B. Levine, S. M. Ringel, and J. M. Cobb, *Chest* **73,** 202 (1978).
45. S. Shadomy, C. J. Utz, and S. White, *Antimicrob. Agents Chemother.* **14,** 95 (1978).
46. N. F. Conant and co-workers, *Manual of Medical Mycology,* 2nd ed., W. B. Saunders Co., Philadelphia, Pa., 1954, p. 298.
47. *Ibid.,* pp. 191 and 300.
48. *Ibid.,* pp. 302 and 401.
49. *Ibid.,* pp. 298 and 428.
50. Ref. 27, p. 10.
51. *Ibid.,* p. 163.
52. Ref. 2, p. 409.
53. M. S. Silva, *Rev. Brasil Med.* **2,** 918 (1945).
54. Ref. 46, p. 91.
55. J. W. Rippon, *Medical Mycology, The Pathogenic Fungi and the Pathogenic Actinomycetes,* W. B. Saunders Co., Philadelphia, Pa., 1974, p. 398.
56. A. C. Curtis and E. R. Harrell, *AMA Arch. Dermatol. Syphilol.* **66,** 676 (1952).
57. Ref. 2, p. 78.
58. J. F. Busey in H. A. Buechner, ed., *Management of Fungus Diseases of the Lungs,* Charles C Thomas, Springfield, Ill., 1971, p. 47.
59. R. Duschinsky, E. Pleven, and C. Heidelburg, *J. Am. Chem. Soc.* **79,** 4559 (1957).
60. E. Grunberg, E. Titsworth, and M. Bennett, *Antimicrob. Agents Chemother.* **3,** 566 (1963).
61. B. A. Koechlin and co-workers, *Biochem. Pharmacol.* **15,** 435 (1966).
62. D. C. E. Speller and M. G. Davis, *J. Med. Microbiol.* **6,** 315 (1973).
63. G. E. Wagner and S. Shadomy, *Antimicrob. Agents Chemother.* **11,** 299 (1977).
64. P. D. Hoeprich, *Ann Rev. Pharmacol. Toxicol.* **18,** 205 (1978).
65. Ref. 55, p. 541.
66. A. Polak and H. J. Scholer, *Chemotherapy* **21,** 113 (1975).
67. G. E. Wagner and S. Shadomy, *Chemotherapy,* **24,** (1978).
68. R. B. Diasio, J. E. Bennett, and C. E. Myers, *Biochem. Pharmacol.* **27,** 703 (1978).
69. G. Vandervelde, A. A. Mauceri, and J. E. Johnson, III, *Ann. Int. Med.* **77,** 43 (1972).
70. S. Shadomy, *Appl. Microbiol.* **17,** 871 (1969).
71. J. P. Utz and co-workers, *J. Inf. Dis.* **132,** 368 (1975).
72. H. J. Scholer, *Chemotherapy* **22,** 103 (1976).
73. J. Schönebeck and co-workers, *Chemotherapy* **18,** 321 (1973).
74. R. J. Holt, *Infection* **2,** 95 (1974).

75. H. P. R. Seeliger, *Mykosen* **1**, 162 (1958).
76. L. J. Sorensen and R. J. Robinson in J. C. Sylvester, ed., *Antimicrobial Agents and Chemotherapy-1964,* American Society for Microbiology, Ann Arbor, Mich., 1965, p. 742.
77. M. Plempel and co-workers, *Deut. Medizinische Wochenschr.* **94**, 1356 (1969).
78. S. Shadomy, *Infect. Immun.* **4**, 143 (1971).
79. S. Shadomy in G. L. Hobby, ed., *Antimicrobial Agents and Chemotherapy-1970,* American Society for Microbiology, Bethesda, Md., 1971, p. 169.
80. J. A. Waitz, E. L. Moss, and M. J. Weinstein, *Appl. Microbiol.* **22**, 891 (1971).
81. G. K. Crompton and L. J. R. Milne, *Br. J. Dis. Chest* **67**, 301 (1973).
82. Y. M. Clayton and B. L. Connor, *Br. J. Dermatol.* **89**, 297 (1973).
83. J. M. Van Cutsem and D. Thienpont, *Chemotherapy* **17**, 392 (1972).
84. S. Shadomy and co-workers, *J. Antimicrob. Chemother.* **3**, 147 (1977).
85. H. Van den Bossche, G. Willemsens, and J. M. Van Cutsem, *Sabouraudia* **13**, 63 (1975).
86. R. J. Holt, *J. Cutaneous Pathol.* **3**, 45 (1976).
87. P. J. Lewi and co-workers, *Eur. J. Clin. Pharmacol.* **10**, 49 (1976).
88. P. D. Hoeprich and E. Goldstein, *J. Am. Med. Assoc.* **230**, 1153 (1974).
89. J. F. Fisher and co-workers, *Antimicrob. Agents Chemother.* **13**, 965 (1978).
90. H. B. Levine and co-workers, *J. Inf. Dis.* **132**, 407 (1975).
91. P. R. Sawyer and co-workers, *Med. Prog.,* 25 (May, 1975).
92. D. A. Stevens, *Am. Rev. Resp. Dis.* **116**, 801 (1977).
93. J. Symoens, *Proc. R. Soc. Med.* **70**(Suppl. 1), 4 (1977).
94. J. E. Davis, J. H. Frudenfeld, and J. L. Goddard, *Obstet. Gynecol.* **44**, 403 (1974).
95. H. B. Nield, *N. Engl. J. Med.* **296**, 1479 (1977).
96. H. Brincker, *Proc. R. Soc. Med.* **70**(Suppl 1), 29 (1977).
97. American Medical Association, *AMA Drug Evaluations,* 3rd ed., Publishing Sciences Group, Inc., Acton, Mass., 1977, pp. 821–838.
98. T. Misato in J. R. Plimmer ed., *Pesticide Chemistry in the 20th Century,* American Chemical Society, Washington, D.C., 1977, pp. 170–192.
99. J. C. Snyder and co-workers, *Ann. Intern. Med.* **27**, 1 (1947).
100. T. E. Woodward and W. R. Raley, *South. Med. J.* **41**, 997 (1948).
101. J. Huys and co-workers, *Trans. R. Soc. Trop. Med. Hyg.* **67**, 718 (1973).
102. P. L. Perine and co-workers, *Lancet ii,* 742 (1974).
103. D. W. Krause and co-workers, *East Afr. Med. J.* **52**, 421 (1975).

General References

Human Mycoses

E. S. Beneke, *Scope® Monograph on the Human Mycoses,* The Upjohn Co., Kalamazoo, Mich., 1974, 1–48.
G. S. Kobayashi and G. Medoff, *Ann. Rev. Microbiol.* **31**, 291 (1977).
J. F. Martin, *Ann. Rev. Microbiol.* **31**, 13 (1977).
K. Iwata, ed., *Recent Advances in Medical and Veterinary Mycology,* University of Tokyo Press, Tokyo, Jpn., 1977, 316 pp.
G. E. W. Wolstenholme and R. Porter, eds., *Systemic Mycoses, A Ciba Foundation Symposium,* Little, Brown and Co., Boston, Mass., 1967, 287 pp.
Pan American Health Organization, *Paracoccidioidomycosis, Proceedings of the First Pan American Symposium,* Sc. Publ. 254, WHO, Washington, D.C., 1972, 319 pp.
E. W. Chick, A. Balows and M. L. Furcolow, *Opportunistic Fungal Infection,* Charles C Thomas, Springfield, Ill., 1975, 359 pp.
L. Ajello, ed., *Coccidioidomycosis, Current Clinical and Diagnostic Status,* Symposia Specialists, Miami, Fl., 1977, 475 pp.
N. F. Conant and co-workers, *Manual of Clinical Mycology,* W. B. Saunders, Philadelphia, Pa., 1971, 255 pp.

Rickettsial Infections

F. L. Horsfall, Jr., and I. Tamm, eds., *Viral and Rickettsial Infections of Man,* J. B. Lippincott Co., Philadelphia, Pa., 1965.

P. B. Beeson and W. McDermott, eds., *Textbook of Medicine,* W. B. Saunders Co., Philadelphia, Pa., 1975.

G. W. Thorn and co-eds., *Harrison's Principles of Internal Medicine,* McGraw Hill Book Co., New York, 1977.

P. D. Hoeprich, ed., *Infectious Diseases, A Modern Treatise of Infectious Processes,* Harper and Row, Publishers, Inc., New York, 1977.

J. C. Snyder in F. R. Moulton, ed., *Rickettsial Diseases of Man,* American Association for the Advancement of Science, Washington, D.C., 1948.

M. W. Rytel and J. D. Coonrod, *Wis. Med. J.* **70,** 116 (1971).

M. J. Snyder and T. E. Woodward, *Med. Clin. N. Am.* **54,** 1187 (1970).

H. L. Dupont and co-workers, *N. Engl. J. Med.* **282,** 53 (1970).

M. A. W. Hattwick, R. J. O'Brien, and B. F. Hanson, *Ann. Intern. Med.* **84,** 732 (1976).

W. Burgdorfer, *Acta Tropica* **34,** 103 (1977).

SMITH SHADOMY
C. GLEN MAYHALL
Medical College of Virginia

ANTIPROTOZOAL

Protozoa are single-cell organisms that constitute the most primitive group of the animal realm. About 45,000 species of protozoa have been described. Some of them parasitize higher animals and man. Antiprotozoal chemotherapy was developed in response to health problems of individuals and to economic needs (1–4). Knowledge of the history of antiprotozoal drugs is useful for future development in this area (5). In this article the term chemotherapy is used for protozoocidal and protozoostatic compounds. The protozoocidal drugs are curative in that they eradicate the parasite in all its stages within the host. Protozoostatic drugs suppress the parasite's clinically relevant developmental stages but not certain latent stages. The surviving, suppressed protozoa may cause either clinical relapse of the disease or stimulate immune defenses which in turn may either cure or control the latent infection.

Many of the antiprotozoal drugs have a narrow safety margin, eg, 1:2. The safety margin is determined on a statistical basis, but as the susceptibility to a drug often varies unpredictably from one patient to another, medication always involves some risk. The narrower the safety margin, the greater the risk. The practitioner must weigh the potentialities of toxicity against the seriousness of the protozoal infection and thus evaluate the risk-to-benefit ratio of the medication.

An adequate prediction of a chemical agent's effectiveness against a certain protozoan cannot be made from the present range of knowledge. For some drugs, eg, antifolates, the site of action is well established, yet the reason for better action in some protozoon species than in others, is unknown. *In vitro* studies have shown many compounds to affect one or more biochemical systems, but quite often, *in vitro* activities are not predictive for clinical efficacy and *in vivo* screening is still important in antiprotozoal drug development.

This article describes those drugs that have reached commercial and clinical significance and a few selected experimental drugs that appear promising. Both human and veterinary drugs are described since many of the principal parasitic diseases discussed infect animals of considerable value in the economy (see also Veterinary drugs).

Coccidiosis

The taxonomic classification of *Coccidia* species is still in a state of flux (6–8). *Coccidia* species are cosmopolitan and widespread in the animal kingdom, although most of them are limited to a narrow range of host species and organ systems. Some *Coccidia*, eg, *Toxoplasma,* may pass from one host species to another changing their target organs from host to host. The life cycle of *Coccidia* includes cysts, sporozoites, schizonts, merozoites, and gametocytes. *Eimeria* and *Toxoplasma* are economically and medically important *coccidia*.

Eimeria infect many vertebrates, including fish, poultry, farm animals, dogs, and cats. The parasite first invades the epithelial lining of the digestive tract and may cause diarrhea, sloughing, and ulceration of the intestinal lining, and hemorrhage, leading to possible metastatic spread, malabsorption of nutrients and vitamins, metabolic imbalance, and anemia and bacteremia. Depending on severity and duration, the consequences may range from growth retardation to death.

Eradication of *Eimeria* species with presently available drugs would be impractical because of toxicological and economic considerations; anticoccidials are currently used in animal husbandry as coccidiostats. Mixed with feeds, the coccidiostats serve to minimize the intensity of infection or to reduce clinical symptoms to a nonfatal course. In this way, time is gained for the host to build up immune defenses. *Eimeria* species develop drug resistance quite rapidly so that development of new anticoccidials is economically vital for animal farming (8–9) (Fig. 1). Furthermore, the efficacy of any given anticoccidial against *Eimeria* and the toxicity to the host can vary from one species of either to another. The situation can become even more complicated as mixed infections by several *Eimeria* species may occur, especially in cattle.

Reports on drug efficacy should be evaluated carefully by an analysis of the assay protocol; uncontrolled studies are meaningless. The course of *Eimeria* infection is often self-limited in individual subjects and in epidemics of population groups. If treatment is initiated at the peak of a clinical case or an epidemic, the kind of drug used is irrelevant as the disease would subside in any case. A system known as floor pen is a good standard for drug assays in chicken coccidiosis (10).

For each of the few drugs described below, a large number of congeners are available for both experimental and commercial use. Some of the anticoccidials belong to drug categories with well known biochemical effector systems. The biochemical rationale for others is still uncertain, a failing that does not diminish their practical value. The safety range of anticoccidials varies widely. Contributing variables of toxicity are dosage and duration of the drug administration, species and metabolic condition of the host, environmental conditions, and nutrition. The anticoccidials with defined biochemical targets are thiamine competitors, antifolates, antibiotics, nitrobenzamides, and nitrofurans.

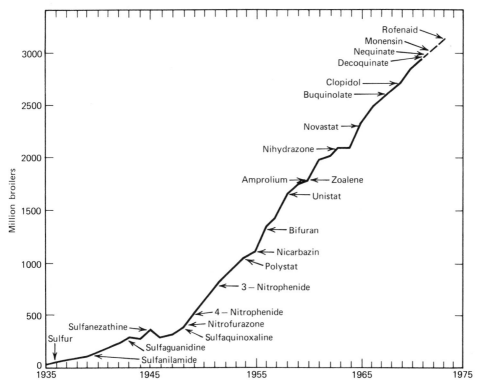

Figure 1. Correlation between growth of the broiler industry and the introduction of coccidiostats (9).

Thiamine Competitors. These are thiamine (**1**) derivatives in which either the side chains are modified, or the thiazolium ring is substituted or opened, or both (11). Examples are amprolium (**2**) and aminoalkenyl sulfides, eg, (**3**).

Amprolium is prepared by reaction of 2-propyl-4-amino-5-chloromethylpyrimidine dihydrochloride with 2-methylpyridine in acetonitrile (12). The synthesis of (**3**) is described in a Japanese patent: a thiamine-type compound is treated with an alkali and the resulting ring-opened thiol is oxidized with potassium iodide to give the disulfide (13).

Toxicity of the thiamine competitors manifests itself as polyneuritis. Administration of thiamine can prevent this condition but will not cure the adverse effects if nerves and their dependent organs have suffered permanent damage (14).

Antifolates. Sulfonamides, pyrimethamine, and *p*-aminobenzoic acid competitors such as Ethopabate (**4**) are in this category (see Antibacterial agents).

Ethopabate is synthesized from the potassium salt of 4-acetamido-2-hydroxybenzoic acid methyl ester and ethyl 4-toluenesulfonate (15).

Antibiotics. Among the various antibiotics, monensin (**5**) has practical relevance (see Antibiotics, polyethers). It is isolated from *Streptomyces cinnamonensis* and is also produced by a fermentation process (16).

Like other monocarboxylic acid antibiotics, monensin increases the monovalent cation permeability of biological membranes. The loss of these cations impairs the enzyme systems that they regulate (17). Information in reports or patents is inadequate

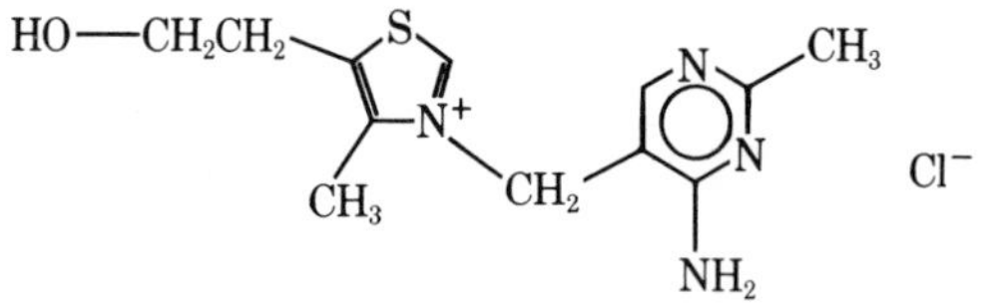

(1) 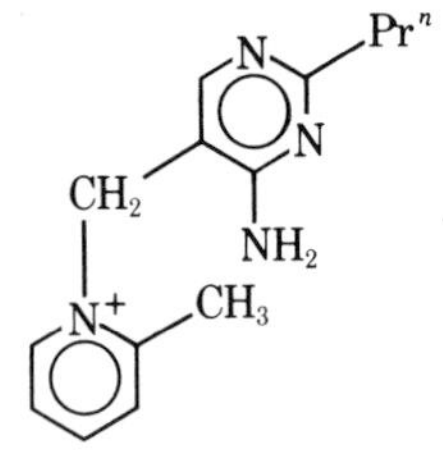   (2)

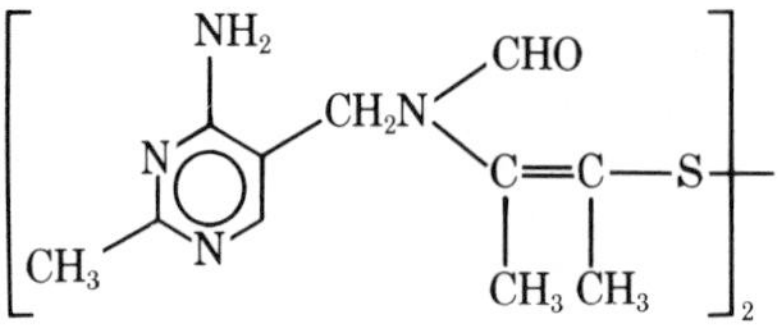

(3) 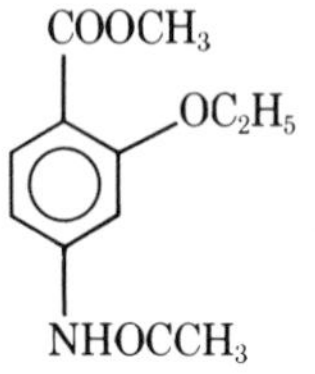   (4)

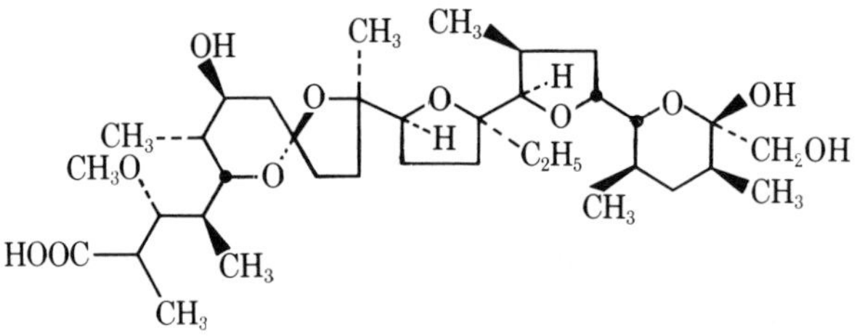

(5)

on the anticoccidial activity of several newer antibiotics. The reported efficacy of oxytetracycline and similar antibiotics in coccidial infections may be explained by their control of secondary infections (see Antibiotics, tetracyclines).

Nitrobenzamides and Nitrofurans. Efforts to develop anticoccidials in these classes seem justified since compounds with a 5-nitro group interfere with the cytochrome system of other protozoa (18) (see Antibacterial agents); however, no satisfactory anticoccidial has as yet been marketed in this class. The available analogues require high dosages for efficacy and have a very narrow safety margin. Information on the mutagenicity of this class will also be needed.

Reports which dealt with relevant biochemical targets of the following drugs could not be located: Robenidine (6), bisthiosemicarbazones (7), Clopidol (8), quinolones (9,10), and quinazolinones (11).

Robenidine (6) is a very effective compound. However, birds whose diet has contained Robenidine, produce tainted eggs, and their flesh reportedly has an unpleasant taste. Compound (6) is 1,3-bis[(4-chlorobenzylidene)amino]guanidine and is obtained by the reaction of 4-chlorobenzaldehyde with 1,3-diaminoguanidine nitrate (19).

Bitipazone (7) is an example of a bisthiosemicarbazone (20). In this class a basic side chain seems to be necessary for activity, and asymmetric compounds are more efficacious than symmetrical ones. The safety margin in this class is very narrow.

Clopidol (8) is thus far the only simple pyridone derivative with good anticoccidial activity. It has been synthesized by chlorination of 2,6-dimethyl-4-pyridinol in aqueous hydrochloric acid (21).

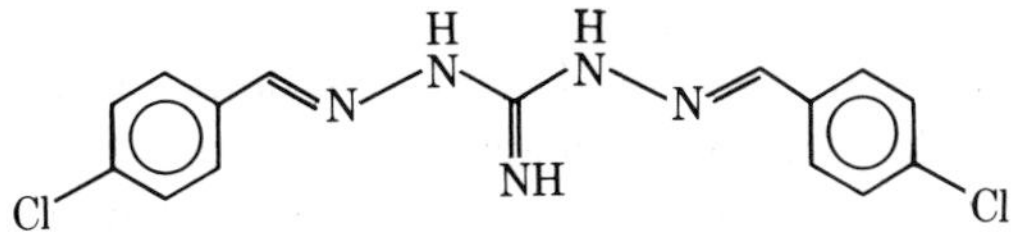

(6)

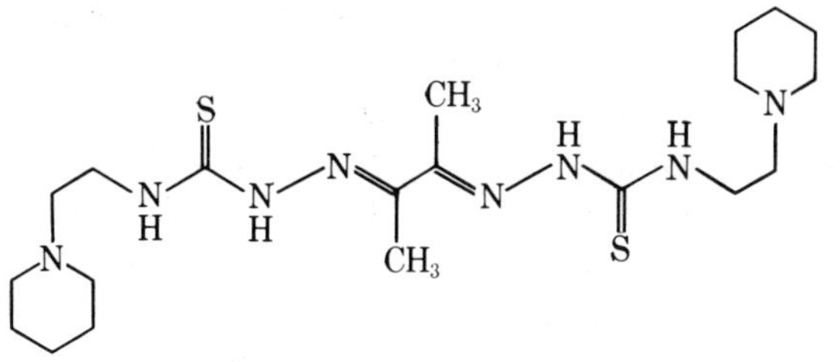

(7)

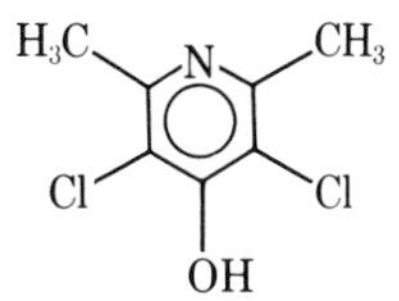

(8)

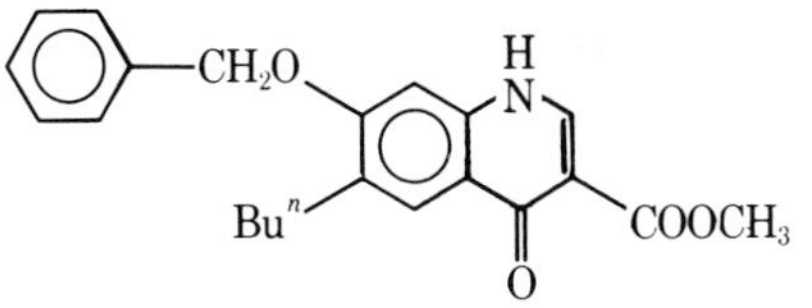

(9)

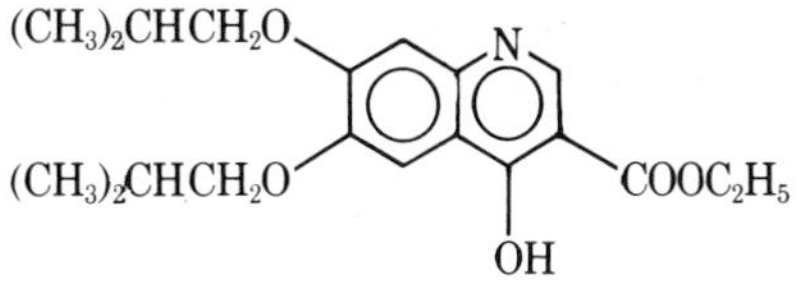

(10)

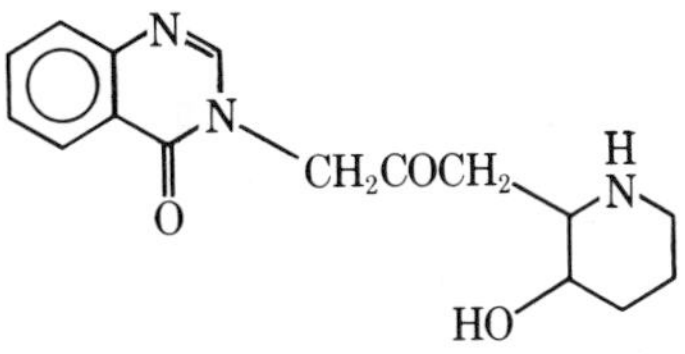

(11)

Among the quinolones, the most active is nequinate (9). Its two-step preparation starts with 4-butyl-3-benzyloxyaniline and diethyl ethoxymethylenemalonate (22).

The quinolones are virtually water-insoluble. For buquinolate (10), the micronized formulation of 1.8 μm particle size was more active than the 6.1-μm milled formulation. Its synthesis starts with catechol diisobutyl ether which is nitrated, catalytically reduced, and the ring closure of an anil diester is accomplished by heating in Dowtherm under reflux (23). Safety studies have not yielded evidence of serious toxicity. But the potential of quinolones for producing drug resistance is very great. Some of the quinazolines are highly active but have a low safety margin. They are compounds with halogen substitutents at positions 6 to 8 derived from the antimalarial febrifugine (11). Febrifugine was isolated from *Dichroa febrifuga* and from the common hydrangea. It was synthesized via the key intermediates 2-methoxy-5-carbobenzoxyaminovaleric acid and 1-carbethoxy-3-methoxy-2-piperidineacetic acid (24).

Drug mixtures including members of the above classes are also successful. Patents have been granted for numerous analogues of each of the above classes but the drugs have not been offered for commercial use. Some new antimicrobials and anthelmintics have anticoccidial potential but often low efficacy or prohibitive toxicity.

Toxoplasmosis. Toxoplasma infections are cosmopolitan and quite common among man and animals (25). Species differentiation between the toxoplasmas of man and other mammals has not been definitely established. According to some estimates one-third or more of human populations may carry a quiescent infection. Though clinical manifestations of toxoplasmosis are relatively rare, they are very serious when they do occur. They are more prevalent in children than in adults and their incidence is increased in immunodeficient individuals (26). In humans, contamination is either transplacental or by consumption of infected meat or animal material. Antifolates are effective in toxoplasmosis chemotherapy. Sulfonamides and pyrimethamine act individually on different steps of the folic acid synthesis and, when combined, they potentiate each other as in Fansidar [37338-39-9] (27).

Sulfonamides that dissolve readily in intracellular fluid are effective against toxoplasmosis, but those distributed mainly extracellularly are not effective (28). The use of antifolates during certain stages of pregnancy can have serious teratogenetic effects. In addition, sulfonamides displace bilirubin from its protein binding which causes the free bilirubin plasma to increase to levels that are toxic to the newborn. Hence the administration of sulfonamides at the end of pregnancy can lead to kernicterus in the newborn.

The antibiotic spiramycin (12) has also been reported to be useful in the treatment of toxoplasmosis (28–31) (see Antibiotics, macrolides).

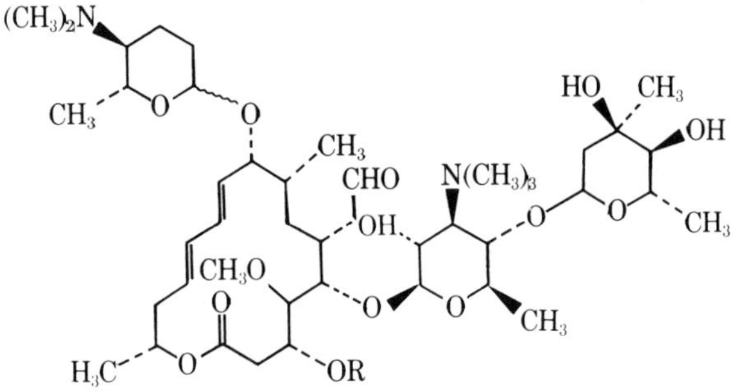

(12)

R = H, COCH₃, COC₂H₅

Anaplasmosis

It has not been established whether the Anaplasma species be classed among protozoa or rickettsia (32). They parasitize the red blood cells of cattle and can cause heavy mortality. Tetracyclines have been found effective by both oral and parenteral administration. Certain dithiosemicarbazones, eg, gloxazone (13), are effective. Its synthesis was accomplished by heating a mixture of crotonaldehyde and ethanol under reflux in the presence of selenium dioxide. The ketoaldehyde obtained was converted to the bisthiosemicarbazone (33). The carbanilide derivative, Imidocarb (14), was found effective (34). It has a very narrow safety margin and anticholinesterase activity in the host, and it can cause adverse neuromuscular and cardiovascular effects.

Babesiasis

Members of the genus *Babesia,* of the order *Haemosporidia,* are transmitted by ticks and parasitize the red blood cells of mammals and birds (3,32). Mortality rates can be higher than 10% in cattle depending on the *Babesia* subspecies. Rare cases of human infection have also been reported (35).

Diamidine and related compounds have proven to be effective in the treatment

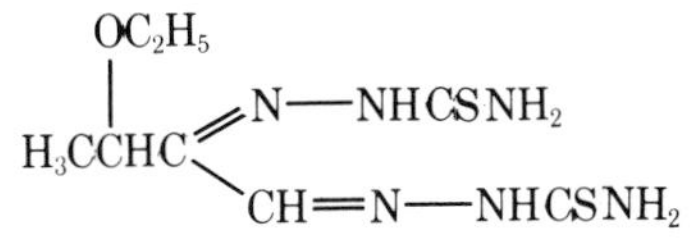

(13) 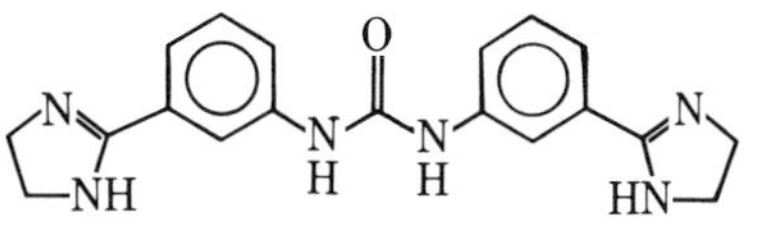   (14)

of babesiasis, eg, (15), (16), and (17).

Pentamidine (15) may be prepared by saturating an anhydrous, alcoholic solution of 1,5-di(4'-cyanophenoxy)pentane with dry hydrogen chloride, and treating the iminoether obtained from the hydrochloride with ammonium β-hydroxyethanesulfonate (36). Amicarbalide (16) is prepared as (15) by the Pinner reaction of the corresponding dinitrile (37). Diminazene aceturate (17), Berenil, is formed via a seven-step synthesis proceeding from 4-toluenesulfonamide through the 4-nitrobenzonitrile, the imidate, amidine and 4-aminobenzamidine with diazotization to the product (38).

Quaternary compounds of the quinuronium class are effective but have a narrow safety range. They are toxic to the parasympathetic nervous system and are potent cholinesterase inhibitors (see Choline; Cholinesterase inhibitors).

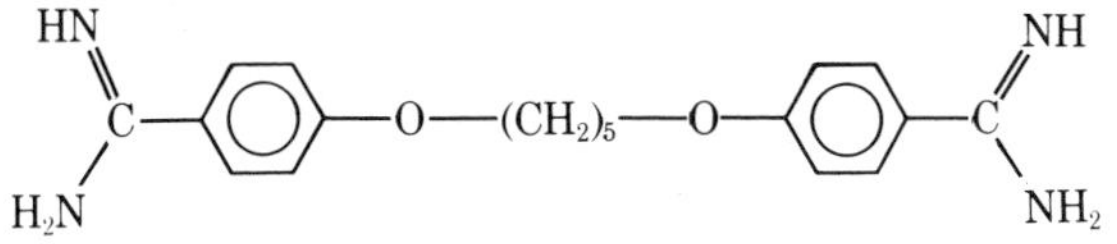

(15)

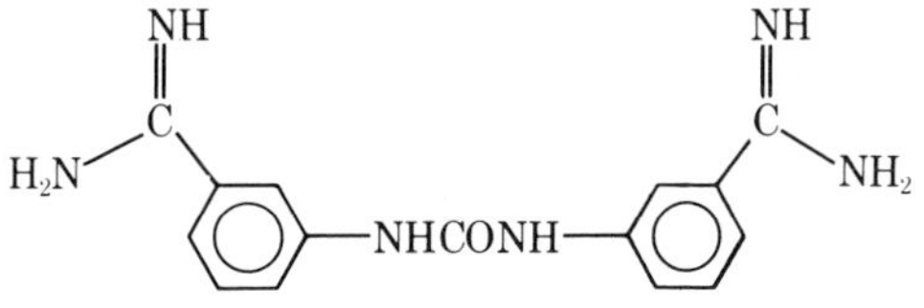

(16)

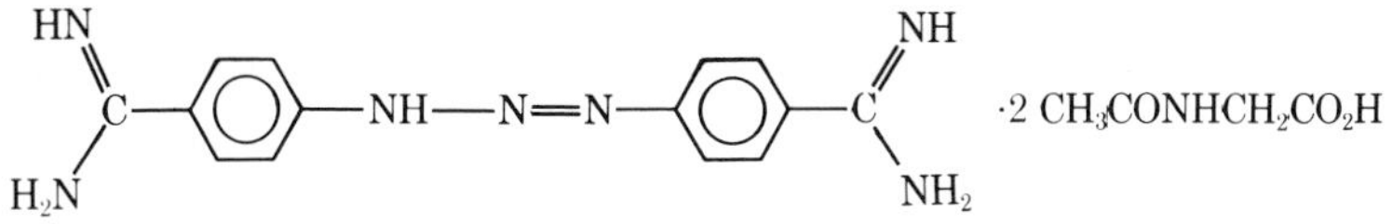

(17)

Theileriasis

Theileria species are transmitted by ticks to cattle and other ungulates (39). Various developmental stages of the parasite are in lymphocytes, histiocytes, and finally erythrocytes. In east and south Africa the species *T. parva* causes considerable damage to herds of farm animals with mortality reaching 90%. Attempts at chemotherapy with almost all known antiparasitic drugs have failed. However, good chemoprophylaxis is obtained when tetracyclines are administered during the period of incubation. This reduces the severity of infection and allows development of immune defenses which keep the infection under clinical control. Another species, *T. annulata*, has a wide geographic distribution. The natural recovery rates from this infection are higher than from *T. parva*. A large number of uncontrolled studies with a variety of drug combinations has been reported.

Trypanosomiasis

Species of *Trypanosoma brucei* cause a variety of diseases, many with serious economic consequences, in wild and domestic animals and in man in tropical and subtropical areas (4,40). *T. cruzi* species cause Chagas' disease which is prevalent in Central and South America.

The trypanosomes are transmitted by insect vectors. They have distinct developmental cycles in the host and in most vectors and the epidemiologic control is difficult since certain wild and domestic animals are disease reservoirs. The available drugs are quite toxic and frequently inadequate for some of the diseases (40c). Retrospective studies *in vitro* showed interference with several enzyme systems or with DNA metabolism of the trypanosomes, or both, although the actual basis for their clinical efficacy has not been established (41).

African Trypanosomiasis.   The African trypanosomes of the brucei type are dreaded scourges for man and animals (42). In man, *T. br. Gambiense* and *T. br. rhodesiense* cause the African sleeping sickness, and various *T. brucei* types cause damage to livestock in endemic areas. Unless treated successfully, the African trypanosomiases are invariably fatal in man. In the mammalian host the trypanosomes progress from blood to lymphatic tissues and, finally, to the central nervous system. Chemotherapy early in the infection is more promising than at the later stages. The available drugs have a narrow safety margin and side effects of some can be fatal. Drug resistance develops readily in African trypanosomiasis (43).

So far two drugs, suramin sodium (**18**) and pentamidine (**15**), have been found promising for safe chemoprophylaxis.

Suramin sodium is prepared by condensing 1-naphthylamine-4,6,8-trisulfonic acid with 3-nitro-4-methylbenzoyl chloride, reducing the product, condensing with 3-nitrobenzoyl chloride, reducing the product, condensing with 3-nitrobenzoyl chloride and reducing again. The product is treated with phosgene and the mixture neutralized with sodium hydroxide (44).

These drugs are firmly bound to tissue proteins from which they are released at a slow rate. Among the hemoflagellates they are effective prophylactics only for African

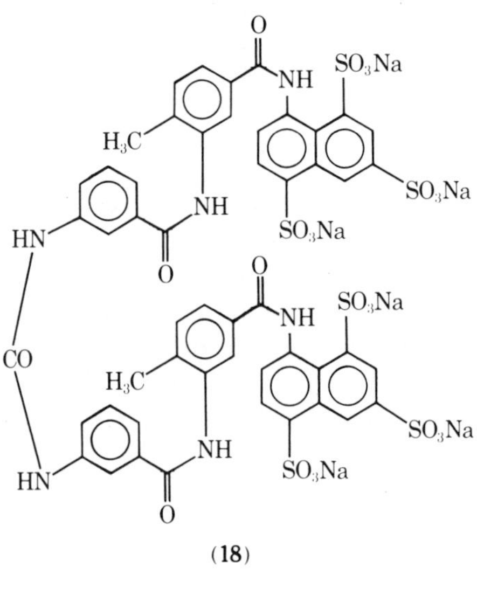

(**18**)

trypanosomiasis. The prophylactic efficacy of (15) exceeds that of (18). It appears to give protection against *T. br. gambiense* for ca 6 mo but its protective efficacy against *T. br. rhodesiense* is not generally accepted. Suramin (18) and pentamidine (15) are quite toxic. Pentamidine in particular is nephrotoxic. Furthermore (18) is teratogenetic in mice and causes abortions in rats (45). Medical field workers have not reported such effects in humans, but the reliability of reporting and patient follow-up in the concerned geographic areas remain to be evaluated. Thus the risk–benefit ratio must be weighed carefully for these drugs.

Pentamidine and suramin are useful in the early stages of African sleeping sickness but they fail to penetrate the blood–brain barrier. At the advanced stages, where parasites have invaded the central nervous system, drugs that can penetrate the blood–brain barrier are used. They are organic arsenicals such as tryparsamide (19), and derivatives of Melarsen oxide (20) such as melarsoprol (21) and melarsonyl potassium (see Arsenic compounds).

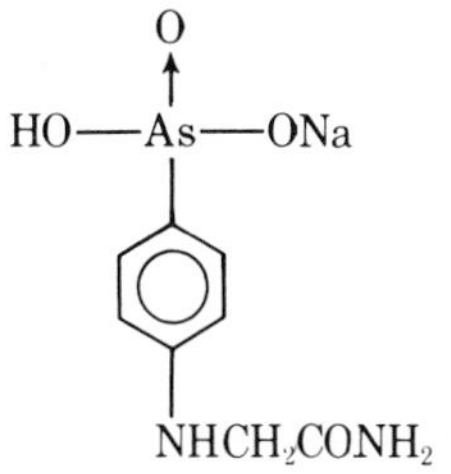

(19)

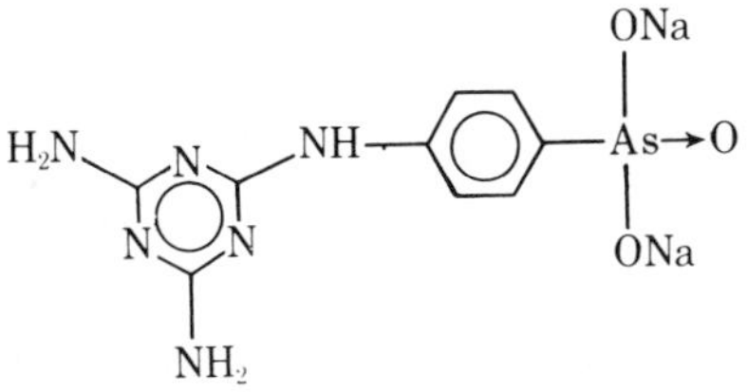

(20)

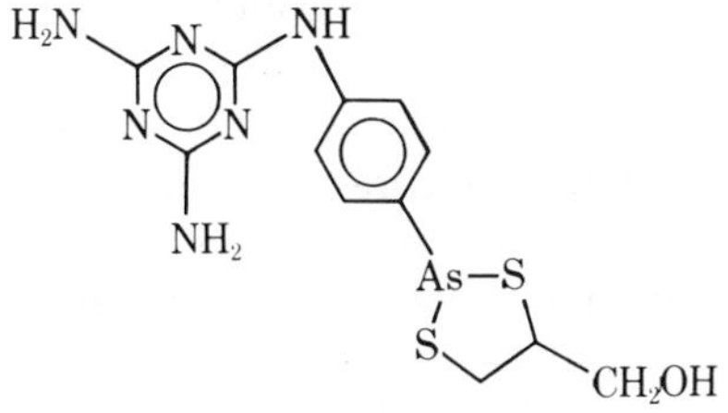

(21)

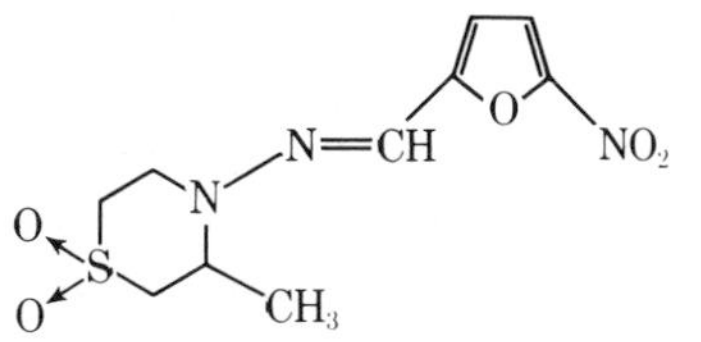

(22)

Tryparsamide (19) is formed by heating a solution of arsanilic acid in aqueous sodium hydroxide, sodium carbonate, and chloracetamide (46). Melarsen (20) may be obtained by the reaction of sodium arsanilate and cyanuric chloride to obtain *p*-(2,4-dichloro-*s*-triazinyl-6)aminophenylarsonic acid. This acid is treated with ammonia under pressure and the sodium salt of the resulting diamine is Melarsen (47). Melarsoprol (21) is prepared from 1-hydroxypropane-2,3-dithiol, *p*-aminophenylarsenic dioxide, and 2-chloro-4,6-diamino-1,3,5-triazine (48). Melarsonyl potassium is a water soluble derivative of melarsoprol.

Other useful drugs in the early stage are the aromatic diamidine, Berenil, which is, however, too toxic for humans; the nitrofuran, nifurtimox (22) (see Antibacterial agents, nitrofurans); the phenanthridines such as homidium bromide (23); quinapyramine (24); and some of their derivatives and antimonials such as ethylstibamine (25) (see Antimony compounds).

Nifurtimox (Lampit) is manufactured by the reaction of 5-nitrofurfural and 4-amino-3-methyltetrahydro-1,4-thiazine-1,1-dioxide (49).

Homidium bromide may be obtained by the reaction of 2,7-bis(carbethoxyam-

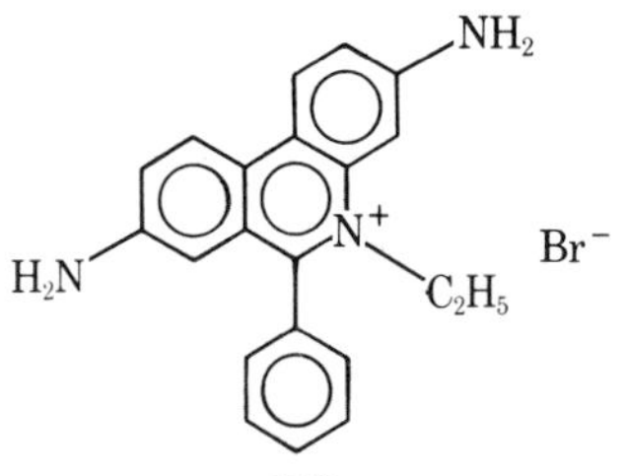

(23)

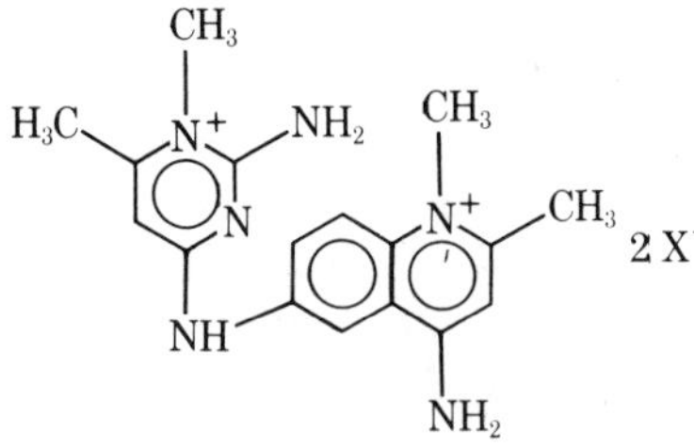

(24)

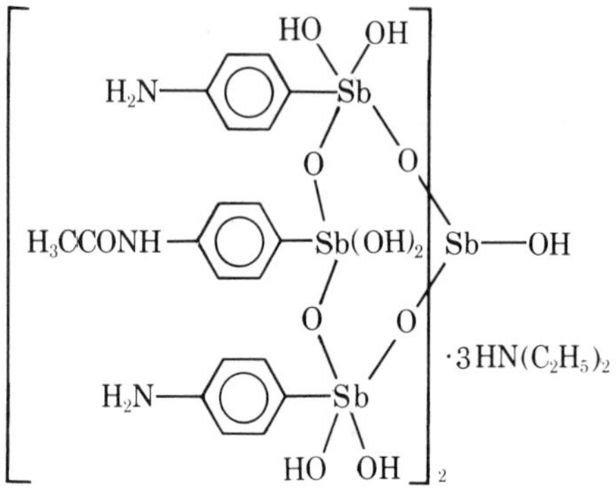

(25)

ino)-9-phenylphenanthridine and the sulfonic acid ester of ethanol. The resulting quaternary salt is hydrolyzed with sulfuric acid, the pH adjusted to 7–7.5 and ammonium bromide added to precipitate the crude quaternary bromide (50). The synthesis of quinapyramine is described in a United States patent (51). Ethylstibamine (Stibosamine, Neostibosan) is a complex of p-aminobenzenestibonic acid (present largely as a tetramer), p-acetylaminobenzenestibonic acid (present largely as a dimer), antimonic acid, and diethylamine in the approximate molar ratio of 1:2:1:3. The manufacture requires special care since the compound is both a colloid and a molecular addition compound, and slight variations greatly affect its toxicity (52).

Structure-activity relationships have been studied under laboratory conditions for the nitroheterocycles (26) (R′ = H [30579-13-6]; R″ = R‴ = H [55330-02-4]) (53).

Similar studies were made on nitrothiazoles (27) (54).

Chagas' Disease. The chemotherapeutic armamentarium against *T. cruzi* is very unsatisfactory (55). This situation has been practically unchanged for many years (56). A large number of compounds, which had been promising when tested on infected laboratory mice, proved inadequate in man. Either they were too toxic or they failed to remove the amastigotes from the tissues. Studies are now under way on 8-aminoquinolines. The nitrofuran (22) gave good results in some but not all clinical trials. Its practicality is questionable since treatment of 120 d is required and side effects can be severe.

A nitroimidazole, Ro-7-1051 (28), showed encouraging results in acute clinical cases but has not been adequately studied in chronic infections. As with other nitro compounds there is concern whether it has mutagenic and carcinogenic potentials. It is prepared by the reaction of the sodium derivative of 2-nitroimidazole with methyl chloroacetate and treatment of the resulting ester with benzylamine (57).

Great circumspection is recommended in appraising reports on the efficacy of

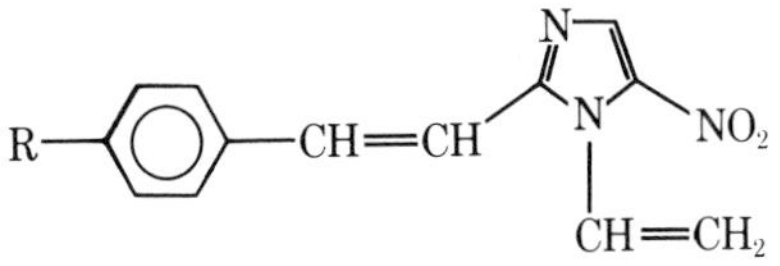

(26) R = CH$_2$R′, C NHR″ NR‴

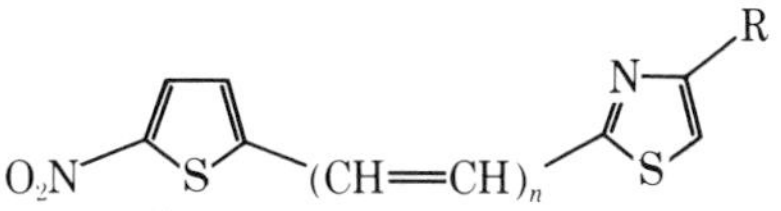

(27)

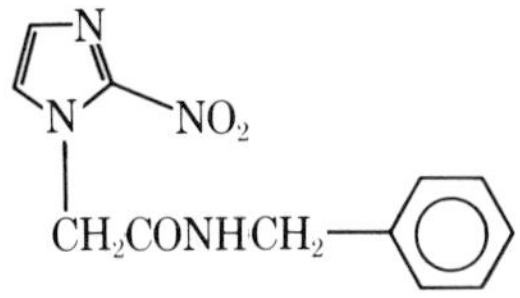

(28)

drugs in Chagas' disease. *T. cruzi* is not a single taxon but a collective term comprising regional varieties of physiologically distinct organisms (58). Hence differences in the clinical course and drug response may occur in different geographic areas.

Leishmaniasis

Members of the genus *Leishmania* have a broad geographic distribution (4,40). They are transmitted by insect vectors, and wild and domestic animals are disease reservoirs. They cause a variety of important diseases in man. *L. donovani, L. tropica,* and *L. brasiliensis* cause visceral cutaneous, and mucocutaneous leishmaniases, respectively. Some species cause chronic progressive diseases, others cause self-limiting conditions. The leishmania amastigote stage presents a particularly serious problem. The parasites invade the reticulo-endothelial system and their amastigotes penetrate and survive in the host's macrophages, thus reducing the host's immune defense capabilities. This sheltered location also interferes with direct drug contact and few drugs, if any, are selective against leishmania. One of the oldest antileishmanials is tartar emetic [*28300-74-5*], antimony potassium tartrate, which is highly toxic.

A number of less toxic, organic antimonials have been developed. These are linear polymers containing pentavalent antimony. Examples are sodium antimonyl gluconate, Pentostam (29), which is prepared from antimony pentoxide, gluconic acid and sodium hydroxide (59); the antimonate of *N*-methylglucamine, Glucantime (30) (60); and ethylstibamine (25). Various investigators differ in their opinions of the efficacy and toxicity of any of these drugs.

Other compounds reportedly effective are amphotericin B [*1397-89-3*] and pentamidine isethionate (15). They may cause severe adverse effects such as thrombophlebitis, abscesses at the respective injection sites, and nephrotoxicity. Hydroxystilbamidine isethionate (31) is also effective. It is prepared via a five-step synthesis starting with 4-methyl-2-nitrobenzonitrile and 4-cyanobenzaldehyde. The subsequent steps involve reduction of the nitro group of 2-nitro-4,4′-dicyanostilbene and diazotization to obtain 2-hydroxy-4,4′-dicyanostilbene. This product is converted to the amidine (31) (61).

Some 8-aminoquinolines seemed promising in tests on the golden hamster but are too toxic for human use. Cycloguanil embonate (32), which may cause necrosis at the injection site, was also reported effective, as were salts of Berberine (33). Cyclo-

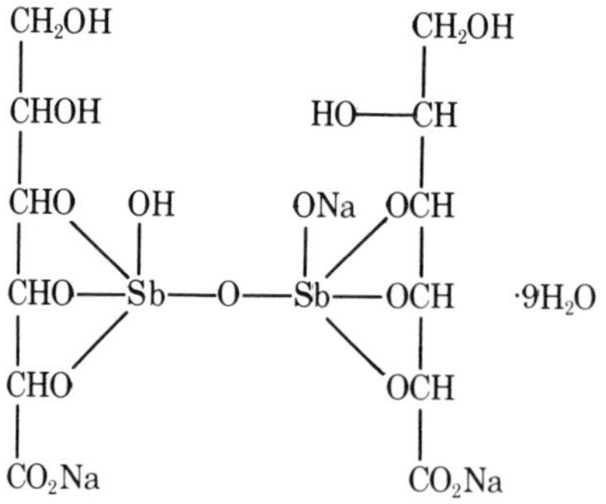

The structures (29), (30), (31), (32), and (33) are chemical diagrams.

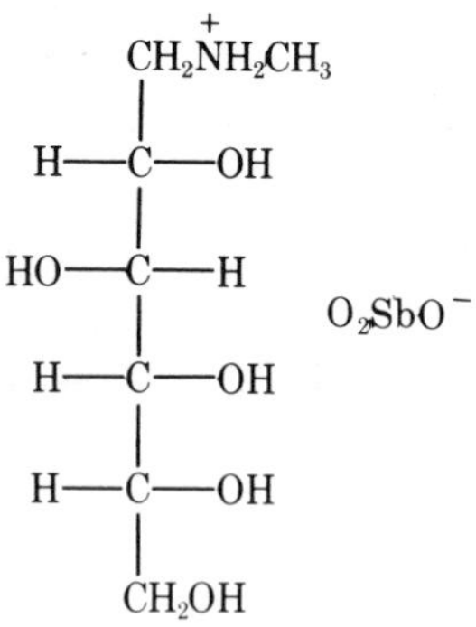

$$
\begin{array}{ccc}
CH_2OH & CH_2OH & \overset{+}{CH_2NH_2CH_3} \\
| & | & | \\
CHOH & HO{-}CH & H{-}C{-}OH \\
| & | & | \\
CHO \quad OH & ONa \ OCH & HO{-}C{-}H \qquad O_2SbO^- \\
| \quad \diagdown \diagup & | \quad | & | \\
CHO{-}Sb{-}O{-}Sb{-}OCH \quad \cdot 9H_2O & H{-}C{-}OH \\
| \quad \diagup & | & | \\
CHO & OCH & H{-}C{-}OH \\
| & | & | \\
CO_2Na & CO_2Na & CH_2OH \\
(29) & & (30)
\end{array}
$$

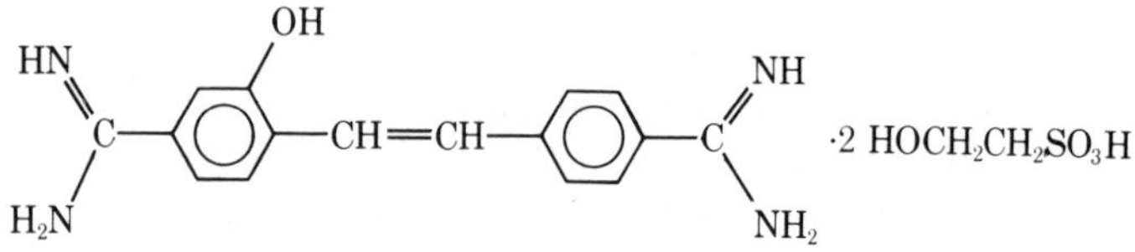

(31)

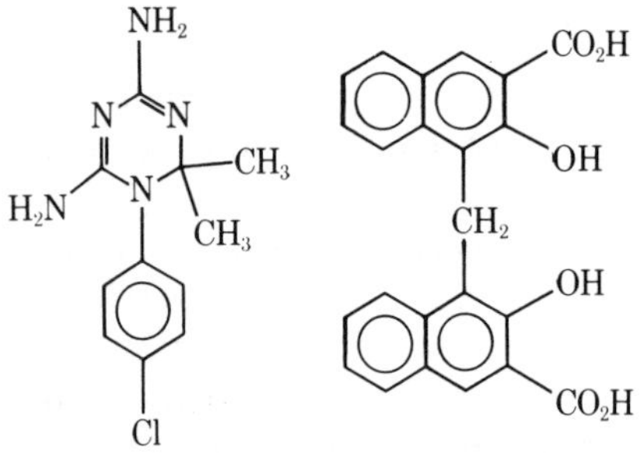

(32)

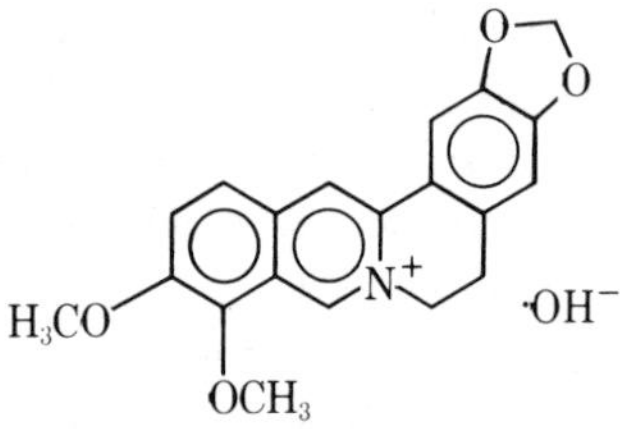

(33)

guanil hydrochloride is produced by condensation of *p*-chloraniline, dicyandiamide, and concentrated hydrochloric acid in acetone. The embonate salt is made from the hydrochloride (62). Berberine is an alkaloid isolated from *Hydrastis canadensis* L., *Berberedaceae*. The total synthesis of berberine iodide was achieved through a very involved route starting with 3,4-methylenedioxyphenethylamine (63) (see Alkaloids).

Leishmania amastigotes can be maintained in tissue culture cells. This system is suitable for rapid and inexpensive mass screening of drugs (64). However, encouraging findings of *in vitro* laboratory methods are not always predictive for the drug effects under clinical conditions.

Pneumocystosis

The infective agent that causes this condition is *Pneumocystis carinii* (65–66). Although this organism has features of both fungi and protozoa, it is treated here as a protozoon (67–68). *P. carinii* is cosmopolitan among man and other vertebrates (69). It has not been established whether the organisms detected in man and various vertebrates are identical. Epidemiologic observations suggest that the parasite is present but clinically silent in most individuals and is transmitted directly. It is an opportunistic pathogen that proliferates and becomes clinically manifest only in individuals whose immune defenses are impaired, eg, cancer patients who have immunosuppressive medications or infants whose immunodefenses are not yet fully developed and are further weakened by malnutrition. Pneumocystosis manifests itself by a particular pneumonitis which, if untreated, has a high mortality. The laboratory drug-testing system uses immunodepressed rats (70). An *in vitro* culture method for *P. carinii* has been recently developed (71). The available drugs are parenteral pentamidine (15) and the oral antifolate combination of a pyrimidine with a sulfonamide such as in Fansidar [37338-39-9] (72) and Bactrim [8064-90-2] (73). They have similar levels of curative efficiency. In the groups of high risk subjects chemoprophylaxis would be important. Fansidar and Bactrim have been reported as being useful for this purpose (72,74). In contrast, (15) as a prophylactic would be risky because of its high incidence of nephrotoxicity and tissue injury at the injection site.

Trichomoniasis

A variety of trichomonad infections occur in vertebrate hosts (2). They are extracellular, flagellated parasites transmitted by direct contact and reside in the superficial layers of the infected organs. *Trichomonad* species that are supposedly innocuous have been found in various cavities of their hosts. But some species are important pathogens of the genitals. In humans, *Trichomonas vaginalis* may cause significant disease in both sexes. The severity of the clinical manifestations may depend on strain differences of the parasite. Symptomless carriers do occur. Various nitroimidazoles are effective against *Trichomonad* species (75), eg, metronidazole (34) and tinidazole (35).

Metronidazole is prepared by heating 2-methyl-5-nitroimidazole with excess 2-chloroethanol to obtain the crude product which is purified by extraction with chloroform and recrystallization from ethyl acetate (76). Tinidazole was obtained by heating a mixture of $4\text{-}CH_3C_6H_4SO_3CH_2CH_2SO_2C_2H_5$ and 2-methyl-5-nitroimidazole under nitrogen at 145–150°C for 4 h (77). The mutagenic and carcinogenic potentials present problems in nitro group-containing drugs. Assay systems for *T. vaginalis* include *in vitro* culture and inoculation of mice.

T. foetus is another important species. It causes abortion in cattle. It is self-limiting in females. Despite the economic importance of the infection there is so far no satisfactory chemotherapy. Nitroimidazoles were used but resistant strains were a problem (75). Bulls can be treated by topical application of trypaflavine (36) and surfen (37) on the penis, a procedure difficult to apply. A species of economic relevance is *T. equi* which can invade the digestive tract and be fatal to horses. No specific chemotherapy is known.

Trypaflavine, acriflavine hydrochloride, is a mixture of 3,6-diamino-10-methylacridinium chloride hydrochloride and 3,6-diaminoacridine dihydrochloride. The 3,6-diaminoacridine is prepared by the condensation of *m*-phenylenediamine and formic acid (78). The synthesis of surfen is described in a German patent (79).

The species *T. gallinae* parasitizes a variety of birds and is of economic significance in domestic fowl. It is transmitted either by drinking water or by direct contact. It invades the upper digestive tract. The virulence of the infection varies with the strain of the protozoon and can be fatal. Enheptin, 2-amino-5-nitrothiazole (38), is therapeutically effective. It is synthesized by deacetylation of 2-acetamido-5-nitrothiazole (80). Screening tests for drugs against *T. gallinae* include culture methods.

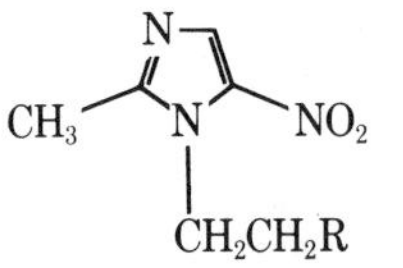

(**34**) R = OH
(**35**) R = SO$_2$C$_2$H$_5$

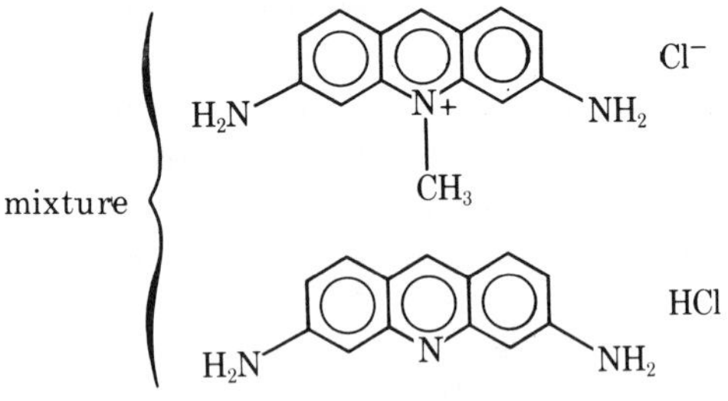

mixture

(**36**)

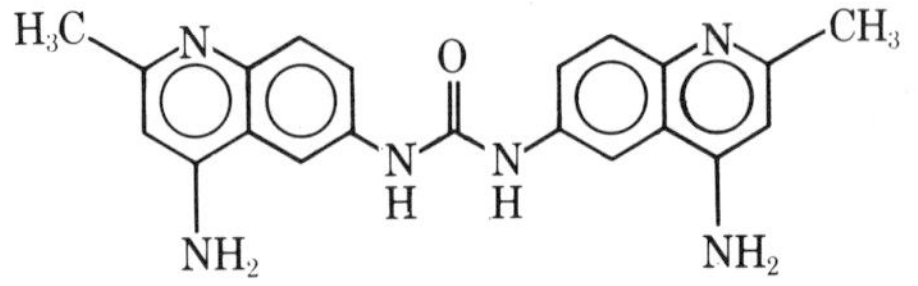

(**37**)

Hexamitosis

The agent of this condition is the flagellate *Hexamita meleagridis* (2,4). It is transmitted by contaminated food and has been reported in Great Britain and the Americas. The parasite lives in the duodenum and small intestines of birds. It is of economic importance in that it may cause up to 80% mortality in young birds. No effective drug is known against this parasite.

Balantidial Dysentery

The agent of this condition, *Balantidium coli,* occurs in man, primates, and several other vertebrates (2,4). It is cosmopolitan and transmitted by contaminated food and beverages. In man the cysts of *B. coli* pass through the small intestines and the trophozoites are found in the large intestines. There they form deep ulcers and can be carried into the mesenteric lymphatic glands. Effective drugs are metronidazole (**34**), tetracycline, and paromomycin (**39**).

(**38**)

Paromomycin is an oligosaccharide antibiotic that was isolated from various *Streptomyces*. It is prepared by a fermentation process and isolated from the broth by resin exchange (81) (see Antibiotics, aminoglycosides).

Giardiasis

The agent of this condition is the flagellate *Giardia lamblia* (82). This parasite lives on the epithelial lining of the human duodenum and jejunum and can cause a variety of digestive disturbances, including malabsorption, though symptom-free carriers are common. The parasite is cosmopolitan and is transmitted by contaminated food and beverages. Drug screening methods include inoculation of mice (83). An *in vitro* culture method has been developed but has not yet been used extensively for

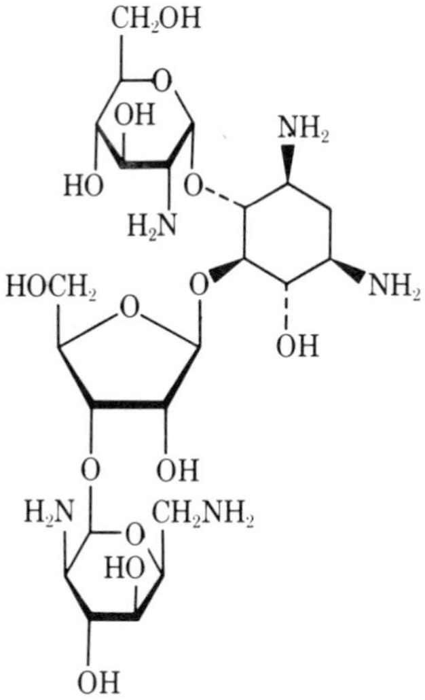

(39)

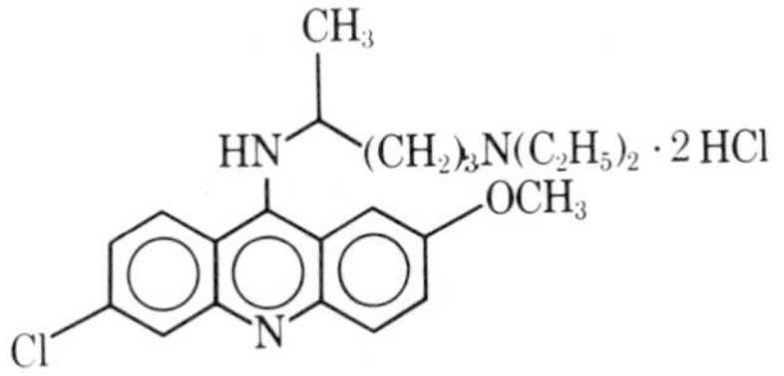

(40)

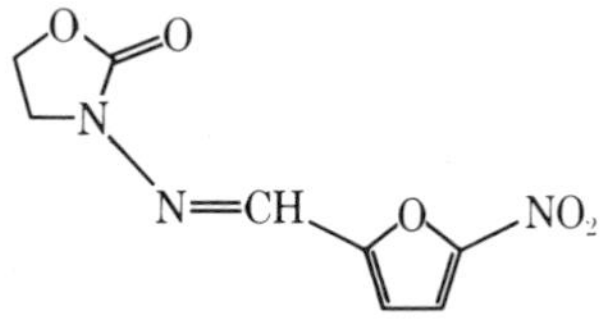

(41)

drug screening (84). There is no specific chemotherapeutic agent for *G. lamblia*. Several antimalarials such as quinacrine (40) are effective, as are the antiamebic drugs metronidazole (34), tinidazole (35), and furazolidone (41).

Quinacrine is obtained by the condensation of 1-diethylamino-4-aminopentane with 3,9-dichloro-7-methoxyacridine (85). The synthesis of furazolidone is accomplished by the reaction of 2-benzylideneamino-2-oxazolidinone and 5-nitro-2-furaldehyde (86).

Amebiases

The agents of these conditions are amebae. They are cosmopolitan and transmitted by ingestion of contaminated material.

Intestinal Amebiasis. The common pathogenic species, *Entamoeba histolytica*, occurs in many vertebrate hosts. It causes amebic dysentery in man although symptomless carriers of the parasite occur. Man becomes infected by ingesting the amebic cysts that descend in the intestinal tract. Amebic trophozoites then develop and reside in the caecum, colon, and sigmoid. They can produce the next generation of infective cysts which are eliminated with the feces. When the trophozoites invade the intestinal wall they cause ulcerations and clinical intestinal symptoms of varying severity. Metastatic amebic lesions may develop in various organs, particularly the liver.

For screening antiamebic drugs, both axenic culture methods and laboratory animals are suitable (87–88). Amebicides have been developed empirically. The nitroimidazoles, metronidazole (34), tinidazole (35), and the more toxic nitro heterocycle niridazole [61-57-4], are effective amebicides at all sites. Parenteral emetine (**42**) and dehydroemetine (**43**) are not effective against cysts, but are effective against amebiasis in the bowel wall and liver.

Emetine (**42**) is the principal alkaloid of ipecac, the ground roots of *Uragoga ipecacuanha* (see Alkaloids). Its total synthesis has been described (89) and a stereospecific synthesis of dehydroemetine has been published (90). Chloroquine (**44**) has been reported effective against liver amebiasis. But amebic abscesses of, eg, liver or brain require surgical treatment in addition to specific chemotherapy. Paromomycin (**39**) which is nonabsorbable from the bowel (41); iodoquinoline analogues, eg, iodochlorhydroxyquin (**45**) (now in disrepute because of toxicity); and various oral arsenical and bismuth preparations such as carbarsone (**46**), Milibis (**47**), and emetine-bismuth iodide [8001-15-8] are effective in the lumen of the bowel against either tropnozoites or cysts, or both.

Chloroquine is prepared by the condensation of 4,7-dichloroquinoline with 1-diethylamino-4-aminopentane (91). The synthesis of (**45**), Entero-Vioform, is accomplished by treating an aqueous solution of an alkali salt of 5-chloro-8-hydroxyquinoline with potassium iodide and a hypochlorite (92). Carbarsone (**46**) is obtained by reaction of the sodium salt of arsanilic acid with potassium cyanate or cyanogen bromide (93), and glycobiarsol is isolated from the reaction of bismuth nitrate and sodium *N*-glycoloylarsanilate (94).

Mebinol (**48**) and diloxanide furoate (**49**) have been reported to be effective against cysts (95).

Among methods of preparing chlorophenoxamide (Mebinol), is the reaction of 4-(4′-nitrophenoxy)benzaldehyde with 2-aminoethanol, reduction of the resulting Schiff base and acetylation of the amine with dichloroacetyl chloride (96). Diloxanide 2-furoic acid ester is prepared from 4-hydroxy-*N*-methylaniline and dichloroacetyl chloride followed by esterification with 2-furoic acid (97).

The antibiotics Fumagillin [23110-15-8] (see Chemotherapeutics, antimitotic)

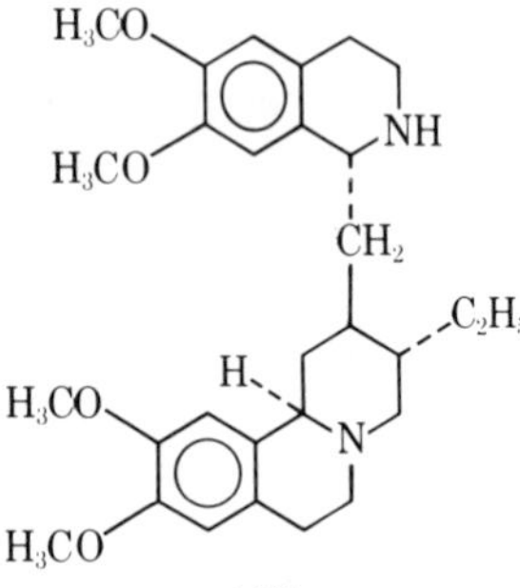

(**42**) 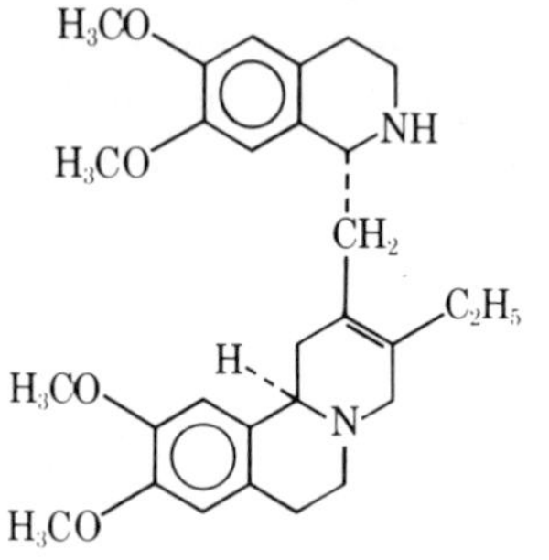   (**43**) 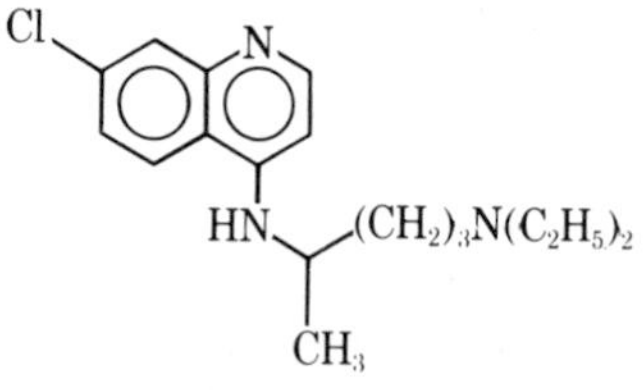   (**44**)

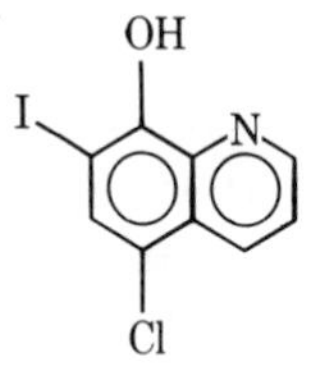

(**45**) 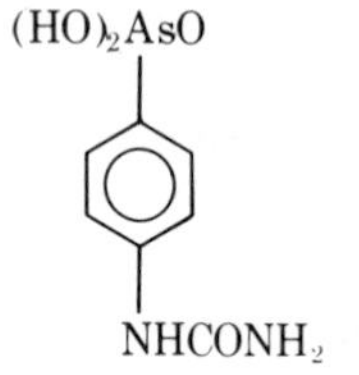   (**46**) 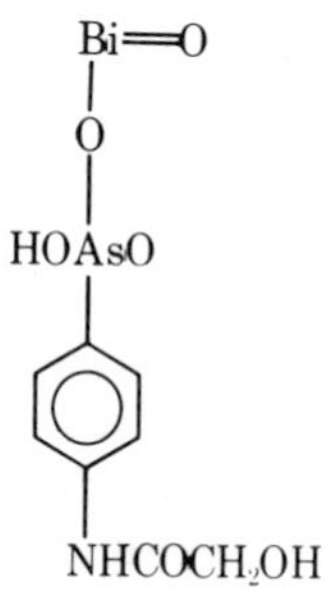   (**47**)

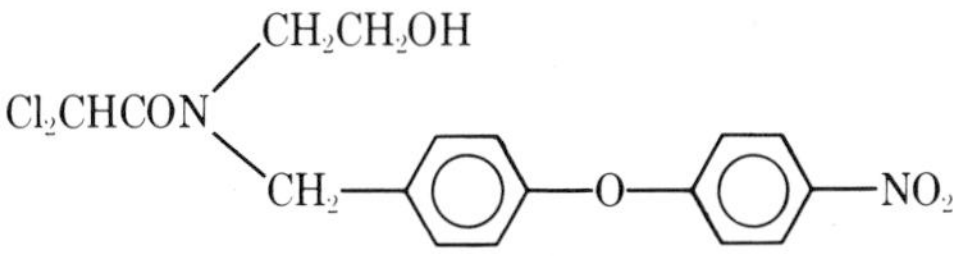

(48) 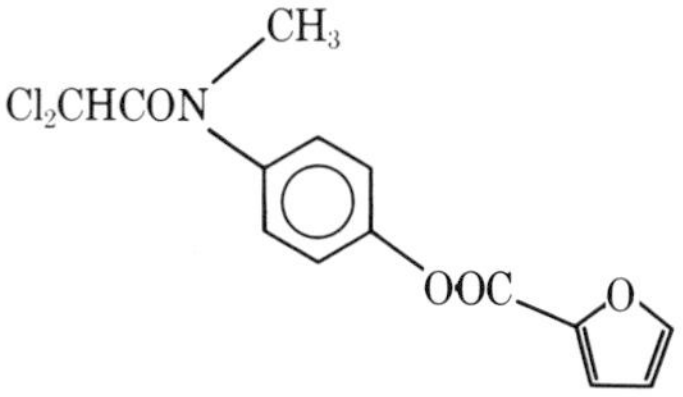   (49)

and tetracyclines (see Antibiotics, tetracyclines) have been reported in conjunction with antiamebic treatment. They act on bacterial associations of the amebic lesions and thus may be adjuvants to antiamebic therapy.

Primary Amebic Meningo-Encephalitis.   This condition is caused by amebae of the genera *Naegleria* and *Hartmanella*. The parasites occur in contaminated mud of ponds and puddles. The incidence of the infection in man is rare, but the disease is invariably fatal. No chemotherapy is available. *Naegleria* can be cultivated *in vitro* (98).

The Malarias

The agents of these infections are intracellular parasites of the genus *Plasmodium* (4,99). They infect a wide variety of vertebrate hosts and are specific for either a host species or a taxonomically narrow category of hosts. Medically and economically important are *P. falciparum, P. vivax, P. ovale,* and *P. malariae*, which cause in man the historically termed malignant, benign, oval tertian, and quartan malaria, respectively. The normal transmission of these plasmodia between host individuals occurs through mosquito vectors. When feeding on an individual with malaria, the mosquito ingurgitates blood containing male and female gametocytes of the plasmodium. In the mosquito they undergo a developmental cycle yielding the infective sporozoites which the mosquito then transmits to a new host. A suitably warm environment is needed for the development of the sporozoites in the mosquito and, thereby, for the endemic prevalence of malaria. In man the malaria parasite develops through sequential stages. Sporozoites find their way into parenchyma cells of the liver where they develop the primary tissue form, the exoerythrocytic, pre-erythrocytic schizonts. Within the schizonts nuclear divisions yield a large number of nucleated parasites. These are eventually released from the limiting membranes as individual merozoites. In *P. falciparum* infection the merozoites get into the blood circulation and penetrate the red cells. In some of the red cells the merozoites develop into the sexual stage, a single gametocyte per red cell, thus closing the chain of the plasmodium life cycle. However, in other red cells the merozoites start asexual blood forms. Erythrocytic schizonts develop, within which nuclear division produces new generations of merozoites. These finally break out and infect new red cells. This erythrocytic circuit of the developmental cycle of *P. falciparum* is repeated at intervals and causes the clinical manifestations of the disease. If adequate host defenses develop, they can stop this cycle. In contrast, *P. vivax* and *P. ovale,* which cause relapsing malaria, have a somewhat more complicated development. While some of the exoerythrocytic schizonts in liver cells release merozoites within a few days (as do those of *P. falciparum*), others remain dormant for extended time periods. When these release their merozoites, clinical relapses can occur even after years of latency. As to *P. malariae* infection, clinically inactive parasitemia may become clinically activated even after years.

Antimalarial drugs, given at their usual dosages, can affect one or more developmental stages of plasmodia species. Only those of clinical relevance to man are considered and they are classified here according to their target stages although some of them act on more than one stage.

Drugs Acting on Asexual Blood Forms.   Drug categories acting primarily on the asexual blood forms of susceptible strains of plasmodia include quinine salts, eg, quinine monohydrochloride (**50**); acridines, eg, (**40**); biguanides, chlorguanide (**51**), dihydrotriazines, eg, cycloguanil (**32**); pyrimidines, eg, pyrimethamine (**52**); sulfones and sulfonamides, eg, dapsone (**53**) (see Antibacterial agents, sulfonamides); antibiotics, eg, tetracycline, clindamycin (**54**) (see Antibiotics, lincosaminides); and 4-aminoquinolines, such as chloroquine (**44**), amodiaquin (**55**); and the promising experimental drugs from the current United States Army antimalarial drug development program, mefloquine HCl (**56**) and WR 030,090HCl (**57**), both quinolinemethanols, and WR 033,063HCl (**58**), a phenanthrenemethanol (**100**). Clindamycin (**54**) is disreputed since it has caused cases of colitis, with some of them being fatal.

Quinine monohydrochloride (**50**) is a salt of one of the cinchona bark alkaloids. The base is obtained by extraction. Synthesis was achieved by two different routes (**101**). However, the natural product is preferred because it is less expensive. Chlorguanide (**51**) is the product of the reaction of 4-chlorophenyldicyandiamine and isopropylamine (**102**). Pyrimethamine (**52**) is prepared by the reaction of guanidine nitrate with 3-isobutoxy-2-(4-chlorophenyl)pent-2-enonitrile in ethanol in the presence of sodium ethoxide (**103**). Dapsone (**53**) is obtained by reaction of 4-acetamidobenzenesulfinic acid sodium salt with 4-chloronitrobenzene followed by reduction with stannous chloride in concentrated hydrochloric acid (**104**). Clindamycin (**54**) is manufactured by modification of lincomycin (**105**), which is produced by *Streptomyces lincolnensis* var. *lincolnensis*, and is prepared by a fermentation process (see Antibiotics, lincosaminides). The pH of the broth is adjusted and the product is isolated by extraction with butanol (**106**). Amodiaquin (**55**) is prepared from 4,7-dichloroquinoline and 4-acetamido-6-diethylamino-*o*-cresol (**107**). One route to the quinolinemethanols related to (**58**) utilizes the appropriate cinchophen and involves the reactions of diazomethylation of the acid chloride to the diazomethyl ketone, hydrobromination, aluminum isopropoxide reduction and condensation with the appropriate amine to obtain the amino alcohol (**108**). The phenanthrenemethanol may be made by this scheme or by a variation as in the original preparation (**109**). The latter involves the bromomethyl ketone as the common intermediate that reacts with diheptylamine, followed by reduction of the aminomethyl ketone. An improvement, devoid of diazomethane usage and suitable for scale-up, is described in a United States patent (**110**). Applicable to a wide variety of acids, the process gives the bromomethyl ketone by way of the acid chloride, the acylmalonate, acylbromomalonate, and the unstable acylbromomalonic acid which undergoes double decarboxylation. Mefloquine (**56**) is prepared by the condensation of the 2,8-bis(trifluoromethyl)-4-quinolinecarboxylic acid ester with 2-pyridyllithium and reduction of the pyridyl quinolyl ketone (**111**).

The drugs that affect the asexual blood form alone can eradicate susceptible strains of *P. falciparum* and can be curative in these infections. However, they can only suppress the relapsing type of infections since they do not affect their exoerythrocytic tissue forms.

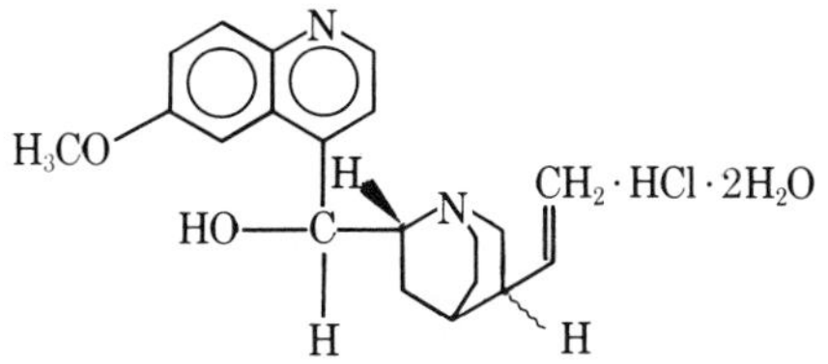

(**50**)

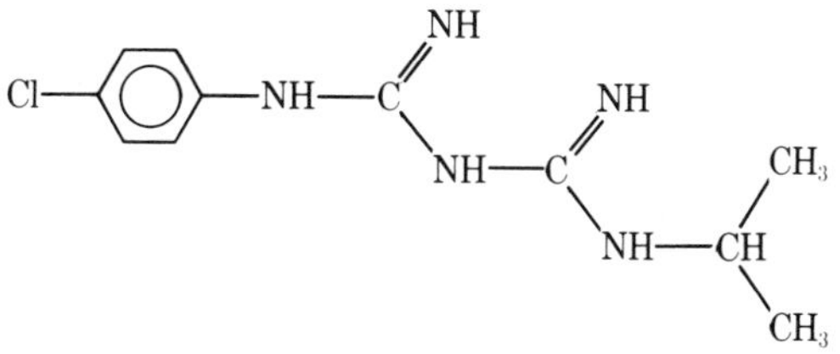

(**51**)

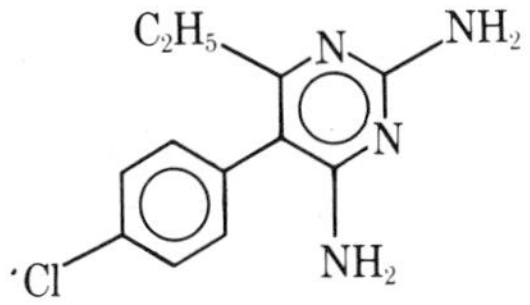

(**52**)

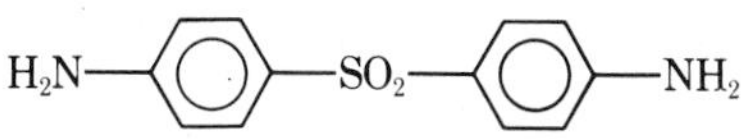

(**53**)

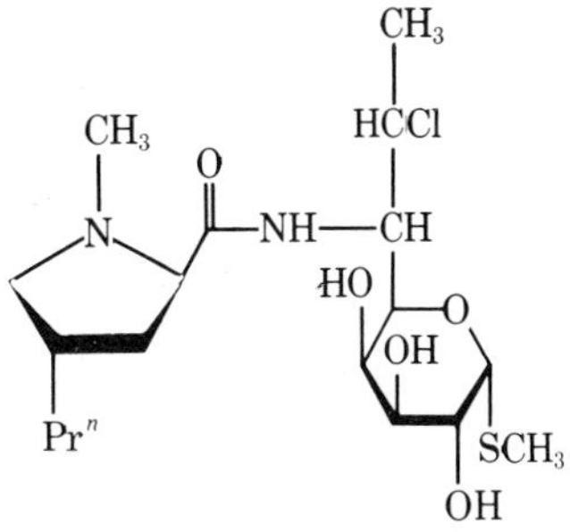

(**54**)

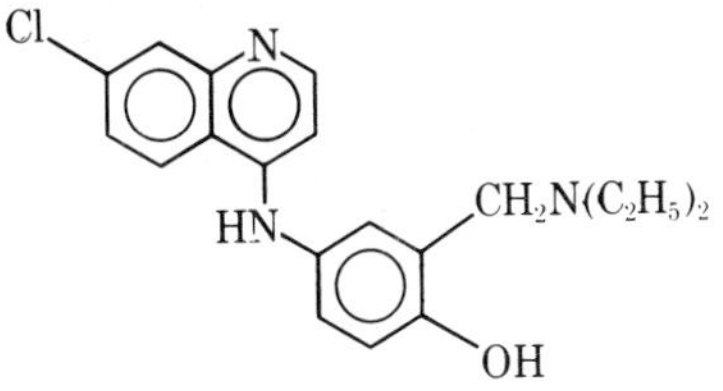

(**55**)

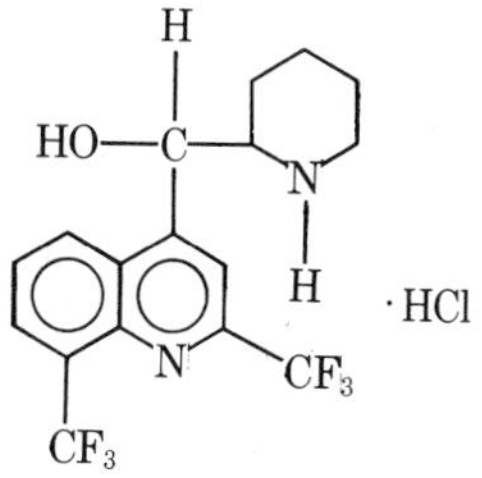

(**56**)

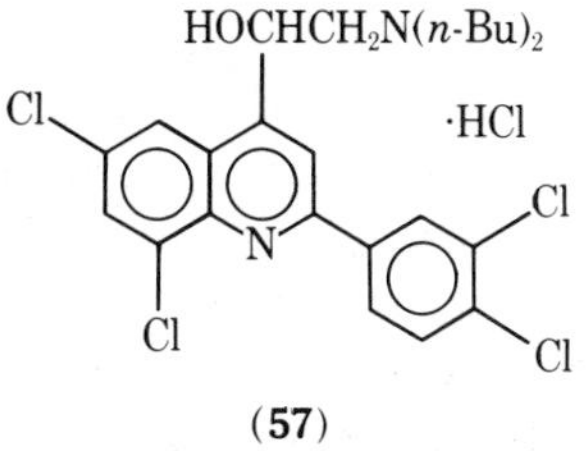

(**57**)

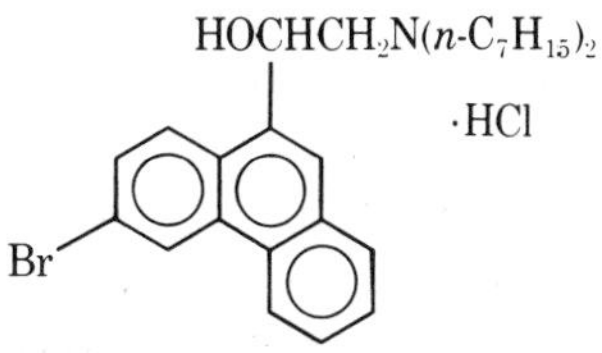

(**58**)

Drugs Affecting Tissue Forms.   Drugs affecting the tissue forms are 8-aminoquinolines, eg, pamaquine (**59**) and primaquine (**60**). Their efficiency is enhanced when given in combination with 4-aminoquinolines. Pamaquine (**59**), plasmoquine, is obtained by reductive condensation of 5-diethylamino-2-pentanone with 6-methoxy-8-aminoquinoline (112). The synthesis of primaquine involves the condensation of 6-methoxy-8-aminoquinoline with 2-bromo-5-(phthalimido)pentane (113).

Drugs Acting on Gametocytes.   Quinacrine (**40**) and 4-aminoquinolines affect the gametocytes of *P. vivax* and *P. malariae* only, chlorguanide (**51**) and 8-aminoquinolines affect those of *P. vivax* and *P. falciparum*.

An important aspect of antimalarial drugs is their use in chemoprophylaxis. Drugs that suppress the merozoites and the asexual blood forms of the plasmodia are commonly used to prevent clinical patency and permit time for immunodefenses to de-

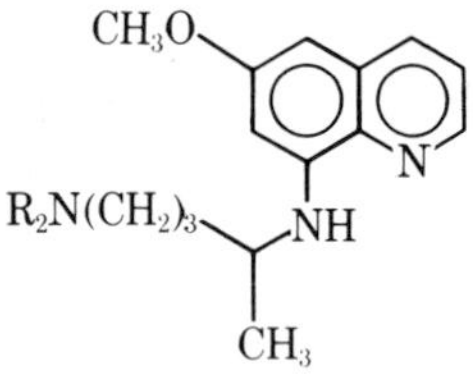

$$CH_3O$$

$$R_2N(CH_2)_3 \quad NH$$

$$CH_3$$

(**59**) R = C_2H_5
(**60**) R = H

velop. Their dose and frequency of administration are far below those used in the treatment of clinical attacks. However, as they are often used for extended periods the only practical ones are those whose chronic administration is least likely to cause adverse effects. Endemic prophylaxis is also obtained with the drugs that antagonize the sexual forms of the plasmodia. An interesting but undeveloped approach would be long-acting drugs against sporozoites (see Pharmaceuticals, sustained-release).

Resistance of plasmodium strains against given drugs poses a serious problem. It appears regionally, can be unique or cross between drugs of apparently different chemical categories, and the proportion of resistant to susceptible strains varies geographically. Owing to these variables, the antimalarial of choice will vary between geographic areas and may change with time in any given area. Certain drugs such as chlorguanide (**51**), pyrimethamine (**52**), and sulfonamides cause higher incidences of resistance than do quinine (**50**), pamaquine (**59**), or quinacrine (**40**). Drug combinations and sequentials seem to reduce the resistance problem (114).

The oldest antimalarial, quinine (**50**), is a herbal product discovered by serendipitous methods. Most of the other antimalarials were developed empirically by screening methods. Information is available on some of their biochemical effects but their mode of therapeutic action is not known. The only categories whose mode of therapeutic actions are well defined are the antifolates and the antibiotics, both spinoffs of antibacterial drug research. In developing antimalarial drugs the initial tests are often done in rodents and birds that are infected with their specific plasmodium species. Information obtained from such tests is often not applicable to human plasmodia. The owl monkey, *Aotus trivirgatus*, is susceptible to *P. falciparum* and *P. vivax,* and the squirrel monkey, *Saimiri sciureus,* to *P. vivax* infection; they are good models for the final drug testing. *In vitro* culture methods, for both plasmodium sporozoites and asexual blood forms, are under development (115–118).

Action Spectra of Antiprotozoal Drugs

Some of the antiprotozoal drugs are effective against more than one protozoal species or nonprotozoal conditions, in fact, some of these drugs, eg, antimetabolites and antibiotics, have been developed primarily against other classes of infective agents and, also, were later found active against protozoa. Within its action spectrum, the efficacy of a drug can vary greatly between classes, species, and strains of the infective agent. Table 1 gives an overview of the action spectra.

Table 1. Clinical Action Spectra of Antiprotozoal Drugs

Class	Group	Drugs	Protozoal infections	Nonprotozoal conditions
Antibiotics		amphotericin B	leish	fung
		clindamycin	mal	bact
		fumagillin	ameb	
		monensin	cocci	
		paromomycin	ameb, giard	bact, helminth
		spiramycin	toxo	bact
		tetracyclines	mal, cocci, ameb, anapl, theileriasis, balant	bact, trachoma, fung, mycoplasma
Antimetabolites	sulfonamides	various congeners	mal, toxo, cocci, pneumocyst	bact, trachoma, fung, lymphogranuloma venerum, dermatitis herpetiforme
	sulfones	dapsone	mal, cocci	bact, leprosy, dermatitis herpetiforme
	pyrimidines	pyrimethamine	mal, cocci, leish, pneumocyst,[b] toxo	bact[b]
		trimethoprim	mal,[b] cocci, leish, pneumocyst[b]	bact[b]
		amprolium, thiamine analogue	cocci	
	biguanide	chlorguanide	mal	
	triazine	cycloguanil	mal, leish	
	guanide	robenidine	cocci	
	thioguanide	bitipazone	cocci	
	PABA analogue	ethopabate	cocci	
Organometallics	As	tryparsamid	Afr tryp	
		melarsoprol (Mel B)	Afr tryp	
		melarsen	Afr tryp	
		carbarsone	ameb, trich, balant	
	Bi	bismuth subgallate	ameb	
		emetine Bi iodide	ameb	
	As + Bi	glycobiarsol	ameb, trich	
	Sb, trivalent	tartar emetic	Afr tryp, leish	filariasis, schistosomiasis, granuloma inguinale, mycosis fungoides,
	Sb, pentavalent	pentostam	leish	
		glucantime	leish, Kala azar	helminth
		neostibosan	leish	helminth, granuloma inguinale

415

Table 1.   (*continued*)

Class	Group	Drugs	Conditions of drug use[a]	
			Protozoal infections	Nonprotozoal conditions
Benzamidines		hydroxystilbam-idine	Afr tryp	fung
		pentamidine	Afr tryp, pneumocyst, bab, leish	
		berenil	Afr tryp, anapl, bab	bact
Anilides	ureas	imidocarb	anapl, bab	
		suramin	Afr tryp	onchocerciasis
	amidine	amicarbalide	bab	
	benzamidine	diloxanide furoate	ameb, giard	
		berenil	Afr tryp, anapl, bab	bact
Halogenated hydrocarbons		clopidol	cocci	
		robenidine	cocci	
	phenanthryls	homidium bromide	Afr tryp, bab	
		WR 033,063	mal	
	quinoline derivatives	mefloquine	mal	
		WR 030,090	mal	
		diiodo–oxy-quinoline	ameb, trich, balant	
	dithiosemi-carbazone	contrapar	anapl	
Quinoline derivatives	alkaloid	quinine	mal	parturition, muscle cramps
	4-aminoquino-lines	chloroquine	mal, ameb, giard, bab	helminth, autoimmune conditions
		amodiaquine	mal, giard	leprosy, autoimmune cond
		quinapyramine	Afr tryp	
	8-aminoquino-lines	pamaquine	mal	
		primaquine	mal	
	ureas	quinuronium sulfate	bab	
		surfen	trich fetus	
	quinazoline	febrifugine	mal, cocci	
	hydroxyquinoline	buquinolate	cocci	
	quinolone	nequinate	cocci	
	halogenated derivatives	mefloquine	mal	
		WR 030,090	mal	
		diiodo–oxy-quinoline	ameb, trich, balant	
	acridinyls	quinacrine	mal, giard	helminth, radiosensitizer
		trypaflavin	trich fetus	bact
Nitro compounds	furans	nitrofurazone	cocci, Afr tryp	bact
		furazolidone	ameb, giard, trich, cocci	bact (incl cholera), fung

416

Table 1. (*continued*)

Class	Group	Drugs	Conditions of drug use[a] Protozoal infections	Nonprotozoal conditions
		nifurtimox	Chagas disease	
	imidazoles	metronidazole	trich, giard, ameb, balant	bact, ulcerative gingivitis radiosensitizer
		tinidazole	trich, giard, ameb	
		RO 7-1051	Chagas disease, leish	
	thiazoles	Enheptin	trich (fowl), histomonas	
		niridazole	ameb	schistosomiasis
	hydrocarbon	Mebinol	ameb	
Alkaloids		emetine	ameb	helminth
		berberine salts	leish	

[a] Abbreviations within the table are: Afr tryp = African trypanosomiasis, African sleeping sickness; ameb = amebiasis; anapl = anaplasmosis; bab = babesiasis; bact = bacterial infections; balant = balantidiasis; cocci = coccidiosis; fung = fungal (mycotic) infections; giard = giardiasis; helminth = helminthiasis; leish = leishmaniasis; mal = malaria; pneumocyst = pneumocystosis; toxo = toxoplasmosis; trich = trichomoniasis.

[b] In these conditions, combination drugs of a pyrimidine with a sulfonamide, eg, Fansidar or Bactrim, are more effective than the single ingredients.

Economic Considerations

References 2, 3, 4, and 7 show the broad geographic distribution of protozoal endemic areas. The *Animal Health Yearbook* gives the annual incidence of protozoal diseases of animals and of those common to animals and man (121). It does not specify, for restricted localities, the density of the incidence and the clinical severity of the diseases. This information may be found after some delay in specialized periodicals (122). The *World Epidemiology Review* gives a monthly report on public health events, some of which are retrospective (123).

For estimating market possibilities of antiprotozoal drugs, the figures of overt disease cases are not the only guide. Equally important are the unknown numbers of individuals with latent nonapparent infections, individuals in endemic areas who take chemoprophylaxis, and individuals who are exposed to infection but take no precautions. As examples, the global incidence of malaria cases in 1974 was estimated to be ca 120 million whereas about 25% of the world population lived in endemic areas (124–125). The global incidence for Chagas' disease was estimated in 1977 at about 8 million cases (125), but for Argentina alone, in 1972, the number of infected individuals was estimated at 2.3 million whereas 12 million people, or about 50% of the nation's population, lived in endemic areas (126). There is a considerable need for new drugs in this market (56). The biggest potential market for antiprotozoal drugs is the developing countries of the tropical and subtropical regions. In many cases, however, reported disease figures are unreliable. The greatest drug needs in the developed countries are for coccidiosis in animal husbandry. However, the use of single anticoccidials can fluctuate widely and rapidly owing to the spreading of drug-resistant protozoal strains and the use of drug combinations (8).

Table 2. Selected Generic and Trade Names with Sources of Antiprotozoal Drugs

WHO proposed name, generic	CAS Registry no.	Structure no.	Trade name	Sources
acriflavine	[8063-24-9]	(36)	Euflavin	Bayer; Imperial Chemical
			Gonacrine	Ind.
			Panflavin	Specia
			Trypaflavine	Hoechst
amicarbalide	[3459-96-9]	(16)	Diampron	May & Baker
aminoalkenyldisulfide	[31482-85-6]	(3)		
aminochinuridum	[3811-56-1]	(37)	Surfen	Hoechst
aminonitrothiazolum	[121-66-4]	(38)	Enheptin T	Lederle
			Nitramin	Ferrosan
amodiaquine	[86-42-0]	(55)	Camoquin Hydrochloride	Parke, Davis
			Flavoquine	Roussel
amprolium	[121-25-5]	(2)	Amprol	Merck
berberine	[2086-83-1]	(33)	Canadine	Merck
bitipazone	[13456-08-1]	(7)	Bitipazone	Burroughs Wellcome
buquinolate	[5486-03-3]	(10)	Bonaid	Eaton
carbarsone	[121-59-5]	(46)	Carbarsone	Lilly
chloroquine salts	[54-05-7]	(44)	Aralen	Sterling-Winthrop-Ross
			Avloclor	Imperial Chemical Ind.
			Nivaquine	Specia; May & Baker
			Resochin	Bayer
clefamide, chlorphenoxamide	[3576-64-5]	(48)	Mebinol	Erba
clindamycin	[18323-44-9]	(54)	Cleocin	Upjohn, USA;
			Sobelin	Upjohn, Germany
clioquinol, iodochlorhydroxyquin	[130-26-7]	(45)	Colicid	Chemedica
			Enteritan	Grossman
			Entero-Vioform	Ciba
clopidol	[2971-90-6]	(8)	Coyden	Dow
cycloguanil	[516-21-2]	(32)	Camolar	Parke, Davis; May &
decoquinate	[18507-89-6]			Baker; Hess and Clark
dehydroemetine	[4914-30-1]	(43)	Dametin	Merck
			Dehydroemetine	Roche
			Mebadine	Glaxo
diloxanide furoate	[579-38-4]	(49)	Furamide	Boots; Clin-Comar
diminazene aceturate	[908-54-3]	(17)	Berenil	Hoechst
diphenyl sulfone,	[80-08-0]	(53)	Alvosulfon	Ayerst; Imperial Chemical
			Dapsone	Ind.
emetine	[483-18-1]	(42)	Emetine	Lilly
ethopabate	[59-06-3]	(4)	Ester Amidobenzoate	Merck
febrifugine	[24159-07-7]	(11)	Febrifugine	Roussel
furazolidone	[67-45-8]	(41)	Enterotoxon	Bieff
			Furazon	Daiko
			Furoxone	Eaton; Norwich; Boehringer
gloxazone	[2507-91-7]	(13)	Contrapar	Burroughs Wellcome

Table 2. (*continued*)

WHO proposed name, generic	CAS Registry no.	Struc-ture no.	Trade name	Sources
glycobiarsol	[116-49-4]	(47)	Amoebicon	Consolidated Midland Corporation
			Broxolin	Breon
			Milibis	Sterling-Winthrop-Ross
homidium bromide	[1239-45-8]	(23)	Ethidium	Boots
hydroxystilb-amidine	[533-22-2]	(31)	Hydroxystilb-amide	May & Baker
imidocarb	[5318-76-3]	(14)	Imizol	Burroughs Wellcome
lincomycin	[154-21-2]		Cillimycin	Hoechst
			Lincocin	Upjohn
			Mycivin	Boots
mefloquine	[51773-92-3]	(56)	Mefloquine	U.S. Army Surgeon General
melarsen	[3599-28-8]	(20)	Melarsen	Hoffmann-La Roche
melarsoprol	[494-79-1]	(21)	Arsobal Mel B	Specia
mepacrine	[69-05-6]	(40)	Atabrine Hydrochloride	Sterling-Winthrop-Ross
			Atebrin	Bayer
			Quinacrine	Specia
			Tenicridine	Norgan
methylgluc-amine, anti-monate	[133-51-7]	(30)	Glucantime	Specia
metronidazole	[443-48-1]	(34)	Clont	Bayer
			Efloran	Kirka
			Elyzol	Dumex
			Flagyl	Specia; May & Baker; Searle
			Metronidal	Kisser
monensin	[17090-79-8]	(5)	Coban; Monelan	Lilly
nequinate	[13997-19-8]	(9)	Statyl	Imperial Chemical Ind.; Ayerst
nifurtimox	[23256-30-6]	(22)	Lampit	Bayer
pamaquine	[491-92-9]	(59)	Plasmochin	Bayer
			Praequine	May & Baker
paromomycin	[7542-37-2]	(39)	Humagel	Parke, Davis
			Pargonyl	Roussel
paromomycin sulfate	[1263-89-4]		Farmiglucina	Farmitalia
			Humatin	Parke, Davis
pentamidine	[140-64-7]	(15)	M&B 800	May & Baker
			Lomidine	Specia
primaquine	[90-34-6]	(60)	Primaquine	Bayer; Sterling-Winthrop-Ross; Imperial Chemical Ind.
proguanil	[500-92-5]	(51)	Chlorguanide	Abbott; Merck
			Guanatol	Lilly
			Paludrine	Ayerst; Imperial Chemical Ind.
pyrimeth-amine	[58-14-0]	(52)	Daraprim	Burroughs Wellcome
			Malocide	Specia
quina-	[20493-41-8]	(24)	Antrycid	Imperial Chemical Ind.

419

Table 2.   (continued)

WHO proposed name, generic	CAS Registry no.	Structure no.	Trade name	Sources
pyramine				
quinine	[130-89-2]	(50)	various quinine salts	Amsterdamsche Chininefabriek
Ro 5-9754	[8076-37-7]		Ormetotrim; Rofenaid	Roche
Ro 7-1051	[22994-85-0]	(28)		
robenidine	[25875-51-8]	(6)	Robenz	Merck
spiramycin	[8025-81-8]	(12)	Rovamycin	Specia; May & Baker
			Selectomycin	Chemie Grunenthal
			Calactin	Leo, Helsingborg
			Suanovil	Biokema, Switzerland
stiboglucon- ate sodium	[16037-91-5]	(29)	Pentostam	Burroughs Wellcome
			Solustibosan	Bayer
stibosamine, ethylstib- amine	[1338-98-3]	(25)	Neostibosan	Bayer
suramine	[129-46-4]	(18)	Antrypol	Bayer; Imperial Chemical Ind.; Sterling-Winthrop-Ross
			Bayer 205, Germanin	Bayer
			Moranyl	Specia
			Naphuride	Sterling-Winthrop-Ross
thiamine	[67-03-8]	(1)	Anevryl	Stella, Belgium
			Benerva	Roche
tinidazole	[19387-91-8]	(35)	Fasigyn, Simplotan	Pfizer
trypars- amide	[554-72-3]	(19)	Tryparsamide	Wallau
WR 030,090	[56162-51-7]	(57)	WR 030,090	U.S. Army Surgeon General
WR 033,063	[58523-33-4]	(58)	WR 033,063	U.S. Army Surgeon General

Sources of Antiprotozoal Drugs

For information on the current status of a drug, the supplier should be consulted. Reference 127 may be useful for locating generic names, trade names, chemical name, and the structural and empirical formula of a drug. The *Index Nominum* gives similar information plus references to monographs, and in many instances names of sources (128). For drugs and sources in the United States consult the *National Drug Code Directory* (129). Table 2 gives an abridged list of generic names, trade names, and sources of antiprotozoal drugs. The listing or omission of a trade name or a source is in no way a recommendation or the reverse.

Notice

The views of the authors in this article do not necessarily represent those of their institutions.

BIBLIOGRAPHY

"Therapeutic Agents, Protozoal Infections" in *ECT* 2nd ed., Vol. 20, pp. 70–99, by Edward F. Elslager, Medical Research and Scientific Affairs Div., Parke, Davis, & Company.

1. E. A. Steck, *Chemotherapy of Protozoon Diseases,* United States Government Printing Office, Washington, D.C., 1972.
2. N. D. Levine, *Protozoon Parasites of Domestic Animals and of Man,* Burgess Publishing Company, Minneapolis, Minn., 1973.
3. L. Hussel and co-workers, *Die Protozoaren Blutparasitosen der Haustiere in Warmen Landern,* S. Hirzel Verlag, Leipzig, GDR, 1966.
4. C. Wilcocks and P. E. C. Manson-Bahr, *Manson's Tropical Diseases,* The Williams and Wilkins Company, Baltimore, Md., 1972.
5. F. Hawking, *Exp. Chemother.* **1,** 1 (1963).
6. L. P. Pellerdy, *Coccidia and Coccidiosis,* Paul Parey Publishing Co., Berlin, 1974.
7. D. M. Hammond and P. L. Long, *The Coccidia,* University Park Press Publishing Co., Baltimore, Md., 1973.
8. J. F. Ryley and M. J. Betts, *Adv. Pharmacol. Chemother.* **11,** 221 (1973).
9. W. M. Reid, *Georgia Agri. Res.* **16,** 4 (1974).
10. J. H. Collins, *Ann. N.Y. Acad. Sci.* **52,** 515 (1949).
11. E. F. Rogers, *Ann. N.Y. Acad. Sci.* **98,** 412 (1962).
12. U.S. Pat. 3,020,277 (Feb. 6, 1962), E. F. Rogers and L. H. Sarett (to Merck and Co., Inc.).
13. Jpn. Pat. 70,34585 (Nov. 6, 1970), I. Uchimi, T. Watanabe, and K. Hayashi (to Tanabe Seiyaku Co., Ltd.).
14. D. A. Roe, *Drug-Induced Nutritional Deficiencies,* The Avi Publishing Company, Inc. Westport, Conn., 1976.
15. U.S. Pat. 3,211,610 (Oct. 12, 1965), E. F. Rogers and R. L. Clark (to Merck and Co., Inc.).
16. M. E. Haney, Jr. and M. M. Hoehn, *Antimicrob. Agents Chemother.* **349,** (1967); W. M. Stark, "Monensin a New Biologically Active Compound Produced by a Fermentation Process" in D. Perlman, ed., *Fermentation Advances,* Academic Press, Inc., New York, 1969, pp. 517–540.
17. D. T. Wong and co-workers, *Biochem. Pharmacol.* **20,** 3169 (1971).
18. D. G. Lindmark and M. Muller, *Antimicrob. Agents Chemother.* **10,** 476 (1976).
19. Ger. Pat. 1,933,112 (Jan. 8, 1970), A. S. Tomcufcik (to American Cyanamid Co.).
20. Fr. Pat. 2,024,194 (Oct. 2, 1970), A. J. S. Evans (to Farbwerke Hoechst A.G.).
21. Neth. Pat. 6,409,766 (Mar. 26, 1965), (to The Dow Chemical Co.).
22. Neth. Pat. 6,602,994 (Sept. 12, 1966), (to Imperial Chemical Industries Ltd.).
23. Belg. Pat. 659,237 (Aug, 3, 1965), E. J. Watson, Jr., (to Norwich Pharmacal Co.).
24. U.S. Pat. 2,651,632 (Sept. 8, 1953), B. R. Baker and M. V. Querry (to American Cyanamid Co.).
25. J. K. Frenkel, *Curr. Top. Pathol.* **54,** 27 (1971).
26. J. K. Frenkel, *Human Pathol.* **6,** 97 (1975).
27. S. R. M. Bushby and G. H. Hitchings, *Br. J. Pharmacol. Chemother.* **33,** 72 (1968).
28. D. E. Eyles, *Exp. Chemother.* **1,** 641 (1963).
29. A. Meyer, *Nouv. Press Med.* **3,** 1383 (1974).
30. J. de Vries and L. E. Francis, *J. Can. Dent. Assoc.* **41,** 101 (1975).
31. J. G. Williams, *J. R. Nav. Med. Serv.* **61,** 44 (1955).
32. L. P. Joyner and D. W. Brocklesby, *Adv. Pharmacol. Chemother.* **11,** 321 (1973).
33. B. D. Tiffany and co-workers, *J. Am. Chem. Soc.* **79,** 1682 (1957).
34. G. Schmidt, R. Hirt, and R. Fischer, *Res. Vet. Sci.* **10,** 530 (1969).
35. A. E. Anderson, P. B. Cassaday, and G. R. Healy, *Am. J. Clin. Pathol.* **62,** 612 (1974).
36. U.S. Pat. 2,410,796 (Nov. 5, 1946), G. Newbery and A. P. T. Easson (to May & Baker Ltd.).
37. J. N. Ashley, S. S. Berg, and J. M. S. Lucas, *Nature* **185,** 461 (1960); S. S. Berg, *J. Chem. Soc.,* 5097 (1961).
38. U.S. Pat. 2,838,485 (June 10, 1958), R. Brodersen, H. Loewe, and H. Ott (to Hoechst A.G.).
39. F. Hawking, *Exp. Chemother.* **1,** 625 (1963).
40. (a) B. A. Newton, *Trypanosomiasis and Leishmaniasis, Ciba Foundation Symposium,* Vol. 20, Associated Scientific Publishers, Amsterdam, 1974, p. 285; (b) E. A. Steck, *Prog. Drug Res.* **18,** 289 (1974); (c) L. G. Goodwin, *Trypanosomiasis and Leishmaniasis, Ciba Foundation Symposium,* Vol. 20, Associated Scientific Publishers, Amsterdam, 1974, p. 303.
41. WHO Technical Report Series No. 411, Geneva, Switz., 1969.

42. J. Williamson, *Trop. Dis. Bull.* **73,** 531 (1976).
43. W. Peters in ref. 40(a), p. 309.
44. E. Fourneau and co-workers, *Compt. Rend.* **178,** 675 (1924).
45. L. Mercier-Parot and H. Tuchmann-Duplessis, *C.R. Soc. Biol.,* **167,** 1518 (1973).
46. W. A. Jacobs and M. Heidelberger, *J. Am. Chem. Soc.* **41,** 1587 (1919); W. A. Jacobs and M. Heildeberger in R. Adams, ed., *Organic Synthesis,* Vol. 8, John Wiley & Sons, Inc., New York, 1928, p. 100.
47. E. A. H. Friedheim, *J. Am. Chem. Soc.* **66,** 1775 (1944).
48. U.S. Pat. 2,659,723 (Nov. 17, 1953), E. A. H. Friedheim.
49. Ger. Pat. 1,170,957 (May 27, 1964), H. Herlinger and co-workers (to Farbenfabriken Bayer A.G.).
50. T. I. Watkins, *J. Chem. Soc.,* 3059 (1952).
51. U.S. Pat. 2,585,917 (Feb. 19, 1952), F. H. S. Curd (to Imperial Chemical Industries, Ltd.).
52. U.S. Pat. 1,988,632 (Jan. 22, 1935), H. Schmidt (to Winthrop Chemical Company, Inc.).
53. W. J. Ross and W. B. Jamieson, *J. Med. Chem.* **18,** 430 (1975).
54. J. P. Verge and P. Roffey, *J. Med. Chem.* **18,** 794 (1975).
55. W. E. Gutteridge, *Trop. Dis. Bull.* **73,** 699 (1976).
56. WHO Technical Report Series No. 202, 1960, p. 14.
57. Brit. Pat. 1,138,529 (Jan. 1, 1969), (to Hoffmann-La Roche A.G.).
58. W. Peters in ref 40(a), p. 311.
59. S. Datta and T. N. Ghosh, *Sci. Cult.* **11,** 699 (1946).
60. P. Karrer, and E. Herkenrath, *Helv. Chem. Acta* **20,** 83 (1937).
61. U.S. Pat. 2,510,047 (May 30, 1950), A. J. Ewins (to May & Baker, Ltd.).
62. E. J. Modest and co-workers, *J. Am. Chem. Soc.* **74,** 855 (1952); U.S. Pat. 2,900,385 (Aug. 18, 1959), E. J. Modest (to Children's Cancer Research Foundation, Inc.).
63. T. Kametani and co-workers *J. Chem. Soc.,* 2036 (1969).
64. N. M. Mattock and W. Peters, *Am. Trop. Med. Parasitol.* **69,** 449 (1975).
65. J. Vanek and O. Jirovec, *Zentralbl. Bakteriol.* **158,** 120 (1952).
66. W. Dutz, *Pathol. Ann.* **5,** 309 (1970).
67. J. Vavra and K. Kucera, *J. Protozool.* **17,** 463 (1970).
68. W. C. Campbell, *Arch. Pathol.* **93,** 312, (1972).
69. F. G. Poelma, *Z. Parasitenk.* **46,** 61 (1975).
70. J. K. Frenkel, J. T. Good, and J. A. Shultz, *Lab. Invest.* **15,** 1559 (1966).
71. L. L. Pifer, W. T. Hughes, and M. J. Murphy, Jr., *Pediat. Res.* **11,** 305 (1977).
72. C. Post and co-workers, *Curr. Ther. Res. Clin. Exp.* **13,** 273 (1971).
73. W. T. Hughes, S. Feldman, and S. K. Sanyal, *Can. Med. Assoc. J.* **112,** 47S (1975).
74. W. T. Hughes and co-workers, *Pediat. Res.* **11,** (776) 501 (1977).
75. C. Rufer and co-workers, *Chim. Ther.* **8,** 567 (1973); D. K. McLoughlin, *J. Parasit.* **53,** 646 (1967).
76. U.S. Pat. 2,944,061 (July 5, 1960), R. M. Jacob, G. L. Regnier, and C. Crisan (to Société Usines Chimiques Rhone-Poulenc).
77. S. Afr. Pat. 66,07,466 (Apr. 25, 1968), K. Butler (to Chas. Pfizer and Co., Inc.).
78. A. Albert, *J. Chem. Soc.* **121,** 484 (1941).
79. Ger. Pat. 591,480 (Jan. 22, 1934), H. Jensch (to I. G. Farbenindustrie A.G.).
80. U.S. Pat. 2,573,641 (Oct. 30, 1951), H. L. Hubbard (to Monsanto Chemical Company); U.S. Pat. 2,573,656 (Oct. 30, 1951), G. W. Steahly (to Monsanto Chemical Company).
81. U.S. Pat. 2,916,485 (Dec. 8, 1959), R. P. Frohardt and co-workers (to Parke, Davis and Company).
82. M. S. Wolfe, *J. Am. Med. Assoc.* **233,** 1362 (1975).
83. C. Rufer, H. J. Kessler, and E. Schroder, *J. Med. Chem.* **18,** 253 (1975).
84. E. A. Meyer, *Exp. Parasitol.* **39,** 101 (1976).
85. U.S. Pat. 2,113,357 (Apr. 5, 1938), F. Mietzsch and H. Mauss (to Winthrop Chemical Company, Inc.).
86. U.S. Pat. 2,759,931 (Aug. 21, 1956) G. D. Drake, G. Gever, and K. J. Hayes (to The Norwich Pharmacal Company).
87. L. S. Diamond, *J. Parasitol.* **54,** 1047 (1968).
88. C. F. T. Mattern and T. B. Keister, *Am. J. Trop. Med. Hyg.* **26,** 393 (1977).
89. E. E. van Tamelen and co-workers, *J. Am. Chem. Soc.* **91,** 7359 (1969); C. Szantay and co-workers, *J. Org. Chem.* **31,** 1447 (1966).
90. D. E. Clark and co-workers, *J. Chem. Soc.,* 2479 (1962).
91. A. R. Surrey and H. F. Hammer, *J. Am. Chem. Soc.* **68,** 113 (1946).

92. U.S. Pat. 641,491 (Jan. 16, 1900), A. Bischler (to Basle Chemical Works).

93. R. W. E. Stickings, *J. Chem. Soc.*, 3131 (1928).

94. B. Reichert, ed., *Hagers Handbook Pharmacological Praxis*, Band I, Suppl. 2, Springer-Verlag, Berlin, 1958, p. 759.

95. G. Woolfe, *Progr. Drug Res.* **8,** 43 (1965).

96. U.S. Pat. 2,824,894 (Feb. 25, 1958), W. Lagemann and L. Almirante (to Carlo Erba).

97. Brit. Pat. 767,148 (Jan. 30, 1957), P. Oxley and co-workers (to Boots Pure Drug Co. Ltd.).

98. L. Cerva, V. Ziman, and K. Novak, *Science* **163,** 575 (1969); L. Cerva and K. Novak, *Science* **160,** 92 (1968).

99. P. E. Thompson and L. Werbel, *Antimalarial Agents and Chemistry and Pharmacology,* Academic Press, Inc., New York, 1972.

100. C. J. Canfield and co-workers, *Antimicrob. Agents Chemother.* **3,** 224 (1973); D. F. Clyde and co-workers, *Antimicrob. Agents Chemotherapy* **9,** 384 (1976).

101. J. Gutzwiller and M. R. Uskokovic, *Helv. Chim. Acta.* **56,** 1494 (1973).

102. F. H. S. Curd and F. L. Rose, *J. Chem. Soc.,* 729 (1946).

103. U.S. Pat. 2,576,939 (Dec. 4, 1951), G. H. Hitchings, P. B. Russell, and E. A. Falco (to Burroughs Wellcome & Co., Inc.).

104. C. W. Ferry, J. S. Buck, and R. Baltzly in L. F. Smith, ed., *Organic Synthesis,* Vol. 22, John Wiley & Sons, Inc., New York, 1942, p. 31.

105. B. J. Magerlein, R. D. Birkenmeyer, and F. Kagan, *Antimicrob. Agents Chemother.* 727 (1966); R. D. Birkenmeyer and F. Kagan, *J. Med. Chem.* **13,** 616 (1970).

106. U.S. Pat. 3,155,580 (Nov. 3, 1964), M. E. Borgy, R. R. Herr, and D. J. Mason (to the Upjohn Company).

107. J. H. Burckhalter and co-workers, *J. Am. Chem. Soc.* **70,** 1363 (1948).

108. R. E. Lutz and co-workers, *J. Am. Chem. Soc.* **68,** 1813 (1946).

109. E. L. May and E. Mosettig, *J. Org. Chem.* **11,** 627 (1946).

110. U.S. Pat. 3,714,168 (Jan. 30, 1973), R. E. Olsen (to United States of America as represented by the Secretary of the Army).

111. C. J. Ohnmacht, A. R. Patel, and R. E. Lutz, *J. Med. Chem.* **14,** 926 (1971).

112. R. C. Elderfield and co-workers, *J. Am. Chem. Soc.* **70,** 40 (1948).

113. R. C. Elderfield and co-workers, *J. Am. Chem. Soc.* **77,** 4816 (1955).

114. R. M. Pinder in A. Burger, ed., *Medicinal Chemistry,* 3rd ed., Vol. 1, Wiley-Interscience, New York, 1970, p. 515; *Chemotherapy of Malaria and Resistance to Antimalarials,* No. 529, WHO Technical Report Series, 1973.

115. H. R. Wolfensberger, *Far East Med. J.* **6,** 48 (1970); A. P. Hall and co-workers, *Br. Med. J.* **1,** 1626 (1977).

116. W. Traeger and J. B. Jensen, *Science* **193,** 673 (1976).

117. R. L. Beaudoin and co-workers, *Exp. Parasitol.* **39,** 438 (1976).

118. J. P. Haynes and co-workers, *Nature* **263,** 767 (1976).

119. M. Windholz, ed., *The Merck Index,* 9th ed., Merck & Co., Inc. Rahway, N. J., 1976.

120. L. S. Goodman and A. Gilman, *The Pharmacological Basis of Therapeutics,* 5th ed., Macmillan Publishing Co., New York, 1975; Martindale, *The Extra Pharmacopeia,* 27th ed., The Pharmaceutical Press, London, Eng., 1977; *United States Dispensatory,* 27th ed., J. B. Lippincott, Co., Philadelphia, Pa., 1973; P. B. Beeson and W. McDermott, *Textbook of Medicine,* 14th ed., W. B. Saunders Co., Philadelphia, Pa., 1975; G. T. Strickland, *Chemotherapy of Parasitic Diseases, CRC Handbook of Clinical Laboratory Science,* Sec. E, Vol. II, Chemical Rubber Company Press, Cleveland, Ohio, 1977.

121. *Animal Health Yearbook FAO-WHO-OIE,* Food and Agricultural Organization of the United Nations, Rome, Italy.

122. *Tropical Diseases Bulletin,* Bureau of Hygiene and Tropical Diseases, London, Eng., *Bulletin of the World Health Organization,* Geneva, Switz.

123. *World Epidemiology Review,* Joint Publications Research Service Publ., Arlington, Va.

124. A. W. A. Brown, J. Haworth, and A. R. Zahar, *J. Med. Entomol.* **13,** 1 (1976).

125. M. G. Schultz, *N. Engl. J. Med.* **297,** 1259 (1977).

126. P. Garaguso, *International Symposium on Chagas' Disease,* Secretario de Estado de Salud Publica, Buenos Aires, Argentina, 1972.

127. M. Negwer, *Organisch-Chemische Arzneimittel u. Ihre Synonyma,* Akademie-Verlag, Berlin, 1971.

128. *Index Nominum,* Société Suisse de Pharmacie, Zurich, Switz., 1975.
129. *National Drug Code Directory 1976,* Vol. 1 and 2, U.S. Department of Health, Education, and Welfare, Public Health Service, Food and Drug Administration, U.S. Government Printing Office, Washington, D.C.

General References

Guidelines: Manufacturing and Controls for IND's and NDA's, FDA Papers, June, 1971, FDA 72-3013, U.S. Government Printing Office, Washington, D.C., 1972-482-082/5.
The United States Pharmacopeia, 20th rev., U.S.P. Convention, Inc., 1975, pp. 707–709.
Remington's Pharmaceutical Sciences, 15th ed., 1975, pp. 1419–1428.
R. M. Bushby, *Exp. Chemother.* **1,** 25 (1963).
B. Basil, *Exp. Chemother.* **1,** 55 (1963).
J. W. Drake and co-workers, *Science* **187,** 503 (1975); R. P. Batzinger and co-workers, *Cancer Res.* **38,** 608 (1978).
J. M. Sontag and co-workers, *Guidelines for Carcinogen Bioassay in Small Rodents, Carcinogenesis Report Series,* No. 1, Nat. Cancer Inst., NCI-CG-TR-1., U.S. Dept. HEW,PHS, 1976.
I. M. Rollo, *Myler's Side Effects of Drugs,* Vol. 8, Excerpta Medica, Amsterdam, 1975, p. 659.

EDGAR J. MARTIN
HOWARD C. ZELL
Food and Drug Administration

BING T. POON
Walter Reed Army Institute of Research

ANTIVIRAL

The search for antiviral agents began at the time when antimicrobial substances were first shown to be effective as prophylactic and therapeutic agents in bacterial diseases (see Antibiotics, nucleosides). Many hundreds of compounds with antiviral activity have been synthesized or isolated from nature over the last three decades, but those available for clinical trials are few. Only three, idoxuridine, adenine arabinoside (ara-A), and amantadine, have been approved by the FDA for use but they are effective in only a few types of viral infections. Idoxuridine and adenine arabinoside are licensed for use only in topical ophthalmic preparations. These limited successes have stimulated the search for other antiviral substances and an increasing number with potential human use are in various stages of conceptual design, development, or evaluation.

The difficulty in designing and developing effective antiviral substances is caused largely by the very nature of viruses. Viruses are a diverse group of infectious agents that differ greatly in size, shape, chemical composition, host range, and effects on hosts. The uniqueness of viruses includes the following characteristics: (*1*) they consist of a genome which is either ribonucleic acid (RNA) or deoxyribonucleic acid (DNA); (*2*) the genome is surrounded by a protein shell (capsid) which protects the genome and provides receptors for recognition of susceptible cells (these capsids are constructed from repeating polypeptide subunits called protomers) (see Biopolymers); (3) viruses replicate only within cells and are entirely dependent upon the host cells' synthetic and energy-yielding apparatuses; (4) replication initially requires the separation of the genome from the capsid so that the genetic material can communicate with the cell; and (5) the parts of the virus replicate individually and then assemble into the finished product, thus they do not grow as do other living things. At times, virions (the name for the mature virus particle) contain an additional external structure referred to as an envelope or peplos. The envelope is derived partly from the cell membrane and contains host lipid with virus induced proteins and glycoproteins. In addition, many viruses contain enzymes that are indispensible in their replication.

Inhibitors of cellular processes will often prevent viral replication but are also toxic for the host. Most of the antiviral drugs that have been discovered cannot be prescribed because of toxicity. Thus the clinical usefulness of idoxuridine is limited to topical application in ophthalmic solution for treatment of herpetic keratitis.

However, many of the inhibitors have been useful in research laboratories and have served as powerful probes for studying the pathways of virus replication. As more is learned about these pathways, and unique processes for virus replication are discovered, it should be possible to design inhibitors that have specific effects upon virus-induced function, eg, RNA viruses either contain or induce a RNA-dependent RNA polymerase (replicase). This enzyme is unique to viruses since cells make their RNA from a DNA template using a DNA-dependent RNA polymerase (transcriptase). Since the viral enzyme is unique, it should be possible to find a chemotherapeutic agent which specifically inhibits its function. Another group of RNA viruses, the retroviruses, contain their own unique enzyme which is a RNA-dependent DNA polymerase (reverse-transcriptase) and should also be amenable to control by chemical substances. Indeed, some rifamycin derivatives inhibit reverse-transcriptase and prevent transformation of cells by retroviruses (1) (see Antibiotics, ansamacrolides).

Methods

Each step in virus replication should be amenable to control. The major systems for screening potential antiviral agents are the use of tissue or cell cultures, the chick embryo, and animals. Cell cultures are very convenient for screening compounds for antiviral activity since viruses readily grow in such cultures and usually demonstrate a cytopathic effect. Compounds are initially selected that prevent the cytopathic effect without inhibiting cell proliferation, and thus have a permissible chemotherapeutic index. The chemotherapeutic index of a compound can be defined as the ratio between the lowest effective antiviral concentration and the highest nontoxic concentration. The spectrum of activity of the compound against various classes of viruses can also be determined in a similar way.

The disease process in animals is much more complex than that in tissue culture and, for practical purposes, a compound should not be considered as a chemotherapeutic agent until efficacy in an animal has been measured. Furthermore, for various reasons, toxicity not apparent in cell cultures may be pronounced in the whole animal. Most animal studies and preliminary studies in humans, after FDA approval, are carried out with challenge infection. In these studies a virus inoculum is introduced into the test animal or human volunteer and the effect of the drug is compared with similarly infected but placebo-treated control groups. Once efficacy is established by such tests, the drug is then evaluated for the prevention or treatment of naturally occurring infections.

Areas of Application

Viral vaccines have been highly successful in controlling many of the more serious viral diseases such as smallpox, yellow fever, rabies, poliomyelitis, and measles. The dramatic success in controlling these diseases by vaccines can partly be attributed to the fact that they are caused by viruses that remain reasonably constant in their chemical composition. In other diseases, however, vaccines have not been as successful for various reasons and control by chemotherapy may be the method of choice. Two major reasons for the inability of vaccines to control some viral diseases are antigenic changes of the virus which occur in nature and the plethora of viral serotypes that may cause some diseases (see also Vaccine technology).

All viral surfaces contain specific antigens which induce the host to make specific antibodies to neutralize the infectivity of the virus. A single antibody molecule is usually sufficient to neutralize one virion; a very effective mechanism for the elimination of extracellular virus. Antibody production either occurs after natural infection or can be induced by vaccines consisting of inactivated or attenuated viruses. With specific antibody, the host will remain resistant to infection by the same virus unless the virus undergoes a change in antigenic structure (antigenic drift). Influenza A viruses undergo a continuous drift and for this reason vaccines have not been very effective. Major antigenic changes (antigenic shift) occur periodically, as in 1957 with the advent of the A2 Asian-type influenza and again in 1968 with the A2 Hong Kong influenza. The efficacy of antiviral compounds is not influenced by these antigenic changes since they do not usually react with the virus surface. Therefore, chemotherapy offers a method of coping with such diseases until a vaccine effective against the new variant is available.

Another difficulty in vaccine production is exemplified by the rhinoviruses which are a major cause of the common cold. These viruses, unlike the influenza viruses, are antigenically stable but over a hundred different antigenic types are known. Thus, to be effective, a vaccine against rhinovirus infection would have to contain each antigenic type and this is not very practical. Laboratory studies show that certain compounds can have activity against all rhinovirus strains. In this case, the use of such compounds would be the method of choice regardless of the strain causing the infection.

A third case for chemotherapy is use against a virus such as herpes simplex which causes disease even in the presence of circulating antibody. These diseases are not amenable to control with vaccines that only stimulate humoral antibody. Of course, cell-mediated immunity is important in some diseases and vaccines may be developed that stimulate this component of the immune system.

Antiviral chemotherapy and prophylaxis would also be useful in those individuals with immunodeficiency disorders, such as hypogammaglobulinemia and Wiskott-Aldrich syndrome, and for those individuals who are immunologically compromised by immunosuppressants following transplantation.

In all instances antiviral drugs have another advantage over vaccines in their immediate action. Vaccines take several days or weeks to induce immunity. Chemical agents can be useful even in cases where very effective vaccines are available. For example, now that smallpox has been virtually eliminated from the face of the earth, vaccination against this disease is no longer required or recommended in the United States. If this virus should emerge again, devastating epidemics could result before the vaccine could be distributed and immunity reestablished in the population. The antiviral drug methisazone could be immediately employed to protect individuals who come in contact with active cases of smallpox.

In addition to the specific immune system, the interferon system is another natural defense mechanism against viral infection. Administered interferon should be an ideal antiviral agent since it is a natural product, relatively nontoxic, and acts against a broad spectrum of viruses. Furthermore, it is effective against replicating viruses that ordinarily evade human defense. To date, it is difficult to purify and concentrate and thus not amenable for general use. Another approach is to induce the body to produce its own interferon: several chemotherapeutic agents owe their antiviral activity to their ability to induce interferon in the recipient. Antiviral antibiotics, such as statalon and helenine, and chemical agents, such as tilorone, and synthetic double-stranded polynucleotides, such as poly (rI:rC) (rI = riboinosinic acid; rC = ribocytidylic acid), are examples. Unfortunately, poly (rI:rC) and others are toxic, causing adverse effects on hematopoiesis and liver function. Thus there is a need to synthesize new interferon inducers with lower toxicity.

Antiviral Agents Effective in Humans

Only the few compounds extensively tested and reported to be effective are described here. A few of the structures are shown in Figure 1 and the major antiviral agents are listed in Table 1. Interferon, the naturally occurring antiviral protein is included since it is currently being extensively studied and shows promise as a prophylactic and therapeutic agent. Many review articles on virus chemotherapy and interferon are available and some are listed in the bibliography.

Thiosemicarbazones. The first report of antiviral activity for this series of compounds was in 1950, when the antituberculosis agent, p-aminobenzaldehyde thiosemicarbazone [7420-39-5], provided protection to chick embryos and mice infected with vaccinia virus (2). A program of analogue synthesis followed, and in 1955 Bauer (3) reported that indole-2,3-dione-3-thiosemicarbazone [487-16-1] (isatin-3-thiosemicarbazone) provided almost complete protection for mice infected with high doses of vaccinia virus. The compound appears to interact with some early product of infection, blocking the translation of late vaccinia messenger-RNA and thereby preventing the formation of some of the virus structural components. The result is that mature virions are not formed. Probably the most effective compound in the series is the methyl derivative methisazone (N-methylisatin 3-thiosemicarbazone, Marboran) (4–5). Methisazone has been shown to exert an effect against variola and vaccinia viruses in both tissue cultures and experimental animals.

Methisazone was shown to have a prophylactic effect against variola in humans in four separate trials (Madras, India, 1963 and 1965–1967; Brazil, 1964–1965; and Pakistan, 1964–1970) (5–8) with a protective effect of 47–83%. It had no therapeutic benefit in the treatment of established clinical disease. In the United States it has been used in the therapy of vaccinia reactions such as eczema vaccinatum and vaccinia gangrenosum but has not been proven effective. The drug is not licensed for use in the United States but is available as Marboran for experimental use.

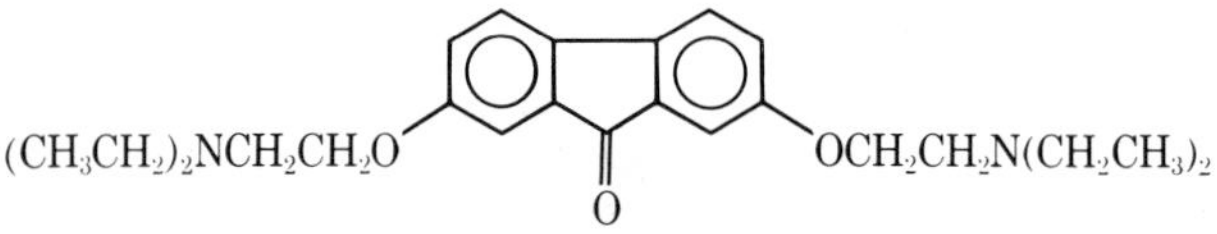

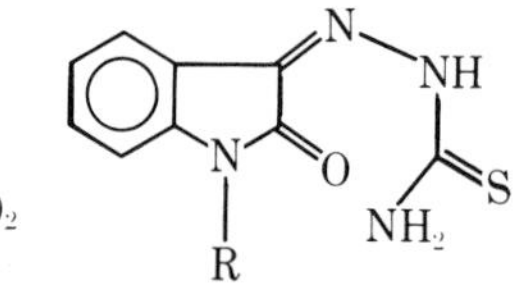

(1)
Tilorone

(2)
Isatin-3-thiosemicarbazone, R = H
Methisazone, R = CH₃

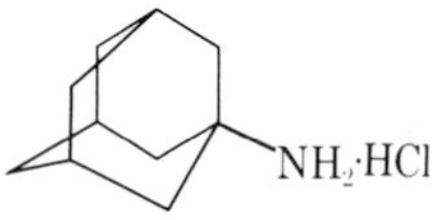

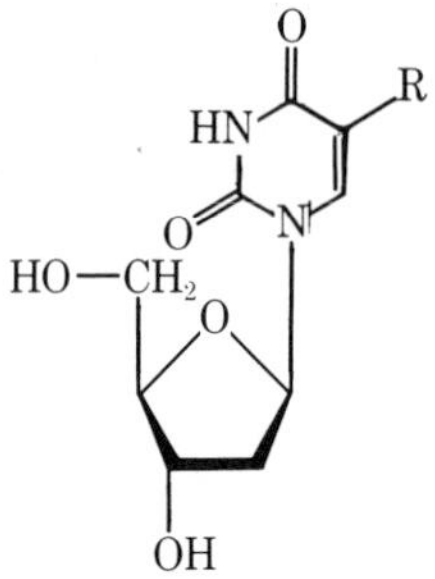

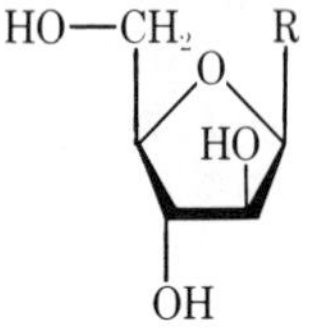

(3)
Amantadine hydrochloride

(4)
Idoxuridine, R = I
Trifluorothymidine, R = CF₃

(5)

Ara-A, R =

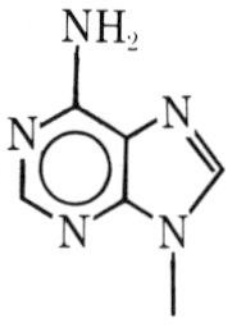

Ara-C, R =

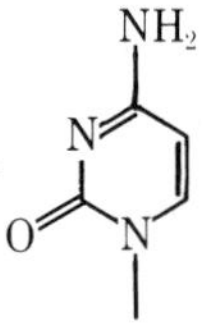

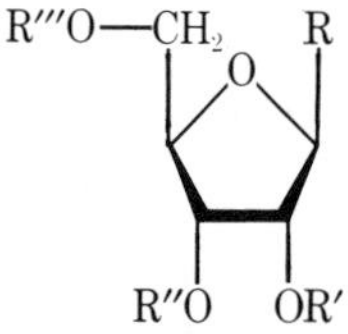

(6)

Ribavirin, R = 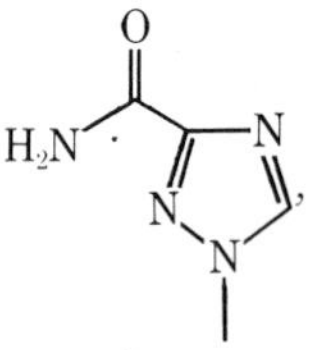 , R′ = R″ = R‴ = H

Isoprinosine, R = · 3CH₃CHOHCH₂N(CH₃)₂

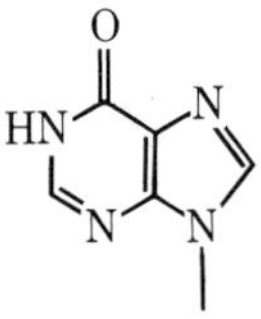

·3CH₃CONH— —CO₂H, R′ = R″ = R‴ = H

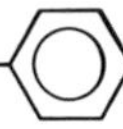

5′-Inosinic acid[131-99-7], R = 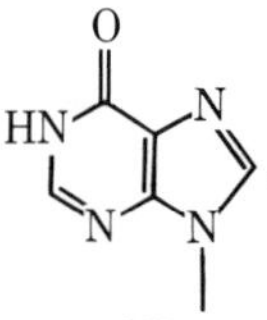 , R′ = R″ = H, R‴ = PO₃H₂

5′-Cytidylic acid[85-94-9], R = 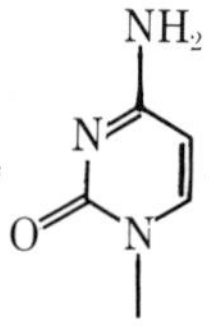 , R′ = R″ = H, R‴ = PO₃H₂

Figure 1. Antiviral agents.

428

Table 1. Antiviral Agents

Drug	CAS Registry Number	Structure number	mp, °C	Manufacturer
amantadine hydrochloride	[665-66-7]	(3)	360 (dec)	DuPont
ara-A	[5536-17-4]	(5)	257–257.5	Parke Davis Div., Warner Lambert
ara-C	[147-94-4]	(5)	212–213	Upjohn
helenine	[1407-14-3]			Merck, Sharp, and Dohme
idoxuridine	[54-42-2]	(4)	240 (dec)	Smith Kline and French
interferon	[9008-11-1]			Calbio; HEM Research, Inc.
isoprinosine	[36703-88-5]	(6)		Newport Pharmaceutical
levamisole	[14769-73-4, 53631-68-8]		60–61.5	Lederle Div., American Cyanamid
methisazone	[1910-68-5]	(2)	245 (dec)	Burroughs Wellcome; Aldrich
poly(rI:rC)	[24939-03-5]	(6) (monomers)		Miles
ribivarin	[36791-04-5]	(6)	174–176	ICN Pharmaceuticals
statolon	[11006-77-2]			Lilly
tilorone	[27591-97-5]	(1)	235–237	Richardson-Merrell
trifluorothymidine	[70-00-8]	(4)	169–172	Heinrich Mack

More recently, methisazone has been shown to have antitumor activity in experimental animals. Transformation of chicken cells by Rous sarcoma virus (RSV) and inhibition of its reverse transcriptase have been reported. Three other derivatives, 2-formylpyridine thiosemicarbazone [3608-75-1], 1-formylisoquinoline thiosemicarbazone [2365-26-6], and diphenyl ketone thiosemicarbazone [7341-60-8], also inhibit transformation by the virus (9). Since the need of these compounds for poxviruses has essentially been eliminated owing to the eradication of smallpox, the use of this series of agents may have a future as antitumor drugs.

Amantadine Hydrochloride. In 1963 it was shown that amantadine hydrochloride (1-adamantanamine hydrochloride, aminoadamantane hydrochloride, Symmetrel) influenced the course of influenza A2 infections in humans (10). In 1964 amantadine hydrochloride was reported to be effective against infections with influenza A, A1, and A2 in tissue culture, in ovo, and in mice (11). In addition to its protective effect against influenza A infections of humans, amantadine hydrochloride has also shown an antiviral effect against equine influenza in horses and avian influenza A strains in quail and turkeys. There is also evidence for *in vitro* activity against a number of other viruses such as rubella, parainfluenza, and vaccinia. More recently, the replication of the arenaviruses in cell cultures have been reduced in the presence of amantadine (12). The compound seems to act at an early stage in the influenza replication cycle by blocking or slowing the penetration of virus into the host cell. In the case of arenaviruses, the drug also seems to affect late viral synthesis and release of progeny virus from the cell (12).

In 1966 amantadine hydrochloride was licensed by the FDA for use in the prevention of respiratory illness owing to influenza A viruses by prophylactic treatment of contacts of patients and when index cases appear in the area (13–14).

The results of representative double-blind studies designed to assess the role of amantadine against influenza A2 in humans under natural conditions indicated a protective efficacy of approximately 66%. Amantadine may be more effective in the prevention of clinical disease when a significant preexisting antibody is present (15–19). Amantadine has also been shown to have a therapeutic effect if given early to persons with clinical disease caused by influenza A2 virus (20–21).

Side effects include nervousness, insomnia, depression, confusion, hallucinations, and drowsiness, although some studies have reported no adverse side reactions.

5-Iodo-2′-deoxyuridine.   5-Iodo-2′-deoxyuridine (idoxuridine, IDU, IUDR, Stoxil) is a halogenated pyrimidine originally synthesized in 1958 as an experimental drug for the inhibition of tumors. In 1961 it was shown that IDU inhibited plaque formation because of herpes simplex virus in tissue culture (22). It is also effective against varicella-zoster virus, cytomegalovirus, and vaccinia in tissue culture. In 1962 the successful treatment with IDU of herpes simplex corneal infections (herpetic keratitis) in humans was reported (23). It has now been used in thousands of patients against acute herpetic keratitis with favorable results but with less significant results in chronic and recurrent herpetic keratitis. Therapeutic success rates with idoxuridine have ranged 47–92% in seven studies (24). An overall success of ca 71% resulted in these studies as compared to 24% for placebo-control groups. Treatment of cutaneous herpetic lesions with topical IDU has yielded conflicting results probably owing to the insolubility of the drug. Addition of dimethylsulfoxide (DMSO) increases the solubility of IDU and the combination has been reported to be effective against cutaneous herpes simplex and herpes zoster. DMSO is not licensed for use and cannot be given in any form to humans in the United States. IDU is licensed for the topical treatment of herpetic keratitis and is available as an ophthalmic solution as Stoxil.

In cells, idoxuridine is phosphorylated and converted to the triphosphate. It acts as a thymidine analogue and is incorporated into both host and viral DNA in place of thymidine. Since both herpes and vaccinia viruses induce a thymidine kinase, more of this analogue may be incorporated into infected cells than in uninfected cells. The resultant DNA is thus altered and can neither be replicated with fidelity nor transcribed into functional mRNA. Defective virions and partially assembled components result. Host cell DNA is also adversely affected, especially rapidly proliferating cells such as in the bone marrow and gastrointestinal tract. Leukopenia, thrombocytopenia, stomatitis, and alopecia result from intravenous administration. Consequently, use of the drug is limited to topical application. Heroic attempts have been made to use the drug in herpetic encephalitis, a serious disease with high mortality. However, it has been clearly shown that idoxuridine is both ineffective and overly toxic in the treatment of herpes encephalitis (25).

Trifluorothymidine.   A related thymidine analogue, trifluorothymidine (5′-trifluoromethyl-2′-deoxyuridine) has been reported to be a significantly superior alternative to iododeoxyuridine for the treatment of human ocular infections with herpes simplex virus (26). It is more soluble than idoxuridine and the resultant higher concentration and greater potency results in more rapid healing of the lesion.

Arabinosylcytosine.   This pyrimidine nucleoside analogue (1-β-D-arabinofuranosylcytosine, ara-C) has arabinose in place of 2-deoxyribose. It has a similar, but not identical, antiviral spectrum to idoxuridine and is equally effective in treating herpetic and vaccinial infections of the eye. However, it is more toxic to the epithelium and is rapidly deaminated to an inactive form *in vivo*.

Arabinosyladenine. This purine nucleoside analogue (9-β-D-arabinofuranosyl-adenine, ara-A, Vidarabine) is virtually identical in potency and activity to idox-uridine and cytosine arabinoside (27). It is not as readily deaminated as arabinosyl-cytosine. It is also less toxic to host cells than either ara-C or idoxuridine. The lesser toxicity is caused by not being incorporated into cellular DNA but it seems to inhibit viral DNA polymerase activity. In systemic administration in therapeutically active doses, it does not suppress the hematopoietic system nor does it have immunosup-pressive effect on antibody formation or on cellular immunity and produces only minimal systemic symptoms. At high doses it causes vomiting, nausea, weight loss, weakness, and megaloblastosis in the erythroid series. Its primary drawback is its low solubility; large volumes of fluid must be administered. Adenine arabinoside is slowly deaminated *in vivo* to the hypoxanthine derivative which is less effective but does retain some antiviral activity. New derivatives are being developed that are more soluble and not so readily deaminated.

Adenine arabinoside has been licensed by the FDA for topical use in ophthalmic ointments. Topical treatment of primary or recurrent herpetic genital infection with 3% ara-A failed to influence the course of the disease (28). However, treatment of herpes zoster in immunosuppressed patients by intravenous administration has shown some success without serious side effects (29). More recently, it was evaluated for treatment of herpes simplex encephalitis in a placebo-controlled study (30). In 28 cases proved by isolation of type 1 herpes simplex virus from brain biopsy, treatment reduced mortality from 70–28% and over 50% of treated survivors had no or only moderately debilitating neurological sequelae. Thus this drug seems to be the first antiviral drug for systemic treatment of herpetic infections.

Ribavirin. Ribavirin (1-β-D-ribofuranosyl-1,2,4-triazole-3-carboxamide, Virazole) is a ribose containing synthetic purine nucleoside which is active *in vitro* and *in vivo* against a number of RNA and DNA viruses including influenza, viral hepatitis, and herpes viruses (31).

The prophylactic effectiveness of ribavirin against challenge with types A and B influenza viruses was evaluated in double-blind clinical trials (32–33). Ribavirin did not affect the development of type A influenza illness and showed only minimal effectiveness in suppressing type B influenza illness in humans. A more recent study, however, using a different strain of influenza A and different treatment regimen in-dicates a significant reduction in clinical manifestations and virus in ribavirin-treated young individuals (34). Caution should be used in giving the drug to women of child bearing age since congenital anomalies of limbs, ribs, eyes, and central nervous system, as well as fetal deaths, have occurred when the drug was given to pregnant hamsters (35).

Interferon. Interferon was discovered in 1956 by Isaacs and Lindenmann (36). It is a glycoprotein produced by cells in response to most viral infections and plays an important role in host defense during viral disease. Interferon has a broad spectrum of antiviral activity and can prevent the replication of most viruses in pretreated cells. More recently, it has been shown that interferon synthesis is also induced by a variety of other substances ranging from bacteria and their products to synthetic poly-mers.

The expression of the antiviral activity of interferon is a two-step process; in-terferon is not active directly but induces the antiviral state in treated cells by the synthesis of a short-lived antiviral protein. A great deal of evidence suggests that the antiviral protein interferes with the translation of viral messenger-RNAs. Being a natural product it has the advantage over chemical agents in that it is relatively nontoxic to normal cells, although when used *in vivo* at high doses it may be immunosuppressive. Prolonged interferon treatment is well tolerated. Low-grade fever and mild malaise may occur and a transient depression in white cell counts as well as platelets and reticulocyte counts occur during therapy with interferon (37). All hematologic measurements promptly reverted to normal when interferon therapy was stopped. It is not clear whether the hematopoietic suppression is an intrinsic property of interferon or caused by a contaminating protein.

Two approaches have been utilized to investigate the efficacy of interferon use in humans: (*1*) the use of inducers to cause the host to make its own interferon and antiviral protein, and (*2*) the direct application of interferon. Synthetic double-stranded RNA polymers, such as polyriboinosinic acid-polyribocytidylic acid complexes [poly(rI:rC)], have been used with some success (38). However, many of these inducers are toxic and studies in humans are usually limited to topical application. Thus topical application of poly(rI:rC) has been shown to prevent illness from rhinovirus challenge (39). It has also been shown to have a definite but slight therapeutic effect in herpetic keratitis (40).

Initially the results from the direct use of human interferon in human disease was discouraging probably due to the low activity of the preparations. Recently, high-titer human interferon (10^7 units/mL) has become available and encouraging results are being obtained (37,41–42).

Immunopotentiating Agents. Another more recent approach is to use chemicals that augment or modulate immune responses of the host. Inosiplex (Isoprinosine) the *p*-acetamidobenzoic acid salt of inosine *N,N*-dimethylaminoisopropanol, has shown antiviral activities in tissue culture, animal models, and human studies but the results have been contradictory. Controlled human-challenge studies with rhinovirus and influenza virus using the drug in a prophylactic fashion have been disappointing. Clinical studies have suggested that the drug may be more effective when used therapeutically instead of prophylactically and it has been suggested that the antiviral effect is caused by its immunopotentiating action (43–45). Levamisole, the levoisomer of tetramisole, may act in a similar manner (see Chemotherapeutics, antihelmintic) (44).

Future of Antiviral Chemotherapy

After some three decades of study, the limited number of antiviral agents available for the treatment and prevention of human disease appears to be discouraging. Furthermore, because of their toxicity, many of them are limited to topical application. However, as more information becomes available about the mechanisms of virus replication, it may be possible to synthesize substances that specifically interfere with unique viral function. Indeed, some drugs seem to act in this way and therefore should be less toxic to the host. The success with vidarabine in systemic treatment of herpes encephalitis gives encouragement for the future. The success with interferon trials also indicate that virus-specific functions can be specifically inhibited without being detrimental to the host. Its wide-spectrum activity would also indicate that drugs might also be developed that will have similar activity.

BIBLIOGRAPHY

"Viral Infections, Chemotherapy" in *ECT* 2nd ed., Vol. 21, pp. 452–460, by Conrad E. Hoffmann, E. I. du Pont de Nemours & Co., Inc.

1. T. E. O'Connor, C. D. Aldrich, and V. S. Sethi, *Ann. N.Y. Acad. Sci.* **284,** 544 (1977).
2. D. Hamre, J. Bernstein, and R. Donovick, *Proc. Soc. Exp. Biol. Med.* **73,** 275 (1950).
3. D. J. Bauer, *Br. J. Exp. Pathol.* **36,** 105 (1955).
4. D. J. Bauer and P. W. Sadler, *Br. J. Pharmacol.* **15,** 101 (1960).
5. D. J. Bauer and co-workers, *Lancet ii,* 494 (1963).
6. A. R. Rao and co-workers, *Indian J. Med. Res.* **57,** 477 (1969).
7. L. A. R. DoValle and co-workers, *Lancet ii,* 976 (1965).
8. G. G. Heiner and co-workers, *Am. J. Epidemiol.* **94,** 435 (1971).
9. W. Levinson and co-workers, *Ann. N.Y. Acad. Sci.* **284,** 525 (1977).
10. G. G. Jackson, R. L. Muldoon, and L. W. Akers, *Antimicrob. Agents Chemother.,* 703 (1963).
11. W. L. Davies and co-workers, *Science* **144,** 862 (1964).
12. R. Welsh and co-workers, *Virology* **45,** 679 (1971).
13. *J. Am. Med. Assoc.* **201,** 374 (1967).
14. *Med. Lett.* **9**(2), 5 (1967).
15. J. J. Quilligan, M. Hirayama, and H. D. Baerstein, *J. Pediatr.* **69,** 572 (1966).
16. A. W. Galbraith and co-workers, *Lancet ii,* 1026 (1969).
17. N. Oker-Blum, *Br. Med. J.* **3,** 676 (1970).
18. A. W. Galbraith and co-workers, *Bull. W.H.O.* **41,** 677 (1969).
19. A. A. Smorodintsev, *Ann. N.Y. Acad. Sci.* **173,** 44 (1970).
20. R. B. Hornick and co-workers, *Bull. W.H.O.* **41,** 671 (1969).
21. A. W. Galbraith and co-workers, *Lancet ii,* 113 (1971).
22. E. C. Herrmann, Jr., *Proc. Soc. Exp. Biol. Med.* **107,** 142 (1961).
23. H. E. Kaufman, A. B. Nesburn, and E. D. Maloney, *Arch. Ophthalmol.* **67,** 583 (1962).
24. R. Jawetz and co-workers, *Ann. N.Y. Acad. Sci.* **173,** 282 (1970).
25. Boston interhospital virus study group and the NIAID-Sponsored Cooperative Antiviral Clinical Study Group, *N. Engl. J. Med.* **292,** 599 (1975).
26. P. C. Wellings and co-workers, *Am. J. Ophthalmol.* **73,** 932 (1972).
27. H. E. Kaufman, E. D. Ellison, and W. M. Townsend, *Arch. Ophthalmol.* **84,** 783 (1970).
28. H. G. Adams and co-workers, *J. Infect. Dis.* **133**(Suppl.), A151 (1976).
29. L. T. Ch'ien and co-workers, *J. Infect. Dis.* **133**(Suppl.), A184 (1976).
30. R. J. Whitley and co-workers, *N. Engl. J. Med.* **297,** 289 (1977).
31. R. W. Sidwell and co-workers, *Science* **177,** 705 (1972).
32. A. Cohen and co-workers, *J. Infect. Dis.* **133**(Suppl.), A114 (1976).
33. Y. Togo and E. A. McCracken, *J. Infect. Dis.* **133**(Suppl.), A109 (1976).
34. F. Salido-Rengell, H. Nassen-Quinones, and B. Briseno-Garcie, *Ann. N.Y. Acad. Sci.* **284,** 272 (1977).
35. L. Kilham and V. H. Ferm, *Science* **195,** 413 (1977).
36. A. Isaacs and J. Lindenmann, *Proc. R. Soc. London Ser. B* **147,** 258 (1957).
37. H. B. Greenberg and co-workers, *N. Engl. J. Med.* **295,** 517 (1976).
38. G. P. Lampson and co-workers, *Proc. Nat. Acad. Sci. U.S.A.* **58,** 782 (1967).
39. C. Panusarn and co-workers, *N. Engl. J. Med.* **291,** 57 (1974).
40. H. E. Kaufman, E. D. Ellison, and S. R. Waltman, *Am. J. Ophthalmol.* **68,** 486 (1969).
41. B. R. Jones and co-workers, *J. Infect. Dis.* **133**(Suppl.), A169 (1976).
42. B. R. Jones and co-workers, *Lancet ii,* 128 (1976).
43. T. Ginsberg and A. J. Glasky, *Ann. N.Y. Acad. Sci.* **284,** 128 (1977).
44. J. W. Hadden and co-workers, *Ann. N.Y. Acad. Sci.* **284,** 139 (1977).
45. R. H. Waldman and R. Ganguly, *Ann. N.Y. Acad. Sci.* **284,** 153 (1977).

434 CHEMOTHERAPEUTICS (ANTIVIRAL)

General References

Review Articles

W. H. Prusoff and B. Goz, "Potential Mechanisms of Action Antiviral Agents," *Fed. Proc.* **32,** 1679 (1973).
R. A. Bucknall, "The Continuing Search for Antiviral Drugs," *Adv. Pharmacol. Chemother.* **11,** 295 (1973).
D. Parkes, *Adv. Drug. Res.* **8,** 11 (1974).
J. P. Luby, M. T. Johnson, and S. R. Jones, "Antiviral Chemotherapy," *Ann. Rev. Med.* **25,** 251 (1974).
D. Pavan-Langston, R. A. Buchanan, and C. A. Elford, Jr., eds., *Adenine Arabinoside: An Antiviral Agent,* Raven Press, New York, 1975.
J. P. Luby, M. T. Johnson, and S. R. Jones, "Antiviral Chemotherapy," *Ann. Rev. Med.* **25,** 251 (1974).
M. Ho and J. A. Armstrong, "Interferon," *Ann. Rev. Microbiol.* **29,** 131 (1975).
N. B. Finter, *Interferon and Interferon Inducers,* American Elsevier Publishing Co., Inc., New York, 1973, pp. 598.
S. Baron and F. Dianzani, eds., "The Interferon System: A Current Review," *Texas Rep. Biol. Med.* **35,** (Oct. 1977).
C. E. Hoffman, "Virus Chemotherapy," *Chemtech.* **8,** 726 (1978).

Symposia

Symposium on Clinical Use of Interferon, Ninth International Immunobiological Symposium, Zagreb, Yugoslavia, Izdavacki zavod, Jugoslovenske academe, Zagreb, Yugoslavia, 1975, 262 pp.
T. Merigan, ed., "Antivirals with Clinical Potential, A Symposium at Stanford University, Aug. 1975," *J. Infect. Dis.* **133**(Suppl.), A1 (1976).
E. C. Hermann, Jr., ed., "Third Conference on Antiviral Substances," *Ann. N.Y. Acad. Sci.* **284,** (1977).

GEORGE E. GIFFORD
University of Florida

DISINFECTANTS AND ANTISEPTICS

The procedures that are currently described as antiseptic or disinfectant began at the dawn of recorded history when food was preserved by smoking, on the application of essential oils and spices for embalming, or by burning of aromatic woods for protection against the plague. The Bible commands the burning of clothes worn by the diseased. Boiling of drinking water and its preservation by storage in silver or copper vessels was known to the Persians as well as to the army of Alexander the Great.

The bubonic plague was fought in medieval Europe by burning sulfur, cedar, or juniper wood in affected houses. Although a connection between pathogenic microorganisms and contagious disease was not established for another several centuries, several early students of disease, including Fracastorius in the 16th, and Robert Boyle in the 17th century clearly suspected the existence of pathogens.

Even before the publication of Pasteur's definitive work on transmission of disease (in 1860 and thereafter), Labarraque used a hypochlorite solution in the treatment of wounds (1825), Alcock recommended it for the purification of drinking water (1827), Lefevre extolled its virtues as a disinfectant (1843), and Semmelweis used it to inactivate the "cadaveric poisons" carried on the hands of physicians attending puerperal fever patients (1846).

Some twenty years later, Lister took up the use of phenol [*108-95-2*] in surgery. In this he was probably stimulated by Pasteur's demonstration of the ubiquity of germs and their involvement in putrefaction, which Lister assumed, resembled suppuration in wounds. At first he applied phenol in concentrated form, and later in an aqueous solution because of the corrosive action of the pure chemical upon tissue. In 1870, in an effort to decontaminate the ambient air, Lister introduced the carbolic acid (phenol) spray and used it for another fifteen years thereafter. It is noteworthy that both hypochlorite and phenol solutions were used for years on an essentially conjectural basis, that is, without any evidence of the actual causes of infection (see also Antibacterial agents; Antibiotics; Chemotherapeutics; Fungicides; Industrial antimicrobial agents; Sterile techniques).

Definitions

The Food and Drug Administration (FDA) has adopted the following definitions (1) for antimicrobial (active) ingredient and antimicrobial preservative (inactive) ingredient:

Antimicrobial (active) ingredient: A compound or substance that kills microorganisms or prevents or inhibits their growth and reproduction and that contributes to the claimed effect of the product in which it is included.

Antimicrobial preservative (inactive) ingredient: A compound or substance that kills microorganisms, or that prevents or inhibits their growth and reproduction, and that is included in a product formulation only at a concentration sufficient to prevent spoilage or prevent growth of inadvertently added microorganisms, but does not contribute to the claimed effects of the product to which it is added.

The Environmental Protection Agency (EPA) has adopted the following definitions (2) for antimicrobial agents:

Disinfectants destroy or irreversibly inactivate infectious or other undesirable bacteria, pathogenic fungi, or viruses on surfaces or inanimate objects.

Sanitizers reduce the number of living bacteria or viable virus particles on inanimate surfaces, in water, or in the air.

Bacteriostats inhibit the growth of bacteria in the presence of moisture.

Sterilizers destroy viruses and all living bacteria, fungi, and their spores on inanimate surfaces.

Fungicides and *fungistats* inhibit the growth of or destroy fungi (including yeasts) pathogenic to man or other animals on inanimate surfaces.

ANTISEPTICS

Antiseptics are generally understood to be agents applied to living tissue and are considered to be drugs. Therefore they may be inactivated by contact with body fluids, such as blood or serum.

The methods prescribed by Ruehle and Brewer for the examination of antiseptics, liquids, ointments, powders, oils, etc, enjoyed a quasi-official status for some time, having originated with a governmental authority (3). These tests are still useful for screening new preparations designed as antiseptics that are preliminary to more extensive clinical tests under conditions of intended use. However, the FDA no longer sponsors these methods; according to its present position, no standard or official tests for the evaluation of antiseptics exist, and no single *in vitro* test is considered sufficiently informative to serve as a criterion of practical performance.

To the extent that *Staphylococcus aureus* represents the most common cause of suppuration and exhibits marked resistance to both physical and chemical factors, its use as a test organism is logical in one of the several applicable screening tests. However, for antiseptics applied to prevent infection through a break in the skin, an *in vivo* method (4–6) yields more relevant results.

Klarmann and co-workers (7) reported a semimicro method that furnishes more information about the performance of liquid antiseptics likely to come in contact with tissue fluids. One of the features of this technique is control of the random-sampling error inherent in methods that depend upon loop transfers from the medication mixture to the subculture. In addition, this method incorporates the following premises: (1) The criterion of fitness of any antiseptic that is likely to come in contact with tissue fluids should be its demonstrated capacity for permanent suppression of bacterial activity under the conditions of use. (2) If an antiseptic that has prevented bacterial proliferation in a nutrient medium does not continue to prevent it upon contact with physiological material such as blood or serum, then its fitness for use as a preoperative or wound antiseptic is open to question.

Although the so-called degerming agents are not, strictly speaking, skin antiseptics, the *in vivo* testing method developed for the evaluation of degerming agents furnishes comparative information about their practical performance. This method has been devised by Price and is known as the serial basin test (8); later modifications were suggested to simplify the procedure (9–10). The procedure recognizes the fact that the skin cannot be disinfected in the true sense of the term, but that it is possible to reduce the "resident" potentially pathogenic bacterial flora for reasons of safety as required, for example, in surgery. With other factors being equal, the more valuable the degerming agent is, the better it depresses the bacterial count.

The glove juice test, ie, the procedure used to determine the effectiveness of surgical scrubs has, since 1973, been part of the guidelines of the Bureau of Drugs for evaluating compounds recommended for the surgical scrub. With some modification, this test was adopted by the OTC Antimicrobial I Panel and published in the Federal Register (11).

Since *in vivo* degerming tests are often cumbersome, an *in vitro* screening test such as the calf-skin disk test may be employed for the preliminary estimation of the effectiveness of antimicrobial soaps or detergents under actual conditions of use (12).

Although various test methods for the determination of tissue toxicity have been suggested in the practical screening of antiseptics (13–14), their results cannot be used as a rational basis of a comparative evaluation of such agents. The problem of tissue toxicity is actually of considerably greater importance in chemotherapy than in antisepsis. However, an antiseptic with lower tissue toxicity should not be given preference over a more toxic one.

DISINFECTANTS

Analytical and Test Methods

Disinfectants are generally understood to be agents suitable for application to inanimate objects. Environmental surfaces are deemed to be contaminated, not infected. Disinfectants kill the growing forms but not necessarily the resistant spore forms of microorganisms (2b).

Rideal and Walker were the first to recognize the need for standardizing a number of factors in the methodology of the evaluation of disinfectants (15). Perhaps their most fundamental requirement was that of determining the resistance of the test organisms to pure phenol at the time when the disinfectant sample was being tested with the same bacterial culture. Of course, this is not to minimize the importance of standardizing other details of the testing technique, without which reproducibility of results would be impossible.

The Rideal-Walker method has been revised and its application extended several times, both in Great Britain and the United States, during the 76 years since its introduction. The most important British revisions were those of the Lancet Commission in 1909 (16), by Rideal and Walker themselves in 1921 (17), and by the British Standards Institution in 1934 (18). In the United States revisions were undertaken by Anderson and McClintic on behalf of the Hygienic Laboratory in 1912 (19), by a committee of the American Public Health Association in 1918 (20), by Brewer and Reddish in 1929 (21), by Ruehle and Brewer in 1931 (3) on behalf of the FDA, and finally, by the Association of Official Agricultural Chemists (AOAC) in 1960 (22). This last method, designated the AOAC Phenol Coefficient Method, although patterned along the lines of the FDA method, provides for special formulas of subculture media designed to suspend bacteriostasis in order to distinguish between germicidal and inhibitory action. Thus, the addition of thioglycolate is specified for testing preparations containing heavy metals (eg, mercury), and lecithin (qv) is used in testing products containing quaternary ammonium compounds (22).

The phenol coefficient is a number obtained by dividing the greatest dilution of the disinfectant under test capable of killing *Salmonella typhosa* at room temperature by the greatest dilution of phenol showing the same result. According to the EPA, any phenol coefficient claim requires testing by the AOAC Phenol Coefficient Method from duplicate samples of one batch against *Salmonella typhosa*. The classic Ruehle and Brewer Circular No. 198 (3) added the requirement for the use of a second test organism, *Staphylococcus aureus* in 1931. This requirement serves to extend the method to testing antiseptics as well as disinfectants. The AOAC test for fungicidal action of environmental disinfectants call for the use of *Trichophyton interdigitale* as the test organism (22).

Methods such as the AOAC phenol coefficient method serve as screening procedures to yield a general idea as to whether or not a given product is of potential value as a germicide, but no single testing procedure is an adequate substitute for a comprehensive inquiry into the total antimicrobial spectrum of a given disinfectant used for pathogens of epidemiological and clinical significance.

The phenol coefficient test has lost some significance today and has been replaced by the AOAC Use-Dilution Test to measure the efficacy of disinfectants. The use-dilution procedure (23–24) differs from the phenol coefficient methods in that it employs bacteria deposited on carriers such as polished stainless steel rings (penicillin cups) rather than their suspensions in nutrient broth. Two test organisms are specified, *Staphylococcus aureus* and *Salmonella choleraesuis* which replaces *Salmonella typhosa* of the phenol coefficient method because the latter does not resist drying on the steel rings. The phenol resistance of a 48-h culture of *Salmonella choleraesuis* should fall within the range specified for a 24-h culture of *Salmonella typhosa*.

The use-dilution test distinguishes between two general classes of disinfectants, those for janitorial or household uses directed especially against enteric organisms, and those for medical, veterinary, hospital, and surgical uses directed against both enteric and pyogenic bacteria. The former must be germicidal for *Salmonella choleraesuis*, and the latter must be effective against both *Salmonella choleraesuis* and *Staphylococcus aureus* in their recommended use-dilutions under the conditions of the ring-carrier testing procedure (25). Supplementary confirmatory tests on floors and surgical instruments have been developed (25).

All disinfectant products must be formally registered with the EPA, according to the Federal Insecticide, Fungicide, and Rodenticide Act of 1947 and the Federal Environmental Pesticide Control Act of 1972 and registrations must be accompanied by efficacy data based on the use-dilution test.

Square Diluent Test. This test has acquired some importance in connection with a Federal specification for disinfectants (26). It recognizes the need for a broad spectrum antimicrobial (bactericidal and fungicidal) performance by requiring tests with three microorganisms representative of pathogenic types, that is *Staphylococcus aureus*, *Salmonella schottmuelleri*, and *Trichophyton interdigitale*. In this method test organisms are employed in mixture rather than individually.

Long-lasting disinfectants that persist in residual quantities on disinfected surfaces obviously have the advantage of inactivating infectious materials that may be later deposited on such surfaces (27).

Chemical Sterilization of Instruments. The tests described thus far relate to disinfection rather than to sterilization. That is, they assess the destruction of vegetative microorganisms but not of bacterial spores. Different chemicals have been claimed to possess sporicidal action. Disregarding those that would be too corrosive for practical use as instrument germicides, direct claims for sporicidal action at room temperature are being made today mostly for ethylene oxide [75-21-8] and aldehyde preparations. Hydrogen peroxide [7722-84-1], some iodophors and some quaternary ammonium compounds (qv) are also being credited with sporicidal potency, but several quaternary ammonium compounds tested are incapable of killing the spores of *Clostridium welchii*, *tetani* and *sporogenes*, and *Bacillus anthracis* even in 24 h (28).

Friedl (29) has reported a sporicidal test "applicable for use with germicides to determine presence or absence of sporicidal activity and potential effectiveness in disinfecting against specified spore-forming bacteria." The test is based on a procedure for obtaining spores of the desired resistance and exposing them to the action of disinfectants. The method provides for standardization by means of 20% hydrochloric acid of the spores of two test organisms, *Bacillus subtilis* and *Clostridium sporogenes*, although it may be carried out also with *Bacillus anthracis*, *Clostridium tetani*, and other species of *Bacilli* or *Clostridia* (30).

With a formaldehyde [50-00-0] germicide, for which sporicidal claims had been made, the spores of *Bacillus subtilis* were killed in 10–30 min, but the product did not kill the spores of *Clostridium sporogenes* in 2 h, the longest period of exposure employed in this study (31–32). These findings were subsequently extended to longer periods of exposure and the control of sporostasis in subcultures.

Steam under pressure, properly applied in an autoclave, is the sterilizing agent *par excellence* for instruments and appliances. Equivalent results, particularly with resistant bacterial spores, can be produced in a short period of time by exposure to boiling dilute aqueous solutions of certain disinfectants, preferably synthetic phenolics that exhibit low volatility with water vapors (31).

Proper sterilization of syringes and needles is important for the prevention of infection with hepatitis viruses A and B carried by human blood, serum, plasma, fibrinogen, etc, when administered by transfusion or injection (33) (see Blood). Since, at present, only man is known to be susceptible to infection by either virus, there is no laboratory method available for the evaluation of the sterilizing effectiveness of chemical disinfectants for these viruses. The Expert Committee on Hepatitis of the WHO considers the following procedures to be adequate: boiling in water for at least 10 min; autoclaving; or treatment in a hot-air oven for $\frac{1}{2}$ h at 170–180°C. No chemical disinfectants acting at room temperature are considered acceptable for this purpose (34).

In the cold sterilization of chemical thermometers and of instruments that cannot be subjected to heat treatment, tuberculocidal potency should be part of the nonspecific bactericidal spectrum of a disinfectant. The confirmatory *in vitro* tests require the use of a virulent culture of *Mycobacterium tuberculosis*; *in vivo* verification of the results obtained is carried out by inoculations in guinea pigs.

Virucidal Action.   A nonspecific disinfectant is not necessarily a nonspecific virucide, some authoritative opinion to the contrary notwithstanding (35). Some of the most valuable germicides are not effective against important viruses, such as that of poliomyelitis, under practical conditions of use. Moreover, the differences in susceptibility of viruses to antiviral agents appear to be as great as, or even greater than, the corresponding differences in bacteria (see also Chemotherapeutics, antiviral).

Unlike bacteria, viruses are metabolically inert entities in the absence of a susceptible host cell and depend upon the living host cells to supply the wherewithal of viral multiplication. They accomplish this by altering the metabolism of the parasitized cell to force the production of new viral material. But here the uniformity among viruses comes to an end. The great chemical differences among them are illustrated by the finding that, in the case of influenza virus, protein material accounts for less than 50% of the dry weight, whereas of rabbit papilloma virus protein makes up over 90%. Although some 50% of influenza virus consists of lipids, less than 6% of the dry weight of vaccinia virus is of this character (36). Such differences in composition must be expected to find expression in the wide variations in susceptibility to chemical and physical agents (37).

Influenza virus may be readily inactivated by different substances, as shown by a variety of testing methods (38–40). This is in contrast to poliomyelitis virus whose inactivation presents a more difficult problem (41).

The EPA (42) has published *Methods for Evaluating the Virucidal Activity of Disinfectants;* however, this agency, in cooperation with other laboratories concerned, is continuing work on improved methods for testing virucides. Apparently, there is not yet a standard or official federal test for virucidal disinfection. Some of the difficulties encountered were described (43–44).

Role of Neutralizers.   The testing methods mentioned occasionally call for the use of neutralizers. Their purpose is to inactivate the residual amounts of antimicrobial agent carried with the microorganisms into the subculture media. Otherwise, bacteriostasis might be mistaken for bactericidal action. These media must contain materials suppressing bacteriostasis by the disinfectant being tested. The character of these neutralizers depends on the antibacterial agent under test. For instance, Tween 80 with lecithin is a satisfactory neutralizer for quaternary ammonium compounds, sodium thiosulfate is effective for chlorine, and iodine compounds and sodium thioglycolate for mercurials.

Alcohols

The antibacterial effectiveness of several of the aliphatic alcohols has been known for a long time (45). In a study of their mode of action, the capacity of the monohydric alcohols from methyl to octyl to serve as substrates for *Escherichia coli* was investigated (46). Methyl alcohol [67-56-1] and the alcohols from butyl through octyl were unable to function as substrates; moreover, they inhibited the dehydrogenation of other substrates, the amount of inhibition increasing with the chain length of the alcohol. However, ethyl and propyl alcohols are capable of playing a dual role in that they act as substrates at low concentrations and as dehydrogenation inhibitors at high concentrations. By far the greatest amount of work has been done on the bactericidal action of ethyl alcohol [64-17-5] (47–50). In the proper concentration, ethyl alcohol is an effective germicide for vegetative pathogens as shown in Table 1.

The transmission of infectious or homologous serum hepatitis cannot be prevented by exposing virus-contaminated surgical instruments to the action of alcohol in any concentration or for any length of time. Only heat properly applied may be relied upon to produce inactivation of both types of hepatitis virus (34).

Isopropyl alcohol [67-63-0] appears to be somewhat more effective as an antimicrobial agent than ethyl alcohol. *Staphylococcus aureus* is reported to be killed by 50–91% isopropyl alcohol in 1 min at 20°C (58). However, earlier reports claim that 90% isopropyl alcohol fails to kill this organism in 2 hours (59). Isopropyl and ethyl alcohol are essentially similar in tuberculocidal performance when acting upon dried sputum smears (52).

In the homologous series of primary normal alcohols, the germicidal action increases with increasing molecular weight from methyl to octyl alcohol as shown in tests with *Salmonella typhosa* and *Staphylococcus aureus* (50). Moreover, there exists a fairly constant ratio between the molecular coefficients of successive members of the series as defined by the equation:

$$\text{molecular coefficient} = \frac{\text{mol wt alcohol}}{\text{mol wt phenol}} \times \frac{\text{phenol}}{\text{coefficient}}$$

Primary alcohols with 6 to 16 carbon atoms inhibit *Mycobacterium tuberculosis* and *Trichophyton gypseum*, but not *Staphylococcus aureus* (60). Ferguson's principle of relating thermodynamic activity to cytostatic activity accounts satisfactorily for many regularities encountered in homologous series of alcohols.

Vapors of propylene glycol [57-55-6] and triethylene glycol [112-27-6] can protect animals against airborne bacteria and influenza virus under controlled conditions of temperature and humidity (61–62) (see Alcohols; Glycols).

Halogens

Chlorine and Hypochlorites. Although the use of chlorinated lime as deodorant for sewage goes back to a report of the Royal Sewage Commission of Great Britain in 1854, it was R. Koch who in 1881 first referred to the bactericidal properties of hypochlorites. Calcium hypochlorite [7778-54-3] has now largely replaced the older chlorinated lime mostly for large-scale usage, and sodium hypochlorite [7681-52-9] is the

Table 1. Bactericidal and Virucidal Action of Ethanol

Organism	Effective conc, %	Time required	Reference
Salmonella typhosa	21.6	5 min	47
	17.3	10 min	47
	40–100	10 s	48
Staphylococcus aureus	34.5	5 min	47
	60–95	10 s	48
	100	50–90 s	48
Staphylococcus albus	70–80	5 min	49
	15	24 h	8
Streptococcus pyogenes	100	50–90 s	48
	50–100	30 s	48
	40	4 min	48
	30	45 min	48
	20	60 min	48
Escherichia coli	60	1–5 min	50
	70	40 s	51
	80	30 s	51
	60	5 min	51
	40–100	10 s	48
Pseudomonas aeruginosa	30–100	10 s	48
	20	30 min	48
Mycobacterium tuberculosis	95	15 s	52
aqueous suspension	100	30 s	52
	70	60 s	52
Mycobacterium tuberculosis			
in dry sputum, thin smears	70	1–5 min	52
thick smears	95	30 min	52
Trichophyton mentagrophytes	50	5 min	53
	25	20 min	53
Trichophyton rubrum	50	5 min	53
	25	20 min	53
Microsporum canis	50	5 min	53
	25	20 min	53
Microsporum audouini	70	24 h	53
fowl pox virus	70–95	10 min	54
	50	30 min	54
Newcastle virus	70–95	3 min	55
vaccinia virus	50	60 min	56
foot and mouth disease virus,	50	15–20 min	57
filtered (Berkefeld)	60	1–15 min	57
foot and mouth disease virus,			
unfiltered	20–60	6 h	57

active principle of many household products and of some hospital specialties (63). A number of organic chlorine compounds have been introduced; their antibacterial action is dependent upon their capacity for releasing "active" chlorine. In various areas of disinfection and sanitization, elementary chlorine [7782-50-5] is employed directly.

The bactericidal action of hypochlorites is caused primarily by the release of hypochlorous acid [7790-92-3], HOCl; however, the hypochlorite ion [13675-18-8], OCl⁻, may be a contributory factor since even distinctly alkaline hypochlorite solutions show some antibacterial potency (64). The pH of the hypochlorite solution has a marked effect on its germicidal activity in tests employing various test organisms (65–67).

The action of chlorine dioxide [10049-04-4], ClO_2, is more sporicidal than that of hypochlorous acid (68).

Although ordinarily all disinfectants suffer impairment of their activity in the presence of organic matter, the hypochlorites particularly lose much of their bactericidal potency under practical conditions of disinfection owing to the intense reactivity of both the hypochlorous acid and the hypochlorite ion. For this reason use of hypochlorites generally calls for prior removal of organic contamination (69).

The hypochlorites are subject to gradual deterioration over a period of time. The rate of deterioration depends upon several factors; the most important of which are the type of product, its pH, and the temperature of storage. The lower the pH, the more germicidal, but the less stable is the solution. A number of hypochlorite preparations available in dry form are quite stable if kept dry and cool (see Bleaching agents; Chlorine oxygen acids and salts).

Dakin's solution, which was used extensively during World War I for the irrigation of wounds, contained in its original form, sodium hypochlorite (0.45–0.5%) and boric acid [11113-50-1]. However, the success of the Carrel-Dakin surgical irrigation treatment is not caused by its antibacterial aspect, instead its action increases transudation from the wound which produces a drainage of stagnated fluid and causes replacement by fresh lymph (70).

N-Chloramines. This group comprises the derivatives of amines in which one or two valences of trivalent nitrogen are taken up by chlorine.

In comparison with hypochlorous acid, monochloramine [10599-90-3], NH_2Cl, requires more time and a higher concentration to produce sporicidal action. Table

Table 2.   Available Chlorine Content of Some N-Chloramines

Name and CAS Registry No.	Structure	Available Cl, %
chloramine T [127-65-1]	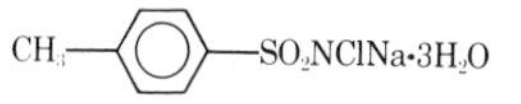 CH_3—⬡—$SO_2NClNa \cdot 3H_2O$	23–26
dichloramine T [473-34-7]	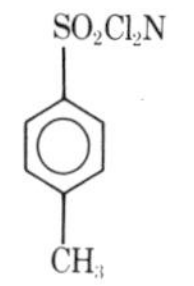 SO_2Cl_2N ⬡ CH_3	56–60
halazone [80-13-7]	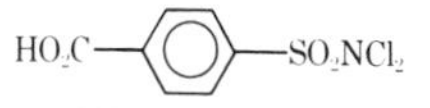 HO_2C—⬡—SO_2NCl_2	48–52.5
succinchlorimide [128-09-6]	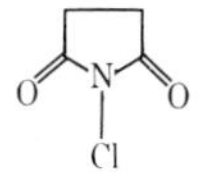 O=⬠N(Cl)=O	50–54
chloroazodin [502-98-7]	$H_2NCN=NCNH_2$, $\|$ NCl $\|$ NCl	75–79
trichlorocyanuric acid [87-90-1]	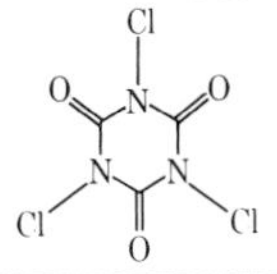 (triazine ring with Cl, O substituents)	88–90

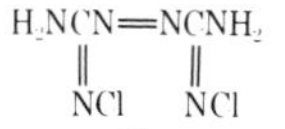

2 lists several other chloramines and gives their available chlorine content (see Chloramines).

Chloramine-T (sodium *N*-chloro-*p*-toluenesulfonamide) was widely used during World War I for the treatment of infected wounds and subsequently for hygienic purposes such as mouthwashes, douches, etc. It can be used for sanitizing food-handling equipment, but its activity is considerably slower than that of hypochlorites.

Dichloramine-T (*N,N*-dichloro-*p*-toluenesulfonamide) is insoluble in water, but soluble in a number of organic solvents, including chlorinated paraffin. Its medical usage appears to have declined.

Halazone (*N,N*-dichloro-*p*-carboxybenzenesulfonamide) is suitable for the decontamination of water, as is also succinchlorimide (*N*-chlorosuccinimide).

Chlorinated cyanuric acid derivatives consist of dichloroisocyanuric acid [2782-57-2], their sodium [2893-78-9] and potassium [2244-21-5] salts, and trichloroisocyanuric acid [87-90-1]. These compounds can be used in sanitation as such or formulated into various products (see Bleaching agents; Cyanuric and isocyanuric acids).

Several commercial cleaner-sanitizer products contain 1,3-dichloro-5,5-dimethyl hydantoin [118-52-5] as antibacterial component. In a pH range of 5.8–7.0 it is found to have similar antimicrobial activity to hypochlorite; it is less effective under alkaline conditions.

Chloromelamine [7673-09-8] is a chlorination product of 1,3,5-triaminotriazine. Formulated with a suitable anionic surfactant, it has been considered as a bactericidal rinse for mess kits and also for the treatment of contaminated fruits and vegetables (71) (see Cyanamides).

Chloroazodin (azochloramide, *N,N*-dichloroazodicarbonamidine) is claimed to be relatively nontoxic to tissue. Applied to a wound it acts as a mild and slow oxidant (72).

N-Trichloromethylmercapto-4-cyclohexene-1,2-dicarboximide [133-06-2] (Captan) was recommended as degerming agent for incorporation in liquid or bar soap (73).

Iodine.   Although bromine is of little significance as an antibacterial agent, iodine [7553-56-2] has held and even expanded its position, especially in the field of antisepsis. Like chlorine, iodine is a highly reactive substance combining with proteins partly by chemical reaction and partly by adsorption. Therefore its antimicrobial action is subject to substantial impairment in the presence of organic matter such as serum, blood, urine, milk, etc. However, where there is no such interference, nonselective microbicidal action is intense and rapid.

A saturated aqueous solution of iodine exhibits antibacterial properties. However, owing to the low solubility of iodine in water (33 mg/100 mL at 25°C), reaction with bacteria or with extraneous organic matter rapidly depletes the solution of its active content.

Iodide ion is often added to increase solubility of iodine in water. This increase takes place by the formation of triiodide, $I_2 + I^- = I_3^-$. An aqueous solution of iodine and iodide at a pH of less than 8 contains mainly free diatomic iodine I_2 and the triiodide [14900-04-0] I_3^-. Their ratio depends upon the concentration of iodide.

A quantitative investigation of the relative bactericidal activities of diatomic iodine and triiodide revealed a negligible effect of the latter upon the test organisms *Staphylococcus aureus* and *Escherichia coli* (74). Similar findings were reported for their sporicidal performance (75).

As a bactericidal antiseptic, iodine is used most frequently in the form of a 2% tincture. Stronger iodine preparations are employed occasionally, for example for preoperative antisepsis. The degerming capacity of iodine tinctures of different concentrations are compared to those of organomercuric and quaternary ammonium antiseptics by the serial basin test (76). The results of this test indicate that the iodine tinctures, within the range of 2–7% of iodine, can reduce the bacterial count of the skin by 97.5–100%; in this respect they appear to be markedly superior to the other antiseptics tested.

Because of the tuberculocidal action of iodine, its solutions are suitable for the disinfection of clinical thermometers (77–78) and for emergency sterilization of surgical appliances (79). Other uses include the sanitization of eating and drinking utensils (80) and the emergency treatment of contaminated drinking water (81–83). In most natural waters, 8 ppm of iodine will reduce a count of one million enteric bacteria per milliliter to less than 5/100 mL within 10 min. The same dosage of iodine will destroy thirty cysts of *Endamoeba histolytica* per milliliter in the same period of time.

Heliogen [127-65-1] contains potassium iodide [7681-11-0] and chloramine-T; free (diatomic) iodine is released upon addition of water (84).

Iodophors are combinations of iodine with suitable solubilizing organic compounds (usually nonionic surfactants) (41,85). Their effectiveness is caused primarily by the free, or the available iodine they contain (86).

Several disinfectant, antiseptic, and sanitizing agents have been formulated on the iodophor principle (63,87–89), among them Wescodyne, Iosan, and Iobac (all products of West Chemical Products, Inc.) (90).

An important solubilizing agent and carrier for iodine is polyvinylpyrrolidinone (PVP). Povidone–iodine (PVP–iodine), to be used externally on humans as an antiseptic, is marketed as Betadine and Isodine (The Purdue-Frederick Co.); other products are commercially available. The history of PVP–iodine, its toxicity and therapeutic uses have been described (91). PVP–iodine has been recommended as a topical antiseptic (92).

Iodine can also be solubilized by quaternary ammonium compounds with formation of complexes said to be nonirritating to the skin and mucous membranes (93–94). In contrast to the complexes produced with nonionic surfactants, those obtained with the cationic ammonium compounds are claimed to have all of their iodine available for antibacterial action. Surprisingly, such complexes do not precipitate with anionic surfactants, even when the original quaternary ammonium compounds would have reacted in such a manner; moreover, the bactericidal action of the iodine–quaternary complex is not abolished in the presence of the anionic surfactant (95–96).

Bisglycine hydriodide–iodine [69943-48-2], $(HO_2CCH_2NH_2)_2.2HI.I_2$ (Bursoline), contains 30.5–32.0% active iodine. It is used mostly for the disinfection of drinking water, reducing a count of 100 million of enteric pathogens per 100 mL of water to an average of 1–5 organisms per 100 mL in 5 min at normal temperatures.

Some other water-disinfecting preparations contain tetraglycine hydroperiodide [7097-60-1] (Globaline), potassium tetraglycine triiodide [55115-56-5] (Potadine), aluminum hexaurea sulfate triiodide [15304-14-0] (Hexadine-*S*), and aluminum hexaurea dinitrate triiodide [69943-58-4] (Hexadine-*N*) as active ingredients.

Organic Iodine Compounds. Iodoform [75-47-8], CHI_3, enjoyed considerable favor as an antiseptic wound powder for a long time; today its use is rather limited. Iodol (2,3,4,5-tetraiodopyrrole) [87-58-1] is still used.

Aristol consists mostly of dithymol diiodide [552-22-7], in addition to other iodine compounds. It formerly served as a substitute for iodoform because it is free from odor.

Iodonium 235 is bis(p-chlorophenyl) iodonium chloride [34220-01-4]. In a suitable detergent base, it provides satisfactory degerming action because of its bacteriostatic effect upon both gram-negative and gram-positive microorganisms (97). It is ten times more inhibitory for *Salmonella typhosa* and 100 times more so for *Staphylococcus aureus* than for *Pseudomonas aeruginosa*.

Metals, Their Salts and Other Compounds

Inorganic Mercurials.   Mercuric chloride [7487-94-7] (bichloride of mercury, $HgCl_2$) is one of the earliest antibacterial agents known. It was studied and credited by R. Koch with exceptional bactericidal and sporicidal potency. Only several years later did Geppert recognize the antibacterial action of mercuric chloride as primarily inhibitory rather than bactericidal in character, by observing that anthrax spores retained their infectiousness following exposure to mercuric chloride even though they did not germinate when subcultured. Moreover, he showed that ammonium sulfide eliminated the inhibitory effect of mercury with the result that a 0.1% solution of mercuric chloride was incapable of killing anthrax spores in 24 h. Similar findings were made subsequently with other pathogens such as *Streptococci* (98), *Staphylococci* (99), *Coli bacilli* (100), and influenza virus (101).

Organic Mercurials.   Organic mercurials are mainly used as antiseptics rather than disinfectants. Here the mercury is linked directly with carbon and is not released in solution as an ion. If ionization takes place, organomercuric ions, RHg^+, are formed. Although the literature is replete with references to the antibacterial action of organic mercurials, most of the published information lacks the clear distinction between bacteriostatic and bactericidal action of the compounds studied. Pathogenic microorganisms in a state of bacteriostasis induced by organomercurials may continue to be infectious for the animal body (4,6,98,102). *In vitro* blood can reverse the action of inorganic and organic mercurials often after prolonged contact with the bacteria (7,103–104).

The inactivation of bacteria by mercurials may be caused by a blocking of cellular enzymatic thiol reception by formation of mercaptide bonds and without any other demonstrable cell injury (105–108). Because the mercaptides formed are dissociable, as a rule, the inhibition of enzyme activity by mercury compounds is reversible. The two reactions involved are illustrated below for a mercuric salt:

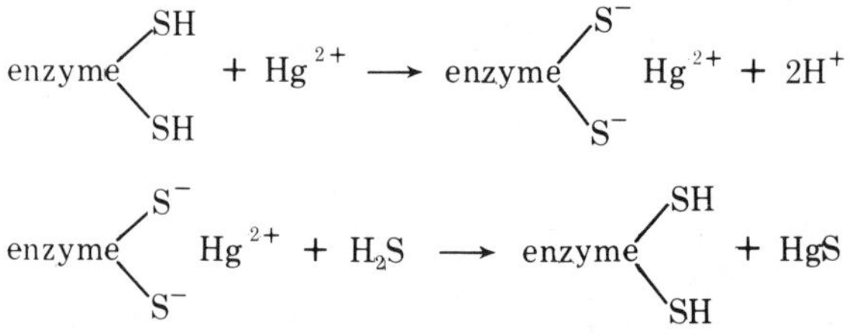

$$\text{enzyme}\begin{array}{c}\diagup\text{SH}\\\diagdown\text{SH}\end{array} + Hg^{2+} \longrightarrow \text{enzyme}\begin{array}{c}\diagup\text{S}^-\\\diagdown\text{S}^-\end{array}Hg^{2+} + 2H^+$$

$$\text{enzyme}\begin{array}{c}\diagup\text{S}^-\\\diagdown\text{S}^-\end{array}Hg^{2+} + H_2S \longrightarrow \text{enzyme}\begin{array}{c}\diagup\text{SH}\\\diagdown\text{SH}\end{array} + HgS$$

Over a period of time, a number of organic mercurials have been adopted for antiseptic usage. Some of the more important ones are listed in Table 3.

Many reports on the *in vitro* antiseptic performance of the aqueous organomer-

Table 3. Organic Mercurials Used as Antiseptics

Chemical name	CAS Registry Number	Nonproprietary name	Proprietary name
phenylmercuric nitrate	[55-68-5]	phenylmercuric nitrate	Merphenyl nitrate, Merphene (Hamilton)
2,7-dibromo-4-hydroxymercuri-fluorescein, sodium salt	[129-16-8]	merbromin	Mercurochrome (Hynson)
4-nitro-3-hydroxymercuri-o-cresol anhydride	[133-58-4]	nitromersol	Metaphen (Abbott)
sodium ethylmercurithiosalicylate	[54-64-8]	thimerosal	Merthiolate (Lilly)
o-hydroxyphenylmercuric chloride	[90-03-9]		Mercarbolide
acetoxymercuri-2-ethylhexylphenol-sulfonate	[1301-13-9]		Mertoxol
sec-amyl tricresols and o-hydroxy-phenylmercuric chloride	[8063-33-0]	mercocresol	Mercresin (Upjohn)
2-acetoxymercuri-4-(1,1,3,3-tetra-methylbutyl)phenol	[584-18-9]	acetomeroctol	Merbak (Schieffelin)
2,4-dihydroxy-3,5-dihydroxymercuri-benzophenone-2'-sulfonate, sodium salt	[6060-47-5]		

curials are controversial. More consistent results are obtained with tinctures. The solvent usually employed is a mixture of alcohol 50 parts, acetone 10 parts, and water qs 100 parts. However, this solvent alone exhibits significant antibacterial potency against *Staphylococcus aureus*. The usefulness of organomercurials for preoperative application has been considered on several occasions.

Elkhouly and Yousef (109) made a detailed study, using *Staphylococcus aureus* and *Pseudomonas aeruginosa*, of the antibacterial efficacy of mercuric chloride, thimerosal, and three salts of phenylmercury. Against *S. aureus* the organic mercurials are much more active than mercuric chloride; there is no significant difference in regard to *Ps. aeruginosa*.

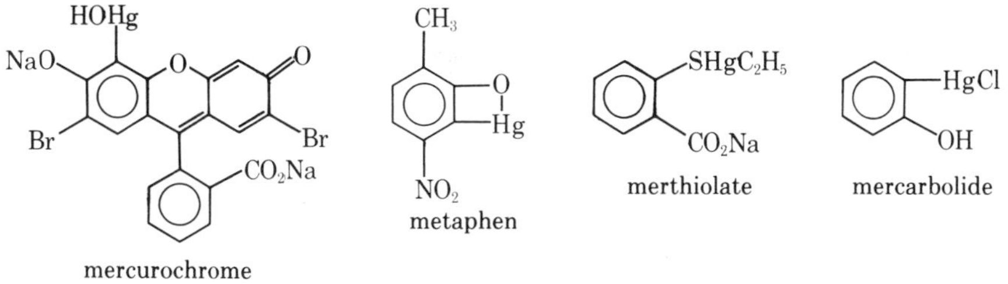

mercurochrome   metaphen   merthiolate   mercarbolide

Silver Compounds. Silver [7440-22-4] both free and in salts produces antimicrobial effects. Colloidal dispersions of metallic silver display oligodynamic action owing to the formation of silver ions which are adsorbed by the bacterial cell with cytotoxic results. Even insoluble silver chloride [7783-90-6] and silver iodide [7783-96-2] show some antibacterial action when dispersed in colloidal form and applied in fairly high concentrations (110).

The dependence of the degree of antibacterial action upon the number of free silver ions present is illustrated by the comparatively high effectiveness of silver nitrate [7761-88-8] as against the low value of an ammoniacal silver complex. Silver nitrate is still used occasionally for routine prophylactic instillation into the eyes of newborn infants, although it has been displaced largely by other more effective and less irritant antimicrobial agents, especially penicillin. Dressings with 0.5% silver nitrate solution were found useful to protect against gram-negative infections in burns (111). Silver sulfadiazine [21548-73-2] is a nonionized water-insoluble powder; it shows an excellent antibacterial spectrum and high potency (112–113). As a 1% cream, it is used in burns for the prevention of bacterial infection.

Several colloidal silver preparations continue in moderate use; they may contain, in addition to the colloidal metal, silver oxide [20667-12-3] or insoluble silver-protein reaction products in colloidal form. Colloidal silver iodide is listed in the *National Formulary* (NF), as are two colloidal silver-protein preparations.

Introduced in 1928, Katadyn Silver consisted originally of metallic silver in spongy form with an added activating metal, such as gold or palladium, which is below silver in the electromotive series. When deposited on filter elements, on sand, etc, Katadyn Silver slowly but continuously reduces the bacterial count of *Escherichia coli*, eg, from 500,000 to 0 within several hours. More intensive antibacterial performance is delivered by the Electro-Katadyn process which has been recommended for the purification of water in swimming pools (see Water). It operates by means of a battery of silver plates with a direct current induced across them (114). Unfortunately, some important pathogens, including *Staphylococci*, appear to resist the action of ionic silver. A more recent modification of Katadyn is Movidyn; it is claimed to possess a wider bactericidal spectrum which includes staphylocidal action (115).

Other Metals and Their Compounds.   Metals and compounds other than those of mercury and silver are of lesser importance as antibacterial agents. Several salts of heavy metals are bactericidal under the conditions of the FDA method (116); Table 4 indicates the minimum concentrations that kill *Salmonella typhosa* and *Staphylococcus aureus* in 10 min.

Mixed oxidized and reduced salts, such as ferric and ferrous chlorides or stannic and stannous chlorides, are more active as bactericidal agents than the oxidized or

Table 4.   Minimum Germicidal Concentrations of Metal Salts (10 min)

Salt	CAS Registry Number	*Salmonella typhosa*	*Staphylococcus aureus*
$ZnCl_2$	[7646-85-7]	1:8	
ZnI_2	[10139-47-6]	1:30	1:10
$Zn(C_2H_3O_2)_2.2H_2O$	[5970-45-6]	1:3	
$ZnSO_4.7H_2O$	[7446-20-0]	1:3	
$NiCl_2.6H_2O$	[7791-20-0]	1:5	1:3
$Ni(NO_3)_2.6H_2O$	[13478-00-7]	1:3	1:3
$CoCl_2.6H_2O$	[7791-13-1]	1:20	1:6
$Co(NO_3)_2$	[14216-74-1]	1:5	1:5
$CoCl_2.2H_2O$	[16544-72-6]	1:300	1:7
$Co(NO_3)_2.6H_2O$	[10026-22-9]	1:50	1:6
$Pb(NO_3)_2$	[18256-98-7]	1:3	
$Pb(C_2H_3O_2)_2.3H_2O$	[10025-69-1]	1:3	
$SnCl_2.2H_2O$	[10025-77-1]	1:350	1:70
$FeCl_3.6H_2O$	[16547-58-3]	1:200	1:10
$Fe_2(SO_4)_3$	[10028-22-5]	1:500	1:30

reduced salts applied individually (117). Substantial enhancement of the germicidal action of such antiseptics as iodine, phenol, cresol [1319-77-3], hexylresorcinol [136-77-6] is observed in the presence of such oxidation-reduction systems.

The germicidal action of the chlorides of several rare earth metals (Y, La, Ce, Pr, Nd, Sm, Eu, and Yb) increases generally with increasing atomic weight of the cation (118), except in the case of yttrium chloride [10361-92-9] which is more effective than the chlorides of the other rare earth metals in spite of its lower atomic weight. Of all the rare earth chlorides only ytterbium chloride [10361-91-8] is more bactericidal than copper sulfate [7758-98-7].

Peroxides and Other Oxidants

The antibacterial potency of some representatives of this group depends primarily upon the reactivity of free OH radicals. Although different microorganisms vary considerably in their susceptibility to oxidizing agents, the obligate anaerobic bacteria are most sensitive to oxidation. Of these, the species capable of forming hydrogen peroxide metabolically, but incapable of producing catalase to decompose it, are damaged and eventually killed by exposure to molecular oxygen (see Peroxides).

Hydrogen peroxide (qv) is used as an antiseptic in a 3% solution; concentrates of 30% or stronger are corrosive to skin and denuded tissue. Hydrogen peroxide solutions, containing as little as 0.1 and 0.25% H_2O_2, kill *Salmonella typhosa*, *Escherichia coli*, and *Staphylococcus aureus* in 1 h but not in 5 min (119). Addition of ferric or cupric ions, potassium dichromate [7778-50-9], cobaltous sulfate, or manganous sulfate (120), enhances the bactericidal action of hydrogen peroxide.

Synergism between ultrasonic waves and hydrogen peroxide in the killing of microorganisms has been reported (121) (see Ultrasonics).

With urea, hydrogen peroxide forms a solid compound capable of yielding over 35% of H_2O_2. A solution of this substance in anhydrous glycerol and stabilized with 8-hydroxyquinoline has been found effective in the treatment of certain eye and ear infections.

Zinc peroxide [1314-22-3], as used for medical purposes, consists of a mixture of this chemical with zinc carbonate [3486-35-9] and zinc hydroxide [20427-58-1]. Especially effective against anaerobic and microaerophilic bacteria (122), it is applied in the treatment of wound infections in the form of a thick suspension, diluted with talc in a dusting powder, or incorporated in an ointment vehicle.

Benzoyl peroxide [94-36-0], applied as an antiseptic dressing, is said to be particularly useful in treating wounds infected with gas-forming anaerobes (123). Peracetic acid [79-21-0] has been used both in aqueous solution and as an aerosol or vapor in germ-free or gnotobiotic research (124–125).

Potassium permanganate [7722-64-7] is no longer used for disinfection of drinking water because of the toxicity of the manganese residue. Different bacteria vary greatly in their resistance to permanganate and other oxidizing agents (126). Thus, *Staphylococcus aureus* and *Proteus vulgaris* are killed in 1 h by a dilution of 1:4000, whereas *Escherichia coli* is killed by 1:16,000 and *Pseudomonas aeruginosa* by 1:64,000 in the same period of time.

Ozone [10028-15-6] (qv) is actively germicidal in the presence of moisture (127). It has been used mainly for the disinfection of water in swimming pools, but chlorine is cheaper for this purpose. The ozone generators introduced for the purification of air do not provide efficient means of control of airborne pathogens; moreover, they may create a toxicological hazard.

Phenolic Compounds

As a disinfectant or antiseptic, phenol (carbolic acid) is mostly of historical interest; however, its extensive use continues in both investigative and analytical microbiology, eg, as in the AOAC phenol coefficient and use-dilution methods described above.

The bactericidal effectiveness of several phenol derivatives has been correlated with their respective partition ratios between oil and water; a high lipophilic character has been found to be associated with greater antibacterial activity (128–129). However, the surface activity of the phenol derivatives plays an important part in their total antibacterial performance by altering the permeability of the cell wall. In this respect their behavior resembles that of other antibacterial surfactants.

There are probably several steps involved in the mode of the antibacterial action of phenol, beginning with adsorption upon the bacterial cell, going through the inactivation of certain essential enzymes, and terminating with lysis and death of the cell. The distinctiveness of these steps depends upon the concentration of phenol present. In high concentrations, phenol acts as a gross protoplasmic poison, rapidly penetrating and rupturing the cell wall. Low concentrations act by causing the leakage of such cell constituents as glutamic acid and other metabolites (130–132) and inactivation of specific enzyme systems. Increased permeability is shown by enhanced penetration of certain dyes (133), and by a release of radioactivity from cells (*Escherichia coli*) incubated with carbon 14-labeled glutamate (134).

A 0.1% solution of phenol destroys the enzyme systems of *Staphylococcus aureus* that activate succinate, fumarate, pyruvate, and glutamate; the lactate, formate, glucose, and butanol systems suffer partial inactivation (135). In *Escherichia coli,* with sodium acetate providing the only source of energy in a synthetic medium, phenol at the retarding concentration of 0.075%, had little damaging effect upon dehydrogenase, oxidase, or catalase activity. At the inhibitory concentration of 0.15%, it inactivated oxidase but not dehydrogenase. At the lethal concentration of 1.2% both oxidase and dehydrogenase virtually ceased to function whereas catalase was inhibited only partially (136).

The effects of lethal and sublethal concentrations of phenol are irreversible by dilution with water. Moreover, unlike inhibitory agents such as sulfanilamide or bacteriostatic dyes, it was not possible to train or adapt microorganisms to grow in the inhibitory concentrations of several phenol derivatives. This is accepted as evidence that the phenols exert their bactericidal effect by a nonspecific mechanism (137–138). Certain phenol homologues, particularly those of higher molecular weight, display a selective (quasispecific) efficacy against different bacterial categories (139).

Coal Tar Disinfectants.   Until recently, coal tar disinfectants constituted the most important category of disinfectants for environmental use. From raw materials obtained by distillation of coal tar, two groups of products, ie, the soluble and the emulsifiable types are produced. The soluble coal tar disinfectants are formulated with tar acids consisting essentially of low molecular weight phenol homologues (cresols, xylenols). The emulsifiable disinfectants are formulated with coal-tar fractions containing varying proportions of neutral oil, which consists mostly of methyl- and dimethylnaphthalenes and other hydrocarbons, organic bases, sulfur compounds, etc, in addition to phenol derivatives.

Technical cresol [1319-77-3], consisting of the three cresol isomers, is only slightly soluble in water; however, when combined with a soap in suitable proportions, it becomes completely and rapidly miscible, forming clear solutions in distilled or demineralized water. This principle is applied in preparing saponated cresol solution which contains 46–52% of cresol rendered soluble by means of a potassium or sodium soap.

Different soaps, including resin soaps, are used to formulate emulsifiable disinfectants which are characterized by the milky appearance of their dilutions. Because of the crude, unrefined character of the coal-tar fractions entering into their composition, these disinfectants emit a rather pungent, disagreeable odor (see Soap).

Phenol Homologues. In a homologous series of monoalkyl phenol derivatives, certain regularities are found in the dependence of bactericidal action upon chemical constitution (see Alkylphenols). As shown in Table 5, the potency against all four test organisms increases with the increase in molecular weight until the n-amyl derivative is reached. Further increase in molecular weight engenders a substantial increase of germicidal potency against three of the microorganisms, and a decline with respect to *Salmonella typhosa*. The term quasispecific has been proposed to describe the action of a disinfectant such as n-heptylphenol which is extremely effective against *Staphylococcus aureus*, but only slightly so against *Salmonella typhosa* (139).

The homologous series of alkylchlorophenol derivatives show a regularity like that of the phenol derivatives. The regularities noted in the series of o- [95-57-8] and p-chlorophenol [106-48-9] and o- [95-56-7] and p-bromophenol [106-41-2] derivatives (139–140) are as follows:

(1) Halogen substitution intensifies the microbicidal potency of phenol derivatives; halogen in the para position to the hydroxyl group is more effective than in the ortho position. (2) Introduction of aliphatic or aromatic groups into the aromatic

Table 5.   Microbicidal Action of Phenol Derivatives (Phenol Coefficients, 37°C)

Substituting radical	CAS Registry No.	Salmonella typhosa	Staphylococcus aureus	Mycobacterium tuberculosis	Candida albicans
none	[108-95-7]	1.0	1.0	1.0	1.0
2-methyl	[95-48-7]	2.3	2.3	2.0	2.0
3-methyl	[108-39-4]	2.3	2.3	2.0	2.0
4-methyl	[106-44-5]	2.3	2.3	2.0	2.0
4-ethyl	[123-07-9]	6.3	6.3	6.7	7.8
2,4-dimethyl	[105-67-9]	5.0	4.4	4.0	5.0
2,5-dimethyl	[95-87-4]	5.0	4.4	4.0	4.0
3,4-dimethyl	[95-65-8]	5.0	3.8	4.0	4.0
2,6-dimethyl	[576-26-1]	3.8	4.4	4.0	3.5
4-n-propyl	[645-56-7]	18.3	16.3	17.8	17.8
4-n-butyl	[99-71-8]	46.7	43.7	44.4	44.4
4-n-amyl	[1322-06-1]	53.3	125.0	133.0	156.0
4-t-amyl	[80-46-6]	30.0	93.8	111.1	100.0
4-n-hexyl	[61902-50-9]	33.3	313.0	389.0	333.0
4-n-heptyl	[26997-02-4]	16.7[a]	625.0	667.0	556.0

[a] Approximate figure.

nucleus of halogenated phenols increases the bactericidal potency up to certain limits, depending in the case of alkyl substitution upon the number of carbon atoms present in the substituting group or groups. (3) A normal aliphatic chain with a given number of carbon atoms generally exerts a greater intensifying effect upon the bactericidal potency than that of a branched chain or of two alkyl groups with the same total number of carbon atoms. (4) o-Alkyl derivatives of p-chlorophenol are more actively germicidal than the corresponding p-alkyl derivatives of o-chlorophenol.

In the case of the higher homologues, the germicidal action manifests the quasispecific character referred to before, as illustrated in Figure 1 which relates to the homologous series of o-alkyl derivatives of p-chlorophenol. Many instances of the same effect have been established also in the group of polyalkyl-, and of aryl- and aralkylchlorophenol derivatives (see also Chlorocarbons).

It is significant that the increase in molecular weight that accompanies the increase in the antimicrobial potential is also accompanied by a decrease in toxicity to animals (mice). Table 6 illustrates this condition for the three homologous series of alkyl derivatives of phenol, p-chlorophenol, and o-chlorophenol.

Several synthetic phenol derivatives have found use as disinfectants or antiseptics. 3,5-Dimethyl-4-chlorophenol [88-04-0] is used in Liquor Chloroxylenolis of the British Pharmacopoeia. p-Chloro-o-benzylphenol [120-32-1] is widely used as an ingredient of disinfectant formulas. o-Phenylphenol [90-43-7] plus xylenols or pine oil is present

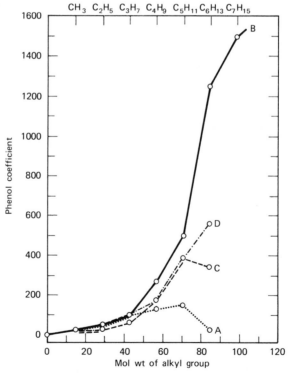

Figure 1.   The quasispecific effect in the homologous series of o-alkyl-p-chlorophenol derivatives. A = *Salmonella typhosa;* B = *Staphylococcus aureus;* C = *Mycobacterium tuberculosis;* and D = *Candida albicans.*

Table 6.   Toxicological Data for Phenols, mg/g, on Subcutaneous Injection in Mice

	p-Alkyl derivatives of phenol	o-Alkyl derivatives of p-chlorophenol	p-Alkyl derivatives of o-chlorophenol
phenol	0.45		
p-chlorophenol		0.6	
o-chlorophenol			0.7
methyl	0.5	2.0	1.5
ethyl	1.0	4.0	4.0
n-propyl	2.0	6.0	6.0
n-butyl	3.0	15.0	15.0
n-amyl	5.0	>20.0	20.0
n-hexyl	6.0	>20.0	>20.0
n-heptyl	10.0	>20.0	>20.0

in two versions of Lysol (Lehn & Fink); with p-tert-amylphenol [80-46-6] it is used in the composition of Amphyl (Lehn & Fink).

Properly formulated phenolic disinfectants are capable of yielding nonspecific or broad-spectrum microbicidal performance. These disinfectants offer considerable advantage over products such as the soap-containing solution of cresol in that they are virtually free of toxicity and corrosiveness to tissue; moreover, they are practically odorless when diluted for use.

Thymol [89-83-8], carvacrol [499-75-2], chlorothymol [89-68-9], and chlorocarvacrol [5665-94-1] have been used for antiseptic and disinfectant purposes (see Terpenoids), whereas polyhalogenophenol derivatives such as trichloro- or pentachlorophenol are useful as fungicides (qv).

A high phenol coefficient need not indicate the exceptional fitness of a given phenol derivative for all practical uses, particularly if protein is present to a significant degree. The microbicidal performance of phenol derivatives with high phenol coefficients is impaired by serum to a greater extent than that of analogues with low phenol coefficients. Some of these variables can be equalized, for practical screening purposes, by confirmatory testing methods, such as the AOAC use-dilution tests and the pertinent validation procedures (141).

Dihydric and Trihydric Phenols.   Although resorcinol [108-46-3] is a comparatively weak bactericide, several of its nuclear-substituted alkyl derivatives are effective microbicidal agents. One of these, n-hexylresorcinol [136-77-6], has gained considerable reputation as a topical antiseptic. The study of the antibacterial properties of resorcinol derivatives dates back to the fundamental work of Johnson and co-workers (142–143) which was extended by others (144–145).

There exists a close quantitative resemblance of the bactericidal properties of the nuclear-substituted resorcinol derivatives and those of the corresponding monoethers. Apparently one free hydroxyl group of the resorcinol derivative is required for initiation of the antibacterial effect, and it matters little to the microbicidal potential whether the substituting radical is attached to an oxygen atom or to the carbon atom in the positions ortho–para to the two hydroxyl groups. The phenomenon of quasispecificity occurs in both series of resorcinol derivatives, as exemplified by the two n-octyl derivatives, 4-(n-octyl)resorcinol [6565-70-4] and 3-(n-octyloxy)phenol [34380-89-7], which combine high potency against Staphylococcus aureus with virtual impotence against Salmonella typhosa (146).

In the homologous series of alkyl monoethers of hydroquinone and catechol (47), a number of effective antibacterial agents have been found, some of which exhibit quasispecific character. However, they are less effective than the corresponding resorcinol monoethers. The same is true for several aromatic monoethers.

Several nuclear dialkylresorcinol derivatives have been studied bacteriologically (147). Although 4,6-diethylresorcinol [52959-32-7], with a phenol coefficient of 10, compared closely to the isomeric 4-n-butylresorcinol [18979-61-8] with a phenol coefficient of 8, the 4,6-di-n-propylresorcinol [69943-49-3] was less effective than the corresponding 4-n-hexylresorcinol [136-77-6], the phenol coefficients being 18 and 45, respectively.

As with alkylphenols, chlorine substitution in the nucleus of the alkylresorcinols intensifies the antibacterial potential, especially against *Staphylococcus aureus* (148–150). As with the higher alkylphenols and alkylchlorophenols, organic matter or soaps markedly depress the antibacterial performance of the higher alkylresorcinols (145).

2,4,4′-Trichloro-2′-hydroxydiphenyl ether [66943-50-6] (Irgasan DP300, Ciba-Geigy, S. A.) shows good activity against gram-positive and gram-negative microorganisms, also against yeasts (qv) and fungi. It had been recommended as an additive for soaps and washing products (151). A broad-spectrum soap contains a mixture of hexachlorophene (see below), triclocarban [101-20-2], and Irgasan DP300 (152).

Hydroxybenzoic Acids. The antibacterial and antifungal properties of the hydroxybenzoic acids depend primarily upon the reactivity of their phenolic hydroxy group. It is masked by intramolecular hydrogen bonding in o-hydroxybenzoic (salicylic) acid which is unimportant as an antimicrobial agent (see Salicylic acid and related compounds). On the other hand, salicylanilides with halogens as substituents have commercial use as antimicrobials. One of the first compounds to be employed as a soap additive was 3,3′,4,5′-tetrachlorosalicylanilide [1322-37-8] (Anobial) (73); however, the initial success of this compound did not last when it was found to cause primary photodermatitis; 53 cases of photosensitization by the use of a soap containing tetrachlorosalicylanilide were confirmed (153–155). Brominated salicylanilides, such as 4,5′-dibromosalicylanilide [87-12-7] (158), 3,5-dibromo-3′-trifluoromethyl salicylanilide [4776-06-1] (fluorosalan) (157), and 3,4,5′-tribromosalicylanilide [87-10-5] (tribromsalan) (158–159) were also found to be photosensitizers (154) and withdrawn from use in soaps and cosmetics.

p-Hydroxybenzoate esters (parabens) play an important role in the preservation of different perishable organic materials against attack and destruction by airborne bacteria, fungi, and yeasts. Among the materials requiring such preservation are those based upon carbohydrates, gums, and proteins, and their many industrial, pharmaceutical, and cosmetic combinations with fats, oils, waxes, surfactants, etc.

The inhibitory capacity of the methyl [99-76-3], ethyl [120-47-8], propyl [94-13-3], and butyl p-hydroxybenzoates [94-26-8] is shown in Table 7 (160–161). The low order of toxicity of these esters (162–163), their lack of irritation, and their absorption and excretion characteristics both in men and animals indicate that the compounds approximate the ideal for a pharmaceutical preservative (164–166). Their application in antimycotic therapy has been considered by several investigators (167).

Bacteriological information on the activity of substituted salicylic and hydroxynaphthoic acids is also available (168).

Table 7. Percentage Inhibition of Bacterial and Fungal Growth by Esters of *p*-Hydroxybenzoic Acid

Microorganism	Methyl	Ethyl	Propyl	Butyl
Salmonella typhosa	0.2	0.1	0.1	0.1
Escherichia coli	0.4	0.1	0.1	0.4
Staphylococcus aureus	0.4	0.1	0.05	0.0125
Proteus vulgaris	0.2	0.1	0.05	0.05
Pseudomonas aeruginosa	0.4	0.4	0.8	0.8
Aspergillus niger	0.1	0.04	0.02	0.02
Rhizopus nigricans	0.05	0.025	0.0125	0.00625
Chaetomium globosum	0.05	0.025	0.00625	0.003125
Trichophyton interdigitale	0.008	0.008	0.004	0.002
Candida albicans	0.1	0.1	0.0125	0.0125
Saccharomyces cerevisiae	0.1	0.05	0.0125	0.00625

Bis(Hydroxyphenyl) Alkanes. Dichlorophene (G-4, Givaudan Corporation) is 2,2'-methylenebis(4-chlorophenol) [*97-23-4*]. Although this compound is active against bacteria, its special merit lies in the mildew proofing of textiles (see Textiles).

The most important member of the series is 2,2'-methylenebis(3,4,6-trichlorophenol) [*70-30-4*], also named bis(3,5,6-trichloro-2-hydroxyphenyl)methane (hexachlorophene, G-11, Givaudan Corporation) (169). It has found extensive use as an antibacterial soap additive as it does not lose activity in presence of soap, as most phenolic compounds do. Such soaps are able to reduce the bacterial skin flora to a small fraction of the original (170–171). Hexachlorophene has also been incorporated in soapless detergent bases (pHisoHex, Winthrop Laboratories, and other preparations). Such combinations of hexachlorophene and detergent or soaps are used for surgical scrub, in nurseries to prevent the spread of staphylococcal infections, and for other therapeutic purposes. Hexachlorophene acts as an inhibitory and slow germicidal agent since it is retained in very small quantities by skin that is repeatedly washed with a soap or detergent containing it (172). Extremely low amounts of hexachlorophene suffice to produce inhibition of *Staphylococcus aureus,* eg, dilutions from $1:10^6$ to $1:5 \times 10^6$, depending on the size of the inoculum (172–173). Hexachlorophene is considerably less active against *Escherichia coli;* the bacteriostatic concentration is in the range of 1:10,000 to 1:50,000 (174).

The action of hexachlorophene is reversed upon contact with blood; this is deemed significant for any prophylactic application to the broken skin against infection in injury, or for preoperative use. Skin that has been "degermed" with hexachlorophene is not proof against subsequent contamination with transient pathogens or against lesions of bacterial origin (174–175).

Hexachlorophene has been used successfully in deodorant soaps and cosmetics; here it controls the proliferation of cutaneous bacteria that cause perspiration malodor by decomposition of apocrine sweat (176) (see Soap; Cosmetics).

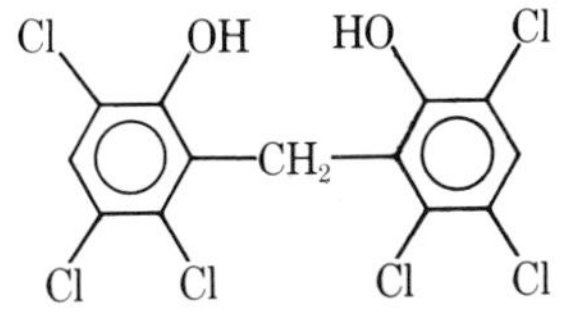

hexachlorophene

Although the extensive use of hexachlorophene over the years has not shown toxic symptoms in humans (177–178), neurotoxicity has been demonstrated in rats with large doses (179–180), also in monkeys (181) and in premature infants (182). In view of these findings, the FDA (183) banned the over-the-counter sale of soaps, cosmetics, and drugs containing an amount of hexachlorophene exceeding 0.1%. All products with a higher percentage were put on a prescription basis.

Bacteriological data for hexachlorophene and its isomers (184) are presented in Table 8. A series of 2,2'-methylenebis(dichlorophenols) has also been described (185).

Although 2,2'-thiobis (4,6-dichlorophenol) [97-18-7], bithionol, is not a substituted diphenylalkane, it is structurally and functionally related to hexachlorophene. Like hexachlorophene, it shows a greater inhibitory effect upon *Staphylococcus aureus* than upon *Salmonella typhosa*, the respective concentrations being 1:10^6 and 1:10^3

Table 8.   Antimicrobial Activity of Methylenebis (Trichlorophenol) Isomers[a]

Organism	Inhibitory concentration, µg/mL (geometric mean, $n = 3$) isomers[b]							
	A	B	C	D	E	F	G	H
S. aureus	0.93	0.61	0.39	10	2.5	20	1.56	25
S. epidermidis	0.93	0.78	0.23	12.5	2.4	20	1.56	25
B. subtilis	0.19	0.39	0.19	3.9	1.9	9.9	1.56	15.6
B. ammoniagenes	0.39	0.48	0.19	15.6	2.4	40	1.56	31.5
P. vulgaris	3.9	1.9	3.9	25	c	63	10	63
E. coli	25	c	12.5	c	c	c	c	c
S. typhosa	40	c	10	c	c	c	c	c
Ps. aeruginosa	25	c	50	c	c	c	c	c
Ps. fluorescens	0.23	0.61	0.19	12.5	2.4	31.5	1.56	25
Sh. sonnei	40	c	9.9	c	c	c	c	c
K. pneumoniae	50	c	15.6	c	c	c	c	c
T. mentagrophytes	1.74	3.12	3.12	8.9	8.9	6.25	4.4	6.25
T. rubrum	4.4	3.12	8.9	8.9	3.1	1.56	1.74	9.9
M. audouini	3.12	1.74	3.12	3.12	4.4	3.12	8.9	4.4
C. albicans	c	c	c	c	c	c	c	c
Cl. tetani	0.19	0.39	0.09	1.56	0.27	1.74	0.19	4.4
Cl. perfringens	0.78	0.39	0.55	1.74	0.55	6.25	0.39	6.25
Cl. sporogenes	0.78	0.55	0.55	1.56	0.55	6.25	0.55	6.25
C. vulgaris	3.12	4.4	8.9	c	c	17.8	4.4	17.8

[a] Ref. 186.

[b] A 2,2'-methylenebis(3,4,6-trichlorophenol) [70-30-4], B 2,2'-methylenebis(4,5,6-trichlorophenol) [584-57-6], C 2,2'-methylenebis(3,4,5-trichlorophenol) [584-33-8], D 3,3'-methylenebis(2,4,6-trichlorophenol) [584-32-7], E 3,3'-methylenebis(2,4,5-trichlorophenol) [70495-29-3], F 3,3'-methylenebis(2,5,6-trichlorophenol) [70495-30-6], G 3,3'-methylenebis(4,5,6-trichlorophenol) [70495-31-7], H 4,4'-methylenebis(2,3,6-trichlorophenol) [70495-32-8].

[c] Denotes growth at 100 µg/mL.

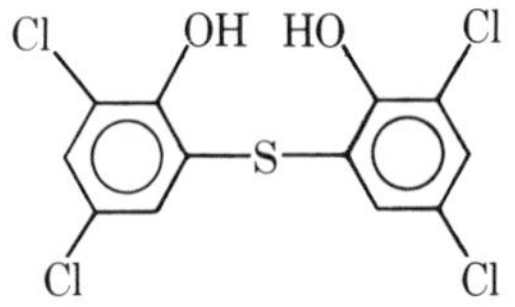

bithionol

(187). It has been used as a soap additive (188) and for other purposes (189), but such use was discontinued when it showed photosensitivity in humans (190). In a series of eight thiobisphenols tested against *Trichophyton gypseum,* it exhibited the greatest fungistatic potency (191).

The antibacterial action of hexachlorophene and bithionol may be associated with their capacity to inactivate iron-containing enzyme systems of the microbial cell since iron and other metals are chelated by either compound (192).

Bacteriologic information is available for other bis(hydroxyphenyl)methane and sulfide derivatives (193–194) as well as for a number of bis(hydroxyphenyl)alkanes in which the two benzene rings are linked by aliphatic chains of greater length (129,195–196).

8-Hydroxyquinoline and Derivatives. Of the seven isomeric hydroxyquinolines, only 8-hydroxyquinoline [148-24-3] exhibits an antimicrobial character; this is ascribed to its capacity to chelate metals that constitute an integral part of some essential biological system of the microbial cell (197–199). 8-Hydroxyquinoline (8-quinolinol, oxine) used either by itself or as a salt such as the sulfate (chinosol) [134-31-6] or benzoate [86-75-9], is the active ingredient of several antiseptics whose effect is bacteriostatic and fungistatic rather than microbicidal. Inhibitory action upon gram-positive microorganisms is more pronounced than upon gram-negative ones, as illustrated by the following growth-preventing concentrations: for staphylococci 1: 100,000; for streptococci 1:50,000; for *Salmonella typhosa* and *Escherichia coli* 1: 10,000; for *Salmonella schottmuelleri* 1:5,000 (200–201).

However, 8-acetoxyquinoline [40245-26-9], which has no free hydroxyl group and is therefore incapable of chelation, also shows high antimicrobial activity (202). It is one of a group of 120 quinoline derivatives several of which were found to have comparatively high bacteriostatic potential.

Certain halogen derivatives of 8-hydroxyquinoline have a record of therapeutic efficacy in the treatment of cutaneous fungus infections and also of amebic dysentery. Among them are 5-chloro-7-iodo-8-quinolinol [130-26-7] (iodochlorhydroxyquin, Vioform), 5,7-diiodo-8-hydroxyquinoline [83-73-8] (diiodohydroxyquin), and sodium 7-iodo-8-hydroxyquinoline-5-sulfonate [885-04-1] (chiniofon) (203–205).

The copper compound of 8-hydroxyquinoline (copper 8-quinolinolate) [10380-28-6] is employed as an industrial preservative for a variety of purposes, including the protection of wood and textiles against fungus-caused rotting.

Quaternary Ammonium and Related Compounds

The antibacterial precursor of the quaternary ammonium compound (quat) is the primary aliphatic long-chain ammonium salt. In this category there are potent antibacterial agents that compare in effectiveness with some of the more active quaternary ammonium compounds. The primary ammonium salt may be regarded as the direct counterpart of soap. Both are surface-active substances; In soap, the anion contributes the hydrophobic principle, whereas in the primary ammonium salt the cation is hydrophobic. By way of illustration, the dissociation equations of potassium laurate (a type of soap) and of dodecylammonium chloride [929-73-7] (a type of primary ammonium salt) are given below:

$$C_{11}H_{23}CO_2K \rightarrow (C_{11}H_{23}CO_2)^- + K^+$$
$$C_{12}H_{25}NH_3Cl \rightarrow (C_{12}H_{25}NH_3)^+ + Cl^-$$

It is apparent that the designation invert soap could have been applied more properly to this type of primary ammonium salt although it was originally used for a quaternary ammonium compound (206) (see Ammonium compounds; Surfactants).

The primary long-chain ammonium salts are derived from the weakly basic aliphatic amines. Hence, their aqueous solutions require a pH low enough to counteract hydrolysis and partial liberation of the amine base. By contrast, because the quaternary ammonium compounds are salts of strong bases, they remain in solution in acidic as well as in basic media. Quaternary ammonium salts owe their surface activity and antibacterial quality primarily to the presence of certain aliphatic long-chain amino groups which, by themselves, or rather in the form of their soluble ammonium salts, display surface-active and antibacterial properties, often of a comparable order of magnitude (207–210).

Generally, the long-chain alkylammonium and the quaternary ammonium salts, like other cation-active compounds, are incompatible with soaps or other anion-active materials. Mutual precipitation usually occurs when aqueous solutions of the representatives of the cation-active and anion-active classes are brought into contact, except where the molecular weights of the cations and anions are sufficiently low.

The long-chain aliphatic amines combine readily with alkyl halides, sulfates, etc, to form quaternary ammonium compounds. In view of the advantages of the latter as outlined above, most of the cation-active antibacterials available today consists of quats, although some of the N-alkylammonium salts have also achieved importance.

The first quaternary ammonium compound to be tested for antiseptic activity was obtained by the reaction of hexamethylenetetramine [100-97-0] with chloroacetamidomethanol (211). Subsequently, other quaternary salts of hexamethylenetetramine were prepared and studied (212–213). These compounds are no longer of any practical importance and they bear only a remote structural resemblance to the important classes of modern quaternary ammonium compounds (206,214).

In the germicidal quaternary ammonium salts, at least one of the four organic radicals must be of such character as to impart surface activity to the compound. Since the activity of the members of this class resides in the cation, they are sometimes referred to as cationic germicides although in reality they constitute only a subgroup of the cationic group, the latter comprising "-onium" compounds other than ammonium-based ones.

The quaternary ammonium salts produce bacteriostasis in very high dilutions; this property is associated with the inhibition of certain bacterial enzymes, especially those involved in respiration and glycolysis (215–217). On the other hand, some microorganisms (*Serratia marcescens*, but not *Staphylococcus aureus* and *Escherichia coli*) may be adapted to grow in many times the originally inhibitory concentrations of the quats after a comparatively small number of transfers (218–220).

Although efforts have been made to explain the mode of antimicrobial activity of quats on the basis of inactivation of enzymes (221), their bactericidal effect appears to be owing to their ability to cause release of the bacterial cell content into the surrounding medium (222–224).

Of the numerous quaternary ammonium salts investigated (225), only a comparatively small number have retained importance as antibacterial agents. Among them are: benzalkonium chloride, ie, alkylbenzyldimethylammonium chloride, in which

$$\overset{+}{C_6H_5CH_2N(CH_3)_2R}\ Cl^-$$

benzalkonium chloride

$$(CH_3)_3CCH_2\overset{\displaystyle CH_3}{\underset{\displaystyle CH_3}{\overset{|}{\underset{|}{C}}}}\!\!-\!\!\langle\bigcirc\rangle\!\!-\!\!O(CH_2)_2O(CH_2)_2\overset{\displaystyle CH_3}{\underset{\displaystyle CH_3}{\overset{|}{\underset{|}{N^+}}}}\!\!-\!\!CH_2C_6H_5\ Cl^-$$

benzethonium chloride

$$\langle\bigcirc\rangle\!\!N^{\pm}(CH_2)_{15}CH_3\cdot H_2O$$ with Cl^-

hexadecylpyridinium chloride
hydrate

R is a mixture of alkyls from C_8H_{17} to $C_{18}H_{37}$, with $C_{12}H_{25}$ predominating; benzethonium chloride [121-54-0], ie, benzyldimethyl [2-[2-(p-1,1,3,3-tetramethyl-butylphenoxy)ethoxy]ethyl] ammonium chloride; methylbenzethonium chloride [106-45-0] with the cresoxy group replacing the phenoxy group of benzethonium chloride; hexadecylpyridinium chloride [25155-18-4], and alkylisoquinolinium bromide. Cetrimide (of the British Pharmacopoeia) is hexadecyltrimethylammonium bromide [57-09-0], $C_{16}H_{33}\overset{+}{N}(CH_3)_3Br^-$.

Although the quaternary ammonium compounds have an extensive record of satisfactory performance, pertinent quantitative bacteriological information is rather contradictory. A number of older papers require cautious reinterpretation in the light of more recent findings, since they tended to ascribe to the quats a disinfectant effectiveness and a broad microbicidal spectrum to which these compounds do not appear to be entitled. Therefore, the older phenol coefficient figures reported for the different quats must be regarded with reservations, especially if they have been obtained without regard to controlling the bacteriostatic action of the quaternary ions in tests for bactericidal potency (210,226–228). As to limitations of the microbicidal spectrum of the quats, *Mycobacterium tuberculosis, Pseudomonas aeruginosa, Trichophyton interdigitale* and *rubrum* are particularly resistant to these agents (225,229–234). However, in contrast to the quaternary ammonium salts, the primary tetradecylamine is credited with antituberculous properties, and *N*-dodecyl-1,3-propanediamine [5538-95-4], $C_{12}H_{25}$-NH(CH$_2$)$_3$NH$_2$, is held to offer possibilities as a surface disinfectant for tuberculosis hygiene (235).

Stuart and co-workers have shown that the phenol coefficient of the quaternary ammonium compounds as obtained, for example, by the AOAC method, cannot serve as a guide for the preparation of solutions that would provide adequate margins of safety for disinfection (228). The data that indicate the bacteriostatic action of the quats are more useful for this purpose. The inhibitory dilutions of benzalkonium chloride as observed with a variety of microorganisms are given in Table 9.

Soaps or other anionic surfactants must be removed by thorough rinsing from surfaces to be treated with quaternary ammonium germicides. The hardness of water can also affect the antibacterial performance of the quats (236–237). However, within these limitations the quaternaries render satisfactory service in the sanitization of eating and drinking utensils, the disinfection of equipment used in dairies and in other food processing plants, the cleaning of eggs, etc.

Mixtures of different quaternary ammonium compounds with hexachlorophene show a loss of antibacterial activity that is greatest at an equimolecular ratio (238).

An important application of quaternary ammonium compounds is the impregnation of fabrics to control the spread of infection from this source (239). Control of diaper rash, for example, is achieved by using a quat solution in the final rinse for the

Table 9.   Bacteriostatic Dilutions of Benzalkonium Chloride

Microorganism	Dilution $\times 10^3$
Salmonella typhosa	1:256
Shigella dysenteriae	1:512
Escherichia coli	1:64
Aerobacter aerogenes	1:16
Salmonella paratyphi	1:64
Salmonella enteritidis	1:32
Proteus vulgaris	1:16
Pseudomonas aeruginosa	1:32
Vibrio cholerae	1:512
Staphylococcus aureus	1:800
Pneumococcus II	1:200
Streptococcus pyogenes	1:800
Clostridium welchii	1:200
Clostridium tetani	1:200
Clostridium histolyticum	1:200
Clostridium oedematiens	1:200

suppression of bacteria that attack the urinary urea with liberation of ammonia (240).

When used for strictly antiseptic purposes, such as the control of skin bacteria at the site of an operation, the quaternary ammonium compounds are more satisfactory in the form of tinctures (diluted with 50% alcohol–10% acetone), rather than in aqueous solution. This conclusion is based upon the results of the serial basin test, as employed in a comparative evaluation of the degerming effectiveness of several hospital antiseptics (76). A 1:1000 solution of benzalkonium chloride in water applied after thorough rinsing to remove soap reduced the bacterial count by 40%, whereas no significant reduction was observed after a superficial rinse. By contrast, the tincture of benzalkonium chloride produced reductions of 85 and 80%, respectively, under the corresponding test conditions. However, the solvent (50% alcohol–10% acetone) alone reduced the bacterial count by 70%, and 70% alcohol delivered an even superior performance of an 88% reduction. Similar results were obtained with cetrimide (241).

Amphoteric Surfactant Disinfectants

In Europe, a group of amphoteric surfactants are marketed as disinfectants under the trade name Tego (242–244). Chemically, they are amino acids, usually glycine, substituted with a long-chain alkylamine group. Table 10 gives the structure of some of the more widely used compounds.

The Tego disinfectants are claimed to be bactericidal, fungicidal, and virucidal, nontoxic and safe, and have been recommended for the surgical scrub, floor disinfection in hospital, and food plants, cleanup in dairies, breweries, and bottling plants, etc. However, contradictory reports on the activity of these compounds leave their effectiveness in doubt (see Surfactants).

Table 10.   Composition of Tego Disinfectants[a]

Tego	Active ingredient	Composition	pH
103S	$RNH(CH_2)_2NH(CH_2)_2NHCH_2CO_2H \cdot HCl$	15% aqueous solution	7.7
103G or MHG	$R'NH(CH_2)_2NH(CH_2)_2NHCH_2CO_2H \cdot HCl$ $+ [R'NH(CH_2)_2]_2NCH_2CO_2H \cdot HCl$	10% aqueous solution	7.7
51	$RNH(CH_2)_2NH(CH_2)_2NHCH_2CO_2H +$ $RNH(CH_2)_3NHCH_2CO_2H$	9% aqueous solution	8.1
51B	$R'NH(CH_2)_2NH(CH_2)_2NHCH_2CO_2H$ $R = C_{12}H_{25}$ $R' = C_8H_{17}$ to $C_{16}H_{33}$	22.5% aqueous solution	8.0

[a] Ref. 186.

Pine Oil Compounds

Pine oil is obtained from waste pine wood by destructive distillation or by distillation with superheated steam. Sometimes solvent extraction is added as a supplementary step, in which case a liquid hydrocarbon mixture is introduced into the retort after it has cooled and heat is applied again until extraction has been completed. The solvent extract is subjected to fractionation for rosin, pine oil, and recovery of the solvent. The volatile fraction obtained by any of these processes is separated into pine oil and turpentine. Although technical pine oil may vary considerably in composition depending upon its distillation range (from 170–350°C), a more uniform product is assured if it answers the distillation requirements of the *National Formulary* (NF), namely that 95% should distill between 200 and 225°C. In this case, the fraction consists mostly of isomeric terpineols, with the α-isomer predominating. The other constituents are dihydro-α-terpineol, borneol, and fenchyl alcohol (see Tall oil; Terpenoids).

Pine oil is insoluble in water but is readily emulsifiable when combined with a soap, a sulfonated oil, or other suitable dispersing agents. Most pine oil disinfectants contain from 60–65 vol % of pine oil. Diluted with water such preparations yield white, milky emulsions, with a characteristic, pungent odor.

A pine oil disinfectant prepared according to the hygienic laboratory formula may have a phenol coefficient against *Salmonella typhosa* of 3.5–4.5; higher coefficients (6 or more) may be obtained by using certain emulsifying agents other than the resin soap specified by the hygienic laboratory. However, the lack of ability to kill *Staphylococcus aureus* disqualifies the pine oil-based products for use as disinfectants for hospital, medical, veterinary, and related purposes where pyogenic cocci play a significant role. Thus, the use of pine oil disinfectants is limited to janitorial activities where a supplementary advantage is offered by their deodorant and odor-masking action (see Odor counteractants).

In recent years a serious problem has been created in the hospital field, owing to the emergence of antibiotic-resistant strains of staphylococci; however, these are susceptible, eg, to the action of most phenolic disinfectants (31). Combinations of pine oil or α-terpineol with phenolic broad-spectrum bactericides can be used for formulations with a range of antibacterial potential warranting a wider disinfectant use (245–246).

Carbamic Acid and Urea Derivatives

The class of dithiocarbamates was previously studied for its capacity to control fungus diseases of tomatoes, beans, potatoes, etc (see Fungicides). More recently some dithiocarbamates were found to exert powerful inhibitory action upon fungi pathogenic for man (*Trichophyton mentagrophytes*, *Epidermophyton floccosum*, *Microsporum audouini*, and *Torula histolytica*) (see Chemotherapeutics, antibacterial and antimycotic). Bacteria, especially those of the gram-positive variety, were also found to be susceptible, as illustrated by disodium bisdithiocarbamate [69943-51-7] whose inhibitory concentration for *Staphylococcus aureus* is 1:100,000. The corresponding dilutions for the gram-negative *Salmonella typhosa* and *Escherichia coli* are 1:5,000 and 1:10,000, respectively (247). In another investigation correlating the chemical structure of dithiocarbamic acid derivatives with their *in vitro* antibacterial and antifungal activity, it was found that within each category of dithiocarbamates, thiuram monosulfides, and methyl and ethyl esters were the most active whereas the higher alkyl derivatives were comparatively inactive (248). Tetramethylthiuram disulfide [137-26-8] (TMTD) was the most active of the compounds tested against pathogenic fungi as well as against bacteria; *Streptococcus pyogenes*, *Streptococcus faecalis*, and *Staphylococcus aureus* show a markedly greater susceptibility to its action than *Escherichia coli* and *Pseudomonas aeruginosa* (see also Rubber chemicals).

$$(CH_3)_2NC\overset{\overset{\text{S}}{\|}}{} SS\overset{\overset{\text{S}}{\|}}{C} N(CH_3)_2$$

tetramethylthiuram disulfide

Systematic investigation of over 200 urea and thiourea derivatives revealed several compounds with high bacteriostatic potency (249). Inhibitory dilutions for *Staphylococcus aureus* of the order of $1{:}3 \times 10^7$ have been established for 3,4,3'-trichloro- and 3,4,4'-trichlorocarbanilide [101-20-2], whereas inhibitory action in a dilution of $1{:}10^7$ was observed with 3,3',4,4'-tetrachloro- [1300-43-0] and 3,3',4,5,5'-pentachlorocarbanilides [69943-52-8], and with 3,4,4'-trichlorothiocarbanilide [5109-07-9], and N-formyl-3,4-dichloroaniline [5470-15-5].

3,4,4'-Trichlorocarbanilide (TCC, triclocarban, Monsanto Chemical Co.) has been introduced commercially as a soap additive for its effective skin degerming and deodorant action. In addition to *Staphylococcus aureus,* it inhibits *Diplococcus pneumoniae, Corynebacterium diphtheriae, Bacterium ammoniagenes,* and *Streptococcus viridans* in a dilution of $1{:}10^7$. *Beta-* and *gamma-hemolytic streptococci* require a dilution of $1{:}10^6$ for suppression of growth. However, most gram-negative bacteria and pathogenic fungi are not inhibited by a 1:1000 dilution. The combination of TCC with hexachlorophene exhibits antibacterial synergism (249).

Another commercial carbanilide is 3-(trifluoromethyl)-4,4'-dichlorocarbanilide [369-77-7] (Cloflucarban, Irgasan CF$_3$, Ciba-Geigy), also used as soap additive. The halogenated carbanilides continue to be approved by the FDA for use in bar soaps pending further studies on their toxicity.

1,6-Bis(4-chlorophenyl)diguanidinohexane [14007-07-9] (Chlorhexidine, Hibi-

3,4,4'-trichlorocarbanilide

tane, Imperial Chemical Industries Ltd.) (250) is a topical antiseptic. It reduces the bacterial flora of the hands when applied in a cream or other vehicle (251).

There are a number of substituted biguanides that are antibacterial and antimycotic and that are not inactivated by serum proteins (252) (see Cyanamides).

Nitrofuran Derivatives

Nitro-substituted furans possess antiseptic properties. The nitro group is essential for antibacterial action, as shown by a bacteriological comparison with the nonnitrated analogues (253–254). Of the many derivatives tested (58,255) a few have achieved practical importance. Among them is 5-nitro-2-furaldehyde-2-ethylsemicarbazone [5579-89-5] (nitrofurazone, Furacin, Eaton Laboratories) which is credited with antibacterial action upon both gram-positive and gram-negative microorganisms. Thus, *Salmonella typhosa* and *schottmuelleri*, and *Shigella dysenteriae* are inhibited in broth by a dilution of $1:10^5$ and *Staphylococcus aureus* by a dilution of 1:80,000 of nitrofurazone. On the other hand, *Streptococcus pyogenes* required the much higher inhibitory concentration of 1:10,000, and the still higher concentration of 1:5000 (at the limit of solubility of nitrofurazone) is needed for the inhibition of *Streptococcus viridans* and of *Pseudomonas aeruginosa*.

$$O_2N\diagdown\diagup O\diagdown\diagup CH=NNHCONH_2$$

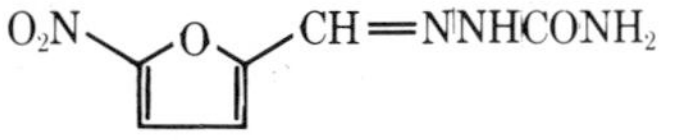

nitrofurazone

Nitrofurazone is reduced by *Aerobacter aerogenes* to 5-amino-2-furaldehyde semicarbazone. The structure of this compound was confirmed by comparison with a sample made by catalytic hydrogenation of nitrofurazone. The bacterial reduction of nitrofuran semicarbazone derivatives in which the NH group of the semicarbazone grouping is blocked by an alkyl group or by involvement in a ring leads to reduction of the nitro group accompanied by furan ring cleavage (256) (see Furan derivatives).

Nitrofurazone has been found useful as a topical prophylactic and therapeutic agent in mixed infections common to contaminated wounds, burns, pyodermas, and the like, and also in the management of purulent otitis and conjunctivitis (257).

Furazolidone (Tricofuron, Eaton Laboratories) 3-(5-nitro-2-furfurylidene)amino-2-oxazolidone [67-45-8], is an antiprotozoan as well as an antibacterial agent. The range of its inhibitory effectiveness for a variety of pathogens extends from less than 0.5 mg/L for *Salmonella pullorum* to more than 99 mg/L for *Pseudomonas aeruginosa* (258). It is used mostly in treating the gynecological infection caused by *Trichomonas vaginalis*.

Another nitrofuran derivative N-(5-nitro-2-furfurylidene)-1-aminohydantoin [67-20-9] (nitrofurantoin, Furadantin, Eaton Laboratories) is also credited with a wide spectrum of antibacterial activity. It is administered orally in the treatment of bacterial infections of the urinary tract (see Chemotherapeutics; Antibacterial agents, synthetic-nitrofurans).

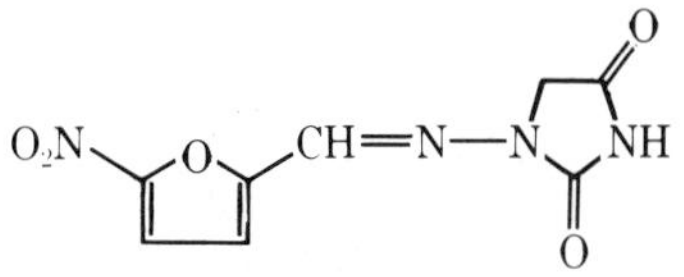

$$O_2N\diagdown\diagup O\diagdown\diagup CH=N-N\diagdown NH$$

nitrofurantoin

Dyes

Those dyes that exhibit an antibacterial action are bacteriostatic rather than bactericidal, as a rule. Although it has been assumed that the basic dyes with their electropositive character are specific for gram-positive microoganisms, and the electronegative acid dyes, for gram-negative bacteria (259), the quantitative determination of the uptake of crystal violet by bacterial cells has failed to show any correlation with their gram character (260) (see Dyes; Triphenylmethane and related dyes; Azine dyes; Azo dyes).

The inhibitory action of basic dyes such as triphenylmethane [519-73-3] and acridine [260-94-6] derivatives is attributed to the tendency of their basic ions to form nonionizing or feebly ionizing complexes with the acidic groups of some cellular constituents of bacteria, probably a nucleoprotein in the cytoskeleton (261). Similarly in acid dyes such as fuchsin, the acidic ion is believed to react with some basic bacterial cell receptor, forming a nondissociating complex (262). These reactions are favored, respectively, by high and by low pH values. Bacteria become increasingly sensitive to basic dyes as the pH is increased, and to acidic dyes as it is decreased.

Thus, the bacteriostatic effectiveness of a dye should be a function of the strength of its ionization; the stronger the ionization, the greater should be the resistance to hydrolysis of the complexes formed with the reactive bacterial constituents. The basic strength of the isomeric aminoacridine dyes has been determined by potentiometric titration. Proceeding from the weakest members (1-amino- or 1,9-diaminoacridine [578-06-3]) to the strongest (5-amino- or 5-amino-1-methylacridine [23015-11-6]), there is a progressive increase in antibacterial potency for several test organisms (263). The relationship between ionization and antibacterial activity holds also in other series of related heterocyclic dyes, such as the benzacridines, benzoquinolines, and phenanthridines (264).

At one time the organic dyes were widely used for chemotherapy of infectious diseases. Several organic dyes are still in use, albeit to a minor extent; following is a selective listing:

Brilliant Green [633-03-4] is the quinonoid, bis(p-diethylamino)triphenylcarbinol anhydride. Tested by the semimicro method indicated a bactericidal capacity for *Staphylococcus aureus* in a dilution of 1:50,000. However, using 10% blood broth as reversing agent, the dye is not germicidal at 1:2000.

Gentian violet [548-62-9] (crystal violet) is essentially hexamethylpararosaniline hydrochloride. It suppresses the growth of *Lactobacillus acidophilus* and of *Micrococcus citreus* in a dilution of $1:10^6$ or higher (265). It has been recommended as a topical antiseptic for the prevention of secondary infection of war wounds and burns (266).

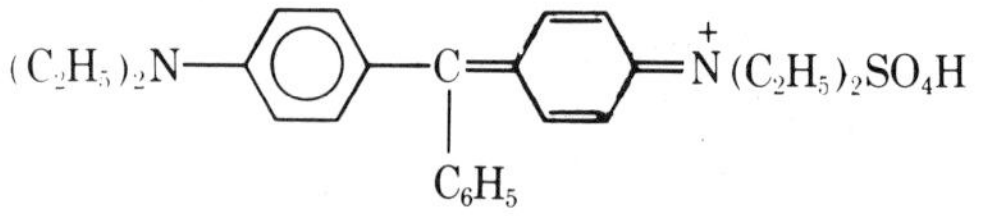

$$(C_2H_5)_2N-\!\!\bigcirc\!\!-\overset{\displaystyle |}{\underset{\displaystyle C_6H_5}{C}}\!\!=\!\!\bigcirc\!\!=\!\overset{+}{N}(C_2H_5)_2SO_4H$$

Brilliant Green

$$p\text{-}[(CH_3)_2NC_6H_4]_2C=\!\!\bigcirc\!\!=\overset{+}{N}(CH_3)_2Cl^-$$

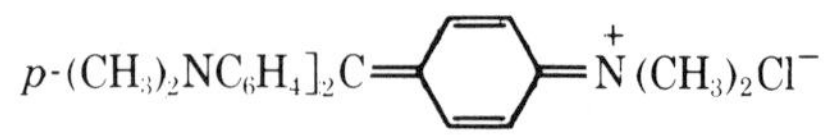

gentian violet

Methylene blue [61-73-4] stains plasmodia and is inhibitory for several pathogens including *Mycobacterium tuberculosis* (266).

Acriflavine is 3,6-diamino-10-methylacridinium chloride [6034-59-9]. Originally considered by Ehrlich for the treatment of trypanosomiasis, it gained importance subsequently as a topical antiseptic with bacteriostatic action. It enjoys limited use as a systemic drug (268). Rivanol, 2-ethoxy-6,9-diaminoacridine lactate [1837-57-6], exhibits antibacterial action *in vitro* that compares favorably with that of acriflavine (269).

Flavicid [525-12-2], 8-amino-2-dimethylamino-3,7,10-trimethylacridinium chloride, has been used as a surgical germicide for wound dressing as well as topically in gonorrhea (270).

Dimazon [83-63-6], diacetamidoazotoluene [83-63-6] is chemically related to scarlet red. It is applied in powder or ointment form to denuded areas as a means of controlling bacterial multiplication and of stimulating epithelization.

2,6-Diamino-3-phenylazopyridine hydrochloride [136-40-3], phenazopyridine hydrochloride, (Pyridium, Warner-Lambert Co.), is used primarily as a urinary antiseptic because of its claimed ability to exert bacteriostatic action in both acid and alkaline urine. It is inhibitory for *staphylococci, streptococci, gonococci,* and *coli bacilli* (271).

Two compounds in the sulfonamide series are dyes: sulfamidochrysoidine [103-12-8], p-[(2,4-diaminophenyl)azo] benzenesulfonamide (Prontosil rubrum) (272), and salicylazosulfapyridine [599-79-1], 5-[p-(2-pyridylsulfamoyl)phenylazo]salicylic acid (273).

The pigments produced by some chromogenic bacteria are inhibitory for other species. The antibiotic effect upon staphylococci and streptococci of pyocyanin [85-66-5], the pigment of *Pseudomonas aeruginosa,* has stimulated a systematic investigation of the series of phenazines to which pyocyanin belongs (274). Several of these dyes exhibited bacteriostatic effectiveness in the dilution range of $1:10^3$ to $1:10^4$ against *Staphylococcus aureus;* by contrast much higher dye concentrations, of the order of 5%, were required to inhibit *Escherichia coli* or *Proteus vulgaris.*

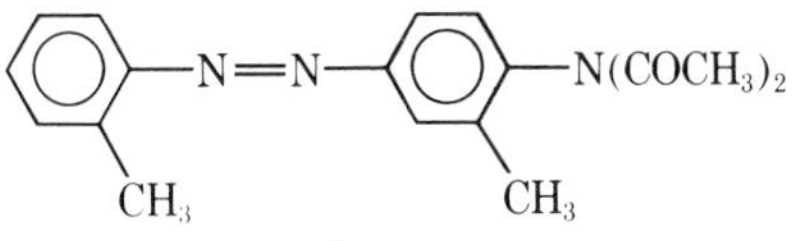

dimazon

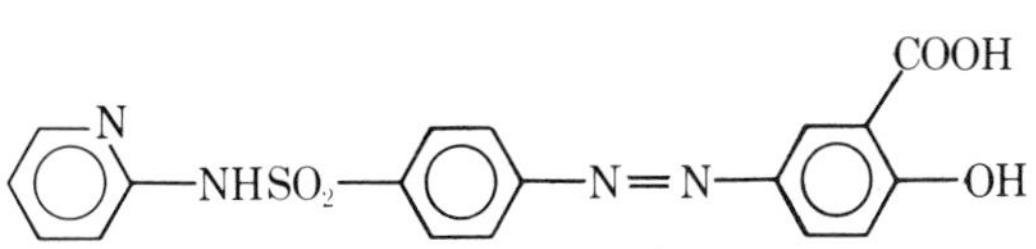

salicylazosulfapyridine

Formaldehyde and Other Aldehydes

At one time gaseous formaldehyde [50-00-0] was used to treat the premises, furniture, and objects exposed to patients with contagious illness. Fumigation with formaldehyde is now practiced only rarely since it has been found to be of little value as a disinfectant procedure. When used for sterilization of enclosed spaces, gaseous formaldehyde requires a very high humidity, approaching saturation (275) (see Sterile techniques).

Solutions of formaldehyde with soap are used as disinfectants, mostly outside the United States. Formaldehyde in hydroalcoholic solution is used widely for the "sterilization" of surgical instruments. Although it has been credited with sporicidal potency when employed for this purpose, its practical sporicidal effectiveness appears to be somewhat questionable (7,29,276). A mixture of formaldehyde and hexachlorophene has been recommended for cold sterilization of surgical instruments (276).

Hexamethylenetetramine [100-97-0], $C_6H_{12}N_4$ (methenamine), is still used as a urinary antiseptic, but to a lesser extent than prior to the advent of sulfonamides and antibiotics (qv). Its antibacterial action depends upon the slow liberation of formaldehyde in acid urine at a pH below 5.6 (see Antibacterial agents).

The slow release of formaldehyde from a new series of quaternary ammonium compounds, prepared by the reaction of hexamethylenetetramine with certain halohydrocarbons, furnishes the reason for their antimicrobial activity which renders them suitable for use in cutting-oil emulsions, latexes, and the like (277).

Methenamine mandelate [587-23-5] (Mandelamine, Warner-Chilcott Laboratories) utilizes the urinary antiseptic action of both methenamine and mandelic acid [90-64-2] ($C_6H_5CHOHCO_2H$). In concentrations of 35–50 g/100 liters of urine it is inhibitory to *Staphylococcus aureus, Bacillus proteus, Escherichia coli,* and *Aerobacter aerogenes* (278–279).

Recently, certain saturated dialdehydes and particularly glutaraldehyde [111-30-8], $OCH(CH_2)_3CHO$, have been found to possess a capacity for sterilizing (including sporicidal) action if employed in a hydroalcoholic solution, and in the presence of an alkalinizing agent, such as sodium bicarbonate. Sonacide is an aqueous 2% solution of glutaraldehyde with a nonionic ethoxylate of isomeric linear alcohols (280). The bactericidal effect upon vegetative pathogens (including *Mycobacterium tuberculosis* and *Pseudomonas aeruginosa*) is claimed to take place within 10 min, immersion for 3 h is required to destroy resistant bacterial spores. This type of preparation is suitable especially for the treatment of surgical instruments. The physical advantage of glutaraldehyde over formaldehyde is that in its use-dilution, the glutaraldehyde (unlike formaldehyde) has a mild odor and a low irritation potential for the skin and mucous membranes (281) (see Aldehydes).

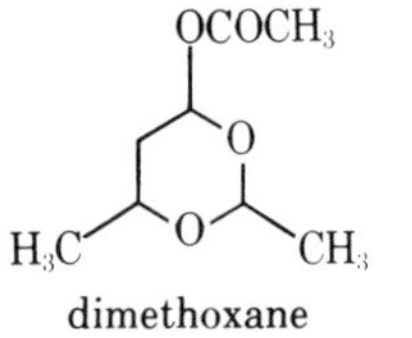

dimethoxane

Dimethoxane (6-Acetoxyl-2,4-dimethyl-*m*-dioxane [828-00-2] (Giv-Gard DXN, Givaudan Corp.) is a bacteriostat and fungistat (282), to be used as preservative for aqueous systems and various types of industrial emulsions. It hydrolyzes in water to form active aldehydic compounds plus some acetic acid.

Ethylene Oxide and Other Alkylating Agents

As indicated above, true sterilization requires destruction of resistant bacterial spores and of all types of viruses, including those of infectious and serum hepatitis; it requires exposure to steam under pressure (autoclaving) for a sufficient period of time (283). Alternatively, such sterilization can be produced by suitable dilute solutions of certain phenolic disinfectants, eg, 2% aqueous Amphyl heated to the boiling point (284). Either treatment is suitable only for objects that tolerate heat (see Sterile techniques).

Important advances have been made in the cold sterilization of a variety of materials of low thermostability, based upon the discovery of the intensive microbicidal action of ethylene oxide [75-21-8] (qv) (285–286), which is extremely reactive in both the liquid and the gaseous states. Although there are a number of references to the bactericidal as well as the virucidal action of liquid ethylene oxide (287–288), the practical application of this chemical calls for its employment as a gas, in specially constructed autoclaves (289–293). Because of its flammability and explosiveness, gaseous ethylene oxide is not used as such; instead, it is diluted with an inert gas such as carbon dioxide or certain fluorohydrocarbons. Thus, the commercially available Carboxide R represents a mixture of 10% ethylene oxide and 90% carbon dioxide.

The bactericidal activity of ethylene oxide is thought to be the result of direct ethoxylation of functional groups of bacterial proteins, as illustrated below:

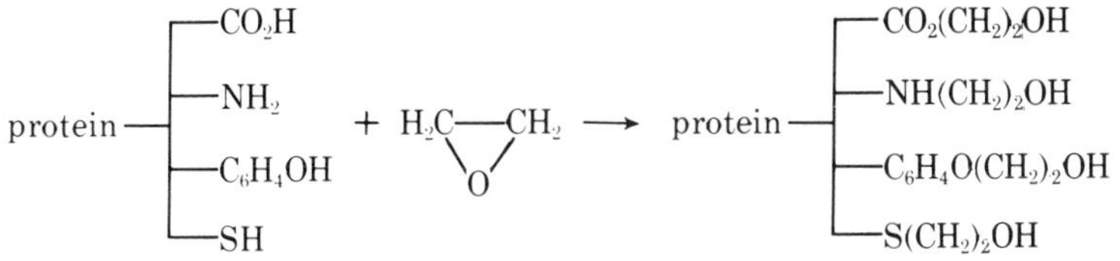

$$\text{protein}\begin{cases}-CO_2H\\-NH_2\\-C_6H_4OH\\-SH\end{cases} + H_2C\overset{\displaystyle\diagdown\!\diagup}{\underset{O}{\quad}}CH_2 \longrightarrow \text{protein}\begin{cases}-CO_2(CH_2)_2OH\\-NH(CH_2)_2OH\\-C_6H_4O(CH_2)_2OH\\-S(CH_2)_2OH\end{cases}$$

Bacterial spores are considerably more resistant to chemical disinfectants than vegetative bacteria, and the two categories differ also in their susceptibility to ethylene oxide (294).

Although most of the basic work on the sporicidal action of ethylene oxide was carried out with the spores of *Bacillus globigii*, Friedl and co-workers (295) extended these studies to include the spores of five anaerobes (*Clostridium botulinum, lentoputrescens, perfringens, sporogenes, tetani*) and of five aerobes (*Bacillus anthracis, coagulans, globigii, stearothermophilus,* and *subtilis*). When exposed to ethylene oxide at room temperature, the dry spores of *Bacillus subtilis* and *Clostridium sporogenes* survived for several hours, whereas those of the other test organisms were killed after shorter periods of time. None survived an 18-h exposure. Spores of pathogenic fungi have also been studied (296). The sporicidal action of ethylene oxide is affected by the factors of concentration, temperature, and humidity (98). At a relative humidity of less than 25%, it is not reliably effective.

Vaccinia virus and Columbia-SK-encephalomyelitis virus are inactivated by ethylene oxide in 8 h at room temperature (297). Ethylene oxide also lends itself to mold control (298) and offers promise in certain areas of sterilization of foods (299–301) and drugs (302–303).

Propylene oxide [75-56-9] (qv) was found similar in properties to ethylene oxide, but less volatile and less active biologically (304). Interest in propylene oxide was revived when the FDA restricted use of ethylene oxide in the food industry because of the toxicity of ethylene glycol, a hydrolytic product found in small amounts (305). Propylene oxide hydrolyzes to nontoxic propylene glycol (see Glycols). Liquid propylene oxide has been suggested for sterilizing borated talc (306).

Other three-membered heterocyclic compounds also exhibit sporicidal action, in some instances superior to that of ethylene oxide (304). Among them are ethyleneimine [151-56-4], $(CH_2)_2NH$, its N-aminoethyl derivative, $(CH_2)_2$-$NCH_2CH_2NH_2$, and ethylene sulfide [420-12-2], $(CH_2)_2S$. Epichlorohydrin [106-89-8] and epibromohydrin [3132-64-7] are more effective than ethylene oxide but less so than either ethylene sulfide or ethylene imine (see Chlorohydrins). All of them are flammable as well as toxic, hence unsuitable for the sterilization of occupied premises.

β-Propiolactone [57-57-8] also exhibits sporicidal action. This chemical is applied usually in aqueous solution. Although stable in nonaqueous media, it hydrolyzes slowly in the presence of water to form 3-hydroxypropionic acid which is nontoxic. For this reason β-propiolactone is suitable for the sterilization of water and milk, of nutrient broth, and of biologicals such as vaccines. β-Propiolactone is active also against vegetative bacteria, as well as pathogenic fungi and viruses (307–312). It has been suggested for the sterilization of operating rooms and of enclosed spaces in general (313–315). As β-propiolactone is under suspicion as a carcinogen, it has been banned in interstate shipping by EPA for use as a pesticide.

$$\begin{array}{ccc} CH_2 & \!\!\!\!\!-\!\!\!\!\! & CH_2 \\ | & & | \\ O & \!\!\!\!\!-\!\!\!\!\! & CO \end{array}$$

β-propiolactone

BIBLIOGRAPHY

"Antiseptics, Disinfectants, and Fungicides" in *ECT* 1st ed., Vol. 2, "Survey," pp. 77–91, by W. C. Tobie, American Cyanamid Company; "Methods of Testing," pp. 91–105, by G. F. Reddish, Lambert Pharmacal Company; "Antiseptics and Disinfectants," in *ECT* 2nd ed., Vol. 2, pp. 604–648, by Emil G. Klarmann, Lehn & Fink, Inc.

1. *Fed. Reg.* **43**, 63771 (Jan. 6, 1978).
2. *Fed. Reg.* **40**, 28270 (July 3, 1975); **40**, 26808 (June 25, 1975).
3. G. L. A. Ruehle and C. M. Brewer, *U.S. Dept. Agric. Circ.* **198**, (1931).
4. W. J. Nungester and A. H. Kempf, *J. Infect. Dis.* **71**, 174 (1942).
5. W. J. Nungester and A. H. Kempf, *J. Am. Med. Assoc.* **121**, 593 (1945).
6. R. W. Sarber, *J. Pharmacol. Exp. Ther.* **75**, 277 (1942).
7. E. G. Klarmann, E. S. Wright, and V. A. Shternov, *Am. J. Pharm.* **122**, 5 (1950).
8. P. B. Price, *J. Infect. Dis.* **63**, 301 (1938).
9. A. R. Cade, *J. Soc. Cosmet. Chem.* **2**, 281 (1951).
10. A. R. Cade, *Am. Soc. Test. Mater., Spec. Tech. Publ.* **115**, 33 (1952).
11. *Fed. Reg.* **39**, 33103 (Sept. 13, 1974).
12. L. J. Vinson and co-workers, *J. Pharm. Sci.* **50**, 827 (1961).
13. A. J. Salle and co-workers, *J. Bacteriol.* **37**, 639 (1939).
14. E. H. Spaulding and J. A. Bondi, *J. Infect. Dis.* **80**, 194 (1947).
15. S. Rideal and J. T. A. Walker, *J. R. Sanit. Inst.* **24**, 424 (1903).
16. Lancet Commission, *Lancet* **177**, 1459, 1516, 1612 (1909).
17. S. Rideal and J. T. A. Walker, *Approved Technique of the Rideal-Walker Test*, Lewis, London, Eng., 1921.

18. *Br. Standards Inst. Bull.* **541,** 113 (1934).

19. J. F. Anderson and T. B. McClintic, *Hyg. Lab. Bull. (U.S. Treas. Dept.)* **82,** (1912).

20. American Public Health Association, *Am. J. Public Health* **8,** 506 (1918).

21. C. M. Brewer and G. F. Reddish, *J. Bacteriol.* **17,** 44 (1929).

22. *Official and Tentative Methods of Analysis,* 9th ed., Association of Official Agricultural Chemists, Washington, D.C., 1960.

23. Association of Official Analytical Chemists, *J. Assoc. Off. Anal. Chem.* **53,** 61 (1970).

24. L. S. Stuart, L. F. Ortenzio, and J. L. Friedl, *J. Assoc. Off. Agric. Chem.* **36,** 466 (1953).

25. E. G. Klarmann, *Am. J. Hosp. Pharm.* **15,** 795 (1958).

26. R. L. Steadman, E. Kravitz, and H. Bell, *Appl. Microbiol.* **2,** 119, 322 (1954); **3,** 71 (1955).

27. E. G. Klarmann, E. S. Wright, and V. A. Shternov, *Appl. Microbiol.* **1,** 19 (1953).

28. E. G. Klarmann and E. S. Wright, *Am. J. Pharm.* **122,** 330 (1950).

29. J. L. Friedl, *J. Assoc. Off. Agric. Chem.* **38,** 280 (1955).

30. L. F. Ortenzio, L. S. Stuart, and J. L. Friedl, *J. Assoc. Off. Agric. Chem.* **36,** 480 (1953).

31. E. G. Klarmann, *Am. J. Pharm.* **129,** 42 (1957).

32. *Ibid.* **131,** 86 (1959).

33. E. G. Klarmann, *Hosp. Top.* **35**(8), 90 (1957).

34. *W.H.O. Tech Rep. Ser.* **62,** (1953).

35. A. J. Rhodes and C. E. van Rooyen, *Textbook of Virology,* Williams and Wilkins, Baltimore, Md., 1953, p. 29.

36. C. L. Hoagland, *Ann. Rev. Biochem.* **12,** 615 (1943).

37. W. B. Dunham and W. J. MacNeal, *J. Immunol.* **49,** 123 (1944).

38. V. Groupe and co-workers, *Appl. Microbiol.* **3,** 333 (1955).

39. M. Klein and D. A. Stevens, *J. Immunol.* **50,** 265 (1945).

40. E. R. Parker, W. B. Dunham, and W. J. MacNeal, *J. Lab. Clin. Med.* **29,** 37 (1944).

41. N. A. Allawala and S. Riegelman, *J. Am. Pharm. Assoc. Sci. Ed.* **42,** 396 (1953).

42. *DIS-13,* Environmental Protection Agency, Washington, D.C., 1973.

43. H. S. Wright, *Appl. Microbiol.* **19,** 92 (1970).

44. J. H. Blackwell and J. H. Chen, *J. Assoc. Off. Anal. Chem.* **53,** 1229 (1970).

45. J. Christiansen, *Z. Physiol. Chem.* **102,** 275 (1918).

46. J. H. Quastel and M. D. Whetham, *Biochem. J.* **19,** 520 (1927).

47. E. G. Klarmann, L. W. Gates, and V. A. Shternov, *J. Am. Chem. Soc.* **54,** 3315 (1932).

48. H. E. Morton, *Ann. N.Y. Acad. Sci.* **53,** 191 (1950).

49. P. B. Price, *Arch. Surg.* **38,** 528 (1939).

50. F. W. Tilley and J. M. Schaffer, *J. Bacteriol.* **12,** 303 (1926).

51. P. B. Price, *Arch. Surg.* **38,** 528 (1929); **60,** 492 (1950).

52. C. R. Smith, *Public Health Rep. (U.S.)* **62,** 1285 (1947).

53. H. Neves, *Arch. Dermatol.* **84,** 132 (1961).

54. E. C. McCulloch, *Disinfection and Sterilization,* Lea and Febiger, Philadelphia, Pa., 1945, p. 319.

55. C. H. Cunningham, *Am. J. Vet. Res.* **9,** 195 (1948).

56. M. H. Gordon, *Med. Res. Council Spec. Rep. Ser.* **98,** (1925).

57. S. Stockman and F. C. Minett, *J. Comp. Pathol. Therap.* **39,** 1 (1926).

58. H. E. Paul and co-workers, *Proc. Soc. Exp. Biol. Med.* **79,** 199 (1952).

59. M. L. Tainter and co-workers, *J. Am. Dental Assoc.* **31,** 479 (1944).

60. G. Weitzel and E. Schraufstätter, *Z. Physiol. Chem.* **285,** 172 (1950).

61. O. H. Robertson and co-workers, *Science* **97,** 142 (1943).

62. O. H. Robertson and W. Lester, Jr., *Am. J. Hyg.* **53,** 69 (1951).

63. V. A. Chandler, R. E. Pepper, and L. E. Gordon, *J. Pharm. Sci.* **46,** 124 (1957).

64. C. K. Johns, *Sci. Agric.* **14,** 585 (1934).

65. S. M. Costigan, *J. Bacteriol.* **34,** 1 (1937).

66. M. Levine and A. S. Rudolph, *Iowa State Coll. Eng. Exp. Stn. Bull.* **150,** (1941).

67. H. C. Marks and F. B. Strandskov, *Ann. N.Y. Acad. Sci.* **53,** 163 (1950).

68. G. M. Ridenour, R. S. Ingols, and E. H. Armbruster, *Water Sewage Works* **96,** 279 (1949).

69. E. C. McCulloch and S. M. Costigan, *J. Infect. Dis.* **59,** 281 (1936).

70. A. Fleming, *Chem. Ind. (London),* 18 (1945).

71. S. L. Chang and G. Berg, *U.S. Armed Forces Med. J.* **10,** 33 (1959).

72. F. C. Schmelkes and E. S. Horning, *J. Bacteriol.* **29,** 323 (1935).

73. H. Lemaire, C. H. Schrammy, and A. Cahn, *J. Pharm. Sci.* **50,** 831 (1961).

74. B. Carroll, *J. Bacteriol.* **69**, 413 (1955).

75. O. Wyss and F. B. Strandskov, *Arch. Biochem.* **6**, 261 (1945).

76. P. B. Price, *Drug Stand.* **19**, 161 (1951).

77. M. Frobisher, Jr., L. Sommermeyer, and M. L. Blackwell, *Appl. Microbiol.* **1**, 187 (1953).

78. L. Gershenfeld, W. B. Flagg, and B. Witlin, *Mil. Surg.* **114**, 172 (1954).

79. L. Gershenfeld and B. Witlin, *J. Am. Pharm. Assoc. Sci. Ed.* **41**, 451 (1952).

80. L. Gershenfeld and B. Witlin, *Am. J. Pharm.* **123**, 87 (1951).

81. C. W. Chambers and co-workers, *Soap Sanit. Chem.* **28**, 149 (1952).

82. S. L. Chang and J. C. Morris, *Ind. Eng. Chem.* **45**, 1009 (1953).

83. J. C. Morris and co-workers, *Ind. Eng. Chem.* **45**, 1013 (1953).

84. L. Gershenfeld and B. Witlin, *Am. J. Pharm.* **125**, 129, 258 (1953).

85. P. G. Bartlett and W. Schmidt, *Appl. Microbiol.* **5**, 355 (1957).

86. R. Blatt and J. V. Maloney, Jr., *Surg. Gynecol. Obstet.* **113**, 699 (1961).

87. J. A. Boswick, E. Kissell, and W. I. Metzger, *J. Abdom. Surg.* **3**, 157 (1961).

88. L. Gershenfeld and B. Witlin, *Am. J. Pharm.* **128**, 335 (1956).

89. B. Witlin and L. Gershenfeld, *J. Milk Food Technol.* **32**, 155, 167 (1956).

90. C. K. Johns, *Can. J. Technol.* **32**, 71 (1954).

91. H. A. Shelanski and M. V. Shelanski, *J. Int. Coll. Surg.* **25**, 727 (1956).

92. L. Gershenfeld, *Am. J. Surg.* **94**, 938 (1957); *Am. J. Pharm.* **134**, 278 (1962).

93. A. W. Frisch, G. H. Davies, and W. Kreppachne, *Surg. Gynecol. Obstet.* **107**, 442 (1958).

94. C. A. Lawrence, *Am. J. Hosp. Pharm.* **17**, 100 (1960).

95. U.S. Pat. 2,679,533 (May 25, 1954), J. L. Darragh and R. House (to California Research Corp.).

96. U.S. Pat. 2,746,928 (May 22, 1956), J. L. Darragh and G. B. Johnson (to California Research Corp.).

97. W. E. Engelhard and A. W. Worton, *J. Am. Pharm. Assoc. Sci. Ed.* **45**, 402 (1956).

98. F. B. Engley, Jr., *Ann. N.Y. Acad. Sci.* **53**, 197 (1950).

99. H. Engelhardt, *Desinfektion* **7**, 63, 81 (1922).

100. J. M. McCalla, *J. Bacteriol.* **40**, 33 (1940).

101. M. Klein and co-workers, *J. Immunol.* **59**, 135 (1948).

102. H. E. Morton, L. L. North, and F. B. Engley, *J. Am. Med. Assoc.* **136**, 37 (1948).

103. L. Banti, *J. Am. Med. Assoc.* **140**, 404 (1948).

104. E. G. Klarmann, *Ann. N.Y. Acad. Sci.* **53**, 123 (1950).

105. E. S. G. Barron and G. Kalnitsky, *Biochem. J.* **41**, 346 (1947).

106. E. S. G. Barron and T. P. Singer, *J. Biol. Chem.* **157**, 221 (1945).

107. P. Fildes, *Br. J. Exp. Pathol.* **21**, 67 (1940).

108. J. A. de Loueiro and E. Lito, *J. Hyg.* **44**, 463 (1946).

109. A. E. Elkhouly and R. T. Yousef, *J. Pharm. Sci.* **63**, 681 (1974).

110. H. Kliewe, F. Steyskal, and K. Steyskal, *Z. Hyg. Infektionskrankh.* **127**, 110 (1947).

111. C. E. Hartford and S. E. Ziffren, *J. Trauma* **12**, 682 (1972).

112. H. S. Carr, T. J. Wodkowski, and H. S. Rosenkranz, *Antimicrob. Agents Chemotherap.* **4**, 585 (1973).

113. C. L. Fox, *Arch. Surg.* **96**, 184 (1968).

114. C. H. Brandes, *Ind. Eng. Chem.* **26**, 962 (1934).

115. R. K. Hoffman and co-workers, *Ind. Eng. Chem.* **45**, 287 (1953).

116. J. B. Sprowls and C. F. Poe, *J. Am. Pharm. Assoc.* **32**, 41 (1943).

117. H. L. Guest and A. J. Salle, *Proc. Soc. Exp. Biol. Med.* **51**, 572 (1942).

118. A. P. Muroma, *Ann. Med. Exp. Biol. Fenniae* (*Helsinki*) **31**, 432 (1953).

119. Th. Kunzman, *Fortschr. Med.* **52**, 357 (1934).

120. H. R. Dittmar, J. L. Baldwin, and S. B. Miller, *J. Bacteriol.* **19**, 203 (1930).

121. F. I. K. Ahmed and C. Russell, *J. Appl. Bacteriol.* **39**, 31 (1975).

122. F. L. Meleney, *J. Am. Med. Assoc.* **149**, 1450 (1952).

123. C. D. Leake, *J. Am. Med. Assoc.* **119**, 101 (1942).

124. J. P. Doll and co-workers, *Midl. Natural* **69**, 23 (1963).

125. F. P. Greenspan, M. A. Johnson, and P. C. Trexler, *Proc. 42nd Annual Meeting Chem. Spec. Manf. Assoc.*, 59 (1955).

126. S. Kojima, *J. Biochem.* (*Tokyo*) **14**, 95 (1931).

127. M. Ingram and R. B. Haines, *J. Hyg.* **47**, 146 (1949).

128. A. H. Fogg and R. M. Lodge, *Trans. Faraday Soc.* **41**, 309 (1945).

129. E. M. Richardson and E. E. Reid, *J. Am. Chem. Soc.* **62,** 413 (1940).
130. E. F. Gale and E. S. Taylor, *J. Gen. Microbiol.* **1,** 77 (1947).
131. D. A. Haydon, *Proc. R. Soc. (London) Ser. B* **145,** 583 (1956).
132. R. J. V. Pulvertaft and G. D. Lumb, *J. Hyg.* **46,** 62 (1948).
133. P. Maurice, *Proc. Soc. Appl. Bacteriol.* **15,** 144 (1952).
134. J. Judis, *J. Pharm. Sci.* **51,** 261 (1962).
135. D. Bach and J. Lambert, *Compt. Rend. Soc. Biol.* **126,** 298 (1937).
136. M. H. Roberts and O. Rahn, *J. Bacteriol.* **52,** 639 (1946).
137. J. H. Quastel and W. R. Wooldridge, *Biochem. J.* **21,** 148, 689 (1927).
138. G. Sykes, *J. Hyg.* **39,** 463 (1939).
139. E. G. Klarmann, V. A. Shternov, and L. W. Gates, *J. Lab. Clin. Med.* **19,** 835; **20,** 40 (1934).
140. E. G. Klarmann and co-workers, *J. Am. Chem. Soc.* **55,** 2576, 4657 (1933).
141. L. F. Ortenzio, C. D. Opalsky, and L. S. Stuart, *Appl. Microbiol.* **9,** 562 (1961).
142. T. B. Johnson and W. W. Hodge, *J. Am. Chem. Soc.* **35,** 1014 (1913).
143. T. B. Johnson and F. W. Lane, *J. Am. Chem. Soc.* **43,** 348 (1921).
144. A. R. L. Dohme, E. H. Cox, and E. Miller, *J. Am. Chem. Soc.* **48,** 1688 (1926).
145. B. Hampil, *J. Infect. Dis.* **43,** 25 (1928).
146. E. G. Klarmann, L. W. Gates, and V. A. Shternov, *J. Am. Chem. Soc.* **54,** 298, 1204 (1932).
147. E. G. Klarmann, *J. Am. Chem. Soc.* **48,** 2358 (1926).
148. E. G. Klarmann and J. Von Wowern, *J. Am. Chem. Soc.* **51,** 605 (1929).
149. M. L. Moore, A. A. Day, and C. M. Suter, *J. Am. Chem. Soc.* **56,** 2456 (1934).
150. R. R. Read, G. F. Reddish, and E. M. Burlingame, *J. Am. Chem. Soc.* **56,** 1377 (1934).
151. R. Zinkernagel and M. Koenig, *Seifen-Öle Fette-Wachse* **93,** 670 (1967).
152. E. Jungermann and D. Taber, *J. Am. Oil Chem. Soc.* **48,** 318 (1971).
153. P. S. Herman and W. M. Sams, *Soap Photodermatitis and Photosensitivity to Halogenated Salicylanilides,* Charles C Thomas, Springfield, Ill., 1972.
154. L. J. Vinson and R. S. Flatt, *J. Invest. Dermatol.* **38,** 327 (1962).
155. D. S. Wilkinson, *Br. J. Dermatol.* **73,** 213 (1961); **74,** 302 (1962).
156. A. Kraushaar, *Arzneim. Forsch.* **4,** 548 (1954).
157. U.S. Pat. 2,745,874 (May 15, 1956), G. Schetty, W. Stammbach, and R. Zinkernagel (to J. R. Geigy A.G.).
158. U.S. Pat. 2,906,711 (Sept. 29, 1959), H. C. Stecker.
159. U.S. Pat. 3,041,236 (June 26, 1962), H. C. Stecker.
160. T. R. Aalto, M. C. Firman, and N. E. Rigler, *J. Am. Pharm. Assoc. Sci. Ed.* **42,** 449 (1953).
161. H. Sokol, *Drug. Stand.* **20,** 89 (1952).
162. H. F. Cremer, *Z. Untersuch. Lebensm.* **70,** 136 (1935).
163. K. Schubel and I. Manger, Jr., *Münch. Med. Wochschr.* **77,** 13 (1929).
164. L. Gershenfeld and D. Perlstein, *Am. J. Pharm.* **111,** 227 (1939).
165. N. S. Gottfried, *Am. J. Hosp. Pharm.* **19,** 310 (1962).
166. C. Mathews and co-workers, *J. Am. Pharm. Assoc. Sci. Ed.* **45,** 260 (1956).
167. M. Huppert, *Antibiot. Chemother.* **7,** 29 (1957).
168. H. Gershon and R. Parmegiani, *Appl. Microbiol.* **10,** 348 (1962).
169. U.S. Pat. 2,250,408 (July 29, 1941), W. S. Gump (to Burton T. Bush, Inc.).
170. W. S. Gump, *Soap Sanit. Chem.* **21,** 36 (1945).
171. U.S. Pat. 2,535,077 (Dec. 26, 1950), E. C. Kunz and W. S. Gump (to Sindar Corp.).
172. C. V. Seastone, *Surg. Gynecol. Obstet.* **84,** 355 (1947).
173. P. B. Price and A. Bonnett, *Surgery* **24,** 542 (1948).
174. I. H. Blank and M. H. Coolidge, *J. Invest. Dermatol.* **15,** 257 (1950).
175. P. B. Price, *Ann. Surg.* **134,** 476 (1951).
176. W. B. Shelley, H. J. Hurley, and A. C. Nichols, *Arch. Dermatol. Syphilol.* **68,** 430 (1953).
177. W. S. Gump, *J. Soc. Cosmet. Chem.* **20,** 173 (1969).
178. B. P. Vaterlaus and J. J. Hostynek, *J. Soc. Cosmet. Chem.* **24,** 291 (1973).
179. R. D. Kimbrough and T. B. Gaines, *Arch. Environ. Health* **23,** 114 (1971).
180. T. B. Gaines, R. D. Kimbrough, and R. E. Linder, *Toxicol. Appl. Pharmacol.* **25,** 332 (1973).
181. J. A. Santolucito, *Toxicol. Appl. Pharmacol.* **22,** 276 (1972).
182. H. M. Powell, *J. Indiana State Med. Assoc.* **38,** 303 (1945).
183. *Fed. Reg.* **37,** 160, 219 (Jan. 7, 1972).
184. W. S. Gump, *J. Soc. Cosmet. Chem.* **14,** 269 (1963).

185. *Ibid.* **15,** 717 (1964).
186. S. S. Block, *Disinfection, Sterilization, and Preservation,* 2nd ed., Lea & Febiger, Philadelphia, Pa., 1977.
187. R. S. Shumard, D. J. Beaver, and M. C. Hunter, *Soap Sanit. Chem.* **29**(1), 34 (1953).
188. U.S. Pat. 2,353,735 (July 18, 1944), E. C. Kunz, M. Luthy, and W. S. Gump (to Burton T. Bush, Inc.).
189. K. M. Wood and S. H. Hopper, *J. Am. Pharm. Assoc. Sci. Ed.* **47,** 317 (1958).
190. O. F. Jillson and R. D. Baughma, *Arch. Dermatol.* **88,** 409 (1963).
191. R. Pfleger and co-workers, *Naturforsch.* **46,** 344 (1949).
192. J. B. Adams and M. Hobbs, *J. Pharm. Pharmacol.* **10,** 507 (1958).
193. W. S. Gump and G. R. Walter, *J. Soc. Cosmet. Chem.* **11,** 307 (1960).
194. G. R. Walter and W. S. Gump, *J. Soc. Cosmet. Chem.* **13,** 477 (1962).
195. W. C. Harden and E. E. Reid, *J. Am. Chem. Soc.* **54,** 4325 (1932).
196. B. Heinemann, *J. Lab. Clin. Med.* **29,** 254 (1944).
197. A. Albert, M. I. Gibson, and S. D. Rubbo, *Br. J. Exp. Pathol.* **34,** 119 (1953).
198. S. D. Rubbo, A. Albert, and M. I. Gibson, *Br. J. Exp. Path.* **31,** 425 (1950).
199. E. D. Weinberg, *Fed. Proc.* **20,** 132 (1961).
200. W. Liese, *Zentr. Bakteriol.* **105**(I), 137 (1927).
201. K. A. Oster and M. J. Golden, *J. Am. Pharm. Assoc. Sci. Ed.* **37,** 283 (1947).
202. S. M. Bahal, M. R. Baichwal, and M. I. Khorana, *J. Pharm. Sci.* **50,** 127 (1961).
203. W. Jadassohn and co-workers, *Schweiz. Med. Wochschr.* **74,** 168 (1944).
204. *Ibid.* **77,** 987 (1947).
205. K. Sigg, *Schweiz. Med. Wochschr.* **77,** 123 (1947).
206. M. Hartmann and H. Kägi, *Z. Angew. Chem.* **41,** 127 (1928).
207. P. M. Borick and M. Bratt, *Appl. Microbiol.* **9,** 475 (1961).
208. D. N. Eggenberger and co-workers, *Ann. N.Y. Acad. Sci.* **53,** 105 (1950).
209. P. H. H. Gray and L. J. Taylor, *Can. J. Botany* **30,** 674 (1952).
210. E. G. Klarmann and E. S. Wright, *Soap Sanit. Chem.* **22**(1), 125; **23**(7), 151 (1947).
211. A. Einhorn and M. Göttler, *Ann. Chem.* **343,** 207 (1908).
212. W. A. Jacobs, *J. Exp. Med.* **23,** 563 (1916).
213. W. A. Jacobs, M. Heidelberger, and C. G. Bull, *J. Exp. Med.* **23,** 577 (1916).
214. G. Domagk, *Dtsch. Med. Wochschr.* **61,** 829 (1935).
215. H. A. Krebs, *Biochem. J.* **43,** 51 (1948).
216. E. J. Ordal and A. F. Borg, *Proc. Soc. Exp. Biol. Med.* **50,** 332 (1942).
217. M. G. Sevag and O. A. Ross, *J. Bacteriol.* **48,** 677 (1944).
218. C. E. Chaplin, *Can. J. Bacteriol.* **29,** 373 (1951).
219. C. K. Crocker, *J. Milk Food Technol.* **14,** 138 (1951).
220. R. Fischer and P. Larose, *Nature* **170,** 175 (1952).
221. W. E. Knox and co-workers, *J. Bacteriol.* **58,** 443 (1949).
222. R. D. Hotchkiss, *Ann. N.Y. Acad. Sci.* **46,** 479 (1946).
223. M. R. J. Salton, *J. Gen. Microbiol.* **5,** 391 (1951).
224. M. R. J. Salton, R. W. Horme, and V. E. Cosslett, *J. Gen. Microbiol.* **5,** 405 (1951).
225. C. A. Lawrence, *Surface-Active Quaternary Ammonium Germicides,* Academic Press, New York, 1950.
226. G. R. Goetchius and H. Grinsfelder, *Appl. Microbiol.* **1,** 271 (1953).
227. E. G. Klarmann and E. S. Wright, *Am. J. Pharm.* **120,** 146 (1948).
228. L. S. Stuart, J. Bogusky, and J. L. Friedl, *Soap Sanit. Chem.* **26**(1), 121 (1950); **26**(2), 127 (1950).
229. W. A. Altemeier, *Ann. Surg.* **147,** 773 (1958).
230. H. Dold and R. Gust, *Arch. Hyg. Bakteriol.* **141,** 321 (1957).
231. J. G. Hirsch, *Am. Rev. Tuberc.* **70,** 312 (1954).
232. E. G. Klarmann, *Am. J. Pharm.* **126,** 267 (1954).
233. C. R. Smith, *Soap Sanit. Chem.* **27**(9–10), (1951).
234. C. R. Smith and co-workers, *Public Health Rep.* (*U.S.*) **65,** 588 (1950).
235. A. Hoyt, A. H. K. Djang, and C. R. Smith, *Public Health Rep.* (*U.S.*) **71,** 1097 (1956).
236. C. W. Chambers and co-workers, *Public Health Rep.* (*U.S.*) **70,** 545 (1955).
237. E. W. Dennis, *Soap Sanit. Chem.* **27,** 117 (1951).
238. G. R. Walter and W. S. Gump, *J. Pharm. Sci.* **51,** 707 (1962).
239. C. A. Lawrence and A. J. Maffia, *Bull. Am. Soc. Hosp. Pharm.* **14,** 164 (1957).

240. R. A. Benson and co-workers, *J. Pediat.* **31,** 369 (1947); **34,** 49 (1949).
241. P. Story, *Br. Med. J.,* 1128 (Nov. 22, 1952).
242. Th. Goldschmidt A. G., *Ned. Tijdschr. Geneeskd.* **3,** 234 (1967).
243. A. Schmitz and W. S. Harris, *Manuf. Chem.* **29,** 51 (1958).
244. A. Schmitz, *Milchwissenschaft* **7,** 250 (1952).
245. U.S. Pat. 2,253,182 (Aug. 19, 1941), E. G. Klarmann (to Lehn & Fink Products Corp.).
246. U.S. Pat. 2,359,241 (Sept. 26, 1944), A. M. Partansky (to The Dow Chemical Co.).
247. A. M. Kligman and W. Rosenzweig, *J. Invest. Dermatol.* **10,** 59 (1947).
248. C. R. Miller and W. O. Elson, *J. Bacteriol.* **57,** 47 (1949).
249. D. J. Beaver, D. P. Roman, and P. F. Stoffel, *J. Am. Chem. Soc.* **79,** 1236 (1957).
250. F. L. Rose and G. Swain, *J. Chem. Soc.,* 4422 (1956).
251. J. Murray and R. M. Calman, *Br. Med. J.* (I), 81 (1955).
252. E. D. Weinberg, *Antibiot. Chemotherapy* **11,** 572 (1961).
253. M. C. Dodd and W. B. Stillman, *J. Pharmacol. Exp. Therap.* **82,** 11 (1944).
254. U.S. Pat. 2,319,481 (May 18, 1943), W. B. Stilman, A. B. Scott, and J. M. Clampit (to Norwich Pharmacol Co.).
255. M. C. Dodd, D. L. Cramer, and W. C. Ward, *J. Am. Pharm. Assoc. Sci. Ed.* **39,** 313 (1950).
256. A. H. Beckett and A. E. Robinson, *Chem. Ind.* (*London*), 523 (1957).
257. M. C. Dodd, *J. Pharmacol. Exp. Therap.* **86,** 311 (1946).
258. J. A. Yourchenco, M. C. Yourchenco, and C. R. Piepoli, *Antibiot. Chemother.* **3,** 1035 (1953).
259. E. R. Kennedy and J. F. Barbaro, *J. Bacteriol.* **65,** 678 (1953).
260. J. W. Bartholomew and H. Finkelstein, *J. Bacteriol.* **67,** 689 (1954).
261. A. Albert, *Lancet,* 278 (1942).
262. T. M. McCalla, *Stain Technol.* **16,** 27 (1941).
263. A. Albert and co-workers, *Br. J. Exp. Pathol.* **26,** 60 (1945).
264. A. Albert, S. D. Rubbo, and M. Burvill, *Br. J. Exp. Pathol.* **30,** 159 (1949).
265. J. E. Weiss and L. F. Rettger, *J. Bacteriol.* **28,** 501 (1934).
266. C. P. G. Wakeley, *Practitioner* **146,** 27 (1941).
267. B. E. Greenberg and M. L. Brodney, *New Engl. J. Med.* **209,** 1153 (1933).
268. A. Albert and R. J. Goldacre, *Nature* **101,** 95 (1948).
269. G. R. Goetchius and C. A. Lawrence, *J. Lab. Clin. Med.* **29,** 134 (1944).
270. R. Wagner and A. Pohlner, *Z. Immunitätsforsch.* **94,** 171 (1938).
271. A. Goerner and F. L. Haley, *J. Lab. Clin. Med.* **16,** 957 (1931).
272. U.S. Pat. 2,085,037 (June 29, 1937), F. Mietzsch and J. Klarer (to Winthrop Chemical Co.).
273. U.S. Pat. 2,396,145 (Mar. 5, 1946), E. E. A. Askelöf, N. Svartz, and H. C. Willstaedt (to Akticbolaget Pharmacia).
274. G. Proske, *Arch. Hyg. Bakteriol.* **136,** 74 (1952).
275. G. Nordgren, *Acta Pathol. Microbiol. Scand.* **40**(Suppl. 1), (1939).
276. U.S. Pat. 2,519,565 (Aug. 22, 1950), H. T. Hallowell (to Bard-Parker Co., Inc.).
277. R. C. Scott and P. A. Wolf, *Appl. Microbiol.* **10,** 211 (1962).
278. J. V. Scudi and C. J. Duca, *J. Urol.* **61,** 459 (1949).
279. I. Simons, *J. Urol.* **64,** 586 (1950).
280. R. M. S. Boucher, *Am. J. Hosp. Pharm.* **29,** 660 (1972).
281. U.S. Pat. 3,016,328 (Jan. 9, 1962), R. E. Pepper and R. E. Lieberman (to Ethicon, Inc.).
282. U.S. Pat. 3,167,477 (Jan. 26, 1965), W. S. Gump and G. R. Walter (to Givaudan Corp.).
283. J. J. Perkins, *Principles and Methods of Sterilization,* Charles C Thomas, Springfield, Ill., 1956; *Sterilization of Surgical Materials, Symposium,* Pharmaceutical Press, London, Eng., 1961, p. 76.
284. E. G. Klarmann, *Am. J. Pharm.* **128,** 4 (1956).
285. C. W. Bruch, *Ann. Rev. Microbiol.* **15,** 245 (1961).
286. U.S. Pat. 2,037,439 (Apr. 14, 1936), H. Schrader and E. Bossert (to Union Carbide and Carbon Corp.).
287. H. S. Ginsberg and A. T. Wilson, *Proc. Soc. Exp. Biol. Med.* **73,** 614 (1950).
288. A. T. Wilson and P. Bruno, *J. Exp. Med.* **51,** 449 (1950).
289. S. Kaye, *J. Lab. Clin. Med.* **35,** 823 (1950).
290. S. Kaye and C. R. Phillips, *Am. J. Hyg.* **50,** 296 (1949).
291. C. R. Phillips, *Am. J. Hyg.* **50,** 280 (1949).
292. C. R. Phillips and S. Kaye, *Am. J. Hyg.* **50,** 270 (1949).
293. C. W. Walter, *Hosp. Top.* **35,** 104 (1957).

294. C. R. Phillips, *Bacteriol. Rev.* **16,** 135 (1952); *Sterilization of Surgical Materials, Symposium,* Pharmaceutical Press, London, Eng., 1961, p. 59.
295. J. L. Friedl, L. F. Ortenzio, and L. S. Stuart, *J. Assoc. Off. Agric. Chem.* **39,** 480 (1956).
296. J. D. Fulton and R. B. Mitchell, *U.S. Armed Forces Med. J.* **3,** 425 (1952).
297. A. Klarenbeck and H. A. E. Tongeren, *Reports on Virucidal Action of Gaseous Ethylene Oxide,* Netherlands Institute for Preventive Medicine, Leiden, The Netherlands, 1950.
298. G. W. Kirby, L. Atkin, and C. N. Frey, *Food Ind.* **8,** 450 (1936).
299. J. S. Barlow and H. L. House, *Science* **123,** 229 (1956).
300. E. A. Hawk and O. Mickelson, *Science* **121,** 442 (1955).
301. H. J. Pappas and L. A. Hall, *Food Technol.* **6,** 456 (1952).
302. S. Kaye, H. F. Irminger, and C. R. Phillips, *J. Lab. Clin. Med.* **40,** 67 (1952).
303. L. C. Miner, *Am. J. Hosp. Pharm.* **16,** 284 (1959).
304. S. Kaye, *Am. J. Hyg.* **50,** 289 (1949).
305. H. T. Gordon, W. W. Thornburg, and L. N. Werum, *Agric. Food Chem.* **7,** 196 (1959).
306. U.S. Pat. 2,809,879 (Oct. 15, 1957), J. N. Masci (to Johnson & Johnson Inc.).
307. F. Bernheim and G. R. Gale, *Proc. Soc. Exp. Biol. Med.* **80,** 162 (1952).
308. F. W. Dawson, H. J. Hearn, and R. K. Hoffman, *Appl. Microbiol.* **7,** 199 (1959).
309. F. W. Dawson, R. J. Janssen, and R. K. Hoffman, *Appl. Microbiol.* **8,** 39 (1960).
310. F. W. Hartman, S. L. Piepes, and A. M. Wallbank, *Fed. Proc.* **10,** 358 (1951).
311. A. R. Kelley and F. W. Hartmann, *Fed. Proc.* **10,** 361 (1951).
312. *Ibid.* **11,** 419 (1952).
313. G. H. Mangun and co-workers, *Fed. Proc.* **10,** 220 (1951).
314. C. W. Bruch, *Am. J. Hyg.* **73,** 1 (1961).
315. R. K. Hoffman and B. Warshowsky, *Appl. Microbiol.* **6,** 358 (1958).
316. D. R. Spiner and R. K. Hoffman, *Appl. Microbiol.* **8,** 152 (1960).

WILLIAM GUMP
Consultant

INDEX

C

treatment, 151, 171
Diphyllobothrium latum, 340
Diplococcus pneumoniae, 82, 462
4,6-Di-*n*-propylresorcinol [*69943-49-3*]
  phenol coefficient, 454
Dirocide, 332
Disinfectants
  EPA registration, 439
  evaluation of, 437
  pine oil, 461
  TEGOS, 460
Disinfectants and antiseptics, **435**
Disodium bisdithiocarbamate [*69943-51-7*]
  antibacterial, 462
Distamycin B [*62851-60-9*], 281
Dithiocarbamates
  antifungals, 462
Dithymol diiodide [*552-22-7*]
  antiseptic, 446
Dixiben, 3
DJ-400 B$_2$
  polyene, 286
D. latum, 341
DNA synthesis
  inhibition by quinolone carboxylic acids, 6
Dodecylammonium chloride [*929-73-7*], 457
N-Dodecyl-1,3-propanediamine [*5538-95-4*]
  antituberculous disinfectant, 459
Dowtherm, 399
Doxorubicin [*23214-92-8*], 360
Doxycycline [*564-25-0*], 29, 318, 392
D. perstans, 346
Dracunculus medinensis, 337, 346
Droncit, 341
Droxacin sodium [*57363-13-0*], 3, 6
DTIC.   See *Dacarbazine*.
Dubos, Rene, 30
Durhamycin [*11003-68-2*], 281
Dwarf tapeworm, 339, 340
Dyes
  antibacterials, 464
Dynamyxin, 229
Dysentery
  treatment, 457

E

Earle's L cells, 198
E. coli, 194, 195
  KY 8323, 191
Eczema vaccinatum
  treatment, 427
Efloran, 420
Ehrlich ascites cells, 191
Eimeria, 396
Electro-katadyn bactericidal process, 448

Elephantiasis
  treatment, 347
Elyzol, 420
Embden-Meyerhof-Parnas scheme
  of glycolysis, 337
Emetine [*483-18-1*], 410, 420
Emetine-bismuth iodide [*8001-15-8*], 410
Emimycin [*3735-45-4*], 181
E-Mycin, 172
Encephalitis
  treatment, 431
Endemic typhus, 389
Endomycin A (Helixin A) [*1391-41-9*], 278
Endomycin B (Helixin B) [*1391-41-9*], 284
Enheptin, 408
Enheptin T, 420
Enniatin A [*2503-13-1*], 244
Enniatin B [*917-13-5*], 244
Entamoeba histolytica, 292, 409
Enteric bacteria
  disinfectants for, 438
Enteritan, 420
Enteritis
  treatment, 146
Enterobacter aerogenes, 207
Enterobacteriacea, 57
Enterobacter sp, 53
Enterobius, 344, 346
Enterobius vermicularis, 344
Enterotoxon, 420
Entero-vioform, 410, 420
Enzymes
  as antitumor agents, 361
Eosinophilic lung
  treatment, 346
Epicillin [*26774-90-3*], 33
Epidemic typhus, 389
Epidemic typhus fever
  treatment, 146
Epi-17-deoxy-(O-8)-salinomycin [*64129-77-?*]
  312, 313
Epidermophyton, 292
Epidermophyton floccosum, 372, 462
2-Epihydroxyribostamycin [*52248-05-2*], 4?
Epitetracycline [*79-85-6*], 321
4-Epitetracycline [*79-85-6*], 324
6-Epitetracycline [*19369-52-9*], 325
Eprofil, 332
Equine influenza
  treatment, 429
Equizole, 332
Ergosterol [*57-87-4*]
  binding to amphotericin b, 376
Erion, 332
Erypar, 172
Erythrasma
  treatment, 171
Erythrocin, 172
Erythrocin ethyl succinate, 172

Flavicid [525-12-2]
germicide, 465
Flavofungin [11006-22-7], 293
Flavofungin A [29919-25-3], 293
Flavofungin B [29843-28-5], 293
Flavomycin A [57608-58-9], 287
Flavomycin B [57608-59-0], 287
Flavomycoin [11076-76-9], 293
Flavoquine, 420
Flavoviridomycin [51668-32-7], 279
Fleming, Alexander, 30, 92
Flucloxacillin [5250-39-5], 33
Flucytosine, 384
Flukes, 332
Flumequine [42835-25-6], 3, 6
5-Fluorocytosine [2022-85-7], 32, 392
7-Fluoro-6-demethyl-6-deoxytetracycline
[61618-26-6], 323
5-Fluoro-2'-deoxyuridine-5'-monophosphate
[134-46-3], 392
Fluorosalan [4776-06-1], 454
Fluorouracil [51-21-8], 358
5-Fluorouracil [51-21-8], 392
5-Fluorouridine [316-46-1], 385, 392
Folic acid [59-30-3]
related to sulfa drugs, 14
sequestered by fish tapeworm, 342
Folinic acid [58-05-9], 21, 369
Food preservative
use of nitrofurans as, 11
Foot and mouth disease virus, filtered (Berkefeld)
effect of ethanol, 441
Foot and mouth disease virus, unfiltered
effect of ethanol, 441
Formaldehyde [50-00-0]
germicide, 439
Formycin [6742-12-7], 184
Formycin B [13877-76-4], 184
N-Formyl-3,4-dichloroaniline [5470-15-5]
bacteriostat, 462
1-Formylisoquinoline thiosemicarbazone [2365-26-6], 429
2-Formylpyridine thiosemicarbazone [3608-75-1], 429
D-Forosamine [18423-27-3], 160
Fortimicin A [55779-06-1], 67
Fortimicin B [54783-95-8], 67
Fouadin, 332
Fowl cholera
treatment, 146
Fradicin [1403-61-8], 284
Framygen, 40
Franocide, 332
Fructose-1,6-diphosphate [488-69-7], 336
Fructose-6-phosphate [6814-87-5], 336
5-FU. See 5-Fluorouracil.
Fuadin, 332
Fulvicin, 380

Fulvomycin A [57608-60-3] B, 287
Fumagillin [23110-15-8], 410
Fumanomycin [50925-98-9], 281
Fumarylcarboxamido-L-2,3-diaminopropionyl-L-alanine, 246
Fungal infections
treatment, 284
Fungal plant pathogens, 388
Fungichromin [6834-98-6], 279, 293
Fungicides, 436
antibiotic, 32
polyenes, 291
Fungillin, 378
Fungimycin [11016-07-2], 293
Fungistats, 436
Fungizone, 293, 377
Fungus infections
treatment with nucleosides, 199
5-FUR. See 5-Fluorouridine.
Furacin
antibacterial activity, 463
Furadantin, 463
Furalazine hydrochloride [3012-10-0], 12
Furaltadone [139-91-3], 10
Furamide, 420
2-Furanacetic acid [2745-26-8], 11
2-Furancarboxaldehyde oxime [1121-47-7], 10
2-Furanmethanol [98-00-00], 11
Furazolidone [67-45-8], 409, 420, 463
Furazolium chloride [5118-17-2], 12
Furazon, 420
2-Furoic acid [88-14-2]
diloxanide from, 410
Furoxone, 420
Furylfuramide [3688-53-7], 11
Fusarium wilt, 388
Fusidic acid [6990-06-3], 29

G

G-4. See Dichlorophene.
G-11. See Hexachlorophene.
Gabbromycin, 40
Gangtokmycin [37220-69-2], 281
Garamine [49751-51-1], 49
Garamycin, 40
Gastrointestinal tract infections
treated with gentamicin, 54
Gauze-Brazhnikova, 232
Geldanamycin [30562-34-6], 72
Gelovermin, 332
Gentacin, 40
Gentamicin [1403-66-3], 29
Gentamicin A [13291-74-2], 47
Gentamicin A$_1$ [55925-13-8], 47
Gentamicin A$_2$ [55715-66-7], 47

M

Pityrosporum, 292
Pityrosporum orbiculare, 373
Plague
treatment, 146
Plasma albumin, 361
Plasmid
of drug resistant organisms, 6
Plasmochin, 420
Plasmodium
life cycle, 412
Plasmodium falciparum, 411, 412
Plasmodium malariae, 411, 414
Plasmodium ovale, 411
Plasmodium vivax, 411, 414
Platenomycin A₁ [40615-47-2], 158
Platenomycin A₃ [16846-24-5], 158
Platenomycin Ao [52310-62-0], 158
Platenomycin B₁ [35457-80-8], 158
Platenomycin B₃ [18361-48-3], 158
Platenomycin C₁ [35775-82-7], 158
Platenomycin C₂ [35867-32-4], 158
Platenomycin C₄ [35908-45-3], 158
Platenomycin W₁ [35867-31-3], 158
Platenomycin W₂ [52310-61-9], 158
Plath-lyse, 332
Plicacetin [43043-15-8], 185
Plumbomycin A [37199-59-0] and B, 279
Pneumocystosis, 406
Pneumonococcal infections
treatment, 171
Podophyllotoxin [518-28-5], 357
Polifungin B [37371-05-4], 277, 279
Polival, 332
Polyangium cellulosum var. *fulvum*, 381
Polyenes. See *Antibiotics, polyenes.*
Polyether antibiotics. See *Antibiotics, polyethers.*
Polyethers, 301.   (See also *Antibiotics, polyethers.*)
Polymycin [1406-11-7], 30
Polymyxin B sulfate [1405-20-5], 207
Polymyxins, 32
Polymyxin sulfate, 229
Polyoxin A [19396-03-3], 185
Polyoxin B [19396-06-6], 185
Polyoxin C [11043-74-6], 185
Polyoxin D [22976-86-9], 186, 392
Polyoxin E [22976-87-0], 186
Polyoxin F [23116-76-9], 186
Polyoxin G [22976-88-1], 186
Polyoxin H [24695-54-3], 186
Polyoxin I [22886-33-5], 186
Polyoxin J [22976-89-2], 186
Polyoxin K [22886-46-0], 186
Polyoxin L [22976-90-5], 186
Polypeptide synthesis
inhibition by lincomycin, 150
Poly(rI:rC) [24939-03-5], 427, 432
Polystat. See *Sulfanitran.*

Polyvinylpyrrolidinone [9007-92-5]
in I₂ antiseptics, 445
Pork tapeworm, 340
P. oryzae, 191
Potadine, 445
Potassium arsenite [10124-50-2]
antitumor agent, 351
Potassium dichloroisocyanurate [2244-21-5]
as disinfectant, 444
Potassium dichromate [7778-50-9]
in H₂O₂ antiseptic, 449
Potassium iodide [7681-11-0]
as antifungal, 383
generation of I₂, 445
Potassium permanganate [7722-64-7]
as antifungal, 382
effectiveness as bactericide, 449
Potassium tetraglycine triiodide [55115-56-5]
in water treatment, 445
Povan, 332
Povanyl, 332
Povidone–iodine
as antiseptic, 445
Praequine, 420
Prasinomycin [12687-95-5], 32
Praziquantel [55268-74-1], 341
Prednisone [53-03-2]
antimitotic agent, 365
Preservatives
antimicrobial, 436
Prestreptovarone [58074-37-6], 75
Preventol G-D, 334
Primaquine [90-34-6], 413, 421
Pristinamycin, 242
Pristinamycin Iᵦ [57206-54-9], 242
Pristinamycin Iₐ [3131-03-1], 242
Pristinamycin Iᴄ [28979-74-0], 242
Pristinamycin IIₐ [21411-53-0], 242
Procaine [59-46-1], 113
Procaine hydrochloride [51-05-8], 113
Procarbazine
antitumor activity, 364
Prodoxal, 3
Progesterone [57-83-0]
antimitotic activity, 365
Proguanil [500-92-5], 421
Proline [147-85-3], 236, 242
in lincosaminides, 149
Prontosil [103-12-8], 17
Prontosil rubrum, 465
9-Propionylmaridomycin III [35775-84-9], 158
2-Propyl-4-amino-5-chloromethylpyrimidine
dihydrochloride [67466-60-8], 397
Propylene glycol [57-55-6]
as germicide, 441
Propyl *p*-hydroxybenzoate [94-13-3]
pharmaceutical preservative, 454
Propylhygric acid [13380-36-4], 150

S

T

U